Common haematology values

If outside this range, consult:

Haemoglobin	men:	13–18g/dL	p572
	women:	11.5–16g/d	p572
Mean cell volume, MCV		76–96fL	↓p574; ↑p580
Platelets		150–400 × 10⁹/L	p610
White cells (total)		4–11 × 10⁹/L	p578
neutrophils		40–75%	p578
lymphocytes		20–45%	p578
eosinophils		1–6%	p578

KT-463-277

Blood gases

	kPa	*mmHg*	
pH	7.35–7.45		p630
P_aO_2	>10.6	75–100	p630
P_aCO_2	4.7–6	35–54	
Base excess	±2mmol/L		

U & E etc (urea and electrolytes) *If outside this range, consult:*

sodium	135–145mmol/L	p638
potassuim	3.5–5mmol/L	p640
creatinine	70–150µmol/L	p384 & p388
urea	2.5–6.7mmol/L	p384 & p388
calcium	2.12–2.65mmol/L	p642–4
albumin	35–50g/L	p650
proteins	60–80g/L	p650

LFTs (liver function tests)

bilirubin	3–17µmol/L	p484
alanine aminotransferase, ALT	3–35iu/L	
aspartate transaminase, AST	3–35iu/L	p484
alkaline phosphatase	30–300iu/L (*adults*)	p484

'Cardiac enzymes'

creatine kinase	25–195iu/L	p280 (p670)
lactate dehydrogenase, LDH	70–250iu/L	p280

Lipids and other biochemical values

cholesterol	4–<6mmol/L *desired*	p654
triglycerides	0.5–1.9mmol/L " " "	p654
amylase	0–180*somorgyi* u/dL	p116
C-reactive protein, CRP	<10mg/L	p650
glucose, fasting	3.5–5.5mmol/L	p528
prostate specific antigen, PSA	0–4ng/mL	p392, **p653**
T4 (total thyroxine)	70–140mmol/L	p538
TSH	0.5– ~5mu/L	p538

For all other reference intervals, see p753–5

DR SARGENT

OXFORD
HANDBOOK
OF CLINICAL
MEDICINE

Fourth Edition

R. A. HOPE
J. M. LONGMORE
S. K. McMANUS
C. A. WOOD-ALLUM

Oxford   New York   Tokyo
OXFORD UNIVERSITY PRESS
1998

Oxford University Press, Great Clarendon Street, Oxford OX2 6DP
Orders by telephone (UK) +44 (0)1865 242913

Oxford New York
Athens Auckland Bangkok Bogota Buenos Aires Calcutta
Cape Town Chennai Dar es Salamm Delhi Florence Hong Kong Istanbul
Karachi Kuala Lumpur Madrid Melbourne Mexico City Mumbai
Nairobi Paris São Paolo Singapore Taipei Tokyo Toronto Warsaw
and associated companies in
Berlin   Ibadan

Oxford is a trade mark of Oxford University Press

Published in the United States
by Oxford University Press Inc., New York

The moral rights of the authors have been asserted

A catalogue record for this book is available from the British Library.

Library of Congress Cataloging-in-Publication Data available
ISBN 0 19 262 783X

Typeset by JML; film output from AMA Graphics Limited, Preston
Printed in China

Translations and adaptations
French translation 1989, 1995
Spanish translation 1991
German translation 1991, 1994
Hungarian translation 1992
Polish translation 1993
Romanian translation 1995
Czech translation 1995
Slovac translation 1996
Portuguese (Brazilian) 1996
Electronic version—Oxford Clinical Mentor OUP 1997
(with Oxford Handbook of Clinical Specialties
and
Oxford Handbook of Clinical Rarities)
US edition forthcoming 1999

Preface to the fourth edition

Medical texts serve two chief aims: to impart a corpus of ideas and knowledge which is *required* to practise medicine, and to act as a treasure-house for storing the enormous volume of facts which may bear on a patient's illness, but which cannot all be remembered by ordinary mortals. In this edition we make our first attempt to distinguish formally (but not always objectively) between these purposes, by arming our most significant pages with 'Damocles' swords' (†, ††, or †††). Those diseases with most Damocles' swords are those where we would, and indeed have, kicked ourselves hardest on missing the diagnosis—stealthy diseases such as bacterial endocarditis, cranial arteritis, and tuberculosis, for example—which are very treatable, if diagnosed early.

To optimize convenience, and to impress our colleagues, we would all of us like to remember everything, all the time—everything, that is, apart from our mistakes. We started writing this work when we were happy and fresh in the first flush of success as junior doctors taking up first appointments. Now, a decade or so later, we have the opportunity to review our mistakes—those patients we would rather forget, but who are indelibly etched on our minds. All too often, it turns out that these failings stem from a lack of communication with our patients, and from not following the well-worn paths of listening, history-taking, examination, and referral for further care as needed—and not from simple lack of knowledge about a certain list of facts. This leads us towards the important conclusion that it is not only difficult to learn a great many facts, but it is wrong to try—because in doing so we run the risk of changing ourselves from ordinary, caring human beings into insatiable guzzlers of medical garbage.

Naturally we feel very sorry for those many pages whose misfortune it is not to have scored a single Damocles' sword. We are not saying that these topics are unimportant. We are saying that they are not *core* topics. In other words, we are saying that by following those well-worn paths of history-taking, examination, and further referral as required, and by *dipping into* these non-Damocles' sword pages, rather than learning them by heart, there is a good chance that, with the help of your colleagues, you will make the correct diagnosis, and start the right treatment—and still have enough energy left over to explain all this to your patient, and to provide that essential ingredient of sympathy.

There remains one big problem with this approach. How are we to diagnose conditions we have never heard of—if these rare and not so rare topics remain largely unread? We do not have a full answer to this, but with the electronic version of this text (described on p17), and its very many thousands of key-word coded facts, it *is* possible to diagnose conditions you have never heard of. In spite of this, the old adage holds good: *If you don't know, ask.*

Readers of earlier editions will note that paragraphs headed *Signs and symptoms*, and *Clinical features* are now headed *The Patient*—not just because it is shorter, but also because, in these days when medical investigations and science take us ever further from the bedside and the direct contemplation of our patients, it is always as well to be reminded that behind the thousand or so clinical features here described, there lies a patient, who is the person suffering from them, and toward whom all our efforts are directed.

R.A.H.
J.M.L.

From the preface to the first edition

This book, written by junior doctors, is intended principally for medical students and house officers. The student becomes, imperceptibly, the house officer. For him we wrote this book not because we know so much, but because we know we remember so little. For the student the problem is not simply the quantity of information, but the diversity of places from which it is dispensed. Trailing eagerly behind the surgeon, the student is admonished never to forget alcohol withdrawal as a cause of post-operative confusion. The scrap of paper on which this is written spends a month in the white coat pocket before being lost for ever in the laundry. At different times, and in inconvenient places, a number of other causes may be presented to the student. Not only are these causes and aphorisms never brought together, but when, as a surgical house officer, the former student faces a confused patient, none is to hand.

This book is intended for use on the ward, in the lecture-theatre, library, and at home. Each subject only occupies one page, and opposite is a blank page for additions, updatings, and refinements. If they face the relevant page of print, they will be automatically indexed.

Clinical medicine has a habit of partly hiding as well as partly revealing the patient and his problems. We aim to encourage the doctor to enjoy his patients: in doing so we believe he will prosper in the practice of medicine. For a long time now, house officers have been encouraged to adopt monstrous proportions in order to straddle simultaneously the diverse pinnacles of clinical science and clinical experience. We hope that this book will make this endeavour a little easier by moving a cumulative memory burden from the mind into the pocket, and by removing some of the fears that are naturally felt when starting a career in medicine, thereby freely allowing the doctor's clinical acumen to grow by the slow accretion of many, many days and nights.

R.A.H.
J.M.L.

Drugs (and how to keep abreast of changes)

While every effort has been made to check this text, it is still possible that drug or other errors have been missed. Also, dosage schedules are continually being revised and new side-effects recognized. Oxford University Press makes no representation, express or implied, that drug dosages in this book are correct. For these reasons, the reader is strongly urged to check with the most up to date published product information and *data sheets* provided by the manufacturers, and the most recent codes of conduct and safety regulations. The authors and the publishers do not accept responsibility or legal liability for any errors in the text, or for the misuse or misapplication of material in this work.

Except where otherwise stated, drug doses and recommendations are for the **non-pregnant adult** who is **not breast feeding**.

Corrections and peer-reviewed updatings are posted on the Internet at http://www.oup.co.uk/OHCM.

See also http://www.oup.co.uk/scimed. More detailed electronic updatings are an integral part of our *Oxford Clinical Mentor* (see p17).

Readers are also reminded of the need to keep up-to-date, and that this need can only ever be *partly* addressed by printed texts such as this.

Drug nomenclature[1]

This volume uses British[uk] approved names, followed, where there is a difference, by the recommended international non-proprietary name (rINN; usually there is no difference). A European Directive requires use of rINNs throughout the European Community; from 1998 there will be a 5-year change-over period (our next edition will employ only rINNs). Exceptions to our rule of giving both names occur where the change is minute, eg amoxycillin[uk]/amoxicillin, where the rINN is used, to avoid tedious near-duplications. Among the new rINNs used are:

Alimemazine	(trimeprazine[uk])	Epinephrine	(adrenaline[uk])
Amoxicillin	(amoxycillin[uk])	Furosemide	(frusemide[uk])
Bendroflumethiazide	(bendrofluazide[uk])	Lidocaine	(lignocaine[uk])
Ciclosporin	(cyclosporin[uk])	Chlormethine	(mustine[uk])
Clomifene	(clomiphene[uk])	Norepinephrine	(noradrenaline[uk])
Diethylstilbestrol	(stilboestrol[uk])	Sulfonamides (all)	(sulphonamides[uk])
Dosulepin	(dothiepin[uk])	Trihexyphenidyl	(benzhexol[uk])

In addition, rINNs for cefalosporins (formerly cephalosporins) now all start with *cef...* (not *ceph*). For consistency, and to avoid distracting variations in adjacent usages, we have spelt sulphur (and its derivatives) *sulfur* as all *sulphonamides* have a rINN starting *sulf...*

---

1 For a full list of international non-proprietary names see *BNF* 1998 **i** x & *Pharmaceutical J* 1997 **259** 668

Acknowledgements

We would like to record our heartfelt thanks to our advisers on specific sections: Dr C Alcock, Dr C Baigent, Dr M Benson, Ms J Boorman, Dr J Brierley, Mr J Britton, Dr D Chapman, Dr D Cranston, Dr J Firth, Ms P Frith, Miss L Hands, Dr A Holmes, Ms R James, Ms A Jennings, Dr M Johnson, Dr J Kay, Dr T Littlewood, Dr G Luzzi, Dr W McCrea, Dr P Moss, Dr A Neil, Ms S Nicholls, Dr J Olson, Dr A Palfreeman, Dr R Peveler, Dr G Rocker, Dr W Rosenberg, Dr J Reynolds, Dr D Sackett, Dr J Satsangi, Dr D Sprigings, Mr P Stanton, Dr J Trowell, Dr S Vinjamuri, Dr D Walters, Dr J Wee, Ms E Weekes, Dr I Wilkinson, Dr S Winner, and Dr A Zeman.

We here acknowledge the good time we have had discussing our text with Dr David Thaler, the author of its American incarnation, which is being published in 1999, with this edition, by OUP in New York. Total textual interpenetration of these two works has not been our goal—nor the crudities of *cut* and *paste*. But if some of his gems have been left to shine on his native shore, the light of others continues to illuminate this new edition—refracted but, we hope, unattenuated, by its passage through our British minds. A similar substantial contribution has come from Dr Sunil Jain whose generosity in making his extensive knowledge freely available to us we here acknowledge. We also thank Dr Martin Gaba for the original idea and the original draft of *Surviving house-jobs* (p11), and we thank Dr A Hutchings for his *Paracetamol graph* on p797.

For checking the entire text we thank, and admire the fortitude of Dr J Collier, Dr S Mercer, Dr J Reynolds, Dr R Wilkins, and Ms J Whitehouse.

It is impossible to over-estimate our debt to our electronic team: Dr H Thomas, Dr P Scott, Dr J Cox, Dr J Orrell, and Mr C Westerman and others.

For ever-ready solutions to the quirks of Quark®, we thank Simon Mather.

Readers' participation Few authors can have been as fortunate in their readers' generosity and attention to detail as we have been in past editions. Thanks to feedback on our readers' comments cards, we hope that this edition is keeping ever more nearly in step with our readers' needs. We have tried to write to all who have been kind enough to write to us, and apologize to anyone we have missed. In some instances comments were sent but either no name was given or we were unable to decipher the writing. We thank these anonymous people as well as the following for their valuable help in developing this handbook:

D Adams, G Adamson, R Adamson, A Adan, A Adiele, A Agbobu, X Airton, N Ahmad, S Ahmad, M Al-Amin, L Alan, A Aldridge, A Alhashem, M Ali, A Alizai, M Allendorf-Burns, S Al-Motari, R Al-Okaili, A Altaf, H Al-Tuiur, A Alvi, C Antonetti, M Anwar, R Armstrong, A Ashoush, R Asser, P Atack, M Azam, C Bache, D Baddeley, B Badgruddin, A Baig, N Balaswiya, D Bansevicius, M Barkham, M Barry, J Barth, G Baumgartner, M Beirne, J Benbow, M Beranek, E Berinou, A Bhattarai, H Bhatti, A Bishop, J Bishop, I Bleehen, K Boddu, V Bookhan, B Bourke, M Bowen, J Bradshaw, E Brewster, A Broadbent, J Brooks, J Brown, P Brykalski, H Bueckert, K Burn, M and G Butoi, P Buttery, A Byron, E Cameron, J Cameron, P Camosa, C Campbell, N Caporaso, D Carr, R Casson, A Caulea, S Cembrowicz, R Chaira, E Chambers, V Char, M Charter, O Chaudhri, W Chicken, P Chiquito, T Choudhry, G Chowdharay-Best, R Ciobanu, B Cleaver, L D Clark, J Collen, E Collier, M Collins, B Colvin, P Conway-Grim, R Coull, J Cox, G Crockett, T Crockett, P Culliney, E Dankwa, A Das-Gupta, N David, Y de Boer, U Desai, A de Silva,

M de Silva, J Devine, G Dex, D Dey, E Dickinson, A Ditri, J Dobbie, P Dowds, N Duthie, T Eden, V Eden, D Eldridge, N Elkan, D Ellis, R England, M Erlewyn-Lajeunesse, E Ersani, M Essa, G Evans, A Ezigweth, M Faragher, M Farooq, C Finfa, P Fisichella, E Fitzpatrick, P Flanagan, J Foust, M Gagan, J Ganane, I Ganans, M Gardarsdottir, J Germain, S Ghaem, J Gibson, K Gibson, M Gibson, J Gilbody, C Goodwin, S Gott, J Gotz, E Goudsmit, H Gray, J Grimley-Evans, S Gupta, X Gussan, C Haase, D Habart, T Halbert, A Halitsky, J Haller, J Halpern, E Hammond, R Hanlon, C Hanna, R Haynes, J Hays, D Heath, G Heese, W Hell, P Henken, T Hennigan, D Herold, F Heindrichs, M Hewitt, S Hjorleifsson, M Hollinshead, J Hopkinson, K Horncastle, A Houghton, R Houghton, L Houlberg, P Hrincto, Z Htwe, M Hughes, M Huqit, I Ibrahim, J Iglesia, A Iqbal, S Jankovic, N Jayasekera, A Jennings, G Johnson, N Joshi, A Joshua, H Kan, Z Kango, R Karplus, E Katz, A Kelly, A Khalid, I Khan, M Klasa, W Klei, B Koh, Y Kontrobarsky, N Kovacevic, M Kuepfer, H Kuralco, L Kwan, J Lagercranbe, G Lane, F Larkin, R Lawson, S Lee, J Lewis, J Lightowler, J Lima, G Linde, J Linder, D Livingstone, F Lloyd, H Lockner, G Lomax, A Longmore, I Low, M Lowenthal, G Lyons, H MacDonald, P Mackey, C Maddock, P Maher, Y Mahomed, M Malkawi, D Mallett, C Martin, T Matteucci, G Matthes, E Mayer, A McCafferty, D McCandless, F McCormick, C McDaniel, A McDougall, J McGregor, H McIntosh, J McKenzie, F McLellan, D Meeking, B Melrad, E Merrens, W Mgaya, R Miller, K Mitchell, A Mohammed, S Monella, S Morariot, M Morgan, B Morton, D Moskopp, S Moultrie, M Moutoussis, M Muqit, H Mutasa, K Muthe, S Muttu, T Mutwirah, N Naqui, A Naraen, J Nasir, M Nassar, M Nasson, B Naunton, E Neoh, M Nekhaila, M Newell, N Numan, K O'Driscoll, B Olalekan, O Olarinde, J Olson, S Otchirov, B Pait, F Palazzo, L Pantanowitz, P Papanicolaou, B Parkin, N Paros, G Pate, A Patel, K Patel, N Patel, C Paterson, S Petkov, F Phraner, B Piat, F Pilsczek, M Pinto, D Player, D Poppe, M Porter, M Powell, N Prho, E Pringle, M Procopiou, J Pryce, J Pryse, D Puxley, B Pynenburg, M Quaraishi, G Quiceno, H Raeder, R Raeder, H Rahman, A Ramachandran, C Ramyad, R Ranai, A Rasheed, R Rastogi, F Regan, J Revilla, D Rharmi, N Richmond, M Robert, J Roberts, J Robinson, F Rosenberg, A Rosenthal, S Rothery, J Rudd, D Ryms, S-U Safer, J Salama, R Salib, A Samieh-Tucker, L Sarkozi, P Saunders, H Sayanvala, J Schmitt, J Schneider, A Schutte, S Schwarz, F Scrase, M Scrase, P Seeley, F Sellers, V Sepe, Shahnaz-Hayat, T Shaikit, K Sheehan, D Shukla, I Silva, A Silverman, K Simpson, T Singh, S Sivananthan, E Smeland, R Smit, S Soran, G Spencer, P Spranh, K Spreadbury, P Statham, D Stead, J Stern, A Stevenson, J Steyn, D Stredder, A Struber, R Szabo, A Taimoor, H Talat, J Tang, A Tavakkolizadeh, A Taylor, D Taylor, N Taylor, S Taylor, M Tengoe, F Teo, F Thompson, L Thomson, W Thomson, T Toma, B Traynor, L Trieu, J Trois, P Trotman, T Tscherning, D Turner, M Turner, F Uddin, K Umanok, S Vaidya, C Vandenbussche, C van der Worp, J Van-Tam, J Verghese, Y Wahowed, L Walker, S Walker, M Walsh, T Walton, T Wang, L Wasantu, J Watkins, L Watson, K Weerasinghe, H Weerasooriya, W Westall, P Whelan, T Whitehouse, J Wiesenfeldt, T Wiggin, R Williams, J Williamsen, J Williamson, J Winkler, M Wong, J Wood, X Xiong, D Yaniu, Y Yawar, E Yeoh, N Yoo, K Yuet, A Zafiropoulos, R Zajdel, K Zarrabi, M Zein, M Zia.

The British Lending Library, and staff at the *Cairns Library*, Oxford, and at the *Worthing Postgraduate Library* have been most helpful in tracing references.

We thank Faber for permission to quote from Ted Hughes' *Lodger* (p52).

Finally we would like to thank the staff of OUP for their help and support.

Symbols and abbreviations

▶	this fact or idea is important
▶▶	don't dawdle!—prompt action saves lives
◁ 1,2, etc ▷	reference to randomized and other trials blessed by pundits of evidence-based medicine (p742); examples on p98, 255 & 530
†††	don't miss this topic—it is vital
††	don't miss this topic either
†	other core topics—an avowedly arbitrary classification, but the person who is new to medicine needs *some* guidance
🖥	internet link
●̇	incendiary (controversial) topic
🖫	further detail available in this text's electronic version (p17)
♂:♀	male to female ratio: ♂:♀=2:1 means twice as common in males
~	approximately
-ve; +ve	negative and posative, respectively
↑; ↓; ↔	increased, decreased, and normal, respectively (eg serum level)
A₂	aortic component of second heart sound
Ab	antibody
ABPA	allergic bronchopulmonary aspergillosis
ac	*ante cibum* (before food)
ACE(i)	angiotensin-converting enzyme (inhibitors)
ACTH	adrenocorticotrophic hormone
ADH	antidiuretic hormone
ADL	activities of daily living
AF	atrial fibrillation
AFB	acid-fast bacillus
AFP	(and α-FP) alpha-fetoprotein
Ag	antigen
AIDS	acquired immunodeficiency syndrome
Al	aluminium
Alk phos	alkaline phosphatase (also ALP)
ALL	acute lymphoblastic leukaemia
AMA	antimitochondrial antibody
AMP	adenosine monophosphate
ANA	antinuclear antibody
ANAC	anti-neutrophil cytoplasmic antibody
APTT	activated partial thromboplastin time
ARDS	adult respiratory distress syndrome
ASD	atrial septal defect
ASO	antistreptolysin O
AST	aspartate transaminase
ATN	acute tubular necrosis
AV	atrioventricular
AVM	arteriovenous malformation(s)
AXR	abdominal x-ray (plain)
azt	zidovudine
Ba	barium
BAL	bronchoalveolar lavage
BCR	British comparative ratio (≈INR)
bd	*bis die* (twice a day)
BKA	below-knee amputation
BMJ	*British Medical Journal*
BNF	*British National Formulary*
BP	blood pressure
bpm	beats per minute (eg pulse)
Ca	carcinoma
CABG	coronary artery bypass graft
cAMP	cyclic adenosine monophosphate (AMP)
CAPD	continuous ambulatory peritoneal dialysis

A_2 aortic component of second heart sound

CBD	common bile duct
CC	creatinine clearance
CCF	congestive cardiac failure (ie left and right heart failure)
CD	cluster of differentiation surface molecules, eg CD4 lymphocytes
CHB	complete heart block
CHD	coronary heart disease (related to ischaemia and atheroma)
CI	contraindications
CK	creatine (phospho)kinase (also CPK)
CLL	chronic lymphocytic leukaemia
CML	chronic myeloid leukaemia
CMV	cytomegalovirus
CNS	central nervous system
COC	combined oral contraceptive, ie (o)estrogen + progesterone
COPD	chronic obstructive pulmonary disease
CPAP	continuous positive airways pressure
CPR	cardiopulmonary resuscitation
CRF	chronic renal failure
CRP	C-reactive protein
CSF	cerebrospinal fluid
CT	computerized tomography
CVP	central venous pressure
CVS	cardiovascular system
CXR	chest x-ray
d	day(s) (also expressed as x/7)
DIC	disseminated intravascular coagulation
DIP	distal interphalangeal
dL	decilitre
DoH	Department of Health (United Kingdom)
DM	diabetes mellitus
DU	duodenal ulcer
D&V	diarrhoea and vomiting
DVT	deep venous thrombosis
DXT	deep radiotherapy
E-BM	evidence-based medicine (& its journal published by the BMA)
EBV	Epstein–Barr virus
ECG	electrocardiogram
Echo	echocardiogram
EDTA	ethylene diamine tetraacetic acid (full blood count bottle)
EEG	electroencephalogram
ELISA	enzyme linked immunosorbant assay
EM	electron microscope
EMG	electromyogram
ENT	ear, nose, and throat
ESR	erythrocyte sedimentation rate
EUA	examination under anaesthesia
FB	foreign body
FBC	full blood count
FDP	fibrin degradation products
FEV_1	forced expiratory volume in first second
FFP	fresh frozen plasma
F_iO_2	partial pressure of O_2 in inspired air
FROM	full range of movements
FSH	follicle-stimulating hormone
FVC	forced vital capacity
g	gram
GA	general anaesthetic
GB	gall bladder
GC	gonococcus
GC	Glasgow coma scale
GFR	glomerular filtration rate
GGT	gamma glutamyl transpeptidase
GH	growth hormone
GI	gastrointestinal

GP	general practitioner
G6PD	glucose-6-phosphate dehydrogenase
GTT	glucose tolerance test (also OGTT: oral GTT)
GU	genitourinary
h	hour
HAV	hepatitis A virus
Hb	haemoglobin
HBsAg	hepatitis B surface antigen
HBV	hepatitis B virus
Hct	haematocrit
HCV	hepatitis C virus
HDL	high-density lipoprotein, a 'good' form of cholesterol, p654
HDV	hepatitis D virus
HHT	hereditary haemorrhagic telangiectasia
HIDA	hepatic immunodiacetic acid
HIV	human immunodeficiency virus
HOCM	hypertrophic obstructive cardiomyopathy
HONK	hyperosmolar non-ketotic (diabetic coma)
HRT	hormone replacement therapy
HSV	Herpes simplex virus
Ib/ibid	Ibidem, Latin for *In the same place*
ICP	intracranial pressure
IDA	iron-deficiency anaemia
IDDM	insulin-dependent diabetes mellitus
IFN-α	alpha interferon
IE	infective endocarditis
Ig	immunoglobulin
IHD	ischaemic heart disease
IM	intramuscular
INR	international normalized ratio (prothrombin ratio)
IPPV	intermittent positive pressure ventilation
ITP	idiopathic thrombocytopenic purpura
ITU	intensive therapy unit
iu	international unit
IVC	inferior vena cava
IV(I)	intravenous (infusion)
IVU	intravenous urography
JAMA	*Journal of the American Medical Association*
JVP	jugular venous pressure
KCCT	kaolin cephalin clotting time
kg	kilogram
kPa	kiloPascal
L	litre
LBBB	left bundle branch block
LDH	lactate dehydrogenase
LDL	low-density lipoprotein, a 'bad' form of cholesterol, p654
LFT	liver function test
LH	luteinizing hormone
LIF	left iliac fossa
LKKS	liver, kidney (R), kidney (L), spleen
LMN	lower motor neurone
LP	lumbar puncture
LUQ	left upper quadrant
LVF	left ventricular failure
LVH	left ventricular hypertrophy
µg	microgram
MAOI	monoamine oxidase inhibitors
MCV	mean cell volume
MDMA	3,4-methylenedioxymethamphetamine
ME	myalgic encephalomyelitis
MET	maximal exercise test
mg	milligram
MI	myocardial infarction

min(s)	minute(s)
mL	millilitre
mmHg	millimetres of mercury
MND	motor neurone disease
MRI	magnetic resonance imaging
MS	multiple sclerosis (do not confuse with mitral stenosis)
MSU	midstream urine
NAD	nothing abnormal detected
NBM	nil by mouth
ND	notifiable disease
NEJM	*New England Journal of Medicine*
NG(T)	nasogastric (tube)
NIDDM	non-insulin-dependent diabetes mellitus
NMDA	N-methyl-D-aspartate
NNT	numbers needed to treat, for 1 extra satisfactory result (p748)
NR	normal range—the same as reference interval
NSAID	non-steroidal anti-inflammatory drugs
N&V	nausea and/or vomiting
OCP	oral contraceptive pill
od	*omni die* (once daily)
OD	overdose
OGD	oesophago gastro duodenoscopy
OGS	oxogenic steroids
OGTT	oral glucose tolerance test
OHCS	*Oxford Handbook of Clinical Specialties*, 5th ed, OUP
om	*omni mane* (in the morning)
on	*omni nocte* (at night)
OPD	out-patients department
ORh–	blood group O, Rh negative
OT	occupational therapist
OTM	*Oxford Textbook of Medicine* (OUP 3e, 1996)
OTS	*Oxford Textbook of Surgery* (OUP 1e, 1994)
P_2	pulmonary component of second heart sound
P_aCO_2	partial pressure of carbon dioxide in arterial blood
PAN	polyarteritis nodosa
P_aO_2	partial pressure of oxygen in arterial blood
PBC	primary biliary cirrhosis
PCP	*pneumocystis carinii* pneumonia
PCR	polymerase chain reaction
PCV	packed cell volume
PE	pulmonary embolism
PEEP	positive end-expiratory pressure
PERLA	pupils equal and reactive to light and accommodation
PEFR	peak expiratory flow rate
PID	pelvic inflammatory disease
PIP	proximal interphalangeal
PL	prolactin
PND	paroxysmal nocturnal dyspnoea
PO	*per os* (by mouth)
PPF	purified plasma fraction (albumin)
PR	*per rectum* (by the rectum)
PRL	prolactin
PRN	*pro re nata* (as required)
PRV	polycythaemia rubra vera
PSA	prostate specific antigen
PTH	parathyroid hormone
PTT	prothrombin time
PUO	pyrexia of unknown origin
PV	*per vaginam* (by the vagina)
qds	*quater die sumendus* (to be taken 4 times a day)
qid	*quater in die* (4 times a day)
qqh	*quarta quaque hora* (every 4 hours)
R	right

RA	rheumatoid arthritis
RBBB	right bundle branch block
RBC	red blood cell
RFT	respiratory function tests
Rh	Rh; not an abbreviation, but derived fom the rhesus monkey
RhF	rheumatic fever
RIF	right iliac fossa
RUQ	right upper quadrant
RVF	right ventricular failure
RVH	right ventricular hypertrophy
R_x	recipe (treat with)
S or sec	second(s)
S1, S2	first and second heart sounds
SBE	subacute bacterial endocarditis (IE, infective endocarditis, is better)
SC	subcutaneous
SD	standard deviation
SE	side-effect(s)
SL	sublingual
SLE	systemic lupus erythematosus
SOB	short of breath (SOBOE: on exercise)
SR	slow-release (also called modified-release)
stat	statim (immediately; as initial dose)
STD/STI	sexually-transmitted disease or sexually-transmitted infection
SVC	superior vena cava
SXR	skull x-ray
sy(n)	syndrome
T°	temperature
$t_{1/2}$	biological half-life
T3	triiodothyronine
T4	thyroxine
TB	tuberculosis
tds	ter die sumendus (to be taken 3 times a day)
TIA	transient ischaemic attack
tid	ter in die (3 times a day)
TPR	temperature, pulse, and respirations count
TRH	thyroid-releasing hormone
TSH	thyroid-stimulating hormone
U	units
UC	ulcerative colitis
U&E	urea and electrolytes—and creatinine
UMN	upper motor neurone
URT	upper respiratory tract
URTI	upper respiratory tract infection
US(S)	ultrasound (scan)
UTI	urinary tract infection
VDRL	venereal diseases research laboratory
VE	ventricular extrasystole
VF	ventricular fibrillation
VMA	vanillyl mandelic acid (HMMA)
V/Q	ventilation:perfusion ratio
VSD	ventriculo-septal defect
WBC	white blood cell
WCC	white cell count
wk(s)	week(s)
WR	Wassermann reaction
yr(s)	year(s)
ZN	Ziehl–Neelsen (stain for acid-fact bacill, eg mycobacteria)

Note: Other abbreviations are given in full on the pages where they occur.

The old Hippocratic oath ~425BC

I swear by Apollo the physician, and Aesculapius and Health and All-heal, and all the gods and goddesses, that, according to my ability and judgment, I will keep this oath and stipulation—to reckon him who taught me this Art equally dear to me as my parents, to share my substance with him, and relieve his necessities if required; to look upon his offspring in the same footing as my own brothers, and to teach them this Art, if they shall wish to learn it, without fee or stipulation, and that by percept, lecture, and every other mode of instruction, I will impart a knowledge of the Art to my own sons, and those of my teachers, and to disciples bound by a stipulation and oath according to the law of medicine, but to none other.

I will follow that system of regimen, which, according to my ability and judgment, I consider for the benefit of my patients, and abstain from whatever is deleterious and mischievous.

I will give no deadly medicine to anyone if asked, nor suggest any such counsel; and in like manner I will not give to a woman a pessary to produce abortion. With purity and with holiness I will pass my life and practice my Art.

I will not cut persons labouring under the stone, but will leave this to be done by men who are practitioners of this work. Into whatever houses I enter, I will go into them for the benefit of the sick, and will abstain from every voluntary act of mischief and corruption; and, further, from the seduction of females, or males, of freemen or slaves.

Whatever, in connection with my professional practice, not in connection with it, I see or hear, in the life of men, which ought not to be spoken of abroad, I will not divulge, as reckoning that all such should be kept secret.

While I continue to keep this Oath unviolated, may it be granted to me to enjoy life and the practice of the Art, respected by all men, in all times. But should I trespass and violate this Oath, may the reverse be my lot.

A new Hippocratic oath ~1998AD

I promise that my medical knowledge will be used to benefit people's health. Patients are my first concern. I will listen to them, and provide the best care I can. I will be honest, respectful, and compassionate towards patients.

I will do my best to help *anyone* in medical need, in emergencies. I will make every effort to ensure that the rights of all patients are respected, including vulnerable groups who lack means of making their needs known.

I will exercise my professional judgment as independently as possible, uninfluenced by political pressure or by the social standing of my patient. I will not put personal profit or advancement above my duty to my patient.

I recognize the special value of human life, but I also know that prolongation of human life is not the only aim of health care. If I agree to perform abortion,* I agree that it should take place only within an ethical and legal framework.

I will not provide treatments which are pointless or harmful, or which an informed and competent patient refuses. I will help** patients find the information and support they want to make decisions on their care.

I will answer as truthfully as I can, and respect patients' decisions, unless that puts others at risk of substantial*** harm. If I cannot agree with their requests, I will explain why.

If my patients have limited mental awareness, I will still encourage them to participate in decisions as much as they feel able. I will do my best to maintain confidentiality about all patients.

If there are overriding reasons which prevent my keeping a patient's confidentiality I will explain them. I will recognize the limits of my knowledge and seek advice from colleagues when needed. I will acknowledge my mistakes.

I will do my best to keep myself and my colleagues informed of new developments, and ensure that poor standards or bad practices are exposed to those who can improve them.

I will show respect for all those with whom I work and be ready to share my knowledge by teaching others what I know. I will use my training and professional standing to improve the community in which I work.

I will treat patients equitably and support a fair and humane distribution of health resources. I will try to influence positively authorities whose policies harm public health.

I will oppose policies which breach internationally accepted standards of human rights. I will strive to change laws which are contrary to patients' interests or to my professional ethics.

While I continue to keep this Oath unviolated, may it be granted to me to enjoy life and the practice of the Art, respected by all, in all times.

After the BMA's *Revised Hippocratic Oath*, with changes: *The BMA draft did not cater for those believing that abortion is unethical. **The BMA wording was stronger here, requiring us to *ensure* that patients actually *receive* this information (often an impossibility). ***The word *substantial* has been added to prevent a serious breach of confidentiality in the name of a slight benefit to another party. Contrary to the the BMA's version, the last paragraph about enjoying life has been inserted from the old oath. Other changes are minor.

What the doctor said

He said it doesn't look good
he said it looks bad in fact real bad
he said I counted thirty-two of them on one lung before
I quit counting them
I said I'm glad I wouldn't want to know
about any more being there than that
he said are you a religious man do you kneel down
in forest groves and let yourself ask for help
when you come to a waterfall
mist blowing against your face and arms
do you stop and ask for understanding at those moments
I said not yet but I intend to start today
he said I'm real sorry he said
I wish I had some other kind of news to give you
I said Amen and he said something else
I didn't catch and not knowing what else to do
and not wanting him to have to repeat it
and me to have to fully digest it
I just looked at him
for a minute and he looked back it was then
I jumped up and shook hands with this man who'd just given me
something no one else on earth had ever given me
I may even have thanked him habit being so strong.

RAYMOND CARVER: *What the Doctor Said* from A NEW PATH TO THE WATERFALL. First published in Great Britain by Collins Harvill 1989. Copyright Tess Gallagher 1989. Reproduced by permission of The Harvill Press.

Contents

Contents of individual chapters are detailed on each chapter's first page.

This work is dedicated to
Johanna, Miriam, Katy, & Beth

1. Thinking about medicine

Ideals

Decision and intervention are the essence of action: reflection and conjecture are the essence of thought: the essence of medicine is combining these realms of action and thought in the service of others. We offer these ideals to stimulate both thought and action: like the stars, these ideals are hard to reach—but they serve for navigation during the night.

- Do not blame the sick for being sick.
- If the patient's wishes are known, comply with them.
- Work for your patients, not your consultant.
- Use ward rounds to boost the patients' morale, not your own.
- Treat the whole patient, not the disease—or the ward sister.
- Admit people, not 'strokes', 'infarcts' or 'crumble'.
- Spend time with the bereaved; you can help them shed tears.
- Question your conscience—however strongly it tells you to act.
- The ward sister is usually right; respect her opinion.
- Be kind to yourself—you are not an inexhaustible resource.
- Give the patient (and yourself) time: time to ask questions, time to reflect, time to allow healing to take place, and time to gain autonomy.
- Give the patient the benefit of the doubt. If you can, be optimistic, for *optimism* plus *communication* plus x = *cure* (or at least alleviation). Often $x = 0$—ie *inaction* while Nature effects a cure (the danger here is needless meddling). The rest of this book describes other values of x.

How to advise a patient

"What shall I do?" asks Gertrude "Not this, by no means, that I bid you do. . ." answers Hamlet, taking reticence about giving didactic advice almost as far as Oscar Wilde's ". . . It's always a silly thing to give advice, but to give good advice is absolutely fatal. . . " We must accept that even though we spend most of our lives giving advice to patients, they spend most of their lives ignoring it. Perhaps this is as it should be. We rarely check for harmony between our view of what should happen and the patient's. *Concordance* is a better word for this than the more often used term *compliance* (as in 'drug compliance') which implies that we are always right, and in authority. This lack of checking is a pity, as when we *do* take the trouble to negotiate with patients on concordance issues, we often learn new and startling things about them and their view of us. So. . . *how can we increase the chance that our advice is taken?*

Avoid jargon 'Jaundice' meant 'generally sick and unwell with yellow vomit' to 10% of patients in one study.

Avoid vague terms These will mean one thing to us and another to the patient; studies show patients' interpretations will be more pessimistic than doctors'. For example, 'you might possibly need a colostomy' meant that the chance was <50% to the surgeon, but was interpreted by the patient to mean that the chance was >60%. Use figures such as '1 in 10', and check the patient understands them. This can be a difficult undertaking when there are many competing risks with different values (eg with smoking there may be risk of death, worsening angina, and leg gangrene). In an attempt to avoid numerical statistics we are advised to use similies, eg 'as rare as being struck by lightning'. But this also has problems, as this risk is similar, say, to winning a large national lottery prize, which, on one level we know we will not win, but which, on another level, we confidently expect to fall into our laps every week. ▶ *Our own feelings, whether as doctor or patient, affect our estimation of risk; we rarely give unbiased advice.*

Help patients to remember Give the most important instruction first. This will be remembered best. Expect half of all subsequent advice to be forgotten. Two 'tricks' help here:
Explicit categorization: "I will tell you the treatment first, then what is wrong, and then the outcome. First the treatment. . ."
Specific advice: "Drink at least 6 cups of water per day", not "drink more".

Give written facts Use short sentences with short words, more like the *Sun* (the UK's most deceptively 'simple' tabloid) than the *Times*.

Flesch's formula quantifies this: 'reading ease' $= 207 - 0.85W - S$ (W is the mean number of syllables/100 words; S is the mean number of words per sentence). Most prose falls between 0 and 100 (100 is very easy). Aim for >70. Note: *not all patients can read*, and may be shy about revealing this. A tactful way to find out if someone can read is to use the chart on p37. If he cannot read *He moved.* . . in large type but correctly reports that the octopus in the series of pictures is holding a small bucket, then reading *is* a problem, and this fact is ascertained via a non-threatening eye test.

If a video is available, this may be helpful (not just to non-readers) in showing how to use an inhaler in asthma etc. Videos starring well-known comedians are available (*What you really want to know about.* . .) for topics such as asthma, bronchitis, colostomies, Crohn's disease, ulcerative colitis, depression, and glue ear.▪ (Advice may be more readily received if it comes from a well-known, well-loved TV actor.)

Satisfied patients take our advice Be friendly; have pleasant surroundings if possible; avoid long waits. Find out what the patient expects.

Advising patients about drugs See p10.

The bedside manner

Our bedside manner matters because it indicates to patients whether they can *trust* us. Where there is no trust there can be little healing. A good bedside manner is not static: it develops in the light of patients' needs—but it is always grounded in those timeless clinical virtues of honesty, humour, and humility in the presence of human weakness and human suffering.

The following are a few examples from an endless variety of phenomena which may arise whenever doctors meet patients. One of the great skills (and pleasures) in clinical medicine is to learn how our actions and attitudes influence patients, and how to take this knowledge into account when assessing the validity and significance of the signs and symptoms we elicit. The information we receive from our patients is not 'hard evidence' but a much more plastic commodity, moulded as much by the doctor's attitude and the hospital or consulting-room environment as by the patient's own hopes and fears. It is our job to adjust our attitudes and environment so that these hidden hopes and fears become manifest and the channels of communication are always open.

Anxiety reduction or intensification Simple explanation of what you are going to do often defuses what can be a highly charged affair. With children, try more subtle techniques, such as examining the abdomen using the child's own hands, or examining his teddy bear first.

Pain reduction or intensification Compare: 'I'm going to press your stomach. If it hurts, cry out' with 'I'm going to touch your stomach. Let me know what you feel' and 'Now I'll lay a hand on your stomach. Sing out if you feel anything'. The examination can be made to sound frightening, neutral, or joyful, and the patient will relax or tense up accordingly.

The tactful or clumsy invasion of personal space During ophthalmoscopy, for example, we must get much nearer to the patient than is acceptable in normal social intercourse. Both doctor and patient may end up holding their breath, which neither helps the patient keep his eyes perfectly still, nor the doctor to carry out a full examination. Simply explain 'I need to get very close to your eyes for this'. (Not 'We need to get very close for this'—one of the authors was kissed repeatedly while conducting ophthalmoscopy by a patient with frontal lobe signs. There are dangers in suggesting too much familiarity.)

The induction of a trance-like state Watch a skilful practitioner at work palpating the abdomen: the right hand rests idly on the abdomen, far away from the part which hurts. He meets the patient's gaze: 'Have you ever been to the seaside?' (His hand caresses rather than penetrates). . .'Imagine you are back on the beach now, perfectly at ease, gazing up at the blue, blue sky, (He presses as hard as he needs) . . .'Tell me now, where were you born and bred?' If the patient stops talking and frowns only when the doctor's hand is over the right iliac fossa, he will already have found out something useful.

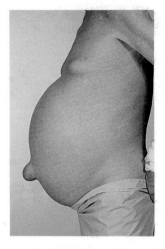

Plate 1
Ascites and
Umbilical
Hernia

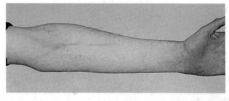

Plate 2
Needle tracks
of an IV drug
user

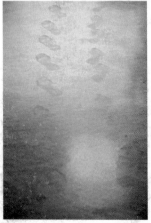

Plate 3
Alcoholic wide based gait

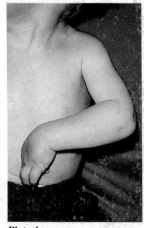

Plate 4
Brachial plexus injury at birth

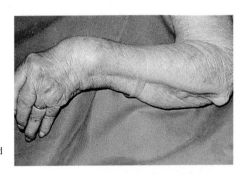

Plate 5
Rheumatoid
Arthritis

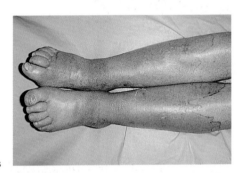

Plate 6
Cellulitis

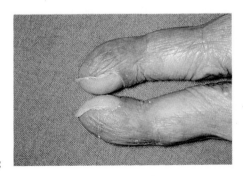

Plate 7
Clubbing

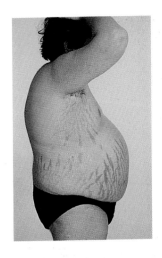

Plate 8
Cushings disease

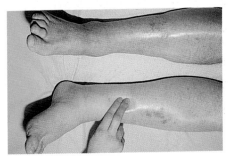

Plate 9
Pitting oedema

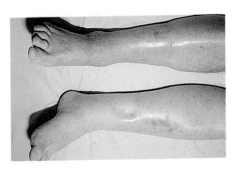

Plate 10
Pitting oedema

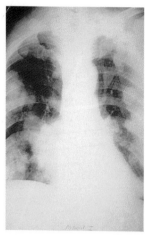

Plate 11
Cannon Ball
metastases

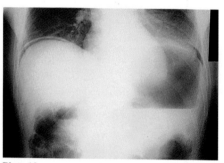

Plate 12
Air under right
diaphragm and
fundal bubble due
to ileus. Typical
post operative
picture

Asking questions

Good diagnosticians ask the most effective questions, a learnable art, given time, practice, and a good supply of patients. The aim of asking questions is to *describe*, not from the point of view of intellectual imperialism ('If you can describe the world, you can have it') but from the point of view of practical help: what cannot be described cannot be cured, and what is described but still cannot be cured can, at least, be shared, mitigated, and so partially overcome. Different kinds of questions either throw light on this issue, or obscure it, as in the two examples below.

Leading questions On seeing a patient's bloodstained handkerchief you ask: "How long have you been coughing up blood for?" "Six weeks, doctor" So you assume that he has been coughing up blood for 6 weeks. In fact, the stain could be due to an infected finger, or to epistaxis (nose bleeds). On finding this out at a later date (and perhaps after expensive and unpleasant investigations), you will be annoyed with your patient for misleading you—whereas he was trying to be polite by giving the sort of answer you were obviously expecting. With such leading questions as these, the patient is not given an opportunity to deny your assumptions.

Questions suggesting the answer "Was the vomit red, yellow, or black—like coffee grounds?"—the classic description of the vomiting of blood. "Yes, black, like coffee grounds, doctor'" The doctor's expectations and hurry to get the evidence he needs into the format of a traditional mould have so tarnished this patient's story as to make it useless.

Open questions The most open of all questions is "How are you?". The question suggests no particular kind of answer, so the direction the patient chooses to take offers valuable information. Other examples are gentle imperatives such as "Tell me about the vomit" "It was dark." "How dark?" "Dark bits in it" "Like . . . ?" "Like bits of soil in it' This information is pure gold, although it is not cast in the form of 'coffee grounds'.

Casting your questions over the whole family This is particularly useful in revealing symptoms are caused or perpetuated by psychological mechanisms. They probe the network of causes and enabling conditions which allow nebulous symptoms to flourish in family life. Until this sort of question is asked these illnesses may be refractory to treatment. Eg: "Who is present when your headache starts? Who notices it first—you or your wife? Who worries about it most (or least)? What does your wife do when (or before) you get it?" Think to yourself: *Who is his headache?* We note with mounting fascination research which shows that in clusters of hard-to-diagnose symptoms it is the *spouse's* view of the symptoms that is the best predictor of outcome 6 months later: if the spouse is determined that the symptoms must be physical, the outcome is worse than if the spouse allows that some or most of the symptoms may be psychological.

Echoes Try repeating the last few words the patient has said, prompting new intimacies, otherwise inaccessible, as the doctor fades into the background and the patient soliloquizes "I've always been suspicious of my wife." "Wife . . ." "My wife . . . and her father together." "Together. . ." "I've never trusted them together." "Trusted them together . . ." "No, well, I've always felt I've known who my son's real father was . . . I can never trust those two together." Without any questions you may unearth the unexpected, important clue which throws a new light on the history.

▶ *If you only ask questions you will only receive answers in reply.* If you interrogate a robin, he'll fly away: treelike silence may bring him to your hand.

Death: diagnosis and management

Death is Nature's master-stroke, albeit a cruel one, because it allows genotypes space and opportunity to try on new phenotypes. The time comes in the life of any organ or person when it is better to start again from scratch rather than carry on with the weight and muddle of endless accretions. Our bodies and minds are these perishable phenotypes—the froth, which always turns to scum, on the wave of our genes. These genes are not really *our* genes. It is us who belong to them for a few decades. It is one of Nature's great insults that she should prefer to put *all* her eggs in the basket of a defenceless, incompetent neonate rather than in the tried and tested custody of our own superb minds. But as our neurofibrils begin to tangle, and that neonate walks to a wisdom that eludes us, we are forced to give Nature credit for her daring idea. Of course, Nature, in her careless way, can get it wrong: people often die in the wrong order (one of our chief rôles is to prevent this mis-ordering of deaths, not the phenomenon of death itself).

So we must admit that, on reflection, dying *is* a brilliant idea, and one that it is most unlikely we could ever have thought of ourselves.

Causes of death Homicide, suicide, misadventure, or natural causes.

Diagnosing death Apnoea with no pulse and no heart sounds, and fixed pupils. If on a ventilator, brain death may be diagnosed even if the heart is still beating, via the *UK brain death criteria* which state that brain death is death of the brainstem, recognized by establishing:
- Deep coma with absent respirations (hence on a ventilator).
- The absence of drug intoxication and hypothermia ($<35°C$).
- The absence of hypoglycaemia, acidosis, and U&E imbalance.

Tests: All brainstem reflexes should be absent.
- Unreactive pupils. Absent corneal response.
- No vestibulo-ocular reflexes, ie no eye movement occurs after or during slow injection of 20mL of ice-cold water into each external auditory meatus in turn. Visualize the tympanic membrane first to eliminate false negative tests, eg due to wax.
- No motor response within the cranial nerve distribution should be elicited by adequate stimulation.
- No gag reflex or response to bronchial stimulation, and no respiratory effort on stopping the ventilator and allowing P_aCO_2 to rise to 6.7kPa.

Other considerations: Repeat the test after a suitable interval—usually 24 hours. Spinal reflexes are not relevant to the diagnosis of brain death. An EEG recording is not required, nor is a neurologist. The doctor diagnosing brain death must be a consultant (or his deputy registered for >5 years). The opinion of one other doctor (any) should also be sought.

USA criteria for brain death are slightly different, eg an EEG is required to confirm the absence of cerebral activity if brain death is to be diagnosed within 6 hours of apparent cessation of brain activity. Diagnosis of brain death is allowed in cases of intoxication if isotope angiography shows absent cerebral circulation, or if the intoxicant has been metabolized.

Organ donation: The point of diagnosing brain death is partly that this allows organs (kidney, liver, cornea, heart, or lungs) to be donated and removed with as little damage from hypoxia as possible. Do not avoid the topic with relatives. Many are glad to give consent and to think that some good can come after the death of their relative, that some part of the relative will go on living, giving a new life to another person.

After death Inform the GP and consultant. See the relatives. Provide a death certificate promptly. If the cause of death is in doubt, or if it is due to violence, injury, neglect, surgery or anaesthesia, alcohol, suicide, or poisoning, inform the Coroner or, in Scotland, the Procurator Fiscal.

Facing death

On most wards death is a daily occurrence, and as helping patients face death is one of our prime functions, this also ought to be a daily occurrence—so if you have not engaged in this activity recently, something, somewhere, may have gone wrong.

Whenever you find yourself thinking: 'It is better for him not to know', suspect that you mean: 'It is easier for me not to tell'. We find it hard to tell for many reasons: it distresses patients; it may hold up the ward round; we do not like acknowledging our impotence to alter the course of diseases; telling reminds us of our own mortality; and it may unlock our previous griefs. We use many tricks to minimize the pain: *rationalization* ('The patient would not want to know'); *intellectualization* ('Research shows that 37% of people at stage 3 survive 2 years. . .'); *brusque honesty* ('You are unlikely to survive 6 months'—and, so saying, the doctor rushes off to more vital things); *inappropriate delegation* ('Sister will explain it all to you when you are calmer').

Why it may help the patient to be told
- He already half knows but everyone shies away so he cannot discuss his fears (of pain, or that his family will not cope).
- There may be many affairs for the patient to put in order.
- To enable him to judge if unpleasant therapy is worthwhile.

▶ *Most patients are told less than they would like to know.*[1]

How and what to tell
- Put yourself in the patient's place. What are his worries likely to be (about himself; his family)?
- Allow the patient to control the information. Give sufficient information, and then the opportunity to ask for more.
- Be sensitive to hints that he may be ready to learn more. 'I'm worried about my son.' 'What is worrying you most?' 'Well, it will be a difficult time for him, (pause) starting school next year.' Silence, broken by the doctor 'I get the impression there are other things worrying you'. The patient now has the opportunity to proceed further, or to stop.
- Ensure that the GP and the nurses know what you have and have not said. Also make sure that this is written in the notes.

Stages of acceptance Accepting imminent death often takes time, and may involve passing through 'stages' on a path. It helps to know where your patient is on this path (but progress is rarely orderly and need not always be forwards: the same ground often needs to be recovered). At first there may be *shock* and *numbness*, then *denial* (which reduces anxiety), then *anger* (which may lead you to dislike your patient, but remember that anger anaesthetizes fear and pain), then *grief*, and then, perhaps, *acceptance*. Finally there may be an intense longing for death as the patient moves beyond the reach of worldly cares.[2]

Recognizing depression which will benefit from antidepressants is difficult in those who are physically ill, because symptoms such as early morning waking and loss of appetite may be due to the physical illness and need not imply depression. Be guided by morbid thoughts, such as undue guilt, low self-esteem, and inability to feel pleasure (anhedonia).

1 A Stedeford 1984 *Facing Death*, Heinemann **2** JS Bach 1727 *Ich habe genug*, Cantata Nᵒ 82 composed for the Feast of the Purification. See also R Buckman 1992 *How to Break Bad News*, Macmillan

Is this new drug any good? (analysis & meta-analysis)

This question frequently arises on reading journals. Not only authors but *all* clinicians have to decide what new treatments to recommend, and which to ignore. In assessing the use of research, ask the following:

8

1 Does it give a clear, clinically significant answer as well as a statistically significant answer in patients similar to those I treat?

2 Does the journal employ 'peer review' (in which so-called 'experts' vet the paper before publication)? Note: *this system is far from perfect!*

3 Are the statistical analyses valid? Much must be taken on trust as many analyses depend on sophisticated computing. Few papers, unfortunately, present 'raw' data. Nevertheless, it is important to look out for obvious faults by asking questions such as:

- Is the sample large enough to detect a clinically important difference, say a 20% drop in deaths from disease X? If the sample is small, the chance of missing such a difference is high. In order to reduce this chance to less than 5%, and if disease X has a mortality of 10%, >10,000 patients would need to be randomized. If a small trial which lacks power (the ability to detect true differences) *does* give 'positive' results, the size of the difference between the groups is likely to be exaggerated. (This is known as a type I error; a type II error applies to results which indicate that there is no effect, when in fact there is.) ►So beware even quite big trials which purport to show that a new treatment is equally effective as an established treatment.
- Were the compared groups chosen randomly, and did the result produce two groups that were well matched?
- Were the treatments being compared carried out by practitioners equally skilled in each treatment?

4 Was the study 'double-blind' (both patient and doctor are unaware of which treatment the patient is having)? Could either have told which was given, eg by the metabolic effects of the drug?

5 Was the study placebo-controlled? Good research can go on outside the realm of double-blind, randomized trials, but you need to be more careful in drawing conclusions—eg for intermittent symptoms, a bad time (prompting a consultation) is followed by a good time, making any treatment given in the bad phase appear effective. *Regression towards the mean* occurs in many areas, eg repeated BP measurement: because of transitory or random effects, most people having a high value today will have a less high value tomorrow—and most of those having a low value today will have a less extreme value tomorrow. This concept works at the bedside: if someone who is drowsy after a head injury has a high BP, and the next measurements are *higher still*, ie no regression to the mean, then this suggests a 'real' effect, such as ICP↑.

6 Has time been allowed for criticism of the research to appear in the correspondence columns of the journal in question?

7 If I were the patient, would I want the new treatment?

Meta-analyses[1] Systematic merging of similar trials, using refined criteria, can help resolve contentious issues and explain data inconsistencies. It is quicker and cheaper than doing new studies, and may establish the generalizability of research findings.[2] *Be cautious!* In one study[3] looking at recommendations of meta-analyses where there was a later 'definitive' big trial, it turned out that meta-analyses got it wrong ~30% of the time.●

►A well-planned clinical trial may be worth centuries of uncritical medical practice; but a week's experience on the wards may be more valuable than years reading journals. This is the central paradox in medical education. How can we trust our own experiences knowing they are all anecdotal; how can we be open to novel ideas but avoid being merely fashionable? A stance of wary open-mindedness may serve us best.

1 JA Turner 1994 *JAMA* 271 1609 2 CD Mulrow 1994 *BMJ* ii 597 3 J LeLorier 1997 *NEJM* (Aug 21)

Prescribing drugs

▶Consult the *British National Formulary* (*BNF*) or your local equivalent before prescribing any drug with which you are not thoroughly familiar.

Before prescribing, ask if the patient is allergic to anything. The answer if often 'Yes', particularly for antibiotics—but do not stop here. Find out what the reaction was, or else you run the risk of denying your patient a possibly life-saving, and very safe drug such as penicillin because of a mild reaction, such as nausea. Categorize the reaction as a *true allergy* (was there anaphylaxis, p766, or a rash?), a *toxic effect* (eg ataxia is inevitable if given large quantities of phenytoin) or a *predictable adverse reaction* (eg GI bleeding from aspirin), or an *idiosyncratic reaction*.

Remember the dictum *primum non nocere*—first do no harm. The more minor the complaint, the more weight this dictum carries. The more serious the complaint, the more this dictum's antithesis comes into play: *nothing ventured, nothing gained*. If someone is dying in front of you from cerebral malaria, it would be quite inappropriate to delay, Hamlet-like, while weighing up the chances of causing harm through a rare side-effect of the quinine you are about to give. But if you are about to give the quinine to someone with night cramps (for which it is also very effective) then it is your duty to allow each of the 10 commandments listed on p10 to filter through your mind. ▶That this advice is obvious does not prevent it from being regularly ignored—with consequences which may be just as dire as when the real 10 commandments are broken.

Prescribing in renal failure Dose modification should be related to creatinine clearance (p632), and the extent to which the drug is renally excreted. This is significant for aminoglycosides (p750), cefalosporins and a few other antibiotics (p177–181), lithium, opiates and digoxin. ▶Never prescribe a drug in renal failure before checking how its administration should be altered. Loading doses should not be changed. If the patient is on dialysis (peritoneal or haemodialysis), dose modification depends on how well it is eliminated by dialysis. Consult the drug's data sheet or an expert. Dosing should be timed around dialysis sessions.

Nephrotoxic drugs include: NSAIDs, aminoglycosides (eg gentamicin), amphotericin B, NSAIDs, frusemide (furosemide), gold, and penicillamine.

The amount by which the dose should be reduced in renal failure (the dose adjustment factor, DAF) depends on the fraction of the drug excreted unchanged in the urine (F) $DAF = 1/(F(kf-1)+1)$, where the kf is the relative kidney function=creatinine clearance/120. The usual dose should be divided by the DAF. In only a few drugs is F large enough to be important.

Note: loading doses should not be modified.

Aminoglycosides*	F=0.9	Cefalosporins	F=1.0
Lithium	F=1.0	Sulfamethoxazole	F=0.3–0.5
Digoxin	F=0.75	Procainamide	F=0.6
Ethambutol	F=0.7	Tetracycline	F=0.4–0.6

*eg gentamicin, netilmicin

Prescribing in liver failure Avoid opiates, diuretics (↑risk of encephalopathy), oral hypoglycaemics, and saline-containing infusions. Warfarin effects are enhanced. Hepatotoxic drugs include: paracetamol, methotrexate, phenothiazines, isoniazid, azathioprine, oestrogen, 6-mercaptopurine, salicylates, tetracycline, mitomycin.

⚕ Ten commandments

▶These 10 commandments should be written on every tablet.

1 Explore any alternatives to a prescription. Prescriptions lead to doctor-dependency, which in turn frequently leads to bad medicine. They are also expensive: £4–5 billion/yr (UK); prices increase much faster than general inflation. There are 3 places to find alternatives:
The larder: lemon and honey for sore throats, rather than penicillin.

The blackboard (eg education about the self-inflicted causes of oesophagitis rather than giving ranitidine, advising against too many big meals, smoking or alcohol excess, and over-tight garments).

Lastly, look to yourself. Giving a piece of yourself; some real sympathy is worth more than all the drugs in your pharmacopoeia to patients who are frightened, bereaved, or weary of life.

2 Find out if the patient wants to take a drug. Perhaps you are pre-scribing for some minor ailment because you want to solve every problem. But the patient may be happy just to know the ailment *is* minor. If he knows what it is, he may be happy to live with it. Some people do not believe in drugs, and you must find this out.

3 Decide if the patient is responsible. If he now swallows *all* the qui-nine pills you have so kindly prescribed, death will be swift.

4 Know of other ways your prescription may be misused. Perhaps the patient whose 'insomnia' you so kindly treated is even now grinding up your prescription prior to injecting himself, desperate for a fix. Will you be suspicious when he returns to say he has lost your prescription?

5 Address these 5 questions when prescribing off the ward:
   ● How many daily doses are there? (≤ 2 is much better than 4.)
   ● Are many other drugs to be taken? Can they be reduced?
   ● The bottle: can the patient read the instructions—and can he open it?
   ● How will you know if the patient forgets to return (follow-up)?
   ● If the patient agrees, enlist the spouse's help in ensuring that he remembers to take the pills. Check, eg by counting the remaining pills at the next visit. List potential benefits of *this* drug to *this* patient.

6 List the risks (side-effects, contraindications, interactions, risk of allergy). Of any new problem, always ask yourself: *Is this a side-effect?*

7 Agree with the patient on the risk : benefit ratio's favourability. Try to ensure there is true concordance (p3) between your ideas and your patient's.

8 Record how you will review the patient's need for each drug.

9 Quantify progress (or lack of it) towards specified, agreed goals, eg pulse rate to mark degree of β-blockade; or peak flow monitoring to guide steroid use in asthma.

10 Make a record of all drugs taken. Offer the patient a copy.

Surviving house jobs

If some fool or visionary were to say that our aim should be to produce the greatest health and happiness for the greatest number of our patients, we would not expect to hear cheering from the tattered ranks of midnight house officers: rather, our ears are detecting a decimated groan— because these men and women know that there is something at stake in house-officership far more elemental than health or happiness: survival. Here we are talking about our own survival, not that of our patients. It is hard to think of a greater peacetime challenge than these first months on the wards. Within the first weeks, however brightly your armour shone, it will now be smeared and splattered if not with blood, then with the fall-out from very many decisions which were taken without sufficient care and attention. Not that you were lazy, but *force majeure* on the part of Nature and the exigencies of ward life have, we are suddenly stunned to realize, taught us to be second-rate: for to insist on being first-rate in all areas is to sign a kind of death warrant for many of our patients, and, more pertinently for this page, for ourselves. Perfectionism cannot survive on the wards or in surgeries. To cope with this fact, or, to put it less depressingly, to flourish in this new world, don't keep re-polishing your armour (what are the 10 causes of atrial fibrillation—or are there 11?), rather furnish your mind—and nourish your body (regular food and drink will make those midnight groans of yours a little less intrusive).

We cannot prepare you for finding out that you do not much like the person you are becoming, and neither would we dream of imposing on our readers a recommended regimen of exercise, diet, and mental fitness. Finding out what can lead you through adversity is the art of living. What will you choose: physical fitness, martial arts, poetry, karate, the sermon on the mount, juggling, meditation, yoga, a love affair—or will you make an art form out of the ironic observation of your contemporaries?

Many nourish their inner person through a religious belief, and attend mosque, church, synagogue, or temple. A multicultural society provides diversity and room for all branches of expression. Bear in mind not to compare yourself with your contemporaries. Those who make the most noise are often *not waving but drowning*. Plan your recreation in advance, and take the opportunity to use any new-found wealth to do new and exciting activities. Start thinking about senior house officer jobs, and speak to the Regional Postgraduate Advisor in the specialty you select. Such enquiries supply energy to get you through the darker hours of house jobs, and may motivate you if the going gets tough. Think about what you are going to need to get through house jobs well in advance, and plan accordingly. Not that this is any guarantee that the plans will work, but if your yoga, your sermons, and your fitness regimens turn to ashes in your mouth, then at least you will know the direction in which to spit.

House jobs are not just a phase to get through and to enjoy where possible (there are frequently *many* such possibilities); they are also the anvil on which we are beaten into a new and perhaps rather uncomfortable shape. Luckily not all of us are made of iron and steel so there is a fair chance that, in due course, we will spring back into something resembling our normal shape, and, in so doing, we may come to realize that it was our weaknesses, not our strengths, which served us best.

House jobs can encompass tremendous up-and-down swings in energy, motivation, and mood which can be precipitated by small incidents. If you are depressed for more than a day, speak to a sympathetic friend, partner, or counsellor to help you put it in perspective.

Quality, QALYs, and the interpretation of dreams

12

Resource allocation: how to decide who gets what Resource allocation is about cutting the health cake—whose size is *given*. What slice should go to transplants, new joints, and services for dementia? Cynics would say that this depends on how vociferous is each group of doctors. But others try to find a rational basis for allocating resources. Health economists (econocrats) have invented the QALY for this purpose.

Making the cake Focusing on how to cut the cake diverts attention from the central issue: how large should the cake be? The answer may be that more needs spending on our health service, not at the expense of some other health gain but at the expense of something else.[1]

What is a QALY? 'The essence of a QALY (Quality Adjusted Life Year) is that it takes a year of healthy life expectancy to be worth 1, but regards a year of unhealthy life expectancy to be worth <1. Its precise value is lower the worse the quality of life of the unhealthy person.'[2] If a patient is likely to live for 8 years in perfect health on an old drug, he gains 8 QALYs; if a new drug would give him 16 years but at a quality of life which is rated by him at only 25% of the maximum, he would gain only 4 QALYs. The dream of health economists is to buy most QALYs for his budget.

Cost per QALY In one study, this was as follows (£):

GP advice to stop smoking	220	Kidney transplant	4710
Preventing stroke by BP treatment	940	Breast cancer screening	5780
Pacemaker implantation	1100	Heart transplant	7840
Valve replaced (aortic stenosis)	1140	Cholesterol screening + R_x	14,150
Hip replacement	1180	Home dialysis	17,260
CABG for LAD stenosis (p311)	2090	Brain tumour surgery	107,780

QALYs are better than raw survival figures for guiding rationing. QALYs counter vested interests, and question assumptions—eg each QALY gained by post-MI thrombolysis costs half as much in those >65 yrs compared with those <55 (in whom there are fewer deaths to prevent).[3] If resources are scarce, should we restrict coronary care to the elderly?

Problems with QALYs •The pricing of QALYs is often problematic.

•Injustice: it is reasonable for *individuals* to choose the treatment most likely to maximize QALYs, but applying QALYs when allocating resources is quite different as it involves choosing between the welfare of different people. Those with mental or physical handicaps will have less claim on resources because their handicap means that each year of their life is given <1 QALY. The old may do badly because palliative intervention is likely to result in fewer QALYs because their life expectancy is less.

•QALYs may not add up. Can one apply valuations made by summing group preferences to individuals who may not share the group's scale of preferences? *Question:* if a vase of flowers is beautiful, are 10 vases of flowers 10 times as beautiful—or might the scent be overpowering?

•Is welfare all important? 1000 people may benefit from constipation treatment—which might give more QALYs for the money it takes to save one person's life. In allocating resources, perhaps the needs of the dying person should come before the benefits to the constipated.

•QALYs do not suggest *who* should choose between treatments of similar QALY value. Doctors do not like deciding (they are put in an invidious position) and polls show that patients do not want to decide—so this leaves only politicians which neither group may be happy to trust.

1 J Bell 1988 *Philosophy and Medical Welfare*, Cambridge University Press   2 A Williams 1985 *Health and Social Service Journal* 3   3 A Renton 1992 *BMJ* i 182

Psychiatry on medical and surgical wards

▶Psychopathology is common in colleagues, patients, and relatives.

▶Seek help for your own problems. Find a sympathetic general practitioner and register with him or her. You may not be the best person to plan your assessment, treatment, and referral if necessary.

Depression This is common, and commonly ignored, at great cost to wellbeing. 'I would be depressed in her situation. . .', you say to yourself, and so you do not think of offering treatment. The usual guides (eg early morning waking, loss of appetite and weight, and loss of interest in sex and other hobbies) are of little help in diagnosing depression as they are very common on general wards. More useful are: persistent *low mood* without moments of happiness and no longer believing in one's capacity to feel pleasure (*anhedonia*); excessive *self-blame*, and thoughts of being *worthless*. ▶*Don't think it's not your job to recognize and treat depression.* It is as important as pain. Try to arrange activities to boost the patient's morale and self-confidence, and keep him in touch with his fellows. Communicate your thoughts to other members of the team looking after the patient: nurses, physiotherapists, and occupational therapists—as well as relatives (if the patient so wishes). Amongst these, your patient may find a kindred spirit who can give real insight and support.

If in doubt, try an antidepressant, and see if it helps—eg lofepramine* 70mg/8–12h PO, if no hepatic or severe renal impairment. For *selective serotonin reuptake inhibitors* (*SSRI*, eg fluoxetine, 20mg/24h PO), see *OHCS* p341.

Alcohol This is a common cause of problems on the ward (both the results of abuse and the effects of withdrawal). See p524.

The violent patient First ensure your own and others' safety. Do not tackle violent patients until adequate help is to hand (eg hospital porters or police). Common causes: *alcohol intoxication*, *drugs* (recreational or prescribed), *hypoglycaemia*, *acute confusional states* (p446).

Once help arrives, try to talk with the patient to calm him—and to gain an understanding of his mental state. If this fails, consider restraining him. English law allows you to do this. Measure blood glucose, or give IV dextrose stat (p784). If not hypoglycaemic, before further investigation is possible, chemical restraint may be needed, eg haloperidol eg 2mg IM (up to 20mg stat, then 5mg/h; monitor vital signs closely).

You can prevent violence by being aware of its early signs, eg restlessness, earnest pacing about in a confined space, clenched fists, morose silences, chanting or shouting. Try to keep your own intuitions alert to developing problems. Liaise with a nurse who knows the patient.

The Mental Health Act (1983, England and Wales) Unlike English common law, this is rarely relevant in general hospitals. Section 5 allows detention of a patient already receiving in-patient treatment—if he is suffering from a mental disorder and is a danger to himself or others. An acute confusional state (p446) is a mental disorder. Application must be made to the hospital managers by the consultant in charge or his deputy. Detention is for <72h. For further details, see *OHCS* p400.

---

*Be cautious if history of heart disease, epilepsy, blood dyscrasias, prostatic hypertrophy, glaucoma, hyperthyroidism or porphyria). SE: drowsiness, confusion, BP↓, pulse↑, vomiting, rashes, LFTs↓, marrow↓, and anticholinergic effects (dry mouth, constipation, blurred vision, urinary retention, sweating, tremor). Interactions: alcohol, anaesthetics (possible arrhythmias), T4. Despite these cautions, lofepramine is usually well-tolerated compared with some of the older tricyclic antidepressants.

What is the mechanism?

Like toddlers, we should always have the question 'Why?' on our lips. The reason for this is not that we are always searching for the ultimate cause of phenomena (although there is a place for this): it is so that we can choose the simplest level for intervention. Some simple change early on in a chain of events may be sufficient to bring about a cure, whereas later on in the chain such opportunities may not arise.

For example, it is not enough for you to diagnose heart failure in your breathless patient. Ask: 'Why is there heart failure?' If you do not, you will be satisfied with giving the patient a diuretic drug—and any side-effects from these, such as uraemia or incontinence induced by polyuria, will be attributed to an unavoidable consequence of necessary therapy.

If only you had asked 'What is the mechanism of the heart failure?' you might have found an underlying cause, such as anaemia coupled with ischaemic heart disease. You cannot cure the latter, but treating the anaemia may be all that is required to cure the patient's breathlessness. But do not stop there. Ask: 'What is the mechanism of the anaemia?' Look at a blood film for the answer. You discover that there is hypochromia and a low serum ferritin (p572)—and at last, you might be tempted to say to yourself, I have the prime cause: iron-deficiency anaemia. Here is the end to my chain of reasoning.

Wrong! Put aside the idea of prime causes, and go on asking 'What is the mechanism?' Return to the blood film to decide if the cause is dietary or bleeding (suggested by polychromasia, p576). You decide that the iron deficiency is dietary and this is confirmed by going over the history again (never think that the process of history taking is over after your first contact with your patient). 'Why is the patient eating a poor diet?' Is he ignorant, or too poor to eat properly? Go back to taking the history again, and perhaps you will find that the patient's wife died a year ago, he is sinking into a depression, and cannot be bothered to eat. He would not care if he died tomorrow. (The social history, often of vital importance, is all too often reduced to questions about alcohol and tobacco.)

You now begin to realize that simply treating the patient's anaemia may not be of much help to him—so go on asking 'Why?': 'Why did you bother to go to the doctor at all if you are not interested in getting better?' It turns out that he only went to see the doctor to please his daughter. Such a patient is most unlikely to take your treatment unless you really get to the bottom of what he cares about. In this case, his daughter is what matters and, unless you can enlist her help, all your therapeutic initiatives will fail. Talk with his daughter, offer help for the depression, teach her about iron-rich foods and, with luck, your patient's breathlessness may gradually begin to disappear. Even if it does *not* start to disappear, you may perhaps have forged a friendship with your patient which can be used to enable him to accept help in other ways—and this dialogue may help you to be a more humane and a kinder doctor, particularly if you are feeling worn out and assaulted by long lists of technical tasks which you must somehow fit into an overcrowded day.

On being busy: Corrigan's secret door

Unstoppable demands, increasing expectations as to what medical care should bring, the rising number of elderly patients, coupled with the introduction of new and complex treatments all conspire, it might be thought, to make doctors ever busier. In fact, doctors have always been busy people. Sir James Paget, for example, would regularly see more than 60 patients each day, sometimes travelling many miles to their bedside. Sir Dominic Corrigan was so busy 140 years ago that he had to have a secret door made in his consulting room so that he could escape from the ever-growing queue of eager patients.

We are all familiar with the phenomenon of being hopelessly over-stretched—and of wanting Corrigan's secret door. Competing, urgent, and simultaneous demands make carrying out any task all but impossible: the house officer is trying to put up an intravenous infusion on a shocked patient when his 'bleep' sounds. On his way to the telephone a patient is falling out of bed, being held in, apparently, only by his visibly lengthening catheter (which had taken the house officer an hour to insert). He knows he should stop to help but, instead, as he picks up the phone, he starts to tell Sister about 'this man dangling from his catheter' (knowing in his heart that the worst will have already happened). But he is interrupted by a thud coming from the bed of the lady who has just had her varicose veins attended to: however, it is not her, but her visiting husband who has collapsed and is now having a seizure. At this moment his cardiac arrest 'bleep' goes off, summoning him to some other patient. In despair, he turns to Sister and groans: "There must be some way out of here!" At times like this we all need Corrigan to take us by the shadow of our hand, and walk with us through his metaphorical secret door, into a calm inner world. To enable this to happen, make things as easy as possible for yourself.

Firstly, however lonely you feel, you are not usually alone. Do not pride yourself on not asking for help. If a decision is a hard one, share it with a colleague. Secondly, take any chance you get to sit down and rest. Have a cup of coffee with other members of staff, or with a friendly patient (patients are sources of renewal, not just devourers of your energies). Thirdly, do not miss meals. If there is no time to go to the canteen, ensure that food is put aside for you to eat when you can: hard work and sleeplessness are twice as bad when you are hungry. Fourthly, avoid making work for yourself. It is too easy for junior doctors, trapped in their image of excessive work and blackmailed by misplaced guilt, to remain on the wards re-clerking patients, rewriting notes, or rechecking results at an hour when the priority should be caring for themselves. Fifthly, when a bad part of the rota is looming, plan a good time for when you are off duty, to look forward to during the long nights.

Finally, remember that however busy the 'on take', your period of duty will end. For you, as for Macbeth:

Come what come may,
Time and the hour runs through the roughest day.

Health and medical ethics

▶ Most consultations have an ethical (ie non-technical) component.

Analysis Our aim is to do good by making people healthy. *Good* is the most general adjective of commendation and entails 4 cardinal duties:
1 Not doing harm. We owe this duty to all people, not just our patients.
2 Doing good. We particularly owe this to our patients.
3 Promoting justice—ie distributing scarce resources fairly (p12) and respecting rights: legal rights, rights to confidentiality, rights to be informed, to be offered all the options, and to be told the truth.
4 Promoting autonomy.[1,2] (This is not universally recognized; in some cultures facing starvation, it may be irrelevant, or even subversive.)

Health entails being sound in body and mind, and having powers of growth, development, healing, and regeneration. *How many people have you made healthy (or at least healthier) today?* And in achieving this, *how many cardinal principles have you ignored?* Herein lies a central facet of medicine. We cannot spend long on the wards or in our surgeries trying to make people healthy without we have breached every cardinal duty—particularly (3) and (4). Does it matter? What is the point of having principles if they are regularly ignored? The point of having them is to provide a context for our negotiations with patients. If we want to be better doctors, there are many worse places to start than by trying to put these principles into action. Inevitably, when we try to, there are times when they conflict with each other. What should guide us when these principles conflict? It is not just a case of deciding off the top of one's head on the basis of the above analysis. It may be worthwhile aspiring to a synthesis—if you have the time (time will so often be what you do *not* have; but so often, in retrospect, when things have gone wrong, you realize that they would not have done so if you had *made* time).

Synthesis When we must act in the face of two conflicting duties, one of the duties is *not* a duty. How do we tell which one? Trying to find out involves getting to know our patients, and asking some questions:
● Are the patient's wishes being complied with?
● What do your colleagues think? You are rarely alone, although pressure of work and isolation may make you feel very much alone.
● What do the relatives think? Ask the patient's permission first. Ask yourself if the relatives have the patient's best interests at heart.
● Is it desirable that the reason for an action be universalizable? (That is, if I say this person is too old for such-and-such an operation, am I happy to make this a general rule for everyone?—Kant's 'law'[?].)
● If an investigative journalist were to sit on a sulcus of mine (so having full knowledge of my thoughts and actions), would she be bored or would she be composing vitriol for tomorrow's newspapers? If so, can I answer her, point for point? Am I happy with my answers? Or are they tactical cerebrations designed to outwit her and to protect me from some unpalatable truth which I am reluctant to define?
● Would bodies such as the General Medical Council approve? One must respect confidentiality but, in some instances, the GMC will approve of breaking confidentiality—eg when instructed by a judge to do so, or when an Act of Parliament requires this (eg notification of some infectious diseases), or if a violent crime has been committed.
● What would a patient's representative think—eg the elected chairman of a patient's participation group (OHCS p440)? These opinions are valuable as they are readily available (if a local group exists) and they can stop decision-making from becoming dangerously medicalized.

1 TL Beauchamp 1989 *Principles of Biomedical Ethics* 3ed, OUP   2 R Gillon 1994 *BMJ* ii 184

Experts and expert systems

The best way to get help with a difficult diagnosis is to ask an expert. But what should you ask her, and how do you decide what the expert should be an expert in? If you end up sending someone to see a dermatologist when he needs a microbiologist, or to a neurologist when he needs a cardiologist, he may die a preventable death. We use the tools that come to hand when there is work to be done. If you only have a hammer, it is all too easy to turn every problem into a nail so that you can get to work on it. Dermatologists provide topical solutions, surgeons provide operative solutions, and psychiatrists provide solutions by listening. Most of the time this works out very well because the doctor who first sees the patient knows in which direction (if any) the patient should be pointed. This doctor might do well to ask 'If I were a dermatologist, what would I do? . . . If I were a were a psychiatrist, what would I do?'—and so on, and then choose what seems to be the best course of action, asking herself: 'If I adopt a surgical solution (if this is what she has chosen), what might I be missing?' And it is here that decision support has its most practical application. Consider a patient who is fed up with his chilblains and headaches. A dermatologist may concentrate on the chilblain, a psychiatrist on the feeling of being fed up, and a neurologist may concentrate on the headache. Each person is doing what he or she thinks is a good job. In fact, what was needed (in this real patient) was either a different specialist—or an electronic system for diagnosis. Headache and chilblains can be fed into an electronic system (eg *Oxford Clinical Mentor*[1]) which, in a second or two, comes up with the idea that the man could have endocarditis if the chilblain is really a vasculitis, and goes on to suggest looking for splenomegaly, murmurs and haematuria; and, if any tests are needed, to include blood cultures. To work this trick what is needed is a list of keywords, preferred terms and synonyms, and a database of a large number of diseases, along with details about mistakes doctors have made so that these too can be taken into account.

It may be irritating to hear that this well-looking man with chilblains and headache could have endocarditis ± a mycotic aneurysm—until your eye strays to Sister's note: 'one plus of haematuria', whereupon irritation turns to a shiver as you realize that you may be sitting next to the embodiment of one of nature's most deadly and stealthy diseases. Mentor-type databases (Iliad and Internist-1/qmr are others[2]) are a powerful (but not unproblematic[2]) way of connecting apparently unrelated phenomena: eg *knee pain* and *constipation* may be explained by pseudogout. The computer postulates hypothyroidism to explain constipation, and hypothyroidism is one of pseudogout's recognized associations.

Another use for databases is for diagnosing very rare diseases. The database referred to above (*Oxford Clinical Mentor*) includes this book (and the *Oxford Handbook of Clinical Specialties*) as well as *The Oxford Handbook of Clinical Rarities*, which only exists electronically.

Keeping up-to-date: 'Do you know, boy, that when they make those maps of the universe, you are looking at the map of something that looked like that six thousand million years ago? You cannot be much more out of date than that, I'll swear.'[3] This edition may not be quite that out of date by the time you read it—but the same principle applies. Our modem-updated electronic database brings you nearer—not to the big bang of oup creation but to the tiny tinkerings of their mundane authors and their latest small, but sometimes not so inconsequential, thoughts, ideas, and updatings.

1 *OXFORD CLINICAL MENTOR*—from OUP: tel. +44 (0)1865 242913 and EMIS: +44 (0)113 2591122, Park House Mews, 77 Back Lane, Off Broadway, Horsforth, Leeds, ls18 4rf UK
2 E Burner 1994 *nejm* 330 1792   3 G Greene 1957 *Under the Garden*, Penguin isbn 0-146-00057-9

2. At the bedside: history and physical examination

Relevant pages in other chapters: Symptoms and signs (p38–58); the elderly patient in hospital (p64); mini-mental test score (p77); pre-operative care (p82); the acute abdomen (p112); lumps (p144–52); hernias (p158 & p160); varicose veins (p162); jugular venous pressure (p258); heart sounds (p260); murmurs (p262); points on examining the chest (p324); urine (p370); testing peripheral nerves (p408); dermatomes (p410); nystagmus (p422).

In OHCS: Vaginal and other gynaecological examinations (*OHCS* p2); abdominal examination in pregnancy (*OHCS* p84); the history and examination in children and neonates (*OHCS* p172–6); examination of the eye (*OHCS* p476); visual acuity (*OHCS* p476); eye movements (*OHCS* p486); ear, nose, and throat examination (*OHCS* p528 and p530); facial nerve lesions (*OHCS* p566); skin examination (*OHCS* p576); examination of joints—see the contents page to Chapter 9 (*Orthopaedics and trauma, OHCS* p604).

▶The way to learn physical signs is at the bedside, with guidance from an experienced colleague. This chapter is not intended as a substitute for this process: it is simply an *aide-mémoire*.

▶We ask questions to get information to help with differential diagnosis. But we also ask questions to find out about the inner life and past exploits of our patients, so that they do not bore us, and so that we can respect them as individuals. The patient is likely to notice and reciprocate this respect, and this reciprocation is the foundation of most of our therapeutic endeavours. One of us (JML) happened to ask a routine 80-year-old 'geriatric' patient with renal failure what he did—meaning *did* in the past, and was surprised to learn that he commuted to London frequently and was a buyer of dried fruits from the Middle East—an area where he had unrivalled business contacts and knowledge of local produce. It was not long before he was having dialysis. The message is not that special people should get special services: rather that it is easy to like, and hence promote the interests of, patients with whom you can identify. The great challenge is to to identify with as broad a range of humanity as possible, without getting exhausted by the scale of this enterprise.

Taking a history

Taking (or receiving) histories is what most of us spend most of our professional life doing: it is worth doing it well. An accurate history is the biggest step in making the correct diagnosis. History-taking, examination, and treatment of a patient begins the moment one reaches the bedside. (The divisions imposed by our page titles are somewhat misleading.) Try to put the patient at ease: a good rapport may relieve distress on its own. It often helps to shake hands. Always introduce yourself. (After a detailed gynaecological examination, a doctor overheard his patient tell her daughter: "it was so kind of the vicar to call"). Check the patient is comfortable. General questions (age, occupation, marital status) help break the ice and help assess mental functions.

Presenting complaint (PC) 'What has been the trouble recently?' Record the patient's own words rather than, eg 'dyspnoea'.

History of presenting complaint (HPC) When did it start? What was the first thing noticed? Progression since then. Ever had it before? Try to characterize pain and symptoms roughly as below:
- Site; Radiation; Intensity; Duration; Onset (gradual, sudden);
- Character (sharp, dull, knife-like, colicky);
- Associated features (nausea, vomiting, etc.);
- Exacerbating and alleviating factors.

Direct questioning (DQ) Specific questions about the diagnosis you have in mind (+ its risk factors, eg travel) & a review of the relevant system.

Past medical history (PMH) Ever in hospital? Illnesses? Operations? Ask specifically about diabetes, asthma, bronchitis, TB, jaundice, rheumatic fever, high BP, heart disease, stroke, epilepsy, anaesthetic problems.

Medications/allergies Any tablets, injections? Any 'off the shelf' drugs? Herbal remedies? Ask the features of allergies; it may not have been one.

Social and family history (SH/FH) Probe without prying. 'Who else is there at home?' Job. Marital status. Spouse's job and health. Housing. Who visits?—relatives, neighbours, GP, nurse. Who does the cooking and shopping? What can the patient not do because of the illness? Age, health, and cause of death, if known, of parents, sibs, children; ask about TB, diabetes mellitus, and other relevant diseases. The social history is all too often seen as a dispensable adjunct, eg while the patient is being rushed to theatre. But vital clues may be missed about quality of life—and it is too late to ask when the surgeon's hand is deep in the belly and he or she is wondering how radical a procedure to perform. It is worth cultivating the skill of asking a few searching questions of the admitting family doctor while you are conversing on the phone. If you are both busy, do not waste time on things you will shortly be verifying for yourself but tap his knowledge of the patient and his 'significant others'. Remember that the GP is likely to be a specialist in his patients, whom he may have known for decades. He may even hold a 'living will' or advance directive to reveal your patient's wishes if he cannot speak for himself.

Areas of the family history may need detailed questioning—eg to determine if there is a significant family history of heart disease you need to ask about grandfathers' and male siblings' health, smoking, and tendency to hypertension, hyperlipidaemia, and claudication before they were 60 years old, as well as ascertaining the cause of death.

Alcohol, 'recreational' drugs, tobacco How much? How long? Smoking is fobidden in the Sikh religion, so make your enquiries tactful.

Functional enquiry (p22) To uncover undeclared symptoms. Some of this may already have been incorporated into the history.

Drawing family trees to reveal dominantly inherited disease*

Advances in genetics will soon touch all branches of medicine. It is increasingly important for doctors to identify patients at high risk of genetic disease, and to make appropriate referrals. The key skill is drawing a family tree to help you structure a family history—as follows:

1 Start with your patient. Draw a square for a male and a circle for a female. Add a small arrow (⬈, see below) to show that this person is the *propositus* (the person through whom the family tree is ascertained).

2 Add your patient's parents, brothers, and sisters. Record basic information only, eg age, and if alive and well (a&w). If dead, note age and cause of death, and pass an oblique stroke through that person's symbol.

3 Ask the key question '*Has anybody else in your family had a similar problem to yourself?*' eg heart attack/angina/stroke, or cancer. Ask only about the family of diseases that relate to your patient's main problem. Do not record a potted medical history for each family member: time is too short.

4 Extend the family tree up to include grandparents. If you haven't revealed a problem by now, go no further. You are unlikely to miss important familial disease. If your patient is elderly it may be impossible to obtain good information about grandparents. If so, fill out the family tree with your patient's uncles and aunts on both the mother's and father's sides.

5 Shade those in the family tree affected by the disease. ● = an affected female; ■ = an affected male. This helps show any genetic problem and, if there is one, will help demonstrate the pattern of inheritance.

6 If you have identified a familial susceptibility, or your patient has a recognized genetic disease, extend the family tree down to include children, to identify others who may be at risk, and who may benefit from screening.

The family tree below shows these ideas at work, and indicates that there is evidence for genetic risk of colon cancer, meriting referral to a geneticist.

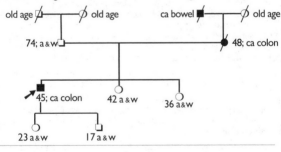

Conventions

□	○	■	⌀
male a&w=alive and well	female	54; ca colon (=male died aged 54yrs and had colon cancer)	73; old age (female died aged 73y from old age)

*Use a different approach in paediatrics, and for autosomal or sex-linked disease. Ask if parents are related (consanguinity ↑risk of recessive diseases).

Acknowledgement: This page owes much to Dr Helen Firth, whom we thank.

Functional enquiry

Just as skilled acrobats are happy to work without safety nets, so older clinicians usually operate without the functional enquiry. But to do this you must be experienced enough to understand all nuances and ramifications of the presenting complaint.

22

General questions may be the most significant, eg in TB or cancer:
- Weight loss
- Night sweats
- Any lumps
- Fatigue
- Appetite
- Fevers
- Itch
- Recent trauma*

Cardiorespiratory symptoms Chest pain (p256). Exertional dyspnoea (quantify exercise tolerance: how many stairs). Paroxysmal nocturnal dyspnoea. Orthopnoea, ie breathlessness on lying flat (a symptom of left ventricular failure). Oedema. Palpitations (awareness of heartbeats). Cough. Sputum. Haemoptysis (coughing up blood). Wheeze.

Gut symptoms Abdominal pain (constant or colicky, sharp or dull; site; radiation; duration; onset; severity; relationship to eating and bowel action; alleviating/exacerbating, or associated features). Other questions:
- Indigestion; nausea/vomiting
- Stool:—colour, consistency, blood, slime
- Swallowing —difficulty flushing away
- Bowel frequency —tenesmus or urgency

Tenesmus is the feeling that there is something in the rectum which cannot be passed (eg due to a tumour). Haematemesis is vomiting blood. Melaena is altered (black) blood passed PR (see p494).

Genitourinary symptoms Incontinence (stress or urge, p74). Dysuria (painful micturition). Haematuria (bloody micturition). Nocturia (needing to micturate at night). Frequency (frequent micturition) or polyuria (passing excessive amounts of urine). Hesitancy (difficulty starting micturition). Terminal dribbling.

Vaginal discharge (p221). Menses: frequency, regularity, heavy or light, duration, painful. First day of last menstrual period (LMP). Number of pregnancies. Menarche. Menopause. Chance of current pregnancy?

Neurological symptoms Sight, hearing, smell, taste. Seizures, faints, funny turns. Headache. 'Pins and needles' (paraesthesiae). Weakness ("Do your arms and legs work?"), poor balance. Speech problems (p430). Sphincter disturbance. Higher mental function and psychiatric symptoms (p34 and p77). The important thing is to assess function: what the patient can and cannot do at home, work, etc.

Musculoskeletal symptoms Pain, stiffness, swelling of joints. Diurnal variation in symptoms (ie with time of day, see p568). Functional deficit.

Thyroid symptoms *Hyperthyroidism:* Prefers cold weather, sweaty, diarrhoea, oligomenorrhoea, weight loss, tremor, visual problems.
Hypothyroidism: Depressed, slow, tired, thin hair, croaky voice, heavy periods, constipation, dry skin.

As set out here, history-taking may seem deceptively easy—as if the patient knew the hard facts and the only problem was extracting them. But what a patient gives you is a mixture of hearsay ('she said I looked very pale'), innuendo ('you know, doctor, down below'), legend ('I suppose I did bite my tongue—it was a real fit, you know'), exaggeration ('I didn't sleep a wink'), and improbabilities ('The Pope put a transmitter in my brain'). The great skill (and pleasure) in taking a good history lies not in ignoring these garbled messages but in making sense of them.

---

*Trauma is not just important because something may be broken, but because even if it seems trivial, it may provide the all-illuminating flash of insight which explains odd CNS features (eg post-traumatic subdural haemorrhage) or the vague prodromes of illnesses such as tetanus. For the significance of the other questions here listed, see p38–60.

2. At the bedside

Presenting your findings—and the rôle of jargon[1,2]

We are forever presenting patients to our colleagues, almost never questioning the mechanisms and unconscious motivations which permeate these oral exchanges—and sometimes send them awry. By some ancient right we assume authority to retell the patient's story at the bedside—not in our own words but in highly stylized medical code: 'Mr Hunt is a 19 year old *Caucasian male*, a *known case of* Down's syndrome with little intelligible speech and an IQ of 60, *who complains of* paraesthesiae and weakness in his right *upper limb*. . . He *admits to drinking 21 units per week* and *other problems* are. . .'

Do not comfort yourself by supposing this ritualistic reinterpretation arises out of the need for brevity. If this were the reason, and we are speaking in front of the patient, all that is in italics above could be omitted, or drastically curtailed. The next easy conclusion to confront is that we purposely use this jargon to confuse or deceive the patient. This is only sometimes the case, and we must look for deeper reasons for why we are wedded to these medicalisms.

We get nearer the truth when we realize that these medicalisms are used to sanitize and tame the raw data of our face-to-face encounters with patients—to make them bearable to us—so that we can *think* about the patient rather than having to *feel* for him or her. This is quite right and proper—but only sometimes. Usually what our patients need is sympathy, and this does not spring from cerebration. These medicalisms insulate us from the horrible unpredictability of experiential phenomena. We need the illusion that we are treading on well-marked-out territory when we are describing someone's pain—a fundamentally problematic enterprise, not least because if the description is objective it is invalid (pain is, *par excellence*, subjective), and if it is subjective it is partly incommunicable.

These medicalisms enrole us into a half-proud, half-guilty brotherhood, cemented by what some call patronage and others call fear. This fear can manifest itself as intense loyalty so that, err as we may, we cling to our medical loyalties unto death (that of the patient, not our own). Language is the tool unwittingly used to defend this autocracy of fear. The modulations of our voice, the stylized vocabulary, and the casual neglect of logic and narrative order ensure, in the above example, that we take on board so little of our patient that we remain upright and afloat, above the whirlpools of our patients' lives. In this case, not a case at all, but a child, a family, a mother worried sick about what will happen to her son when she dies: a son who has never *complained* of anything, has never *admitted* to anything, expresses no *problems*—it is *our* problem that his hand is weak, and his mother's that he can no longer attend riding for the disabled, because she can no longer be away from home and do her part-time job.

So when you next hear yourself declaim in one breath that "Mr Smith is a 50-year-old caucasian male with crushing central chest pain radiating down his left arm", take heed—what you may be communicating is that you have stopped thinking about this person—and pause for a moment. Look into your patient's eyes: confront the whirlpool.

1 R Horton 1998 *Lancet* 351 826   2 WJ Donnelly 1997 *Ann Int Med* 127 1045–8

Physical examination

With a few exceptions (eg BP, breast lumps), physical examination is not a good screening test for detecting undisclosed disease. Plan your examination to emphasize the areas that the history suggests may be abnormal. A few well-directed, problem-orientated minutes can save hours of fruitless, but very thorough, physical examination. You will still be expected to examine all 4 systems (p26–33), but with time you will be adept at excluding any major undisclosed pathology. Practice is the key.

Look at your patient as a whole to decide how sick he seems to be. Is he well or *in extremis*? Try to decide *why* you think so. Is he in pain and does it make him lie still (eg peritonitis) or writhe about (eg colic)? Is his breathing laboured and rapid? Is he obese or cachectic? Is his behaviour appropriate?

Specific diagnoses can often be made from the face and body habitus and these may be missed unless you stop and consider them: eg acromegaly, thyrotoxicosis, myxoedema, Cushing's syndrome, or hypopituitarism. Is there anything about him to trigger thoughts about Paget's disease, Marfan's, myotonia, and Parkinson's syndrome? Look for rashes, eg the malar flush of mitral disease and the butterfly rash of SLE.

Assess the degree of hydration by examining the skin turgor, the axillae, and mucous membranes. Check peripheral perfusion (eg press the nose, and time capillary return). Do temperature, and BP (lying and standing may be compared to detect early signs of shock).

Check for cyanosis (central and peripheral, p42). Is the patient jaundiced? Yellow skin is unreliable and may resemble the lemon tinge of uraemia, pernicious anaemia, carotenaemia (sclerae are not yellow), or caecal carcinoma. The sign of jaundice is yellow sclerae seen in good daylight. Pallor is a nonspecific sign and may be racial, familial, or cosmetic. Anaemia is assessed from the skin creases and conjunctivae (usually pale if Hb <9g/dL: you cannot conclude anything from *normal* conjunctival colour; but if they are pale there is a good chance that the patient is anaemic.[1] Koilonychia and stomatitis (redness around the mouth, particularly at its lateral edge) suggest iron-deficiency. Anaemia with jaundice suggests malignancy or haemolysis. Pathological hyperpigmentation is seen in Addison's, haemochromatosis (slate-grey) and amiodarone, gold, silver, and minocycline therapy.

Palpate for lymph nodes in the neck (from behind), axillae, groins, epitrochlear region, and abdomen (p50). Any subcutaneous nodules (p52)?

Don't forget to look at the temperature chart and the results of urinalysis and urine output where indicated.

1 *Bandolier* 1997 **45** page 6: 55% of 302 patients with Hb <9g/dL had conjunctival pallor and 22 had borderline pallor (TS Sheth 1997 J of *General Internal Medicine* **12** 102–6)

The hands

A wealth of information can be gained from shaking hands and rapidly examining the hands of the patient. Are they warm and well-perfused? Warm, sweaty hands may signal hyperthyroidism while cold, moist hands may be due to anxiety. Are the rings tight with oedema? Lightly pinch the dorsum of the hand—persistent ridging of the skin suggests loss of tissue turgor. Are there any nicotine stains?

Nails The nails are affected by a variety of metabolic disturbances: *Koilonychia (spoon-shaped nails)* suggests iron deficiency but may occur in other conditions such as syphilis or ischaemic heart disease. *Onycholysis (destruction of nails)* is seen with hyperthyroidism, fungal nail infection, and psoriasis. *Beau's lines* are transverse furrows that signify temporary arrest of nail growth and occur with periods of severe illness. As nails grow at roughly 0.1mm/day, by measuring the distance from the cuticle it is often possible to date the stress. *Mees' lines* are paired white, parallel transverse bands sometimes seen in hypoalbuminaemia. *Terry's lines* are white nails with normal pink tips seen in cirrhosis. *Pitting* of the nails is seen in psoriasis and alopecia areata.

Splinter haemorrhages are fine longitudinal haemorrhagic streaks, (under nails) which, in the febrile patient, may suggest infective endocarditis. They may be normal—being caused, for example, by gardening, when their subconjuntival correlates will be *absent*.

Nail-fold infarcts are characteristically seen in vasculitic disorders.

Clubbing (PLATE 7) of the nails occurs with many disorders (see p42). It is not generally seen in simple emphysema. There is an exaggerated longitudinal curvature, loss of the angle between the nail and the nail bed, and the nail feels 'boggy'. Cause unknown but may be due to increased blood flow through multiple AV shunts in the distal phalanges.

Chronic paronychia is a chronic infection of the nail-fold and presents as a painful swollen nail with intermittent discharge. Treatment involves keeping the nail dry and antibiotics, eg erythromycin 250mg/6h PO and nystatin ointment.

Changes occur in **the hands** in many diseases. *Palmar erythema* is associated with cirrhosis, pregnancy, and polycythaemia. *Pallor* of the palmar creases suggests anaemia. *Pigmentation* of the palmar creases is normal in Asians and blacks but is also seen in Addison's. *Dupuytren's contracture* (fibrosis and contracture of palmar fascia, p696) is seen in liver disease, trauma, epilepsy and ageing. Swollen proximal interphalangeal (PIP) joints with distal (DIP) joints spared suggests rheumatoid arthritis; swollen DIP joints suggests osteoarthritis, gout, or psoriasis. Look for *Heberden's* (distal) and *Bouchard's* (proximal) 'nodes' (osteophytes—bone overgrowth at a joint—seen with osteoarthritis).

The cardiovascular system

Presenting symptoms	Risk factors for IHD
Chest pain	Smoking
Dyspnoea—exertional?	Hypertension
orthopnoea? PND?	Diabetes mellitus
Ankle swelling	Hyperlipidaemia
Palpitations; dizziness; blackouts	Family history (stroke; heart disease)

Past history	Past tests and procedures	
Angina or MI	ECG	Echocardiography
Rheumatic fever	Angiograms	Scintigraphy
Intermittent claudication	Angioplasty/stents	CABG (bypass grafts)

Examination *Inspection:* Form a general impression of the patient while taking the above history. Is the patient in distress or pain? Note the general colour and body habitus. Are there features of Marfan's (tall, long-fingered, aortic incompetence), Down's, (ASD, VSD) or Turner's (coarctation of the aorta)? Rheumatological disorders are associated with cardiac lesions (eg ankylosing spondylitis—aortic incompetence).

The face may suggest certain cardiovascular diseases. Mitral stenosis is associated with a characteristic *malar flush*. Examine the eyes for *Argyll Robertson pupils* (p56) which may be seen with syphilitic aortic incompetence. Prosthetic valves can produce *jaundice* from low-grade haemolysis. *Xanthelasma* and *corneal arcus* suggest hyperlipidaemia. *Proptosis, lid lag,* and *lid retraction* may alert you to Graves' disease (p542) as the cause of the irregular rhythm and heart failure. Look at tongue and lips for *cyanosis* (p42); while here, a *high-arched palate* may remind you of Marfan's; *mucosal petechiae* and *dental engineering* suggest endocarditis.

Pick up the patient's *hand*. See p25. Look for the peripheral stigmata of endocarditis: splinter haemorrhages, Osler's nodes (tender lumps in the pulps of fingertips), Janeway lesions (red macules on the wrist and dorsum). Note any tendon xanthomas (≈lipidaemia) and nicotine stains.

Next examine the *pulse.* See p54. Note rate and rhythm at the radial pulse and character and volume at the carotid or brachial pulse. Feel for the peripheral pulses. *Radio-radial delay* and *radio-femoral delay* (ie asynchrony of the two pulses) is seen in coarctation of the aorta. Do *blood pressure* (use a broad cuff for fat arms). Assess *venous pressure* from height of filling of internal jugular vein above the manubrium (at 45°, p258).

Inspect the *praecordium* for *scars* (lateral thoracotomy≈mitral valvotomy; midline sternotomy≈bypass grafts), *deformity, visible pulsations,* and *rectangles* (≈pacemaker). Palpate the *apex beat*—the point furthest from the manubrium where the heart is felt beating, normally in the 5th intercostal space in the mid-clavicular line (= '5th ICS MCL')—see p40. Palpate with the palm and heel of your hand for a *parasternal heave* of right ventricular hypertrophy, and for *praecordial thrills* (palpable murmurs).

Chest Percuss the back to exclude pleural effusions and listen for inspiratory crepitations due to left ventricular failure. Feel for sacral oedema.

Abdomen Lie the patient flat and feel for hepatomegaly (right ventricular failure) and check if it is pulsatile (tricuspid incompetence). Feel for splenomegaly (endocarditis) and for an abdominal aneurysm. Palpate the femoral arteries and auscultate for any bruits.

The extremities Next feel peripheral pulses and look for signs of peripheral vascular disease, oedema, clubbing, xanthomata, and varicose veins (if CABG may be a possibility). Listen over the femoral pulses for bruits.

Examine the *fundi* for hypertensive change (p300) or Roth's spots (in endocarditis, also ward test for haematuria). See *temperature charts*.

Auscultating the heart

Auscultating means listening—generally, but wrongly, held to be the essence of cardiovascular medicine at the bedside. A caricature of cardiology ward rounds is of the anxious junior gabbling through the history, while noting his chief's fingers twisting his stethoscope hotly under his collar, impatient to 'get down to the main business' of listening to the heart—thereby blotting out all talk in favour of a few blissful minutes communing with 'lub' and 'dup'. This is absurd because it is the heart sounds which are repetitive, and the patient's story which is ever-changing, and which is so often the real challenge to elicit and interpret. If you spend time listening to the history, and feeling pulses, auscultation should hold few surprises: you will often already know the diagnosis.

Listen with bell and diaphragm at the apex (mitral area, p26). Identify 1st and 2nd heart sounds: are they normal? Listen for added sounds and murmurs. Repeat at lower left sternal edge and in aortic and pulmonary areas (right and left of manubrium)—and in the left axilla (sounds of mitral incompetence radiate here). Reposition the patient in the left lateral position: again feel the apex beat (?tapping) and listen specifically for a diastolic rumble of mitral stenosis. Sit the patient up and listen at the lower left sternal edge for the blowing diastolic sound of aortic regurgitation—accentuated at the end of expiration.

History Age, race, occupation. *Family history* of atopy*, TB, emphysema?

Presenting symptoms		Past history
Cough	Chest pain	Pneumonia; bronchitis
Sputum	Haemoptysis	Tuberculosis
Dyspnoea	Wheeze	Previous CXR abnormalities
Sinusitis	Hoarseness	Drugs (eg steroids, bronchodilators)
Fevers	Night sweats	Allergies; atopy* (eg eczema)

28

Social history Smoking; occupation (farming, mining); pets.

Examination Undress to the waist, and sit him on the edge of the bed.

Inspection *Assess general health:* is he distressed? Cachetic? Dyspnoeic patients are sitting forward, with elbows supported, using accessory muscles of respiration and often exhibit nasal flaring and intercostal recession with inspiration. Count the respiratory rate and note breathing *pattern*. Look for chest wall deformities (p40). Inspect the chest for *scars* of past surgery, chest drains, or radiotherapy (skin thickening and tattoos demarcating the field of irradiation). Note *chest wall movement:* is it symmetrical? If not, pathology is on the restricted side.

Examine the hands for *clubbing* (p42; PLATE 7), peripheral cyanosis, nicotine staining, and wasting of the intrinsic muscles of the hand—seen in T1 lesions (Pancoast's syndrome p706). Palpate the wrist for tenderness (hypertrophic pulmonary osteoarthropathy, p342). Check for *asterixis* (CO_2 retention flap). Palpate the pulse for obvious *paradox* (weakens in inspiration), take the BP, if necessary, to quantify paradox in mmHg.

Inspect the face Look out for the ptosis and constricted pupil of Horner's syndrome. Are the tongue and lips bluish (central cyanosis)?

Feel the trachea in the sternal notch (it should pass just to the right). If deviated, concentrate on the upper lobes for pathology. Note the presence of *tracheal tug* (descent of trachea with inspiration, suggesting severe airflow limitation). Palpate for **cervical lymphadenopathy**.

Assess chest expansion using hands or tape measure (normal 5cm). Pathology lies on the side with limited movement. Ask the patient to repeat '99' while palpating the chest wall. The differences in vibration or **vocal fremitus** follow the same pattern as for vocal resonance.

Percussion Percuss all areas including axillae, clavicles, and supraclavicular areas. Listen and *feel* for the nature and symmetry of the sound. Distinguish between normal, resonant (hyperexpanded chest or pneumothorax), dull (over liver, consolidated lung), and stony dull (effusion).

Auscultation "Please breath in and out while I listen" (not too deep or fast). Note change in *intensity* ($\uparrow$ or $\downarrow$) or change in *nature* (eg bronchial breathing, high pitched or blowing; symmetrical or asymmetrical). Listen for *added sounds,* eg wheeze (poly- or monophonic; inspiratory or expiratory), crackles (early vs late/pan-inspiratory, fine vs coarse), rub (suggests pleurisy—eg from pulmonary infarct or pneumonia).

Vocal resonance is the auscultatory equivalent of tactile vocal fremitus and is altered similarly by pathology: "Please say '99'." Sounds are muffled over normal lung but *louder* and *clearer* over *consolidated lung*. Whispering may be heard clearly over consolidated lung (*whispering pectoriloquy*).

If an abnormality is detected, try to localize it to the likely segment (see figure opposite). Look at the JVP (p258) and examine the heart for signs of **cor pulmonale** (p366). Look at **temperature charts**. Is the **sputum** clear, white, red, pink, frothy, or green (p56 and p48)?

*Atopy implies predisposition to, or concurrence of, asthma, hay fever & eczema. It is defined as production of specific IgE on exposure to common allergens (from house dust mite, grass, cats); BMJ 1998 i 607

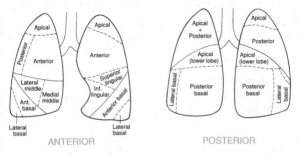

The respiratory segments supplied by the segmental bronchi.

Genitourinary history

Presenting symptoms
Fever, loin pain, dysuria[i], haematuria
Urethral/vaginal discharge (p221)
Sex—any problems? Painful inter-
course (dyspareunia, OHCS p74)
Menstrual history: menarche, meno-
pause, length of periods, amount,
pain? intermenstrual loss? LMP?

Past history
Urinary tract infection
Renal colic
DM, BP↑, gout, analgesic use
Previous operations
Social history
Smoking
Sexual orientation

Detecting outflow obstruction (eg from prostatic hypertrophy). Ask:
On wanting to pass water, is there delay before you start? (*Hesitancy*)
Does the flow stop and start? Do you go on dribbling when you think
you've stopped, even after giving it a good shake? (*Terminal dribbling*)
Is your stream getting weaker? Can you hit the wall OK? (*Poor stream*)
Do you ever pass water when you do not want to? (*Incontinence*)
Do you feel the bladder is not empty after passing water? (*Strangury*[i])
On feeling an urge to pass water, do you have to go at once? (*Urgency*[i])
Do you urinate often at night? *Nocturia*[i] In the day? How often? (*Frequency*[i])

[i] = irritative symptoms; *they can be caused by eg UTI as well as obstruction.*

Gastrointestinal history

Presenting symptoms
Abdominal pain
Nausea, vomiting, haematemesis
Dysphagia (p492)
Indigestion (dyspepsia, p44)
Recent change in bowel habit
Diarrhoea or constipation
Rectal bleeding or melaena
Appetite, weight change
Mouth ulcers; Jaundice
Pruritus; Dark urine, pale stools

Past history
Peptic ulcer
Carcinoma
Jaundice, hepatitis
Blood transfusions, tattoos
Previous operations
Last menstrual period, LMP
Past treatment
Steroids, the Pill
NSAIDs; antibiotics
Dietary changes

Social history
Smoking, alcohol
Overseas travel, tropical illnesses
Contact with jaundiced persons
Occupational exposures
Sexual orientation

Family history
Irritable bowel disease
Inflammatory bowel disease
Peptic ulcer
Polyps, cancer
Jaundice

Examining the gastrointestinal system

Inspect (and smell) for signs of chronic liver disease:
●Hepatic foetor on breath (p504) ●Gynaecomastia ●Clubbing (rare)
●Purpura (purple stained skin, p592) ●Scratch marks ●Muscle wasting
●Spider naevi (fill from the centre) (pruritus) ●Jaundice
●Leuconychia (hypoalbuminaemia) ●Palmar erythema
●Liver flap (asterixis, a coarse irregular tremor)
Inspect for signs of malignancy, anaemia, jaundice, hard Virchow's node
in left supraclavicular fossa (p142). Look at the abdomen. Note:
●Visible pulsation (aneurysm, p118) ●Peristalsis ●Scars ●Masses
●Striae (stretch marks, eg pregnancy) ●Distension ●Genitalia ●Herniae

If abdominal wall veins look dilated, assess *direction of flow*. In IVC
obstruction, flow below the umbilicus is up; in portal hypertension
(*caput medusae*), it is down. *The cough test:* While looking at the face, ask
the patient to cough. If this causes abdominal pain, flinching, or a protective movement of hands towards the abdomen, suspect peritonitis.

Palpating and percussing the abdomen

Adjust the patient so that his head rests on only one pillow, his arms at his side. Make sure that he and your hands are warm. While palpating, be looking at his face to assess any pain. First palpate gently through each quadrant, starting away from the pain. Note tenderness, guarding (involuntary tensing of abdominal muscles because of pain or fear of it), and rebound tenderness (greater pain on removing hand than on gently depressing abdomen: it is a sign of peritoneal inflammation); Rovsing's sign (p114).

Palpating the liver: Begin in the right iliac fossa with the patient breathing deeply. Use the radial border of the index finger to feel the liver edge, moving up 2cm at a time at each breath. Assess its size, regularity, smoothness, and tenderness. Is it pulsatile? Confirm the lower border and define the upper border by percussion (normal upper limit is in 5th intercostal space): it may be pushed down by emphysema. Listen for an overlying bruit. See p48 for causes of hepatomegaly (enlarged liver).

Palpating the spleen: Start in the RIF and move towards the left upper quadrant with each respiration. Features of spleen which differentiate it from kidney: one cannot get above it (ribs overlie its top), overlying percussion note is dull, it moves more with respiration—toward the RIF, it may have a palpable notch on its medial side. If you suspect splenomegaly but cannot detect it, assess the patient in the right lateral position with your left hand pulling forwards from behind the rib cage; also percuss in the mid-axillary line in the 10th interspace: it should be resonant.

Palpating the kidneys: Try bimanually with the left hand under the patient to push it up in the renal angle. Attempt to ballot the kidney (ie bounce it gently but decisively between a hand applied to the loin and the other applied opposite, anteriorly). It moves only slightly with respiration.

Assess other masses by the scheme on p152.

Percuss for the shifting dullness of ascites (p152; also PLATE 1): the level of right-sided flank dullness increases by lying on the right.

Auscultation Bowel sounds: absence implies ileus; they are enhanced and tinkling in bowel obstruction. Listen for bruits.

Examine Mouth, tongue, rectum (p155), genitalia, urine, as appropriate.

The neurological system

History This should be taken from the patient and if possible, from a close friend or relative as well. The patient's memory, perception or speech may be affected by the disorder making the history difficult to obtain. Note the progression of the symptoms and signs: gradual deterioration (eg tumour) vs intermittent exacerbations (eg multiple sclerosis). Ask about age, occupation, ethnic origin. Right- or left-handed?

Presenting symptoms
Headache
Problems with:
  –vision (blurring or double vision)
  –hearing (tinnitus, vertigo)
  –smell, taste
  –speech (dysarthria, dysphasia p430)
Pain
Pins and needles (paraesthesiae)
Numbness or abnormal sensations
Weakness or balance problems
Sphincter disturbance
Abnormal involuntary movements
Fits, faints, or 'turns': –frequency, duration
  –mode of onset, termination ?warning
  –tongue biting? incontinence?
  –time to recovery; confused after?
Cognitive state (p77)

Past history
Meningitis, encephalitis
Head or spine trauma
Seizures
Previous operations
Risks for vascular disease
  (p432, AF, BP↑, lipids↑,
  diabetes mellitus, smoking)

Medications
Current and previous

Social + family history
What can the patient do
  or not do, eg get to pub
Family history of neuro-
  logical or psychiatric
  disease
Consanguinity

The neurological examination

Higher mental function Conscious level, orientation in time, place and person, memory (short- and long-term). See p77.

Speech Dysphasia, dysarthria, dysphonia. See p430.

Skull and spine Malformation. Signs of injury. Palpate scalp. If there is any question of spinal injury, *do not move the spine*. Carotid/cranial bruits.

Sensation Light touch (cotton-wool), pain (pin-prick), vibration (128Hz tuning fork), joint position sense. See dermatomes p410–11.

Motor system *Inspect* for abnormality of posture, or involuntary movement, wasting or fasciculation (visible muscle twitching not moving the limb)? *Drift:* Patient sitting, arms outstretched, eyes closed. Do arms drift? Then do *tone, power* (p402), *reflexes* (remember to test for clonus), *sensation*, and then ask patient to touch nose with index finger (*coordination*). *Tone:* Look for spasticity (pressure fails to move a joint until it gives way—like a clasp-knife), rigidity (lead pipe), rigidity + tremor = cogwheeling, clonus (rhythmic muscle 'beats' on sudden stretching, eg gastrocnemius on ankle dorsiflexion). *Power:* Oppose each movement: see p402; root values: p408. *Coordination:* Finger–nose (touch nose with index finger), rapid alternating movements, rub heel up and down shin. *Reflexes:* Biceps (C5–6), triceps (C7–8), supinator (C5–6), knee (L3–4 ± L2), ankle (S1–2), abdominals (lost in upper motor neurone—UMN—lesions), plantars (up-going in UMN lesions). See myotomes p408. *Gait* (PLATE 3): Have patient walk: normally; heel-to-toe; on heels; then on toes. Ask him to stand feet together. If balance is worse on shutting eyes, Romberg's test is +ve, implying abnormal joint position sense. If he cannot perform this even [wi]th eyes open, this may be cerebellar ataxia, but is not Romberg's+ve. [B]ear in mind books present idealized situations: often one or more sign [eq]uivocal or even contrary to expectation; don't be put off, consider [w]hole picture, including the history; try re-examining the patient.

Examining the cranial nerves

Face the patient (helps spot asymmetry). *For causes of lesions, see p458.*

I   *Smell*—Test ability of each nostril to differentiate floral smells.

II   *Acuity* and its correctability with glasses or pin-hole; use chart on p37. Visual fields: compare during confrontation with your own fields or formally; note losses and any inattention. Tests and sites of lesions are given in full in *OHCS* p492. Pupils (p54): size, shape, symmetry, reactions to light (direct and consensual), and accommodation if reactions to light are poor. *Ophthalmoscopy:* Darken the room. Instil tropicamide 0.5%, 1 drop, if needed. Select the focusing lens for the best view of the optic disc (pale? swollen?). Follow vessels outwards to view each quadrant; rack back through the ophthalmoscope's lenses to inspect lens and cornea. If the view is obscured, examine the red reflex with your focus on the margin of the pupil. You will get a view of the fovea if you ask the patient to look at the ophthalmoscope's finest beam (after drops)—this is the sacred place: the *only* place with 6/6 vision. Any pathology here merits prompt ophthalmic referral.

III, IV, and VI: *Eye movements*—(*OHCS* p486), nystagmus p422.
III palsy: ptosis, large pupil, eye down and out.
IV palsy: diplopia on looking down and in (often noticed on descending stairs)—he may try compensating for this by tilting his head (ocular torticollis).
VI nerve palsy: horizontal diplopia on looking out.

V   *Motor palsy*—'Open your mouth': jaw deviates to side of lesion. *Sensory:* Corneal reflex lost first; check all 3 divisions.

VII *Facial nerve lesions* cause droop and weakness. As the forehead has bilateral representation in the brain, only the lower ⅔ is affected in UMN lesions, but all of one side of the face in LMN lesions. Ask to: 'raise your eyebrows'; 'show me your teeth'; 'puff out your cheeks'. Test taste (rarely done) with salt/sweet solutions; p458–60.

VIII *Hearing*—Ask patient to repeat a number whispered in an ear while you block the other. *Balance:* See p420 & p422.

IX and X *Gag reflex*—Palate pulled to normal side on saying 'Ah'.

XI *Trapezii*—'Shrug your shoulders' against resistance.
Sternomastoid—'Turn your head to the left/right' against resistance.

XII *Tongue movement*—Deviates to the side of the lesion.

The psychiatric assessment

Introduce yourself, ask a few factual questions (precise name, age, marital status, job, and who is at home). These will help your patient to relax.

34 **Presenting problem** Then ask for the main problems which have led to this consultation. Sit back and listen. Don't worry whether the information is in convenient form or not—this is an opportunity for the patient to come out with his or her worries unsullied by your expectations. Ask: 'Are there any other problems?' After 3–5 minutes you should have a list of all the problems (each sketched only briefly). Read them back to the patient and ask if there are any more.

History of presenting problem For each problem obtain details, both current state and history of onset, precipitating factors, and effects on life.

Check of major psychiatric symptoms Check those which have not yet been covered: *depression* (low mood, thoughts of worthlessness, hopelessness, suicidal thoughts and plans: "Have you ever been so low that you thought of harming yourself?", "What thoughts have you had?", sleep disturbance with early morning waking, loss of weight and appetite); *hallucinations* ("Have you ever heard voices when there has not been anyone there, or seen visions?"), and *delusions* ("Have you ever had any thoughts or beliefs which have struck you afterwards as bizarre?"); *anxiety* and *avoidance behaviour* (eg avoiding shopping because of anxiety or phobias); *alcohol* and *other drugs*.

Family history Ask about health, personality and occupation of parents and siblings, and the family's medical and psychiatric history.

Background history Try to understand the presenting problem.
Biography (relationships with family and peers as a child, school and work record, sexual relationships and current relationships and family). Previous ways of dealing with stress and whether there have been problems and symptoms similar to the presenting ones.
Previous personality (mood, character, hobbies, attitudes, and standards).

Past medical and psychiatric history

Mental state examination This is the state *now*, at the time of interview.
- *Observable behaviour:* Eg excessive slowness, signs of anxiety.
- *Mode of speech:* Include the rate of speech, eg retarded or gabbling (pressure of speech). Note its content.
- *Mood:* Note thoughts about harming self or others. Gauge your own responses to the patient. The laughter and grandiose ideas of manic patients are contagious, as to a lesser extent is the expression of thoughts from a depressed person.
- *Beliefs:* Eg about himself, his own body, about other people and the future. Note abnormal beliefs (delusions), eg that thoughts are overheard, and abnormal ideas (eg persecutory, grandiose).
- *Unusual experiences or hallucinations:* Note modality, eg visual.
- *Orientation:* In time, place, and person. What is the date? What time of day is it? Where are you? What is your name?
- *Short-term memory:* Give a name and address and test recall after 5 minutes. Make sure that he has got the address clear in his head before waiting for the 5 minutes to elapse.
- *Long-term memory:* Current affairs recall. Name of current political leaders (p78). This tests many other CNS functions, not just memory.
- *Concentration:* Months of the year backwards.

Note the patient's insight and the degree of your rapport.

Non-verbal behaviour Gesture, gaze and mutual gaze, expressions, laughter, pauses (while listening to voices?), attitude (eg withdrawn).

Assessing the locomotor system

This aims to find any rheumatological conditions, and to assess any motor disability. It is based on the GALS locomotor screen (see below).[1]

▶Don't *just* catalogue muscle function. (Details of testing each muscle may be found on p408.) Find out what she can do—eg with her arthritic fingers, can she do up zips or buttons? Can she open a tin? Is she using any special devices to assist in daily life? What can't she do that she would like? Does she have any comments on her joints? In short, assess disability (and ability) and handicap as well as impairment (p66).

Essence Ask questions, look, compare, move, and palpate. If a joint feels normal to the patient, looks normal to you, and has a full range of movement, it usually *is* normal.

Valgus or varus? In a valgus deformity, the part of the limb distal to the deformity is angled *away* from the midline. (Varus is the other way.)

3 screening questions ●Are you free of muscle pain or stiffness? ●Can you dress all right? ●Can you manage stairs? If 'Yes' to all 3, muscle and joint problems are unlikely. If 'No' to any, go into detail.

Screening examination To be done in light underwear. (No corsets!)

Spine: Observe from behind: Is muscle bulk OK (buttocks, shoulders)? Is the spine straight? Symmetrical paraspinal muscles? Swellings/deformities?
Observe from the side: Normal cervical and lumbar lordosis? Kyphosis?
'Touch your toes, please': Are lumbar spine and hip flexion normal?
Observe from in front for the rest of the examination. Ask him to:
'Tilt head towards shoulders': Is lateral cervical flexion normal?

Arms: 'Arms straight': Tests elbow extension. Also test supination/pronation.
'Put hands behind head': Tests glenohumeral + sternoclavicular movement.
Examine the hands: See p25. Any deformity, wasting, or swellings?
'Put index finger on thumb': Tests pincer grip. Assess dexterity.

Legs: Observe legs: Normal quadriceps bulk? Any swelling or deformity?
Find any knee effusion: Sit the patient down, take the leg on your lap and do the patella tap test (this also tests for patello-femoral tenderness) or, to be more sensitive, watch any fluid moving from compartment to compartment by stroking upwards over the medial side of the knee and then downwards over the lateral side. If there is fluid, consider aspirating it. Any blood, crystals or pus?
Observe feet: Any deformity? Are arches high or low? Any callosities? These may indicate an abnormal gait of some chronicity.

Gait: 'Walk over there please': Is the gait smooth? Good arm swing? Stride length OK? Normal heel strike and toe off? Can he turn quickly? PLATE 3

Other manoeuvres ●Press over the midpoint of each supraspinatus muscle to elicit the tenderness of fibromyalgia (OHCS p675).
●Squeeze across 2nd–5th metacarpals. Any synovitis? Repeat in metatarsals.
●Palpate for crepitus with your palm on his knee (patient supine) while you passively flex knee and hip to the full extent. Is movement limited?
●Internally rotate each hip in flexion.

The GALS system for quickly recording your findings[2]

	Appearance:	Movement:
G (Gait) ✓		
A (Arms)	✓	✓
L (Legs)	✓	✓
S (Spine)	✓	✓

A tick (✓) means normal. If not nor~~ stitute a cross with a footnote to explain what the exac~

1 M Doherty 1992 *Annals of the Rheumatic Diseases* 51 1165–9 2 Ap Arthritis and Rheumatism Council and the UK Society for Rheuma

Method and order for routine examination

We all have our own system, sometimes based on these lines, but sometimes containing elements unique to each doctor, arising from his or her own interaction with countless past patients and their eccentricities. This fact is one reason why it is often so helpful to ask for second opinions: the same field may be ploughed again but yield quite a different harvest.

1 Look at the patient. Is he healthy, unwell, or *in extremis*?

2 Put the thermometer in his mouth.

3 Examine the nails and hands.

4 Work up the arm: pulse rate and rhythm. Keeping your finger on the pulse, count respiratory rate and specifically consider: Paget's, acromegaly, endocrine disease (thyroid, pituitary, or adrenal hypo- or hyper-function), body hair, abnormal pigmentation, skin conditions.

5 Blood pressure.

6 Conjunctivae (anaemia) and sclerae (jaundice).

7 Read thermometer.

8 Examine mouth & tongue (*cyanosed; smooth; furred; beefy*, ie rhomboid area denuded of papillae by candida, eg after much steroid inhaler use).

9 Examine the neck from behind: nodes, goitre.

10 Make sure the patient is at 45° to begin cvs examination in the neck: jvp; feel for character and volume of carotid pulse.

11 The praecordium. Look for abnormal pulsations. Feel the apex beat for character and position. Feel for parasternal heave and thrills. Auscultate the apex (bell) in the left lateral position, then the other three areas (p26) and carotids (diaphragm). Sit the patient forward and listen during expiration.

12 Sit patient forward to find sacral oedema; look for ankle oedema.

13 Now begin the respiratory examination with the patient at 90°. Observe respiration and posterior chest wall. Assess expansion, then percuss and auscultate the chest with the bell.

14 Sit the patient back. Feel the trachea. Inspect again. Assess expansion of the anterior chest. Percuss and auscultate again.

15 Examine the breasts and axillary nodes (p138).

16 Lie the patient flat with only one pillow. Inspect, palpate, percuss and auscultate the abdomen.

17 Look at the legs: swellings, perfusion, pulses, oedema.

18 cns exam: *Cranial nerves:* pupil responses; fundi. Do corneal reflexes. 'Open your mouth; stick your tongue out; screw up your eyes; show me your teeth; raise your eyebrows'. *Peripheral nerves:* Look for wasting and fasciculation. Test tone in all limbs. 'Hold your hands out with your palms towards the ceiling and fingers wide. Now shut your eyes'. Watch for pronator drift. 'Keep your eyes shut and touch your nose with each index finger.' 'Lift your leg straight in the air. Keep it there. Put your heel on the opposite knee (eyes shut) and run it up your own shin'. You have now tested power, coordination, and joint position sense. Tuning fork on toes and index fingers to assess sensation.

19 Examine the gait and the speech.

20 Any abnormalities of higher mental function to pursue?

1 Consider rectal and vaginal examination. Is a chaperone needed?

Examine the urine with dipstick and microscope if appropriate.

...neral, go into detail where you find (or suspect) something to be wrong.

He moved

all the brightest gems

faster and faster towards the

ever-growing bucket of lost hopes;
had there been just one more year

of peace the battalion would have made
a floating system of perpetual drainage.

A silent fall of immense snow came near oily
remains of the recently eaten supper on the table.

We drove on in our old sunless walnut. Presently
classical eggs ticked in the new afternoon shadows.

We were instructed by my cousin Jasper not to exercise by country
house visiting unless accompanied by thirteen geese or gangsters.

The modern American did not prevail over the pair of redundant bronze puppies.
The worn-out principle is a bad omen which I am never glad to ransom in August.

Record the smallest type or object accurately read or named at 30cm

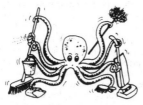

38 Symptoms are features which the patient reports. Physical signs are elicited on examination by the doctor. Together they constitute the clinical features of the condition in that patient. To discuss any single feature in isolation is artificial as each is interpretable only in the context of the others. Nonetheless, it is still valuable to have an understanding of the pathophysiology and significance of individual features. Here we discuss some of the more important symptoms, and signs. Where these are discussed in relevant chapters of this book and the OHCS, reference is given.

This chapter is disappointing in trying to explain *combinations* of symptoms, as illnesses often do not fit into the 80-or-so features given below. It is hard to compare one list with others on separate pages—and the lists are not exhaustive. It was this disappointment which was our stimulus to produce an electronic system (p17), where over 20,000 signs, symptoms and test results can be sifted in devious and diverse ways to help with difficult problems in differential diagnosis. So do not expect too much from this chapter: just a few common causes of common symptoms and signs.

Abdominal distension†† *Causes:* The famous five Fs—*fat, fluid, faeces, fetus,* or *flatus*). Also *food* (eg in malabsorption). Specific groups:

Air:	*Ascites:*	*Solid masses:*	*Pelvic masses:*
Gastrointestinal obstruction (including faecal)	Malignancy*	Malignancy*	Bladder: full or Ca
	Hypoproteinaemia (eg nephrotic)	Lymph nodes	Fibroids; fetus
Aerophagy (air swallowing)	R heart failure	Aorta aneurysm	Ovarian cyst
	Portal hypertension	*Cysts:* renal, pancreatic	Ovarian cancer
			Uterine cancer

*Any intra-abdominal organ, eg colon, stomach, pancreas, liver, kidney.

Air is resonant on percussion. *Ascites* (free fluid in peritoneal cavity, PLATE 1): Signs: shifting dullness (p30); fluid thrill (place patient's hand firmly on his abdomen in sagittal plane and flick one flank with your finger while your other hand feels on the other flank for a fluid thrill). The characteristic feature of *pelvic masses* is that you cannot get below them (ie their lower border cannot be defined). Causes of *right iliac fossa masses:* Appendix mass or abscess (p114); kidney mass; Ca caecum; a Crohn's or TB mass; intussusception; amoebic abscess or any pelvic mass (above).

Causes of *ascites with portal hypertension:* See p152. See causes of hepatomegaly (p48) and splenomegaly (p152).

Abdominal pain††† varies greatly depending on the underlying cause. Examples include: irritation of the mucosa (acute gastritis), smooth muscle spasm (acute enterocolitis), capsular stretching (liver congestion in CCF), peritoneal inflammation (acute appendicitis), direct splanchnic nerve stimulation (retroperitoneal extension of tumour). The *character, duration,* and *frequency* depend on the mechanism of production. The *location* and *distribution* of referred pain depend on the anatomical site. *Time of occurrence* and *aggravating or relieving factors* such as meals, defaecation, and sleep also have special significance related to the underlying disease process. The site of the pain may provide a clue as to the cause. Evaluation of the *acute abdomen* is considered on p112.

Amaurosis fugax See p436.

Anaemia†† may be assessed from the skin creases and conjunctivae (pale if Hb<9g/dL). Koilonychia and stomatitis suggest iron deficiency. Anaemia with jaundice suggests malignancy or haemolysis. See p572.

Apex beat[†] This is the point furthest from the manubrium where the heart can be felt beating—normally the 5th intercostal space in the mid-clavicular line (5th ICS MCL). Lateral displacement may be from cardiomegaly or mediastinal shift. Assess its character: a *pressure loaded* apex is a forceful, sustained undisplaced impulse (eg hypertension or aortic stenosis causing LV hypertrophy with unenlarged cavity). A *volume overloaded* (hyperdynamic) apex is forceful, unsustained, and displaced down and laterally (eg cavity enlargement from aortic or mitral incompetence). It is *tapping* in mitral stenosis (palpable 1st heart sound); *dyskinetic* after anterior MI or with LV aneurysm; *double* or *triple impulse* in HOCM (p316–7).

Backache p661. **Blackouts** p418. **Breathlessness** p44.

Breast pain Often this is premenstrual (*cyclical mastalgia*, OHCS p16)—but the patient is often worried that she has breast cancer. So examine carefully (p138), and refer eg for mammography as appropriate. If there is no sign of breast pathology, and it is not cyclical, think of:
- Tietze's syndrome
- Gall stones
- Angina
- Oestrogens (HRT)
- Bornholm disease
- Lung disease
- Thoracic outlet syndrome[□]

If none of the above, *wearing a firm bra* all day may help, as may *NSAIDs or gamolenic acid* 40mg/4h PO. If there is very local pain, consider injecting it with 2mL of 1% *lignocaine (lidocaine)* with 40mg *methylprednisolone* (1994 *BMJ* ii 866).

Cachexia Severe generalized muscle wasting usually implying malnutrition, neoplasia, Alzheimer's disease, prolonged inanition, or infection—eg TB, enteropathic AIDS ('slim disease', eg from *Cryptosporidium*, p486).

Carotid bruits may signify stenosis (>30%) often near the origin of internal carotid. Heard best behind the angle of jaw. Usual cause: atheroma. The key question is: *is the patient symptomatic?* With symptomless carotid bruits the risk of stroke is too small (<3% over 3 years for non-fatal strokes, and ~0.3% for fatal strokes) to justify the risks of endarterectomy. If symptomatic, consider Doppler (p432–6) + surgery if stenosis >70%. In anyone with a carotid bruit, consider aspirin prophylaxis. Ask a neurologist's advice. (1995 *JAMA* 273 1412 + 1995 *Lancet* 345 209 + 1254).

Chest deformity *Barrel chest*: AP diameter↑, tracheal descent and expansion↓, seen in chronic hyperinflation (eg asthma/COPD). *Pigeon chest (pectus carinatum):* Prominent sternum with a flat chest, seen in chronic childhood asthma and rickets. *Funnel chest (pectus excavatum):* Local sternum depression (lower end). *Kyphosis* is increased forward spinal convexity. *Scoliosis* is lateral curvature (OHCS p620)—both may cause a restrictive ventilatory defect. *Harrison's sulcus* is a groove deformity of lower ribs at the diaphragm attachment site, suggesting chronic childhood asthma or rickets.

Chest pains See p256.

Cheyne–Stokes respiration Breathing becomes progressively deeper and then shallower (± episodic apnoea) in cycles. Causes: brainstem lesions/compression (stroke, ICP↑). If the cycle is long (eg 3 minutes) the cause may be a long lung-to-brain circulation time (eg in chronic pulmonary oedema, poor cardiac output). It is enhanced by narcotics.

Chorea means dance—a continuous flow of jerky movements, flitting from one limb or part to another. Each movement looks like a fragment of a normal movement. *Cause:* Basal ganglia lesion: Huntington's (p700); Sydenham's (p304); SLE (p672); Wilson's (p712); kernicterus; polycythaemia (p612); neuroacanthocytosis (a familial association of acanthocytes in peripheral blood with chorea, oro-facial dyskinesia, and axonal neuropathy); thyrotoxicosis (p542); drugs (L-dopa, contraceptive steroids). The early stages of chorea may be detected by feeling fluctuations in muscle tension while the patient grips your finger. Treat with dopamine antagonists, eg haloperidol 0.5–1.5mg/8h PO, or tetrabenazine 25–50mg/8h PO.

Clubbing† (PLATE 7) Finger nails have exaggerated longitudinal curvature + loss of angle between nail and nail bed, and the nail-fold feels boggy.

Thoracic causes:
- Bronchial carcinoma (usually *not* small cell)
- Chronic lung suppuration
  - empyema, abscess
  - bronchiectasis
  - cystic fibrosis
- Fibrosing alveolitis
- Mesothelioma

GI causes:
- Inflammatory bowel (esp. Crohn's disease)
- Cirrhosis
- GI lymphoma
- Malabsorption, eg coeliac

Rare:
- Familial
- Thyroid acropachy (p678)
- Unilateral clubbing, from:
  - axillary artery aneurysm
  - brachial arterio–venous malformations

Cardiac causes:
- Cyanotic congenital heart disease
- Endocarditis
- Atrial myxoma

Constipation See p488.

Cough†† This symptom is a nonspecific reaction to irritation anywhere from the pharynx to the lungs. The patient can sometimes help with the anatomical localization if it is of proximal origin. Some characteristics of the cough may help diagnostically: even if the patient is not expectorating, listening to the cough may tell you that it is *productive*. Other features may help: a *brassy cough*, described as hard and metallic, may be associated with pressure on the trachea; a cough in which the patient complains of a retrosternal pain like a hot poker occurs in *tracheitis*; a *bovine cough* is prolonged and of deep pitch, and occurs in abductor paralysis of the vocal cords; croup is a harsh and hoarse cough of laryngitis; a hacking, irritating, frequent cough occurs in pharyngitis, tracheobronchitis and early in pneumonia. Some coughs are psychogenic. See also *Haemoptysis* (p48).

Chronic cough: Think of pertussis, TB, foreign body, asthma (eg nocturnal).

Cramp (Painful muscle spasm.) Cramp in the legs is common, especially at night. It may also occur after exercise. It only occasionally indicates a disease, in particular: salt depletion, muscle ischaemia, myopathy. Forearm cramps suggest motor neurone disease. Night cramps in the elderly may respond to quinine bisulfate 300mg at night PO twice weekly. Writer's cramp is a focal dystonia causing difficulty with the motor act of writing. The pen is gripped firmly, with excessive flexion of the thumb and index finger (±tremor). There is normally no CNS deficit. Oral drugs or psychotherapy rarely help, but botulinum toxin (OHCS p522) often helps, sometimes dramatically (it has side-effects—*Lancet* **346** 154). Similar specific dystonias may apply to other tasks.

Cyanosis††† Dusky blue skin (*peripheral*, eg of the fingers) or mucosae (*central*, eg of the tongue, representing ≥2.5g/dL of Hb in its rduced form, hence it occurs more readily in polycythaemia than anaemia). Causes:
1. Lung disease resulting in inadequate oxygen transfer (eg COPD, severe pneumonia)—usually correctable by increasing the inspired O_2.
2. Shunting from pulmonary to systemic circulation (eg R–L shunting VSD, patent ductus arteriosus, transposition of the great arteries)—cyanosis is *not* reversed by increasing inspired O_2.
3. Inadequate oxygen uptake (eg met-, or sulf-haemoglobinaemia).

Peripheral cyanosis will occur in causes of central cyanosis, but may also be induced by changes in the peripheral and cutaneous vascular systems in patients with normal oxygen saturations. It occurs in the cold, in hypovolaemia, and in arterial disease, and is therefore not a specific sign.

Deafness See p424. **Dehydration** See p636. **Diarrhoea** See p486.

Dizziness has 3 versions: 1. *Vertigo* is the sensation of the environment

spinning around the patient (p420) ± an unwilled need to cast oneself into any nearby abyss (OHCS p547). 2. *Imbalance* implies difficulty in walking straight eg from disease of peripheral nerves, posterior columns, cerebellum or other central pathways. 3. *Faintness* is the feeling of being about to pass out. It occurs with some seizure disorders and a variety of non-neurological conditions (p418). Sometimes 2–3 elements co-exist: '. . . At the place where I stood, the hillside was cut away like a cliff, with the sea groaning at its foot, blue and pure. There was no more than a moment to suffer. Oh how terrible was the dizziness of that thought! Two times I threw myself forward, and I do not know what power flung me back, still alive, onto the grass which I kissed. . .' (Gérard de Nerval, 1837, translated by Richard Holmes, 1996, in *Footsteps,* HarperCollins).

Dysarthria See p430. **Dysdiadochokinesis** See p457.

Dyspepsia[††] and **indigestion** These are broad terms, used often by patients to signify epigastric or retrosternal pain (or discomfort) which is usually related to meals. ▸Find out exactly what your patient means. 30% have no real abnormality on endoscopy (p498). Of positive findings:

Oesophagitis alone	24%	Gastritis	9%	≥2 'lesions'	23%
Duodenal ulcer (DU)	17%	Duodenitis	6%	Bile reflux	0.7%
Hiatus hernia	15%	Gastric ulcer 5%		Gastric cancer	0.2%

Can we reduce recourse to endoscopy for dyspepsia in those with *H pylori*-induced peptic ulcers (p490) by using bedside tests for *H pylori*? For odds-ratio, see p744. Experience shows some bedside tests are not quick, cheap, or accurate enough for general use. Helisal® and FlexSure® have been compared (*Lancet* 1996 **348** 617). The latter uses serum, formed by allowing a clotted sample to stand. The Helisal test uses capillary or venous blood. The 'gold standard' was taken to be the combined results of the urease test at endoscopy, and histological analysis. Helisal had a false +ve rate of 33% and a false −ve rate of 25%. FlexSure fared better, but it turns out that you have to leave the serum to form for 3 hours before the accuracy of the test approaches the 'gold-standard'—not ideal for a bedside test.

Dyspnoea[†††] is the subjective sensation of shortness of breath, often exacerbated by exertion. Try to quantify exercise tolerance (eg dressing, distance walked, climbing stairs). May be due to:

●*Cardiac*—eg mitral stenosis or left ventricular failure of any cause; LVF is associated with *orthopnoea* (dyspnoea worse on lying; 'how many pillows?') and *paroxysmal nocturnal dyspnoea* (PND; dyspnoea waking one up). There may be ankle oedema also. ▸Any patient who is shocked may also be dyspnoeic—and this may be shock's presenting feature.

●*Lung*—both airway and interstitial disease. May be hard to separate from cardiac causes; asthma may also wake the patient as well as cause early morning dyspnoea and wheeze. Focus on the circumstances in which dyspnoea occurs (eg on exposure to an occupational allergen).

●*Anatomical*—ie diseases of the chest wall, muscles, or pleura.

●*Others*—thyrotoxicosis, ketoacidosis, aspirin poisoning, anaemia, psychogenic. Look for other clues: dyspnoea at rest *unassociated with exertion* may be psychogenic; look for respiratory alkalaemia (peripheral ± perioral parasthesiae ± carpopedal spasm). Speed of onset helps diagnosis:

Acute	Subacute	Chronic
Foreign body	Asthma	COPD and chronic
Pneumothorax	Parenchymal disease	parenchymal diseases
Acute asthma	eg alveolitis	Non-respiratory cause
Pulmonary embolus	effusions	eg cardiac failure
Acute pulmonary oedema	pneumonia	anaemia

Dysuria[†] is painful micturition (from urethral or bladder inflammation typically from infection; also urethral syndrome, p374). *Strangury* is the distressing desire to pass something that will not pass (eg a stone).

Managing dyspepsia in those ≤45yrs not on NSAIDs,
with no weight loss, dysphagia, bleeding, repeated
vomiting, anaemia, masses, or bowel habit change*

↓

Simple antacids ± anti-reflux
measures (p491) if symptoms
of reflux (eg pain on stooping)

↓

Symptoms still persistent   Symptoms not persistent

↓

Previous peptic ulcer   No past ulcer   **No further action**

↓

Test for *H Pylori*
but see caveats opposite

↓

H Pylori found to be present   *H pylori* absent

Eradicate *H Pylori* (p490)
unless this has already
been done elsewhere

Give H$_2$-blocker for 2 weeks

↓

Review symptoms at about 3–4 weeks

↓

Patient well   Patient still has symptoms

↓

No further action

**Upper GI endoscopy (or barium
meal if very old and frail)**

---

*Do endoscopy urgently in dyspeptic adults not falling into this group, or stop NSAIDs and monitor closely.   (After *Clinical Effectiveness Group*, Queen Mary & Westfield College, London, 1997)

Epigastric pain[†] *Acute causes:* Peritonitis; pancreatitis; GI obstruction; gall bladder disease; peptic ulcer; ruptured aortic aneurysm; irritable bowel syndrome. Distant and disobedient organs frequently complain to the epigastrium (p81): the heart (MI), the pleura, the psyche (depression), and the spine: see p280. *Chronic causes:* Peptic ulcer; gastric cancer; chronic pancreatitis; aortic aneurysm; root pain referred from the spine.

Facial pain can be neurological (eg trigeminal neuralgia, p417) or from any other pain-sensitive structure in the head or neck (opposite). *Post-herpetic neuralgia:* This nasty burning pain (eg ophthalmic division of V) all too often becomes chronic and intractable. It is described as 'constant burning with superimposed stabs'. Skin previously affected by zoster is exquisitely sensitive. Treatment is difficult. Give strong psychological support whatever else is tried. Transcutaneous nerve stimulation, capsaicin ointment, and infiltration of local anaesthetic may be tried. Carbamazepine can help (NNT≈3–4). *Sometimes* the pain resolves. If not, tricyclics ± bedtime sedatives may be of help. Note: there is no evidence that treatment of the acute eruption with antivirals reduces the incidence of post-herpetic neuralgia. *Atypical facial pain:* When all causes have been excluded, a group remains who complain of unilateral pain deep in the face or at the angle of cheek and nose. The pain is typically constant, severe, and unresponsive to analgesia. Patients are commonly young females, and while their pain is often attributed to 'psychological' factors, in reality very few meet diagnostic criteria for hysteria or depression. Such patients should certainly not be exposed to the risks of destructive surgery and while many are prescribed antidepressants, some neurologists advocate no treatment.

Faints See **Blackouts** p418.

Fatigue[†††] This feeling is so common that it is a variant of normality. Only 1 in 400 episodes leads to a consultation with a doctor. ►Do not miss depression which often presents in this way. Even if the patient is depressed, a screening history and examination is important to rule out chronic disease. *Tests* should include FBC, ESR, U&E, plasma glucose, TFTs, and CXR. Arrange follow-up to see what develops. In most, the cause will be emotional problems and these must be addressed (*OHCS* p471).

Fever and night sweats While moderate night sweating is common in anxiety states, drenching sweats requiring several changes of nightclothes is a more ominous symptom associated with infection or lymphoproliferative disease. Patterns of fever may be relevant (see p186). *Rigors* are uncontrolled, sometimes violent episodes of shivering which occur with some causes of fever (eg pyelonephritis, pneumonia).

Flatulence 400–1300mL of gas are expelled PR per day, and if this, coupled with belching (eructation) and abdominal distension, seems excessive to the patient, he may complain of flatulence. Eructation may occur in those with hiatus hernia—but most patients complaining of flatulence have no GI disease. The most likely cause is air-swallowing (aerophagy).

Frequency (urinary) means increased frequency of micturition. It is important to differentiate increased urine production (as in diabetes insipidus p566, diabetes mellitus, polydipsia, diuretics, renal tubular disease, adrenal insufficiency, and alcohol) from frequent passage of small amounts of urine, eg cystitis, urethritis, neurogenic bladder, extrinsic bladder compression (eg pregnancy), bladder tumour, enlarged prostate.

Guarding[†††] Reflex contraction of abdominal muscles, eg as you press (gently!) on the abdomen. It signifies local or general peritoneal inflammation (p112). It is an imperfect sign of peritonism, but is one of the best we have; eg if you decide not to operate on someone with guarding in the RIF, the risk of missing appendicitis is about 1 in 4. If you *do* operate, the chance of finding appendicitis is 1 in 2 (J Dixon 1991 *BMJ* ii 386).

Non-neurological causes of facial pain	
Neck	Cervical disc pathology
Sinuses	Sinusitis; neoplasia
Eye	Glaucoma; iritis; eye strain
Temporomandibular joint	Arthritis
Teeth	Caries; abscess; malocclusion
Ear	Otitis media; otitis externa
Vascular	Giant cell arteritis

Gynaecomastia p556. Haematemesis p494. Haematuria p370.

Haemoptysis[†††] Don't confuse with haematemesis. Haemoptysis is blood coughed up (eg frothy, alkaline, and bright red—usually in the context of known chest disease). It often contains haemosiderin-laden macrophages. Note: melaena occurs if enough blood is swallowed. Haematemesis is acidic and usually dark ('coffee grounds'). Blood not mixed with sputum suggests infarction or trauma. Haemoptysis rarely needs treating in its own right, but if massive, call an anaesthetist and thoracic surgeon (the danger is drowning; lobe resection may be needed); set up IVI, do CXR, blood gases, FBC, INR/APTT, crossmatch. If distressing, consider *prompt* IV morphine, eg if inoperable malignancy.

Halitosis (foetor oris, oral malodour) results from gingivitis (Vincent's angina, p710), metabolic activity of bacteria in plaque, or sulfide-yielding food putrefaction. As well as poor hygiene, also consider causes such as smoking, alcohol, disulfiram, isosorbide. Delusional halitosis is also common. *Treatment:* Try to eliminate anaerobes: ●Stand nearer the toothbrush ●Dental floss ●0.2% aqueous chlorhexidine gluconate. ▣

Heartburn This is an intermittent, gripping, retrosternal pain usually worsened by: stooping, lying down, large meals, and pregnancy. It indicates oesophageal disease—usually reflux oesophagitis.

Hepatomegaly[††] (Big liver) *Causes: Right heart failure* may be pulsatile in tricuspid incompetence. *Infection:* Glandular fever, hepatitis viruses, malaria. *Malignancy:* Metastatic or primary, myeloma, leukaemia, lymphoma. *Others:* Sickle-cell disease, other haemolytic anaemias, porphyria.

Hyperpigmentation See *Skin discolouration* (p56).

Hyperventilation is over-breathing that may be either fast (tachypnoea—ie >20 breaths/min) or deep (hyperpnoea—ie tidal volume ↑). Hyperpnoea may not be perceived by the patient (unlike dyspnoea), and is usually 'excessive' in that it produces a metabolic alkalosis. This may be appropriate (Kussmaul respiration) or inappropriate—the latter results in palpitations, dizziness, faintness, tinnitus, chest pains, perioral and peripheral tingling (plasma Ca^{2+}↓). The commonest cause for hyperventilation is anxiety; others include fever and brainstem lesions.
●*Kussmaul respiration* is deep, sighing breathing that is principally seen in metabolic acidoses—diabetic ketoacidosis and uraemia.
●*Neurogenic hyperventilation* is produced by pontine lesions.

Insomnia When we are sleeping well this is a trivial and irritating complaint, but if we suffer the odd sleepless night, sleep becomes the most desirable thing imaginable and the ability to bestow the best sleep we can do for a patient, second only to relieving pain. But before giving hypnotics ask: *What is the cause? Can it be treated?* *Causes of insomnia:*

Minor, self-limiting:	*Psychological:*	*Some typical organic causes:*		
Travel	Jet lag	Depression	Drugs	Nocturia	Alcoholism
Stress	Shift work	Anxiety	Pain; Itch	Asthma	Dystonias
Arousal	In hospital	Mania, grief	Tinnitus	Apnoea (p362)

Management: 'Sleep Hygiene' ●Do not go to bed until you feel sleepy.
●Avoid daytime naps. Establish regular bed time routines.
●If you can, reserve a room for sleep. Do not eat or watch TV in it.
●Avoid caffeine, nicotine, alcohol—and late-evening hard exercise (sexual activity is the exception: it may produce excellent torpor).
●Consider monitoring with a sleep diary (quantifies sleep pattern and quality), but this could feed insomnia by encouraging obsessions.

Only prescribe hypnotics for up to a few weeks at a time. They are addictive. They may cause daytime somnolence ± rebound insomnia on stopping. Warn about driving and machine working. Example: temazepam 10mg PO.

Causes of haemoptysis

1 Respiratory causes of haemoptysis

Traumatic	Wounds; post-intubation; foreign body
Infective	Acute bronchitis*; pneumonia*; lung abscess; bronchiectasis; TB; fungi; paragonimiasis (p250).
Neoplastic	Primary* or secondary.
Vascular	Lung infarction; vasculitis (Wegener's, RA, SLE, Osler–Weber–Rendu); AV fistula; malformations.
Parenchymal	Diffuse interstitial fibrosis; sarcoidosis; haemosiderosis; Goodpasture's syn; cystic fibrosis.

2 Cardiovascular (pulmonary hypertension) Pulmonary oedema*; mitral stenosis; aortic aneurysm; Eisenmenger's syndrome, p366.

3 Bleeding diatheses

[*Denotes major UK causes; TB and parasites are common abroad.]

Itching† **(Pruritus)** is common and, if chronic, most unpleasant.

Local causes:	Systemic: (Do FBC, ESR, ferritin, LFT, U&E, T4)	
Eczema	Liver disease (bile salt deposition)	
Scabies	Chronic renal failure	
Lichen planus	Lymphomas	
Drug reactions	Polycythaemia	
Atopic dermatitis	Pregnancy	Old age
Dermatitis herpetiformis	Iron deficiency	Thyroid disease

Most drugs are unhelpful but antihistamines may help. Keep the skin well-hydrated (eg with oilatum). ▣

Jugular venous pulse and pressure See p258.

Left iliac fossa pain†† *Acute:* Gastroenteritis; ureteric colic; UTI; diverticulitis; torted ovarian cyst; salpingitis; ectopic; volvulus; pelvic abscess; cancer in undescended testis. *Chronic/subacute:* Constipation; irritable bowel syndrome; colon cancer; inflammatory bowel disease; hip pathology.

Lassitude See *Fatigue* (p46).

Left upper quadrant pain†† *Causes:* Large kidney or spleen; gastric or colonic (splenic flexure) cancer; pneumonia; subphrenic or perinephric abscess; renal colic; pyelonephritis.

Lid lag is the lagging behind of the lid as the eye looks down. **Lid retraction** is the static state of the upper eyelid traversing the eye *above* the iris, rather than transecting it. Causes (both): thyrotoxicosis and anxiety.

Loin pain†† *Causes:* Pyelonephritis; hydronephrosis; renal calculus; renal tumour; perinephric abscess; pain referred from vertebral column.

Lymphadenopathy†† Causes may be divided into:

1 *Reactive: Infective* Bacterial (pyogenic, TB, brucella, syphilis); fungal (coccidiomycosis); viral (EBV, CMV, HIV); toxoplasmosis, trypanosomiasis.
   Non-infective Sarcoid; connective tissue disease (rheumatoid); dermatopathic (eczema, psoriasis); drugs (phenytoin); berylliosis.

2 *Infiltrative: Benign* Histiocytosis (see OHCS p748); lipoidoses. *Malignant* Lymphoma (p606 & p608), metastases.

Musculoskeletal symptoms Chiefly *pain, deformity, reduced function.*
Pain: Degenerative arthritis generally produces an aching pain worse with exercise and relieved by rest. Discomfort may be more in certain positions or motions. Cervical or lumbar spine degeneration may also produce subjective changes in sensation not following dermatome distribution. Both inflammatory and degenerative joint disease produce *morning stiffness* in the affected joints but in the former this generally improves during the day, while in the latter the pain is worse at the end of the day. The pain of *bone erosion* due to tumour or aneurysm tends to be deep, boring, and constant. The pain of *fracture* or *infection* of the bone is severe and throbbing and is increased by any motion of the part. *Acute nerve compression* causes a sharp, severe pain radiating along the distribution of the nerve. Joint pain may be referred, eg that from a hip disorder to anterior and lateral aspect of the thigh or to knee; shoulder to the lateral aspect of the humerus; cervical spine to the interscapular area, medial border of scapulae or tips of shoulders and lateral aspect of arms. (*Back pain*, p661; GALS *locomotor assessment*, p35.)
Reduced function: Causes: pain, bone or joint instability, or restriction of joint movement (eg due to muscle weakness, contractures, bony fusion or mechanical block by intracapsular bony fragments or cartilage).

Nodules *(subcutaneous)* Rheumatoid nodules; PAN; xanthomata; tuberose sclerosis; neurofibromata; sarcoid; granuloma annulare; rheumatic fever.

Oedema†† (p92). Causes: ↑*Venous pressure* (eg DVT or right-heart failure) or *lowered intravascular oncotic pressure* (plasma proteins↓, eg cirrhosis, nephrosis, malnutrition, or protein-losing enteropathy—here

water moves down the osmotic gradient into the interstitium to dilute the solutes there, increasing entropy, according to the laws of thermodynamics). On standing, venous pressure at the ankle rises according to the height of blood from the heart (~100mmHg). This increase is short-lived if leg movement pumps blood through valved veins; but if venous pressure rises, or valves fail, capillary pressure rises, fluid is forced out of them (oedema), the PCV rises locally, and microvascular stasis occurs. *Non-pitting oedema* (ie non-indentible with a finger) implies poor lymphatic drainage (lymphoedema), eg primary (Milroy's syndrome p704) or secondary (radiotherapy, malignant infiltration, infection, filariasis).

Oliguria[†] is defined as a urine output of <400mL/24h. This occurs in extreme dehydration, severe cardiac failure, urethral or bilateral ureteric obstruction, acute and chronic renal failure.

Orthopnoea See **Dyspnoea** above.

Pallor[†] is a nonspecific sign and may be racial, familial, or cosmetic. Pathology suggested by pallor includes anaemia, shock, Stokes–Adams attack, vasovagal faint, myxoedema, hypopituitarism, and albinism.

Palmar erythema Associations: cirrhosis, pregnancy, polycythaemia.

Palpitations represent to the patient the sensation of feeling his heart beat; to the doctor, the sensation of feeling his heart sink—because the symptom is notoriously elusive. Have the patient tap out the rate and regularity of the palpitations. ●Irregular fast palpitations are likely to be paroxysmal AF, or flutter with variable block. ●Dropped or missed beats related to rest, recumbency or eating are likely to be atrial or ventricular ectopics. ●Regular pounding is likely to be due to anxiety. ●Slow palpitations are likely to be due to drugs such as β-blockers, or to bigeminus. Ask about associated pain, dyspnoea, and faints, suggesting haemodynamic compromise. Ask *when* symptoms occur: people often feel their (normal) heart beat in the anxious nocturnal silence of the bedroom:

'At night on my pillow the syncopated stagger
Of the pulse in my ear. Russian roulette:
Every heartbeat a fresh throw of the dice. . .
Hypochondria walked, holding my arm
Like a nurse, her fingers over my pulse. . .
The sudden lapping at my throat of loose blood. . .' Ted Hughes, *Birthday Letters*, Faber & Faber, by kind permission

Often a clinical diagnosis of awareness of normal heart beats may be made—and reassurance is essential. If not, do TSH and transtelephonic event recording[ꞯ] (better than 48h ambulatory ECG which may miss attacks).

Paraphimosis occurs when a tight foreskin is retracted and then becomes irreplaceable as the glans swells. Treat by asking the patient to squeeze the glans for half an hour. Or try soaking a swab in 50% dextrose, and applying it to the oedematous area for an hour, and the oedema may follow the osmotic gradient. (A Coutts 1991 *B J Surg* 252.)

Pelvic pain[†] *Causes:* UTI; urine retention; bladder stones; menses; labour; pregnancy; endometriosis (*OHCS* p52); salpingitis; endometritis (*OHCS* p36); ovarian cyst (eg torted). Cancer of: rectum, colon, ovary, cervix, bladder.

Phimosis The foreskin occludes the meatus, obstructing urine. Time (± trials of gentle retraction) usually obviates the need for circumcision.[ꞯ]

Polyuria is the passing of excessive volumes of urine. Urine output depends on fluid intake and body losses. Up to 3.5 litres per day is typical. Causes of polyuria include diabetes mellitus, cranial diabetes insipidus, nephrogenic diabetes insipidus (inherited or secondary to renal disease), hypercalcaemia, polydipsia, and chronic renal failure.

Prostatism[†] Symptoms of prostate enlargement are often termed 'prostatism', but it is better to use the terms *irritative* or *obstructive* bladder

symptoms. Don't assume the cause is prostatic. 1 *Irritative bladder symptoms:* Urgency, dysuria, frequency, nocturia (the last 2 also caused by UTI, polydipsia, detrusor instability, hypercalcaemia, or uraemia); 2 *Obstructive symptoms* (eg reduced size and force of urinary stream, hesitancy and interruption of stream during voiding)—may also be produced by strictures, tumours, urethral valves, or bladder neck contracture. Maximum flow rate of urine is normally ~18–30mL/sec.

Pruritus See *Itching*, p50.

Ptosis is drooping of the upper eyelid. It is best observed with the patient sitting up, his head held by the examiner. The third cranial nerve innervates the main muscle concerned (levator palpebrae), but nerves from the cervical sympathetic chain innervate the superior tarsal muscle, and a lesion of these nerves will cause a mild ptosis which can be overcome on looking up. *Causes:* 1 *Third nerve lesions* usually causing unilateral complete ptosis. Look for other evidence of third nerve lesion (ophthalmoplegia with outward deviation of the eye, pupil dilated and unreactive to light and accommodation). 2 *Sympathetic paralysis* usually causes unilateral partial ptosis. Look for other evidence of sympathetic lesion (constricted pupil, lack of sweating on same side of the face—Horner's syndrome). 3 *Myopathy* (dystrophia myotonica, myasthenia gravis). These usually cause bilateral partial ptosis. 4 *Congenital* (present since birth). May be unilateral or bilateral, is usually partial and is not associated with other neurological signs. 5 *Syphilis.*

Pulses[†††] 1 *Rate and rhythm* may be assessed at the radial pulse. An irregularly irregular pulse will be AF or multiple ectopics. Regularly irregular: 2° heart block (p287); ventricular bigemini. A bounding pulse occurs in CO_2 retention, liver failure, and sepsis. Shock gives a small volume thready pulse. 2 *Character and volume* are best assessed at the brachials or carotids. Feel the radial and femoral pulse simultaneously if the patient is hypertensive (?radio-femoral delay of coarctation). *Character:*
Small volume, slow-rising pulses are caused by aortic stenosis.
Bisferiens (collapsing + slow-rising) are caused by mixed aortic valve disease.
Collapsing pulses are caused by aortic incompetence, hyperdynamic circulation and patent ductus arteriosus.
Pulsus alternans is caused by left ventricular failure
Jerky pulses are caused by HOCM
Pulsus paradoxus (weakens in inspiration by more than 10mmHg) is caused by asthma, cardiac tamponade and pericarditis.

Pupillary abnormalities[†††]
Are the pupils equal, central, circular, dilated, or constricted? Do they react to light, directly and consensually, and on convergence/accommodation? *Irregular pupils* are caused by iritis, syphilis, or globe rupture.
Dilated pupils Causes: third cranial nerve lesions and mydriatic drugs. But always ask: is this pupil dilated, or is it the other which is constricted?
Constricted pupils are associated with old age, sympathetic nerve damage (Horner's syndrome, p700, and see **Ptosis** above), opiates, miotics (eg pilocarpine eye-drops for glaucoma), and pontine damage.
Unequal pupils (anisocoria) may be due to a unilateral lesion, eye-drops, syphilis, or be a Holmes–Adie pupil (below). Some inequality is normal.
Reaction to light: Test by covering one eye and shining light into the other obliquely. Both pupils should constrict (one by the direct, the other by the consensual or indirect light reflex). Lesion site may be deduced by knowing the pathway: from the retina the message passes up the optic nerve to the superior colliculus (midbrain) and thence to the third nerve nuclei bilaterally. The third nerve causes pupillary constriction. If a light in one eye causes only contralateral constriction, the defect is 'efferent', as the afferent pathways from the retina being stimulated must be intact.

Reaction to accommodation/convergence: If the patient first looks at a distant object and then at the examiner's finger held a few inches away, the eyes will converge and the pupils constrict. The neural pathway involves a projection from the cortex to the nucleus of the third nerve.

Holmes–Adie (myotonic) pupil: This is a benign condition, which occurs usually in women and is unilateral in about 80% of cases. The affected pupil is normally moderately dilated and is poorly reactive to light, if at all. It is slowly reactive to accommodation; wait and watch carefully: it may eventually constrict more than a normal pupil. It is often associated with diminished or absent ankle and knee reflexes, in which case the Holmes–Adie syndrome is present. *Argyll Robertson pupil:* This occurs in neurosyphilis, but a similar phenomenon may occur in diabetes mellitus. The pupil is constricted. It is unreactive to light, but reacts to accommodation. The iris is usually patchily atrophied and depigmented. *Hutchinson pupil:* This refers to the sequence of events resulting from rapidly rising unilateral intracranial pressure (eg in intracerebral haemorrhage). The pupil on the side of the lesion first constricts then widely dilates. The other pupil then goes through the same sequence.

Rebound abdominal pain[†††] is present if, on the sudden removal of pressure from the examiner's hand, the patient feels a *momentary increase* in pain. It signifies local peritoneal inflammation, manifest as pain as the peritoneum rebounds after being gently displaced.

Rectal bleeding[†††] *Causes:* Diverticulitis; colon cancer; polyps; piles; radiation proctitis; trauma; fissure-in-ano; angiodysplasia (this common cause of bleeding in the elderly is due to arteriovenous malformation).

Regurgitation Gastric and oesophageal contents are regurgitated effortlessly into the mouth—without contraction of abdominal muscles and diaphragm (so distinguishing it from true vomiting). Regurgitation is rarely preceded by nausea, and when due to gastro-oesophageal reflux, it is often associated with heartburn. An oesophageal pouch may cause regurgitation. Very high GI obstructions (eg gastric volulus, p126) cause non-productive retching rather than true regurgitation.

Right iliac fossa pain[††] *Causes:* All causes of left iliac fossa pain (see p48) plus appendicitis but usually excluding diverticulitis.

Right upper quadrant (hypochondrial) pain[††] *Causes:* Gallstones; hepatitis; appendicitis (eg if pregnant); colonic cancer at the hepatic flexure; right kidney pathology (eg renal colic; pyelonephritis); intrathoracic conditions (eg pneumonia); subphrenic or perinephric abscess.

Rigors are uncontrolled, sometimes violent episodes of shivering which occur as a patient's temperature rises fast from normal. PUO: p186.

Skin discolouration Generalized hyperpigmentation due at least in part to melanin, may be genetic, or due to radiation, Addison's (p552), chronic renal failure (p388), pregnancy, oral contraceptive pill, any chronic wasting (eg TB, carcinoma), malabsorption, biliary cirrhosis, haemochromatosis, chlorpromazine, or busulfan. Hyperpigmentation due to other causes occurs in jaundice, carotenaemia, and gold therapy.

Splenomegaly[†] Abnormally large spleen. *Causes:* See p152. If massive, think of: leishmaniasis, malaria, myelofibrosis, chronic myeloid leukaemia.

Sputum Smoking is the leading cause of excess sputum production (look for black specks of inhaled carbon). Yellow-green sputum is due to cell debris (bronchial epithelium, neutrophils, eosinophils) and is not *always* infected. Bronchiectasis causes copious greenish sputum. Blood-stained sputum (*haemoptysis*) always needs full investigation. Pink froth suggests pulmonary oedema. Absolutely clear sputum is probably saliva.

Stridor[†††] is an inspiratory sound due to partial obstruction of the upper airways. That obstruction may be due to something within the lumen (eg foreign body, tumour), within the wall (eg oedema, laryngospasm, tumour, croup) or extrinsic (eg goitre, lymphadenopathy). It is a medical (or surgical) emergency if the airway is compromised.

Tactile vocal fremitus See p28.

Tenesmus[†††] This is a sensation felt in the rectum of incomplete emptying following defecation—as if there was something else left behind, which cannot be passed. It is very common in the irritable bowel syndrome (p518), but can be caused by a tumour.

Tinnitus See p424.

Tiredness See *Fatigue* p46.

Tremor[†] is rhythmic oscillation of limbs, trunk, head, or tongue. 3 types:

1 *Resting tremor*—worst at rest; feature of parkinsonism, but the tremor is more resistant to treatment than bradykinesia or rigidity.

2 *Postural tremor*—worst eg if arms outstretched. May be exaggerated physiological tremor (eg anxiety, thyrotoxicosis, alcohol, drugs), metabolic (eg hepatic encephalopathy, CO_2 retention), due to brain damage (eg Wilson's disease, syphilis) or *benign essential tremor* (BET). This is usually a familial (autosomal dominant) tremor of arms and head which may present at any age and is suppressed by moderately large amounts of alcohol. Rarely progressive. Propranolol (40–80mg/12h PO) helps one-third of patients as does primidone (50–750mg/24h PO).

3 *Intention tremor*—is worst during movement and occurs in cerebellar disease (eg in MS). No effective drug has been found.

Trousseau's sign The hands and feet go into spasm (carpopedal spasm) in hypocalcaemia. The metacarpophalangeal joints become flexed and the interphalangeal joints are extended.

Urinary changes[†††] *Cloudy urine* may suggest pus in the urine (infection) but is often normal phosphate precipitation in an alkaline urine. *Pneumaturia* (bubbles in the urine as it is passed) occurs with UTI due to gas-forming organisms or may signal an enterovesical fistula from inflammatory or neoplastic diseases of the gut. *Nocturia* is seen in prostatism, diabetes mellitus, UTI, and reversed diurnal rhythm (p568) as occurs with renal and cardiac insufficiency. *Haematuria* (blood in the urine) must be considered to be due to neoplasm until proven otherwise (p370).

Urinary frequency See *Frequency* p46.

Vertigo See p420.

Visual disturbance may be due to eye disease or drugs; CNS lesions may present with a history of visual field loss (eg stroke), double vision (MS, trauma, tumour, basilar artery insufficiency, chronic basilar meningitis), flashing lights (migraine, seizure disorder), visual hallucinations (seizure disorder, drugs) or transient blindness (vascular lesions, migraine). See OHCS: *Sudden* and *Gradual loss of vision*, p498 & p500.

Voice and disturbance of speech may be noted by the patient or the doctor. Try to assess if difficulty is with articulation (*dysarthria*, eg from muscle or problems) or of word command (*dysphasia*—always central, see p430).

Vocal resonance See p28 and p324.

Vomiting[†††] Ask about amount, colour, sour, old or recent food, blood, 'coffee grounds', relationship to eating (see table).

This can cause metabolic alkalaemia, hyponatraemia, and $K^+\downarrow$—as well as haematemesis from a Mallory–Weiss tear of the oesophagus.

GI causes:	CNS causes:	Metabolic:
Food poisoning (p190)	Intracranial pressure ↑	Uraemia
Gastroenteritis	(tumours, meningoencephalitis)	Pregnancy
GI obstruction (p130)	Motion (eg sea-sickness)	Drugs/toxins, eg
Appendicitis	Migraine	−cytoxics
'Acute abdomen'	Ménière's disease	−alcohol
	Labyrinthitis	−opiates
	Head injury	−antibiotics
	Cerebellar and brain	
	stem disease	
	Psychiatric disorder	

Walking difficulty ('Off my legs')[††] In the elderly, this is a common and nonspecific presentation: the reason may not be local (typically osteo- or rheumatoid arthritis, but remember fractured neck of femur), and it may not even be systemic (eg pneumonia, UTI, anaemia, drugs, hypothyroidism, renal failure, hypothermia)—but it may be a manifestation of depression or bereavement. *It is only rarely a manipulative strategy.*

More specific causes to consider are Parkinson's disease, (p452), polymyalgia (very treatable, p674) and various neuropathies/myopathies. One of the key questions is 'Is there pain?'—another issue to address is whether there is muscle wasting and, if so, is it symmetrical?

If there is ataxia too, the cause is not always alcohol: other chemicals may be involved (cannabis, arsenic, thallium, mercury—or prescribed sedatives), or there may be a metastatic or non-metastatic manifestation of malignancy—or a CNS primary or vascular lesion.

Remember also treatable conditions such as pellagra, $B_{12}\downarrow$, and beriberi, and infections such as encephalitis, myelitis, Lyme disease, brucellosis, or rarities such as botulism (p794).

Bilateral weak legs in an otherwise fit person suggests a cord lesion: see p426. If there is associated incontinence ± saddle anaesthesia, prompt treatment for cord compression may be needed.

Waterbrash Saliva suddenly fills the mouth. It typically occurs after meals, and may denote oesophageal disease. It is suggested that this is an exaggeration of the oesophago-salivary reflex.

Weight loss[†††] is a nonspecific feature of chronic disease and depression—also of malnutrition, chronic infections and infestations (eg TB, enteropathic AIDS), malignancy, diabetes mellitus, and hyperthyroidism (typically in the presence of increased appetite). Severe generalized muscle wasting is also seen as part of a number of degenerative neurological and muscle diseases and in cardiac failure (cardiac cachexia), although in the latter right heart failure may not make weight loss a major complaint.

4. Geriatric medicine

Relevant pages in other chapters:
Stroke (p432); prevention and investigation of stroke (p434).

When I am an old woman I shall wear purple
With a red hat which doesn't go, and doesn't suit me
And I shall spend my pension on brandy and summer gloves
*And satin sandals. . .**

*If our older patients do not conform to our expectations of a dignified, quiet old age, do not be surprised. Their expectations are not quite what we might think! See S Lyon 1995 *Geriatric Medicine* **25** 7 and S Martz 1991 *When I Am an Old Woman I Shall Wear Purple*, Papier-mâché Press

The elderly patient in hospital

An ageing population is a sign of successful social, health, and economic policies.[1]

Beware of ageism Old age is associated with disease but doesn't cause it *per se.*[2] Any deterioration is from treatable disease *until proved otherwise.*

1 Contrary to stereotype, most old people are fit.[1] 95% of those over 65yrs and 80% of those over 85 years old do not live in institutions; about 70% of the latter can manage stairs and can bathe without help.

2 If there is a problem, find the cause. Do not accept problems as the inevitable result of ageing. Look for: disease, loss of fitness, and social factors, which may be amenable to therapy.

3 Do not restrict treatment simply because a person is old. Old people vary. Age alone is a poor predictor of outcome for an individual and should not be used as a substitute for careful clinical assessment of each patient's potential for benefit and risk.[3]

Characteristics of disease in old age There are differences of emphasis in the approach to old people compared with young people.[4]

1 *Multiple pathology:* Several disease processes may coincide: find out which impinge on each complaint (eg senile cataract + arthritis = falls).

2 *Multiple causes:* One problem may have several causes. Treating each alone may do little good; treating all may be of much benefit.[5]

3 *nonspecific presentation of disease:* Some presentations are common in old people. In particular the 'geriatric giants':[6] incontinence (p74); immobility; instability (falls, p68); and dementia/confusion (p76 & p446). Virtually any disease may present with these. Furthermore, typical signs and symptoms may be absent (eg myocardial infarction without chest pain, chest infection without cough or sputum).

4 Rapid deterioration can occur if diseases are untreated.

5 Complications are common.

6 More time is required for recovery. Points 4–6 reflect impairment in homeostatic mechanisms and loss of 'physiological reserve'.

7 Impaired metabolism and excretion of drugs. Doses may need lowering.

8 Social factors are central in aiding recovery and return to home.

Special points *In the history:*

- Assess disability (p66).
- Obtain home details (eg stairs; access to toilet? can alarm be raised?).
- Medication What? When? Assess understanding and concordance (p3). How many different tablets can he cope with? Probably not many more than two. So which are the most important drugs? You may have to ignore other desirable remedies, or enlist the help of a friend, a spouse or a pharmacist (who can batch morning, noon and night doses in compartmentalized containers so complex regimens may be reduced to 'take the morning compartment when you get up, the noon compartment before lunch, and the night compartment before bed').
- Social network (regular visitors; family and friends).
- Care details: what services are in operation?—meals delivered; community psychiatric or distric nurse—who else is involved in the care?
- Speak to others (relatives; neighbours; carers; GP).

On examination: Check BP lying and standing (postural hypotension). Consider a rectal examination (constipation causes incontinence). Detailed CNS examination is often needed, eg if presentation is nonspecific. This may tire the patient, so consider doing in small batches.

1 S Ebrahim 1998 *BMJ* i 148   2 R Doll 1997 *BMJ* ii 1030   3 Royal College Group 1991 *J Roy Col Phys* 25 197   4 After J Grimley Evans 1992 *Oxford Textbook of Geriatric Medicine*, OUP 703   5 D Fairweather 1991 *J Roy Col Phys* 25 105   6 B Isaacs 1992 *The Challenge of Geriatric Medicine* OUP

Impairment, disability, and handicap

►Focus on patients' problems not doctors' diseases.

Doctors are at home with diagnosing disease and identifying impairment. But we are slow to see the patient's perspective. Three key concepts can help: impairment; disability; handicap.

Impairment refers to systems or parts of the body that do not work. 'Any loss or abnormality of psychological, physiological, or anatomical structure or function.'[1] For example, following stroke, paralysis of the right arm or dysphasia would be impairment.

Disability refers to things people cannot do. 'Any restriction or lack (resulting from an impairment) of ability to perform an activity in the manner, or within the range, considered normal for a human being.'[1] For example, following stroke, difficulties in 'activities of daily living' (eg with dressing, walking).

Handicap refers to the inability to carry out social functions. 'A disadvantage for a given individual, resulting from an impairment or disability, that limits or prevents the fulfilment of a rôle. . . for that individual.'[1] For example, following stroke, being unable to go out to work or to go to tea with a friend.

Making use of these distinctions Two people with the same impairment (eg paralysed arm) may have different disabilities (eg one able to dress, the other unable). The disabilities are likely to determine the quality of the person's future. Treatment may usefully be directed at reducing disabilities. For example, Velcro® fasteners in place of buttons may enable a person to dress.

Three stages of management

1 *Assessment of disability and handicap.*[2] Traditional 'medical' clerking focuses on disease and impairment. Full assessment requires, in addition, a thorough understanding of disability and handicap. For structured assessment of disability we recommend the Barthel index (p67). Discuss further detailed assessments with expert therapists, the patient, and relatives to help define their problems.

2 *Who can help?* As a doctor you are part of a team. You may need to inform others that their help is needed, eg nurses (including community liaison nurses), occupational therapists, physiotherapists, speech therapists, social workers, the general practitioner, geriatrician and psychogeriatrician. There are self-help organizations for most chronic diseases aimed at both patients and their carers (p756).

3 *Generate solutions to problems:* A list of disabilities is the key. To plan rehabilitation look at each disability (eg unable to dress). Work out origin of disability (in terms of disease and impairment). Goals need agreeing with patient and relatives in the light of their wishes and professional predictions. Record agreed goals and ensure all work together with mutual understanding. Review, renew, and adapt goals.

1 WHO 1989 Tech Report No 779, *Health of the Elderly*, Geneva 2 E Dickinson 1990 *Lancet* **337** 778 See also: *Equipment for an Easier Life* 1994, RICA, 2 Marylebone Rd London NW1 4DF, UK—free on receipt of a stamped-addressed envelope

Barthel's index of activities of daily living (BAI)

Bowels	0	Incontinent (or needs to be given enemas)
	1	Occasional accidents (once a week)
	2	Continent
Bladder	0	Incontinent, or catheterized but unable to manage it
	1	Occasional accidents (up to once per 24 hours)
	2	Continent (for more than seven days)
Grooming	0	Needs help with personal care: face, hair, teeth, shaving
	1	Independent (implements provided)
Toilet use	0	Dependent
	1	Needs some help but can do some things alone
	2	Independent (on and off, wiping, dressing)
Feeding	0	Unable
	1	Needs help in cutting, spreading butter, etc.
	2	Independent (food provided within reach)
Transfer	0	Unable to get from bed to commode: *the vital transfer* to prevent the need for 24-hour nursing care
	1	Major help needed (physical, 1–2 people), can sit
	2	Minor help needed (verbal or physical)
	3	Independent
Mobility	0	Immobile
	1	Wheelchair-independent, including corners, etc.
	2	Walks with help of one person (verbal or physical)
	3	Independent
Dressing	0	Dependent
	1	Needs help but can do about half unaided
	2	Independent (including buttons, zips, laces, etc.)
Stairs	0	Unable
	1	Needs help (verbal, physical, carrying aid)
	2	Independent up and down
Bathing	0	Dependent
	1	Independent (bath: must get in and out unsupervised and wash self; shower: unsupervised/unaided)

The aim is to establish the degree of independence from any help.
Barthel's paradox The more we contemplate Barthel's eulogy of independence the more we see it as a mirage reflecting a greater truth about human affairs: there is no such thing as *independence**—only *interdependence*, and in fostering this interdependence lies our true vocation.

*No man is an Island, intire of it selfe; every man is a peece of the *Continent*, a part of the *maine*; if a *Clod* bee washed away by the *Sea*, *Europe* is the lesse, as well as if a *promontorie* were, as well as if a *Mannor* of thy *friends* or of *thine owne* were. Any mans *death* diminishes *me*, because I am involved in *mankinde*; And therefore never send to know for whom the *bell* tolls: It tolls for *thee*. *John Donne 1572-1631 (meditation XVII) Selected Prose*, page 101, OUP

✛ Stroke, falls, and postural hypotension

Rehabilitation after stroke (See p432–4 for stroke's acute phase.)
►Good care requires attention to detail. The principles of rehabilitation are those of any chronic disease (p66); they are best carried out in specialist rehabilitation units or by community teams ◁▷ (they reduce morbidity and institutionalization). *Special points in early management:*

- Watch your patient swallow water from a spoon. If he chokes, he may require *nil by mouth* for some days (+IV fluids), then semi-solids (eg jelly; avoid soups and crumbly food). Avoid early NG tube feeds (needed only in those few patients with established chronic swallowing problems).
- Avoid damaging shoulders of patient through careless lifting.
- Ensure good bladder and bowel care through frequent toiletting. Avoid early catheterization which may prevent return to continence.
- Position the patient to minimize spasticity. Get prompt physiotherapy.
- Often 'pseudo-emotionalism' is a problem after stroke, eg sobbing unprovoked by sorrow (failure of limbic system inhibition by cortex). It may respond to tricyclics,[2] fluoxetine (OHCS p341).▣

Special tests: ●Asking to point to a named part of the body tests for *perceptual dysfunction* ●Copying patterns of matchsticks tests *spacial ability.* ●Dressing or drawing a clock face tests for *apraxia.* ●Picking out and naming common objects from a pile tests for *agnosia.*

Falls are common (30% of those >65yrs fall in a year) and this may be the start of a fatal train of events. Causes are many. 10% are related to loss of consciousness or dizziness. For most, there is no clear cause. For the differential diagnosis of 'off my legs', see p60.

History: Exact circumstances of fall. Find out about any CNS, cardiac, or musculoskeletal abnormalities. Drugs, eg causing: postural hypotension (below); sedation; arrhythmia, eg tricyclics; parkinsonism, eg neuroleptics including metoclopramide and prochlorperazine). Alcohol.

Examination—for causes: Postural hypotension; arrhythmias; carotid bruits; detailed neurological examination including cerebellar signs, parkinsonism, proximal myopathy, gait (PLATE 3), watch patient get up from chair, test for Romberg's sign (p32); instability in knees. *For consequences:* Cuts; bruises; fractured ribs (± pneumonia) or limbs, especially neck of femur; head injury (± subdural haematoma).

Management: Confidence may be shattered even if no serious injury. Look for causes and treat. Consider physiotherapy—to include learning techniques to get up from floor. Occupational therapists may advise on reducing household hazards, and adding aids or a personal alarm radio-linked by phone to 24h cover—*so* reassuring to those living alone. Exercising, balance instruction, and Tai Chi can prevent falls.▣

Postural hypotension is important because it is common and a cause of falls and poor mobility. Typical times are after meals, on exercise, and on getting up at night. May be transient with illness (eg 'flu).

Causes: Leg vein insufficiency; autonomic neuropathy (p463; especially diabetes mellitus); drugs (diuretics, nitrates, antihypertensives, antidepressants, sedatives). ↓Red cell mass may be a contributing factor.[3]
Management: Reduce or stop drugs if possible. Counsel patient to stand up slowly in stages. Try compression stockings (OHCS p598). Reserve fluid-retaining drugs (eg NSAIDs, p664) or fludrocortisone 0.1mg/24h PO increasing as needed) in those severely affected, if other measures fail.▣

◁▷ A Rudd 1997 BMJ ii 1039: early dischage works *if there is a good community rehabilitation team in place;* Cochrane Data 1995 No.1 2 J van Gijn 1993 *Lancet* ii 816 3 R Hoeldtke 1993 NEJM 329 611

⚕ Hypothermia

►*Have a high index of suspicion and a low-reading thermometer.* Most patients are elderly and do not complain, or feel, cold—so they have not tried to warm themselves up. In the young, hypothermia is usually either from cold-exposure (eg near-drowning), or it is secondary to impaired conscious level (eg following excess alcohol or drug overdose).

Definition Hypothermia implies a core (rectal) temperature <35°C.

Causes In the elderly hypothermia is often caused by a combination of:
- Impaired homeostatic mechanisms: usually age related.
- Low room-temperature: poverty, poor housing.
- Disease: Impaired thermoregulation (pneumonia, MI, heart failure).
- Reduced metabolism (immobility, hypothyroidism, diabetes mellitus).
- Autonomic neuropathy (p463, eg diabetes mellitus, Parkinson's).
- Excess heat loss (psoriasis). Cold awareness↓ (dementia, confusion).
- Increased exposure to cold (falls, especially at night when cold).
- Drugs (major tranquillizers, antidepressants, diuretics). Alcohol.

The Patient *How frozen I then became: I did not die, yet nothing of life remained.*[1] So don't assume that if vital signs seem to be absent, the patient must be dead: rewarm (below) and re-examine. If T° <32°C this sequence may occur: ↓BP → coma → bradycardia → AF → VT → VF. The abdomen can feel 'colder than clay'. If >32°C, signs may be mild: pallor; apathy; pulse↑.

Diagnosis Check oral or axillary T°. If ordinary thermometer shows <36.5°C, use a low-reading one PR. Is the rectal temperature <35°C?

Tests Urgent U&E, plasma glucose, and amylase. Thyroid function tests; FBC; blood cultures. Consider blood gases. The ECG may show J-waves.

Treatment • Ventilate with O_2 if comatose or respiratory insufficiency.
- IVI (for access or to correct electrolyte disturbance).
- Cardiac monitor (both VF and AF can occur during warming).
- Consider antibiotics for the prevention of pneumonia (p336). Give these routinely in patients over 65 years with a temperature <32°C.
- Consider urinary catheter (to assess renal function).
- *Slowly rewarm.* Do not reheat too fast, causing peripheral vasodilatation, shock, and death. Aim for a rise of ½°C/h. Old, conscious patients should sit in a warm room taking hot drinks. Thermal blankets may cause too rapid warming in old patients. The first sign of too rapid warming is falling BP. Treat by allowing patient to cool down slightly.
- Rectal temperature, BP, pulse, and respiratory rate every ½ hour.

Note: advice is different for victims of sudden hypothermia from immersion. Here, eg if there has been a cardiac arrest and T°<30°C, mediastinal warm-lavage, peritoneal or haemodialysis, and cardiopulmonary bypass (no heparin if trauma) may be needed (OHCS p683). ▣ Because of the danger of circulatory collapse, victims of immersion should be transported in the horizontal position. Get expert advice.

Complications Arrhythmias (if there is a cardiac arrest continue resuscitating until T° >33°C, as cold brains are less damaged by hypoxia); pneumonia; pancreatitis; acute renal failure; intravascular coagulation.

Prognosis Depends on age and degree of hypothermia. If age >70yrs and T° <32°C then mortality >50%.

Before hospital discharge Anticipate problems. *Will it happen again? What is her network of support?* Review medication (could you stop tranquillizers?). *How is progress to be monitored?* Liaise with GP/social worker.

---

1 In the last round of the 9th circle of *Hell*, Dante tells how those betraying their benefactors are encased in ice (*canto XXXIV*) 'Com'io divenni allor gelato e fioco... Io non mori e non rimasi vivo.'

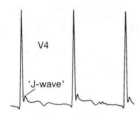

Kindly supplied by Drs Richard Luke and EM McLachlan.

Nicer interventions

The foregoing pages of this chapter paint a bright and optimistic picture of geriatric medicine. The message is: list all disabilities and handicaps, and work down the list curing or ameliorating everything that you can, and avoiding dismissing items on the list as the inevitable consequence of ageing. The trouble is, neither over-pressed doctors nor our bewildered patients may survive this approach, unless something else is added. A true story illustrates this: an old man with chronic but not too severe obstructive airways disease went to hospital for assessment. The doctor was very thorough, and the whole process (including various investigations and waits for these in rather poor surroundings) took more than 3 hours. The exhausted patient returned home rather more breathless than usual. Later he began to cough, and within 48 hours of his appointment he died. The assessment and the doctor's care was in many ways ideal—but not for the patient. It is very easy to over-investigate patients, to raise their expectations—and then to let them down.

A different approach to the exhaustive problem list (if it shows signs of exhausting either the doctor or the patient) is to develop the skill of recognizing opportunities for minimal, highly selected interventions which act as nudges to move the patient in a healthier direction, without interrupting the delicate matrix which allows the patient to function in the first place. For example, if a patient with Parkinson's disease is troubled by insomnia, you could attempt to combine objective assessment of your changes to his anti-parkinsonian treatment (how long does it take you to do X?) with treatment of the insomnia (fresh air) and with attempts to keep him fit (repetitive exercise)—by simply suggesting that he notes down how long it takes him to walk to the letter-box. This intervention will also give you a written record of any tendency to micrographia. So the message is now 'How many nails can I hit on the head with one blow of the hammer?' or 'Of all the interventions which are possible, which is the nicest one?' (using 'nicest' in both its senses).

Only experience can teach when to opt for complete problem lists and multiple interventions, and when to opt for minimalism. The advantages of developing a flair for this is that time will be released for other activities, such as listening to the patient and giving him or her time to share fears. You may also give yourself time for a little rest and recuperation—an exhausted, uncommunicative doctor is usually a bad one. It is by having the time and the inclination to explore patients' fears that you may be of most use to them. Almost any elderly patient coming into hospital will have fears (for example of dying—and in geriatric medicine this fear will often not be groundless). You may vastly reassure the patient if you explain that one of your main jobs is to ensure that when death comes, it is as good a death as possible. The fears will often not centre on the patient himself. His worry may be that his handicapped daughter will be forced out of her lodgings when he is gone, or that his son's marriage will fail again if he is not there. Sympathetic listening may be all you can offer, but do not undervalue how much patients appreciate this.

Urinary incontinence

▶Think twice before inserting a urinary catheter. ▶Carry out rectal examination to exclude faecal impaction. ▶Is the bladder palpable after voiding (retention with overflow)?

Anyone might 'wet themselves' on a long coach ride (we all would if the journey was long enough). Do not think of people as either dry or incontinent but as incontinent in certain circumstances. Attending to these circumstances is as important as focusing on the physiology.

Incontinence in men Enlargement of the prostate is the major cause of incontinence: urge incontinence (see below) or dribbling may result from the partial retention of urine. Transurethral resection of the prostate may weaken the bladder sphincter and cause incontinence. Troublesome incontinence needs specialist assessment.

Incontinence in women (See also *Voiding difficulty, OHCS p71*.)

1 *Functional incontinence* ie when physiological factors are relatively unimportant. The patient is 'caught short' and too slow in finding the toilet because of eg immobility or unfamiliar surroundings.

2 *Stress incontinence:* Leakage of urine due to incompetent sphincter. Leakage typically occurs when intra-abdominal pressure rises (eg coughing, laughing). The key to diagnosis is the loss of small (but often frequent) amounts of urine when coughing etc. Examine for pelvic floor prolapse. Look for cough leak with the patient standing and with full bladder. Stress incontinence is common during pregnancy and following childbirth. It occurs to some degree in about 50% of post-menopausal women. In elderly women, pelvic floor weakness, eg with uterine prolapse or urethrocele (*OHCS p54*) is commonest cause.

3 *Urge incontinence* is the most common type seen in hospital practice. The urge to pass urine is quickly followed by uncontrollable complete emptying of the bladder as the detrusor muscle contracts. Large amounts of urine flow down the patient's legs. In the elderly it is usually related to detrusor instability or organic brain damage. Look for evidence of: stroke; Parkinson's; dementia. Other causes: urinary infection; diabetes; diuretics; 'senile' vaginitis; urethritis.

In both sexes incontinence may result from diminished awareness due to confusion or sedation. Occasionally incontinence may be purposeful (eg preventing admission to an old people's home) or due to anger.

Management *Check for:* UTI; diabetes mellitus; diuretic use; faecal impaction. Do U&E. Pelvic floor exercises may help stress incontinence. A ring pessary may help uterine prolapse eg while awaiting surgical repair (this must be preceded by cystometry and urine flow rate measurement to exclude detrusor instability or sphincter dyssynergia). If urge incontinence, examine for spinal cord and CNS signs (including cognitive test, p77); and for vaginitis (treat with dienoestrol 0.01% cream—consider cyclical progesterone if prolonged use, if no hysterectomy, to avoid risk of uterine cancer). The patient (or carer) should complete an 'incontinence' chart for 3 days to obtain pattern of incontinence. Maximize access to toilet; advise on toiletting regimen (eg every 4 hours). The aim is to keep bladder volume below that which triggers emptying. Drugs may help reduce night-time incontinence (see table opposite) but are generally disappointing. Consider aids (absorbent pad, Paul's tubing).

Do urodynamic assessment before any surgical intervention.

Managing detrusor instability

Agents for detrusor instability:	*Symptoms which they may improve:*
Oxybutynin 2.5mg/12h–5mg/12h SE: dry mouth, vision↓, drowsy abdo pain, flushing, arrhythmias	Frequency, urgency, urge incontinence (beware high doses if: elderly, ischaemic heart disease, glaucoma)
Imipramine 50mg PO at night	Nocturia, enuresis, coital incontinence
Propantheline 15mg/8h PO ≥1h ac	Frequency
Desmopressin nasal spray 20µg as a night-time dose	Nocturia/enuresis (↓urine production) SE: fluid retention, heart failure
Oestrogens	Postmenopausal urgency, frequency + nocturia may be improved by raising the bladder's sensory threshold
Surgery, eg clam ileocystoplasty	The bladder is bisected, opened like a clam, and 25cm of ileum is sewn in
Hypnosis/psychotherapy	(This requires good motivation)

Sources: G Wilcock 1991, *Geriatric Problems in General Practice*, OUP; L Cardoso 1991 BMJ ii 1453

⊹ Dementia

▶Ensure no treatable cause has been missed.
▶Assume confusion is due to acute illness until proved otherwise (p446).

Dementia is a syndrome, with many causes, of global impairment of cognition in clear consciousness (*cf* acute confusional state).

The Patient The key to diagnosis is a good history (usually requiring the help of a spouse, relative or friend) of progressive impairment of memory and cognition together with objective evidence of such impairment. The history should go back at least several months, and usually several years. Typically the patient has become increasingly forgetful, and has carried out the normal tasks of daily living (eg cooking, shopping) with increasing incompetence—for example going to the butcher to buy sausages six times in a day, and then being baffled as to why there was a great mound of sausages in the kitchen. Sometimes the patient appears to have changed personality, eg by becoming uncharacteristically rude and aggressive. For objective evidence, carry out a test of cognitive functioning (p77).

Epidemiology Increasing incidence with age. Rare below 55 years of age. 5–10% prevalence above 65 years. 20% prevalence above 80 years.

Commonest causes *Alzheimer's disease*—see p78. *Vascular dementia:* ~25% of all cases. Essentially multiple small strokes. Usually evidence of vascular pathology (BP↑, past strokes); sometimes of focal neurological damage; onset sometimes sudden and deterioration often stepwise.

Lewy body dementia: Characterized by Lewy bodies* (p452) in brainstem *and* neo-cortex, and a fluctuating but persisting cognitive impairment, parkinsonism (p452), and hallucinations. It is a common form of dementia.

Frontotemporal dementia: Characterized by atrophy of frontal and temporal lobes, without features of Alzheimer's pathology (p78).[1] Signs: early change in personality with disinhibition, hyperorality, stereotyped behaviour, and emotional unconcern. Spatial orientation is preserved.

Rarer causes Chronic alcohol or barbiturate abuse; pellagra (p520); Huntington's (p704); Jakob–Creutzfeldt disease (p702); Parkinson's (p452); Pick's disease; HIV; chronic cryptococcosis (p244); subacute sclerosing panencephalitis (p440); progressive multiple leukencephalopathy.

Ameliorable causes Hypothyroidism; B₁₂/folate↓; syphilis; thiamine deficiency (eg from alcohol abuse); operable cerebral tumour (eg parasagittal meningioma); subdural haematoma; CNS cysticercosis (p248); normal pressure hydrocephalus (dilation of ventricles without signs of ↑pressure, due possibly to partial obstruction of CSF flow from subarachnoid space). A CSF shunt may reverse intellectual deterioration. The diagnosis is suggested by incontinence early in dementia, and gait dyspraxia.

Tests FBC/film; ESR; U&E; Ca²⁺; LFT; syphilis serology; B₁₂; folate; thyroid function; CXR; urine ward test. Consider: CT scan (atypical history, young onset, head injury); EEG. After counselling carers, test for HIV if at risk.

Management There are specific treatments for Alzheimer's (p78), HIV (p218), myxoedema, and dementia associated with low B₁₂ and folate.

Treat concurrent illnesses (these may contribute significantly to confusion). In most people the dementia remains and will progress. The approach to management is that of any chronic illness (p66). Involve relatives and relevant agencies. Alzheimer's Disease Society (p756). Stress in the carer is inevitable: try to ameliorate it by talking through frustrations and offering respite admission. Prepare the spouse for the day when the patient no longer recognizes loved ones.

---

*Lewy bodies are eosinophilic intracytoplasmic neuronal inclusion bodies; there is overlap between Lewy body dementia and Alzheimer's and Parkinson's diseases, making treatment hard as antiparkinsonian drugs can precipitate delusions, and antipsychotic drugs worsen parkinsonism (see S Cercy 1997 *J Int Neurops* 3 179 & I McKeith 1994 *Br J Psych* 165 324) 1 Lund/Manchester group 1994 *J Neurol Nsurg Psy* 57 416

The mini-mental state examination

If dementia is suspected test memory and other intellectual abilities formally. The mini-mental state examination is one of many similar tests; it has been more fully studied than most.

- *What day of the week is it?* [1 point]
- *What is the date today? Day; Month; Year* [1 point each]
- *What is the season?* Allow flexibility when testing during times of seasonal change. [1 point]
- *Can you tell me where we are now? What country are we in?* [1 point]
- *What is the name of this town?* [1 point]
- *What are two main streets nearby?* [1 point]
- *What floor of the building are we on?* [1 point]
- *What is the name of this place?* (or *what is this address?*) [1 point]
- Read the following, then offer the paper: *'I am going to give you a piece of paper. When I do, take the paper in your right hand. Fold the paper in half with both hands and put the paper down on your lap.'* [Give 1 point for each of the three actions.]
- *Show a pencil and ask what it is called.* [1 point]
- *Show a wristwatch and ask what it is called.* [1 point]
- Say (once only): *'I am going to say something and I would like you to repeat it after me: No ifs, ands, or buts.'* [1 point]
- Say: *'Please read what is written here and do what it says.'* Show card with: CLOSE YOUR EYES written on it. Score only if action is carried out correctly. If respondent reads instruction but fails to carry out action, say: 'Now do what it says'. [1 point]
- Say: *'Write a complete sentence on this sheet of paper.'* Spelling and grammar are not important. The sentence must have a verb, real or implied, and must make sense. 'Help!', 'Go away' are acceptable. [1 point]
- Say: *'Here is a drawing. Please copy the drawing.'* [See drawing below.] Mark as correct if the two figures intersect to form a four-sided figure and if all angles are preserved. [1 point]
- Say: *'I am going to name three objects. After I have finished saying all three I want you to repeat them. Remember what they are because I am going to ask you to name them again in a few minutes.'* Name three objects taking 1 second to say each, eg APPLE; TABLE; PENNY. Score first try [1 point each object] and repeat until all are learned.
- Say: *'Now I would like you to take 7 away from 100. Now take 7 away from the number you get. Now keep subtracting until I tell you to stop.'* Score 1 point each time the difference is 7 even if a previous answer was incorrect. Go on for 5 subtractions (eg 93, 86, 79, 72, 65). [5 points]
- Say: *'What were the three objects I asked you to remember a little while ago?'* [1 point each object]

Interpreting the score The maximum is 30; 28–30 does not support the diagnosis of dementia. A score 25–27 is borderline; <25 suggests dementia but consider also *acute confusional state* and *depression*. ~13% of over-75s in the general population have scores <25.

Close your eyes

Alzheimer's dementia (AD)

This is the worst neuropsychiatric disorder of our times, dominating not just psychogeriatric wards, but the lives of thousands of sons, daughters and spouses who have given up work, friends, and all their accustomed ways of life to support relatives through the last long years. The struggle of caring for loved ones through terminal illness always puts us on our mettle: never more so than when that loved one's personality disintegrates, and the person who is loved is gone long before their eventual death.

Suspect Alzheimer's disease in adults with any enduring, acquired deficit of memory and cognition—eg as revealed in the mental test score and other neuropsychometric tests (p77). Onset may be from 40 years (or earlier, eg in Down's syndrome)—so the notions of 'senile' and 'pre-senile' dementia are blurred (and irrelevant). $\female:\male \approx 1.4:1$.

Memory loss is not like loss of land with a rising tide: the last things to be sunk in the sea of forgetfulness are not earliest or latest memories, but the deepest, the most personal, and the most bizarre: prime ministers come and go, but, for dementing British patients of a certain age, the last name to be retained is always that of Mrs Thatcher. When this name sinks into oblivion (fame's eternal dumping ground[1]), often long after that of sovereigns, deities, principalities, spouses and children, one may safely say that the waters have covered the sea.

Risk factors *Defective genes* on chromosomes 1, 14, 19, 21; the apoE4 variant brings forward age of onset. *Insulin resistance* may be important (p529).

Diagnosis is often haphazard, as the exact form of dementia used not to influence outcome, provided B_{12} and TSH were normal. This view is hard to justify now that *specific* treatments are available for Alzheimer's. Specialist assessment with neuroimaging for all would be ideal (this would help rule out frontal lobe dementia and Lewy body dementia, and Pick's disease).

Histology (rarely used) ●Deposition of type Aβ-amyloid protein in cortex (a few patients have mutations in the amyloid precursor protein). ●Neurofibrillary tangles and an increased number of senile plaques. ●A deficit of neurotransmitter acetylcholine from damage to an ascending forebrain projection (nucleus basalis of Meynert; connects with cortex).

Presentation As well as failing memory, there may be cognitive impairment (eg spatial disorientation); behavioural change (eg aggression, wandering); psychosis (hallucinations, persecutory delusions). There is no standard natural history. Cognitive impairment is progressive, but behavioural and psychotic symptoms may go after a few months or years. Towards the end, often but by no means invariably, patients become sedentary, apparently taking little interest in anything. Parkinsonism, wasting, mutism, incontinence, and seizures may occur.

Mean survival 7 years from onset.

Management *Theoretical issues:* Potential strategies—the MRC menu:
●Preventing the breakdown of acetylcholine, eg donepezil, opposite.
●Augmenting nerve growth factor (NGF), which is taken up at nerve endings, and promotes nerve cell repair.
●Stimulating nicotinic receptors which may protect nerve cells.
●Inhibition of the enzymes that snip out β-amyloid peptide from APP (amyloid precursor protein), so preventing fibrils and plaques.
●Anti-inflammatories to prevent activation of microglial cells to secrete neurotoxins (eg glutamate, cytokines) which stimulate formation of APP.
●Regulation of calcium entry (mediates the damage of neurotoxins).
●Preventing oxidative damage by free radicals.

Prevention Keeping alert and engaged with current and family affairs and enjoying education seems sensible. HRT appears to offer some protection.[3]

1 Ambrose Bierce 1967 *Devil's Dictionary* 2 M Tang 1996 *Lancet* **348** 429 3 C Kelly 1997 *BMJ* i 693

Practical issues in managing Alzheimer's disease

- *Exclude treatable dementias* (B$_{12}$, folate, syphilis serology, T$_4$, ?HIV).
- *Treat concurrent illnesses* (many can make dementia worse). In most people the dementia remains and will progress. Involve relatives and relevant agencies. Alzheimer's Disease Society (p756).
- *Avoid drugs which may ↓cognition* (neuroleptics, sedatives, tricyclics).
- In many countries there is *special help* made available for those looking after demented relatives at home—eg if the UK:

Laundry services for soiled linen	Attendance allowance
'Orange badge' giving priority parking	Respite care in hospital
Carers' groups for mutual support	Council tax rebate
Help from occupational therapist	Community nursing input
Help from community psychiatric nurses	Day care/lunch clubs

►See *Living with neurological disease*, p478. *Drugs:* It is too early to give a certain, practical rôle to drugs which ↑acetylcholine availability for synaptic transmission (by inhibiting the enzyme for its breakdown, eg donepezil, sometimes tried in a dose of 5mg/24h PO at night, increasing to 10mg nocte after 1 month). This may marginally delay need for institutional care, but not necessarily its duration.[2] Liaise with a psychiatrist or psychogeriatrician. It is hard to justify its use partly because of incomplete evidence on efficacy, and partly because of cost, particularly if its use diverts more important resources away from others, including those with advanced Alzheimer's disease. ►*In general, when you have to choose between interventions of similar or unknown benefit, choose low-technology over high-technology.* The high-technology option can always be added later, but if the fundamentals of care (such as respite admission to give relatives a break) are ignored even the most vigorously pursued high technology options may fail to produce real benefit.

5. Surgery

(*These are the 3 conditions where the promptest surgery is essential;
► notify the duty surgical registrar or consultant, and theatre, *at once*.)

Relevant pages in other chapters:
► See *Gastroenterology* and *Dictionary of symptoms and signs* (p480 & p38).

Urology: Urine/UTI (p370–4); haematuria (p370); 'prostatism' (p52); urological cancer (p136, p392); gynaecological urology (OHCS p70); incontinence
(p74); retention; BPH/TURP (p134); stones (p376); GU obstruction (p378).

Principle sources: British Medical Journal 1996–7; PJ Morris & RA Malt 1994, *Oxford Textbook of Surgery* OUP

The language of surgery

Incisions have their names

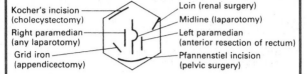

- Kocher's incision (cholecystectomy)
- Right paramedian (any laparotomy)
- Grid iron (appendicectomy)
- Loin (renal surgery)
- Midline (laparotomy)
- Left paramedian (anterior resection of rectum)
- Pfannenstiel incision (pelvic surgery)

Abdominal areas

1,2: Right & left upper quadrants.
3,4: Right & left flanks.
5,6: Right & left iliac fossae.
  7: Epigastrium.
  8: Central abdominal area.
  9: Suprapubic area.

-ostomy An artificial opening usually made to create a new connection either between two conduits or between a conduit and the outside world, eg colostomy: the colon is made to open onto the skin (p96). Stoma means a mouth.

-plasty This is the refashioning of something to make it work, eg pyloroplasty relieves pyloric (gastric outlet) obstruction.

-ectomy Cutting something out, eg appendicectomy.

-otomy Cutting something open, eg laparotomy (opening of abdomen).

-oscope An instrument for looking into the body, eg cystoscope (a device for looking into the bladder).

-lith- Stone, eg nephrolithotomy (cutting kidney open to get to a stone).

-chole- To do with gall or bile.

-cyst- A fluid-filled sac.

-gram A radiological image, eg using a radio-opaque contrast medium.

-docho- To do with ducts.

-angio- To do with tubes or blood vessels.

Per- Going through a structure (invasive).

Stent An artificial tube inserted into a biological tube to keep it open.

Trans- Going across a structure.

Use the above to understand *choledochojejunostomy* and *percutaneous transhepatic cholangiogram*.

A **fistula** is an abnormal communication between two epithelial surfaces (or endothelial in arterio–venous fistulae), eg gastrocolic fistula (stomach/colon). Fistulae commonly close spontaneously but will not do so in the presence of chronic inflammation, distal obstruction, epithelialization of the track, foreign bodies, or malignant tissue. External intestinal fistulae are managed by protection of the skin, replacement of fluid and electrolytes, parenteral nutrition and, if this fails, operation.

A **sinus** is a blind-ending track, typically lined by epithelial or granulation tissue, which opens onto an epithelial surface.

An **ulcer** is an abnormal area of discontinuity in an epithelial surface.

An **abscess** is a cavity containing pus. For different types, consult the *index*. Remember the aphorism: *if there is pus about, let it out.*

Aims ►To ensure that, as far as possible, any fears are addressed and the patient understands the nature, aims and expected outcome of surgery.

1 To ensure that the right patient gets the right surgery. Have the symptoms and signs changed? If so, inform the surgeon.

2 Get informed consent. Explain the 'op' and reasons for it (diagrams help); outline serious/commoner (>1%) complications; allow time for questions.

3 To assess and balance the risks of anaesthesia, and to maximize fitness.

4 To choose type of anaesthesia/analgesia. Aim to allay all anxiety and pain.

Pre-operative checks Assess cardiorespiratory system, exercise tolerance, existing illnesses, drug therapy, and allergies. Assess past history: of myocardial infarction, diabetes mellitus, asthma, hypertension, rheumatic fever, epilepsy, jaundice. Assess any specific risks, eg is the patient pregnant? Is the neck immobile (intubation risk)? Has there been recent anaesthesia? Were there any problems (nausea, DVT)?

Family history Ask questions about malignant hyperpyrexia (p86); dystrophia myotonica (p470); porphyria; cholinesterase problems; sickle-cell disease (test if needed).

Drugs Ask about allergy to any drug, antiseptic, plaster. Inform the anaesthetist about *all* drugs (including over-the-counter medicines).

Antibiotics: Neomycin, streptomycin, kanamycin, polymyxin and tetracyclines may prolong neuromuscular blockade.

Anticoagulants: Epidural, spinal, and regional blocks are contraindicated. Warn both surgeon and anaesthetist.

Anticonvulsants: Give as usual pre-op. Post-op, give drugs IV (or by NGT) until able to take oral drugs. Sodium valproate: an IV form is available (give the patient's usual dose). Phenytoin: give IV slowly (<50mg/min). IM phenytoin absorption is unreliable.

Beta-blockers: Continue up to and including the day of surgery as this precludes a labile cardiovascular response.

Contraceptive steroids: Many doctors stop 6 weeks pre-op but this is not evidence based.[1] If you *do* stop her Pill, will she get pregnant?

Digoxin: Continue up to and including morning of surgery. Check for toxicity (ECG; plasma level); do plasma K^+ and Ca^{2+} (suxamethonium ↑K^+ and can lead to ventricular arrhythmias in the fully digitalized). ▣

Diuretics: Beware hypokalaemia. Do U&E (and bicarbonate).

Hormone replacement therapy: As there is little increased risk of DVT or PE, there is no need to stop these agents.[1]

Insulin: Inform the anaesthetist. See details on p108.

Levodopa: Possible arrhythmias when the patient is under GA.

Lithium: Stop 3 weeks pre-op (arrhythmia risk↑). See OHCS p354.

MAOI: Stop 3 weeks before surgery to avert hypertensive crises.

Glaucoma eye-drops: β-blockers are systemically absorbed and anticholinesterases increase the half-life of suxamethonium.

Oral hypoglycaemics: No chlorpropamide 24h pre-op (long $t_{1/2}$).

Steroids: See p110.

Tricyclics: These enhance adrenaline (epinephrine) and lower BP.

Preparation ►Fast the patient—and nil by mouth for ≥2h pre-op.[2]

• Is any bowel or skin preparation needed—or prophylactic antibiotics?

• Start DVT prophylaxis as indicated, eg heparin 5000U SC pre-op, then every 12h SC until ambulant. Low molecular weight heparin: p278.

• Write up the pre-med (p86); book any pre-, intra-, or post-operative x-rays or frozen sections. Book post-operative physiotherapy.

• Catheterize and insert nasogastric tube (before induction and its attendant risk of vomiting) as indicated.

1 *Scottish Medical Journal* 1994 **36** 165   2 SM Greenfield 1997 BMJ i 16277

Pre-operative examination and tests

It is the anaesthetist's duty to assess suitability for anaesthesia. The ward doctor assists by obtaining a good history and examination—and should also reassure, inform and obtain written consent from the patient (eg remember to get consent for orchidectomy in orchidopexy procedures; also inform thyroidectomy patients of the risk of nerve damage).

Be alert to chronic lung disease, BP↑, arrhythmias, and murmurs (endocarditis prophylaxis needed?—see p312). In rheumatoid arthritis do a lateral cervical spine x-ray to warn about difficult intubations.

Tests Be guided by the history and examination.
● U&E, FBC, and ward test for blood glucose in most patients. If Hb <10g/dL tell anaesthetist. Investigate/treat as appropriate. U&E are particularly important if the patient is on diuretics, a diabetic, a burns patient, or has hepatic or renal diseases, or has starved, has an ileus, or is parenterally fed.
● Crossmatching: group and save for mastectomy, cholecystectomy. Crossmatch 2 units for Caesarean section; 4 units for a gastrectomy, and >6 units for abdominal aortic aneurysm surgery.
● Specific blood tests: LFT in jaundice, malignancy, or alcohol abuse. Amylase in acute abdominal pain.
Blood glucose in diabetic patients (p108).
Drug levels as appropriate (eg digoxin).
Clotting studies in liver disease, DIC, massive blood loss, already on warfarin or heparin. Contact lab as special bottles are needed.
HIV, HBsAg in high risk patients—after appropriate counselling.
Sickle test in those from Africa, West Indies, or Mediterranean—and others whose origins are in malarial areas (including most of India).
Thyroid function tests in those with thyroid disease.
● CXR: if known cardiorespiratory disease, pathology or symptoms or >65 years old.
● ECG: if >65 years old or poor exercise tolerance, or history of myocardial ischaemia, hypertension, rheumatic fever, or other heart disease.

ASA classification (American Society of Anesthesiologists)
1 Normally healthy.
2 Mild systemic disease.
3 Severe systemic disease that limits activity; not incapacitating.
4 Incapacitating systemic disease which poses a threat to life.
5 Moribund. Not expected to survive 24h even with operation.

You will see a space for an ASA number on most anaesthetic charts. It is a health index *at the time of surgery*. The prefix *E* is used in emergencies.

Prophylactic antibiotics in gut surgery

▶*The major error of antibiotic therapy is unnecessary usage.*

Wound infections These occur in 20–60% of those undergoing GI surgery. Sepsis may lead to delayed mobilization, haemorrhage, wound dehiscence and initiate a fatal chain of events.

Prophylaxis substantially reduces infection rates.

Rules for success:
- Give the antibiotic just before (eg 1h) surgery.
- Give it IV or IM (or as a suppository for metronidazole).
- Usually the antibiotic can be stopped after 24h.
- Use antibiotics which will kill anaerobes and coliforms (eg metronidazole and gentamicin, p181 & p750).

Bowel preparation is important before colorectal surgery. Typically the patient is put on a 'low residue' diet for 3 days pre-op. 24h prior to surgery only free fluids are allowed. Mechanical preparation is needed and involves use of laxatives and washouts. One sachet of Picolax® (10mg sodium picosulfate with magnesium citrate) may be given on the morning before surgery and a second sachet during the afternoon before surgery; but these should be used with care if there is any risk of perforation. Washouts (if used) should be continued until evacuation is clear.

Antibiotic regimens There is usually a local preference; examples:
Biliary surgery: Broad spectrum penicillin (eg ampicillin 500mg IV/8h for 3 doses) or cefalosporin (eg cefuroxime 1.5g/8h, 3 doses IV/IM).

Appendicectomy: A 3-dose regimen of metronidazole suppositories 1g/8h, + cefuroxime 1.5g/8h IV or gentamicin IV (p750).

Colorectal surgery: Cefuroxime 1.5g/8h, 3 doses IV/IM plus metronidazole 500mg/8h, 3 doses IV.

Vascular surgery: Co-amoxiclav 1.2g IV on induction; if penicillin-allergic, cefuroxime 1.5g IV/IM plus metronidazole 500mg IV.

Sutures

Sutures (stitches) are central to the art of surgery. The range of types available may appear confusing. Generally they are absorbable or non-absorbable and their structure may be divided into monofilament, twisted, or braided. Examples of absorbable sutures are catgut, polyglactin (Vicryl®), and polyglycolic acid (Dexon®). Non-absorbable sutures include silk, nylon, and prolene. Monofilament sutures are quite slippery but minimize infection and produce less reaction. Braided sutures have plaited strands and provide secure knots, but they may allow infection to occur between their strands. Twisted sutures have 2 twisted strands and similar qualities to braided sutures.

The time of suture removal depends on the site and the general state of the patient. Face and neck sutures tend to be removed after 5 days (may be earlier in children), scalp and back of neck after 5 days, and abdominal incisions after 5–8 days. In patients with poor wound healing, eg on steroids, with malignancy, infection or cachexia (p40), the sutures may need 14 days or longer.

Anaesthesia

Before anaesthesia, explain to the patient what will happen and where he will wake up, otherwise the recovery room or ITU will be frightening. Explain that he may feel ill on waking. The premedication aims to allay anxiety and to make the anaesthesia itself easier to conduct. Examples:

- Temazepam 10–20mg PO.
- The traditional, but now less commonly used pre-med, is papaveretum 15.4mg combined in a 1mL ampoule with 0.4mg hyoscine (also known as scopolamine; it aids amnesia and the drying of secretions). The typical adult dose is ½–1 ampoule IM.
- For children (2–7yrs), trimeprazine tartrate (=alimemazine) 2mg/kg as syrup (30mg/5mL). Try to avoid injections. If essential, morphine 0.15mg/kg IM may be used. Also use Emla® local anaesthetic cream on a few possible sites for the anaesthetist's IVI.

Give oral premedication 2h before surgery (1h if IM route used).

The side-effects of anaesthetic agents
Hyoscine, atropine: Tachycardia, urinary retention, glaucoma.

Opiates: Respiratory depression, cough reflex↓, vomiting, constipation.

Thiopentone (=tiopental): For rapid induction of anaesthesia) Laryngospasm.

Halothane: Vasodilatation, arrhythmias, hepatitis.

The complications of anaesthesia are due to loss of:
Pain sensation: Urinary retention, diathermy burns.

Consciousness: Cannot communicate 'wrong leg'.

Muscle power: Corneal abrasion, no respiration, no cough (leads to pneumonia and atelectasis—partial lung collapse causing shunting ± impaired gas exchange: it starts minutes after induction, and may be related to the use of 100% O_2 as well as to loss of power). Cannot phonate (speak) and is unable to impart vital information—eg 'I am in pain. . .' when paralysed and in pain, and unable to communicate.

Local anaesthesia If unfit for general anaesthesia, local nerve blocks or spinal blocks (contraindication: anticoagulation) using long-acting local anaesthetics (eg bupivacaine) may be indicated. Intercostal blocks aid post-operative pain control.

Drugs complicating anaesthesia ►Inform anaesthetist. See p82 for lists of specific drugs, and actions to take.

Malignant hyperpyrexia This is a rare complication. There is a rapid rise in temperature (eg 1°C every 5 minutes, up to 43°C) and acidosis due to rigidity. It may respond to prompt treatment with dantrolene. Give 1mg/kg every 5 minutes IV—up to 10mg/kg in total. See *OHCS* p722.

For further details see the chapter titled *Anaesthesia* in *OHCS* (p760–78).

Post-operative complications: a guide (see PLATE 12)

Pyrexia Mild pyrexia in the first 24h may be due to tissue damage or necrosis but a raised temperature post-op should stimulate an infection screen. Check the chest for pneumonia, the wound for infection, and the abdomen for signs of peritonism (eg anastomotic leakage) or UTI. Examine sites of IV cannulae and check for signs of meningism and endocarditis. Check the legs for DVT. Send blood for FBC and culture. Consider MSU, CXR and abdominal USS depending on clinical findings.

Confusion This may manifest as agitation, disorientation, and attempts to leave hospital especially at night. Gently reassure the patient in well-lit surroundings. See p 446 for a full work-up: here are the common causes:
  Hypoxia (pneumonia, post-anaesthesic lung collapse/atelectasis, LVF, PE)
  Infection (see above)
  Drugs (opiates, sedatives and any new drugs)
  Alcohol withdrawal
  Urinary retention
  Liver/renal failure
  MI or CVA

Occasionally, sedation is necessary to examine the patient; consider midazolam (see p768; antidote: flumazenil) or haloperidol 0.5–2mg IM. Reassure relatives that post-op confusion is common and reversible.

Shortness of breath or hypoxia Any previous lung disease?
Sit up and give oxygen. Examine for evidence of:
  Pneumonia/pulmonary collapse
  LVF (MI or fluid overload)
  Pulmonary embolism
  Pneumothorax (CVP line; intercostal anaesthetic block)
Do FBC, arterial blood gases, CXR and ECG. Manage according to findings.

BP↓ If severe, tilt bed head down and give O$_2$. Check pulse rate and measure BP yourself; compare it with that prior to surgery. Post-op ↓BP is commonly due to hypovolaemia resulting from inadequate fluid input so check fluid chart and replace losses. Hypovolaemia may also be caused by haemorrhage so review wounds and abdomen. If severe, return to theatre for haemostasis. Beware cardiogenic causes and look for evidence of MI and PE. Consider sepsis and anaphylaxis. Management: p766.

Urine output↓ Aim for output of >30mL/h. Anuria means a blocked or malsited catheter (and never, we hope, an impending lawsuit: both ureters tied). Flush or replace catheter. *Oliguria is usually due to inadequate replacement of lost fluid.* Treat by increasing fluid intake. Acute renal failure may follow shock, nephrotoxic drugs, transfusion, or trauma.
● Review fluid chart and examine for signs of volume depletion.
● Urinary retention is also common, so examine for a palpable bladder.
● Establish normovolaemia (a CVP line may help here, normal is 0–5cmH$_2$O relative to sternal angle); you may need 1L/h IVI for 2–3h.
● Catheterize bladder (for accurate monitoring).
● If intrinsic renal failure is suspected, refer to a nephrologist early.

Nausea/vomiting Any mechanical obstruction, paralytic ileus, or emetic drugs (opiates, digoxin, anaesthetics)? Consider AXR, NGT, and antiemetic.

After day-case surgery Don't discharge until 'LEAP-FROG' is established:
  Lucid, not vomiting, and cough reflex established.
  Easy breathing; easy urination.
  Ambulant without fainting.
  Pain relief+post-op drugs dispensed+given. Does he understand doses?
  Follow-up arranged.
  Rhythm, pulse rate, and BP checked one last time. Is trend satisfactory?
  Operation site checked and explained to patient.
  GP letter sent with patient or carer. He *must* know what's happened.

Post-operative bleeding

- Primary haemorrhage: ie continuous bleeding, starting during surgery. Replace blood loss. If severe, return to theatre for adequate haemostasis. Treat shock vigorously (p766).
- Reactive haemorrhage: haemostasis appears secure until BP rises and bleeding starts. Replace blood and re-explore wound.
- Secondary haemorrhage occurs a week or two post-op and is the result of infection.

Surgical drains in the post-operative period

The decision when to insert and remove drains may seem to be one of the great surgical enigmas—but there are basically two types to get a grip on. Most are inserted to drain the area of surgery and are often put on gentle suction. These are removed when they stop draining. The other type of drain is used to protect sites where leakage may occur in the post-operative period such, as bowel anastomoses. These form a tract and are removed after about one week.

'Shortening a drain' means withdrawing it (eg by 2cm/day). This allows the tract to seal up, bit by bit.

⁘ The control of pain

We humans are the most exquisite devices ever made for the experiencing of pain: the richer our inner lives, the greater the varieties of pain there are for us to feel—and the more resources we will have for mitigating pain. If you can connect with your patient's inner life you may make a real difference. *Never forget how painful pain is*—nor how fear magnifies pain. Try not to let these sensations, so often interposed between your patient and his recovery, be invisible to you as he or she bravely puts up with them.∗

Guidelines for success Assess each pain carefully. This is important as different types of pain respond to different approaches and analgesics.
●Identify and treat the underlying pathology wherever possible.
●Review and chart each pain regularly, eg on a pain score chart.
●Give regular doses rather than on an *as required* basis.
●Choose the best route: oral, PR, IM, epidural, SC, inhalation, or IV infusion.
●Explanation and reassurance contribute greatly to analgesia.

Non-narcotic (simple) analgesia Paracetamol: 0.5–1.0g/4h PO (up to 4g daily). Caution in liver impairment. Non-steroidal anti-inflammatories (NSAIDs), eg ibuprofen 400mg/8h PO or diclofenac 75mg/12h PO, PR (100mg) or IM; these are good for musculoskeletal pain and renal colic. CI: peptic ulcer, clotting disorder, anticoagulants. Cautions: asthma, renal or hepatic impairment, pregnancy, the elderly, and children.[1]

Narcotic ('controlled') drugs for severe pain Morphine (eg 10–15mg/2–4h) or *diamorphine* (5–10mg/2–4h) PO, SC, or slow IV, but you may need much more) are best. For terminal care, see p688).

Side-effects of narcotics: These include nausea (so give with an anti-emetic eg prochlorperazine 12.5mg/6h IM), respiratory depression, constipation, cough suppression, urinary retention, BP↓, and sedation (do not use in hepatic failure or head injury). Dependency is rarely a problem.

How effective are standard analgesics? Pain is subjective, but its measurement by patients is surprisingly consistent and reproducible. The table below gives 'numbers needed to treat' (NNT, p748), that is the number of patients who need to receive the drug for one to achieve a 50% reduction in pain (the range is 95% confidence intervals). Ibuprofen comes out best.[1]

Codeine[60mg]	11–20	Paracetamol[650]/proproxyphene[100]	3–6
Tramadol[50mg]	6–13	Paracetamol[1000mg]	3–4
Paracetamol[300mg]/codeine[60mg]	4–8	Paracetamol[600mg]/codeine[60mg]	2.5–4
Aspirin[650mg]/codeine[60mg]	4–7	Ibuprofen[400mg]	2–3

Epidural analgesia Opioids and anaesthetic are given into the epidural space by infusion or as boluses. Ask the advice of the Pain Service (if available).[1] SE: thought to be less as drug more localised; watch for respiratory depression; local anaesthetic-induced autonomic blockade (BP↓).

Adjuvant treatments Eg radiotherapy for bone cancer pain; anticonvulsants, antidepressants or steroids for nerve pain, antispasmodics eg buscopan 10–20mg/8h for intestinal, renal, or bladder colic. If brief pain relief is needed (eg for changing a dressing or exploring a wound), try inhaled nitrous oxide (with 50% O₂—as Entonox®) with an 'on demand' valve. Transcutaneous electrical nerve stimulation (TENS), local heat, local or regional anaesthesia, and neurosurgical procedures (eg excision of neuroma) may tried but can prove disappointing. Treat conditions which exacerbate pain (eg constipation, depression, anxiety).

∗Compare with Proust's '*egg of pain* . . . this structure. . . interposed between the face of a woman and the eyes of her lover which encases it and conceals it as a mantel of snow conceals a fountain. . .' Marcel Proust 1925 *Remembrance of Things Past* 11; *Albertine Disparue* 30, Chatto

◁1▷Co-codamol 30/500 (codeine phosphate and paracetamol) 2 tablets/6h is a less effective alternative: H McQuay 1997 *BMJ* i 153 & http:www.jr2.ox.ac.uk/Bandolier/painres/MApain.html

Deep vein thrombosis (DVT)

DVTs occur in ~30% of surgical patients (they also often present in non-surgical patients). 65% of below-knee DVTs are asymptomatic (these rarely embolize to the lung—the major complication).

Risk Age↑, pregnancy, synthetic oestrogen, surgery (especially pelvic/ortho-paedic), past DVT, malignancy, obesity, immobility, thrombophilia (p620).

Signs are fickle: ●Calf tenderness ●Mild fever ●Pitting oedema (PLATES 9-10) ●↑Warmth and distended veins ●Calf swelling 2–3cm greater than other side is significant. Homans' sign (↑ resistance to forced foot dorsiflexion, which may be painful) is of dubious value, and may dislodge thrombus.

Differential diagnosis Cellulitis (may co-exist). Ruptured Baker's cyst.

Tests *The Cogo regimen:* compression ultrasound* repeated at 1 week (to catch those with early but propagating DVTs). <0.1% have normal results, but go on to fatal PE.[1] *Venography* isn't usually needed. *Thrombophilia tests:* p620.

Prevention ●Stop the Pill 6 weeks pre-op (p82). ●Mobilize early. ●Heparin 5000u/12h sc; low molecular weight heparin (eg enoxaparin 20mg/24h PO for 7d, starting 2h pre-op, or dalteparin) may be better (less bleeding, no monitoring needed) ●Support hosiery ●Intermittent pneumatic pressure, until 16h post-op ●Aspirin for 3wks gives extra help.[2]

Treatment Calf thrombi <10cm long may be treated with compression stockings and heparin 5000u/12h. Larger thrombi need heparin IVI via a pump, eg 15,000u/12h (as indicated by APTT, p596)—or low molec-ular weight heparin, eg enoxaparin[3] 1mg/kg/12h, and initiation of war-farin. Stop heparin when INR is 2.0–3.0. Treat for 6 weeks if post-op; or long-term if the cause is permanent (eg malignancy). If no cause can be found, or DVT is recurrent, 6 months may be a suitable duration.☞

Swollen legs

(see PLATES 9-10)

Bilateral oedema implies systemic disease with ↑venous pressure (right heart failure) or ↓intravascular oncotic pressure (any cause of albumin↓, so test the urine for protein). It is 'dependent' (distributed by gravity), which is why legs are affected first—but severe oedema extends above the legs. In the bed-bound, or after lying down, fluid relocates to the new depen-dent area, causing a sacral pad. The exception is the local increase in venous pressure occurring in IVC or bilateral iliac vein obstruction: the swelling neither extends above the legs nor redistributes. Causes: ●Right heart failure—also JVP↑ and hepatomegaly. ●Hypoalbuminaemia—liver fail-ure, nephrotic syndrome, malnutrition, malabsorption, and protein-losing enteropathy. ●Venous insufficiency: acute—eg prolonged sitting, or chronic, with haemosiderin-pigmented, itchy, eczematous skin ± ulcers. ●Vasodilators, eg nifedipine[et al] (p276). ●Pelvic mass (p38). ●Pregnancy—if BP↑ + proteinuria, diagnose pre-eclampsia (OHCS, p96): find an obstetrician urgently. *In all the above, both legs need not be affected to the same extent.*

Unilateral oedema: Pain ± redness implies DVT or inflammation, eg celluli-tis or insect bites (any blisters?). Bone or muscle may be to blame, eg trauma (check pulses: a compartment syndrome with ischaemic necro-sis needs prompt fasciotomy▣); tumours; or necrotizing fasciitis, p124.

Impaired mobility suggests trauma, arthritis, or a Baker's cyst (p694).

Non-pitting oedema means you cannot indent it with your fingers. ▶p52.

Treatment Treat the cause. Giving diuretics to everyone is no answer. Ameliorate dependent oedema by elevating the legs (ankles higher than hips—do not just use foot stools); raise the foot of the bed (~30cm). Graduated support stockings (OHCS p598) may help (CI: ischaemia).

---

1 The key question is: *can the ultrasound transducer compress the femoral and popliteal veins?* If not, diagnose DVT. 1 A Cogo BMJ 1998 i 4 & 17 2 Antiplatelet trialists 1994 BMJ i 235 3 Levine 1996 NEJM 334 677

---

9 questions to ask those with swollen legs

–Is it *both* legs?	– Is she pregnant?	– Is she mobile?
–Any trauma?	– Any pitting? (PLATE 10)	–Past diseases/on drugs?
–Any pain?	–Any skin changes?	–Any oedema elsewhere?

When is there a high probability of a DVT?[1]

– 1 calf circumference >3cm than the other*   – Active malignancy
– Immobile (eg in bed, in plaster or paralysed) – Family history of DVT
– Local tenderness over deep venous system   (≥2 close relatives)

---

1 Less telling signs are pitting oedema, dilated superfical veins, erythema, and recent (<6 months) history of being in hospital. See *E-BM* 1998 3 5 *Measure 10cm below tibial tuberosity.

Specific post-operative complications

Laparotomy In the elderly, or the malnourished, the wound may break down from a few days to a few weeks post-op, particularly if infection or haematoma is present, or there has been major surgery in a patient already compromised, eg by cancer, or because this is a *second* laparotomy.

The warning sign of 'burst abdomen' is a pink serous discharge. If you are on the ward when this happens, put the guts back into the abdomen, and place a sterile dressing over the wound. Call your senior. Allay anxiety, give parenteral pain control, set up IVI, and return patient to theatre.

Biliary surgery After exploration of the common bile duct (CBD), a T-tube is usually left in the bile duct draining freely to the exterior. A T-tube cholangiogram is performed at 8–10 days and if there are no retained stones the tube may be pulled out.

Retained stones may be removed by ERCP (p498), further surgery, or instillation of stone-dissolving agents (via T-tube to dissolve the stone). If there is distal obstruction in the CBD, fistula formation may occur with a chronic leak of bile. Other complications of biliary surgery are CBD stricture; cholangitis; bleeding into the biliary tree (haemobilia) which may lead to biliary colic, jaundice and haematemesis; pancreatitis, and leak of bile causing biliary peritonitis. If jaundiced, it is important to maintain a good urine output as the danger is the hepato-renal syndrome (p110).

Thyroid surgery Laryngeal nerve palsy (hoarseness); hypoparathyroidism (p546), causing hypocalcaemia (p642); hypothyroidism; thyroid storm (p786). Tracheal obstruction due to haematoma in the wound may occur. ▶▶Relieve by immediate removal of stitches or clips.

Prostatectomy Retrograde ejaculation (eg in 75%); anorgasmia or altered orgasmic sensation (in 80% of those having a radical prostratectomy: less with transurethral prostastectomies);[1] epididymo-orchitis; impaction of blood clot in the urethra, causing urinary retention ('clot retention'); urethral stricture and incontinence. Urokinase release may promote devastating reactive haemorrhage. Hypervolaemia may be a problem during TURP as >1 litre of irrigating fluid may be absorbed.[2]

Haemorrhoidectomy Constipation; infection; stricture; bleeding. 1 week's lactulose + metronidazole (p181) starting pre-op ↓pain and time off work.[3]

Mastectomy Arm oedema; necrosis of skin edge; "My husband won't cuddle me any more".

Arterial surgery Bleeding; thrombosis; embolism; graft infection. Complications of aortic surgery: gut ischaemia; renal failure; respiratory distress; bleeding into the gut (aorto-enteric fistula); trauma to ureters; and anterior spinal artery (leading to paraplegia).

Colonic surgery Sepsis; ileus; fistulae; anastomotic leaks; obstruction; haemorrhage; trauma to ureters or spleen.

Tracheostomy Stenosis; mediastinitis; surgical emphysema.

Splenectomy Thrombocytosis; pneumococcal septicaemia—prevent with pneumococcal vaccine (p332) pre-operatively if the splenectomy is elective, or post-operatively if an emergency procedure; other infections.

Genitourinary surgery Septicaemia (from instrumentation in the presence of infected urine); urinoma—rupture of a ureter or renal pelvis leading to a mass of extravasated urine.

Gastrectomy See p164.

1 W Dunsmuir 1997 *BMJ* i 319 2 *Lancet* Ed 1991 ii 606 3 E Carapeti 1998 *Lancet* 351 169

95

Nasogastric (Ryle's) tubes

These tubes are passed into the stomach via either the nose or the mouth, and drain externally. Sizes: 16=large, 12=medium, 10=small. Uses:
- To empty the stomach before anaesthesia.

- Bowel obstruction, acute pancreatitis, and paralytic ileus.
- For irreversible dysphagia (eg motor neurone disease).
- For feeding ill patients (use a special fine-bore tube).

Passing the tube Nurses are experts and will ask you (who may never have passed one) to do so only when they fail—so the first question to ask is: "Have you asked the charge-nurse from the ward next door?"
- Don non-sterile gloves and a nurse's apron to protect from those 'rich encrustations' so often found on our clothes after a few days on the wards.
- Explain the procedure. Take a new, cool (hence less flexible) tube.
- Use the tube, by holding it against the patient's head, to estimate the length required to get from the nostril to the back of the throat.
- Place lubricated tube in nostril with its natural curve promoting passage down, rather than up. Advance towards occiput (not upwards).
- When the tip is estimated to be entering the throat, rotate the tube by ~180° to discourage passage into the mouth.
- Advance the tube into the oesophagus during a swallow—and thence into the stomach. *If this fails:* Try the other nostril, then oral insertion.
- Secure with tape to the nose. Use litmus paper (are the contents gastric?)
- Either spigot the tube, or allow to drain into a dependent catheter bag secured to the patient's clothing (zinc oxide tape around tube to form a flap, safety pin through flap). ▶Do not allow plans to pass the tube under anaesthesia: the great danger is fatal inhalation of vomit on induction.

Complications Pain, or, rarely:
- Loss of electrolytes
- Oesophagitis
- Tracheal or duodenal intubation
- Necrosis: retro- or nasopharyngeal
- Perforation of the stomach

Stoma care

A stoma is an artificial union made between two conduits (eg a chole-dochojejunostomy) or, more commonly, between a conduit and the outside—eg a colostomy, in which faeces are made to pass through a hole in the abdominal wall into an adherent plastic bag, hopefully as 1–2 formed motions per day. (Mouths and anuses are natural stomas.) The physical and psychological aspects of stoma care may be undervalued. Many hospitals have a stoma nurse who is expert in fitting secure, odourless devices. Ask her to talk to the patient *before* surgery—or else he may reject his colostomy and never attend to it. He may even take his own life. Explain what a colostomy is, why it is needed, where it will be (she should mark the site), and say what it will look like. Confirm that the patient is unsuited to one of the newer colostomy-preventing operations (eg employing muscle fibres from gracilis muscle).

1 *Loop colostomies:* A loop of colon is exteriorized, opened, and sewn to the skin. A rod under the loop prevents retraction and may be removed after 7 days. This is often called a defunctioning colostomy but this is not strictly true as faeces may pass beyond the loop. A loop colostomy is used to protect a distal anastomosis or to relieve distal obstruction.

2 *End colostomy:* The bowel is divided; the proximal end brought out as a stoma. The distal end may be: •Resected, eg abdominoperineal excision of the rectum. •Closed and left in the abdomen (Hartman's procedure). •Exteriorized, forming a 'mucous fistula'.

3 *Double-barrelled (Paul–Mikulicz) colostomy:* The colon is brought out as a double-barrel. It may be closed using an enterotome.

Ileostomies protrude from the skin and emit fluid motions. End ileostomy usually follows proctocolectomy, typically for UC. Loop ileostomy can be used to protect distal anastomoses. *Complications:* Prolapse, stricture, ischaemia, hernia, K$^+$↓, bleeding, diarrhoea.

Total anorectal reconstruction: an alternative to colostomy
Total anorectal reconstruction uses gracilis muscle disconnected distally and wound round the anus and induced to contract by a pulse generator implanted in the abdomen, with bowel action triggered by a hand-held radiofrequency controller. We regard it as still experimental, but patients will ask about it. Warn them that normal-quality continence cannot be achieved because of lack of sensation of the arrival of stools.[1]

1 D Jack 1997 *Lancet* 349 1750

Placing iv cannulae ('drips') (For cut-downs, see p798)

►Try to avoid ivis, as infections at the ivi site can cause real problems.

1 **Set up a tray** Swab to clean skin. Find: 3 cannulas; syringe + 1mL 1% lignocaine (=lidocaine); 3 fine needles (orange); cotton-wool to stop bleeding from unsuccessful attempts; tape to fix cannula; heparin.

2 **Set up a 'drip-stand'** with first bag of fluid (carefully checked with a nurse); 'run through' a giving set (a nurse will show how).

3 **Ask a nurse to help** until you are experienced. Nurses prefer helping to changing the bed because of spilt blood.

4 **Explain** procedure to patient. Place the tourniquet around the arm.

5 **Search hard for the best vein** (palpable, not merely visible). Don't be too hasty. Rest the arm below the level of the heart to aid filling.

6 **Sit comfortably**—with the patient lying (prevents most faints).[1]

7 **Tapping on the vein** often brings it to prominence. Avoid sites spanning joints: these are uncomfortable and easily 'tissue'.

8 **Place a paper towel** under arm to soak up any blood.

9 **Clean skin** around the chosen site. Use local anaesthetic (or Emla® cream): it is kinder, and it *does* work.[2] Use a fine needle to raise a bleb of lignocaine (lidocaine), like a nettle sting, just to the vein's side. Wait 15sec. Insertion skill is best taught at the bedside by an expert.

After it's in: 1 Connect fluid tube; check flow. 2 Fix cannula firmly with tape. 3 Bandage a loop of the tube to the arm. If the 'drip' is across a joint use a splint. 4 Check the flow chart (p100). Does the nurse understand it? 5 Explain that no needle is left in the arm, but that care needs to be taken. 6 Adding heparin to the ivi fluid makes drips last ~33h longer.[3] (Give 500u/500mL; it is incompatible with phenytoin, aminoglycosides, and amiodarone; se: platelets↓). 7 When the 'drip' comes down remove the cannula. (A patient once asked at follow-up if he still needed 'this green plastic thing on my hand'.)

If you fail after 3 attempts ►Shocked patients need fluid quickly: if you are having trouble putting in a 'drip' call your senior. The advice below assumes that the 'drip' is not immediately life-saving.

Experienced doctors, like drivers, forget they had to learn. Ask to be taught and ask for help when you need it. Is this the right needle for the right job? What is the 'drip' for? If the patient may need blood quickly use a large size (eg brown; green is suitable for slow ivis—or even pink if the veins are fragile). *If the ivi really is needed*, proceed as follows:

1 Explain to the patient that veins are difficult.

2 Fetch a bowl of warm water. This gives you time to calm down.

3 Immerse the patient's arm in the warm water for 2 minutes.

4 Use a blood pressure cuff at 80mmHg as a tourniquet—and try again.

If you still can't get the 'drip' in You are now getting downcast, so call your senior—it may pique your pride but there is nothing that makes your registrar happier than to succeed with a 'drip' where you have failed. Calling him could make both of you and your patient happy. Not many things do that! If you are too frightened of your senior, ask another house-officer—they are much more likely to succeed than you at this juncture. If you can't find another person to help, have a cup of coffee and return an hour later. Veins are capricious: they come and go.

'The drip has tissued' Ask yourself:
●Is there fluid in bag and giving-set?
●Inspect the cannula: take bandage off.
●Is the 'drip' still needed?
●Are the control taps open?
●Are there kinks in the tube?

Inflamed drip sites need prompt resiting of the drip. If site is healthy, gently infuse a 2mL syringe of 0.9% saline through the cannula. If resistance prevents this, the 'drip' needs resiting. (Needle-stick injury: see p216.)

1 S Rapp 1993 *Arch Int Med* **153** 1698 ◄2► J Jones 1994 *B J Anaes* **72** 147 3 M Hervás 1992 *An Phar* **26** 1211 See also Weber 1991 *Ann Pharmacoth* **25** 399-407 and Garrets 1992 *Clin Pharmacy* **11** 797-9

Pre-op fluids Shocked or dehydrated patients should rarely be rushed to theatre before adequate resuscitation. Anaesthesia compounds shock by causing vasodilatation and depressing cardiac contractility. Exceptions are exsanguination from a ruptured ectopic pregnancy, major trauma, or aortic aneurysm, where blood is lost faster than it can be replaced.

Post-operative fluids A normal requirement is 2–3 litres/24h which allows for urinary, faecal, and insensible loss.

A standard regimen: (One of many) 2 litres 5% dextrose with 1 litre 0.9% saline/24h. Add K⁺ post-op (20mmol/L). See p628 for another example.

When to increase the above regimen:
- Dehydration: this may be by ≥5 litres if severe. Replace this slowly.
- Shock (all causes, except for cardiogenic shock).
- Losses from gut: replace NGT aspirate volume with 0.9% saline.
- Transpiration losses: feverish patients and burns.
- Pancreatitis: there are large pools of sequestered fluid which should be allowed for.
- Low urine output (the night after surgery) is almost always due to inadequate infusion of fluid. Check JVP, and review for signs of cardiac failure. Treat by increasing IVI rate unless patient is in heart or renal failure, or profusely bleeding (when blood should be transfused). If in doubt a fluid challenge may be indicated: ½–1L over 30–60 minutes, with monitoring of urine output. Then you may increase IVI rate to 1 litre/h for 2–3h. Only if output does not increase should a diuretic be considered; a CVP line may be needed if estimation of fluid balance is difficult. A normal value is 0–5cm of water relative to the sternal angle.

If not catheterized exclude retention, but otherwise do not catheterize until absolutely necessary.

When to decrease the above regimen: Acute renal failure—give 500mL plus the previous day's output (►with no K⁺).
In heart failure—halve the volume (1–1.5 litres/24h).

Guidelines for success
- Be simple. Chart losses and replace them. Know the urine output. Aim for 60mL/h; 30mL/h is the minimum (½mL/kg/h).
- Measure plasma U&E if the patient is ill. Regular U&Es are not needed on young, fit people with good kidneys.
- Start oral fluids as soon as possible. They are safer.

What fluids to use ►*Haemorrhagic/hypovolaemic shock* (see p766): Insert 2 large IV cannulae, for fast fluid infusion. Start with crystalloid (eg 0.9% saline) or colloid (eg Haemaccel®) until blood is available. The advantage of crystalloids is that they are very cheap—but they do not stay as long in the intravascular compartment as colloids, because they equilibrate with the total extracellular volume (dextrose is useless for resuscitation as it rapidly equilibrates with the enormous intracellular volume). In practice, the best results in resuscitation are achieved by combining crystalloids and colloids. Aim to keep the haematocrit at ~0.3, and urine flowing at >30mL/h. Monitor pulse and BP often.

Septicaemic shock: Use a plasma-like substance (eg Haemaccel®).

Heart or liver failure: Avoid sodium loads: use 5% dextrose.

Excessive vomiting: Use 0.9% saline: replace losses, including K⁺.

Blood transfusion and blood products

▶Know *and use* local procedures to ensure that the right blood gets to the right patient at the right time. See p83 for quantities to request.

- Take blood for crossmatching from only one patient at a time. Label immediately. This minimizes risk of wrong labelling of samples.
- When giving blood monitor TPR and BP every half-hour.
- Do not use giving sets which have contained dextrose or Haemaccel®.

Group-and-save (G&S) requests Find out your local guidelines for elective surgery. Having crossmatched blood to hand may not be needed if a blood sample is already in the lab, with group determined, with any atypical antibodies (ie G&S). **Whole blood** (rarely used) *Indications:* Exchange transfusion; grave exsanguination—use crossmatched blood if possible, but if not, use 'universal donor' group ORh–ve blood, changing to crossmatched blood as soon as possible. ▶Blood >2 days old has no effective platelets. Complications of massive transfusion: platelets↓, Ca^{2+}↓, clotting factors↓, K^+↑, hypothermia.

Red cells (packed to make haematocrit ~70%) Use to correct anaemia or blood loss. 1u ↑Hb by 1–1.5g/dL. If prone to heart failure give each unit over 4h with frusemide (=furosemide, eg 40mg slow IV/PO) with alternate units. Keep a watch on the JVP and listen for pulmonary oedema.

Platelet transfusion (p610) Not usually needed if not bleeding or count is >20 × 10^9/L. If surgery is planned, get advice if <100 × 10^9/L.

Fresh frozen plasma (FFP) Use to correct clotting defects: eg DIC, warfarin overdosage where vitamin K would be too slow, liver disease, thrombotic thrombocytopenic purpura. It is expensive and carries all the risks of blood transfusion. It is probably not needed routinely after large transfusions—only when a suspected clotting defect is confirmed in the lab. FFP should not be used simply as a volume expander.

Human albumin solution (Plasma protein fraction) is produced as 4.5% or 20% protein solution and is basically albumin to use for protein replacement. There are no compatibility requirements. Both of the solutions have much the same Na^+ content and 20% albumin can be used temporarily in the hypoproteinaemic (eg liver disease; nephrotic) who is fluid overloaded, without giving an excessive salt load.

Others Cryoprecipitate (a source of fibrinogen); coagulation concentrates (self-injected in haemophilia); immunoglobulin (anti-D, *OHCS* p109).[1]

Complications of transfusing red cells[3]
- Serious bacterial contamination or ABO incompatibility with a rapid fever spike (>40°C) ± anaphylaxis (p766).
- Mild reactions (eg from HLA antibodies): fever, itch, urticaria, wheeze. *Management:* Give hydrocortisone 100mg IV and chlorpheniramine (=chlorphenamine) 10mg IV. Consider slowing or stopping transfusion.
- Heart failure, if the transfusion is too rapid.
- Transfer of: viruses (hepatitis B/C; HIV); bacteria; protozoa; ?prions (p702: CJD risk is theoretical, some advise removing white cells from all donated blood).

▶What is uncontroversial is that blood should only be given if strictly necessary, and that there is a rôle for patients having their own blood stored pre-op for later use (*autologous transfusion*). In anaemia, transfuse up to 8g/dL. If Hb ≤5g/dL with heart failure, transfusion is vital to restore Hb to safe level, eg 6–8g/dL, but must be done with great care. Give packed red cells slowly with 40mg frusemide IV/PO with alternate units (do not mix with blood). Check for ↑JVP and basal crepitations; consider CVP line. If CCF gets worse, and immediate transfusion is essential, try a 2–3u exchange transfusion, removing blood at same rate as transfused.

Transfusion reactions

A rapid spike of temperature (>40°C) at the start of a bag indicates that the transfusion should be stopped (suggests intravascular haemolysis—see opposite). For a slowly rising temperature (<40°C) slow the IVI—this is most frequently due to antibodies against white cells (if recurrent, use leucocyte depleted blood or white cell filter).

Acute transfusion reactions	*Action*[2]
Acute haemolytic reaction Agitation, fever (often within minutes of starting transfusion), ↓BP, abdominal or chest pain, bleeding from puncture sites, flushing, DIC.	STOP the transfusion. Check patient identity against unit, Inform haematologist and send unit and fresh blood samples (FBC, U&E, clotting and cultures) and urine (haemoglobinuria) to lab. Keep IV line open with 0.9% saline.
Anaphylaxis Bronchospasm, cyanosis, ↓BP, soft tissue swelling.	SLOW or STOP the transfusion. Maintain airway and give oxygen. Contact anaesthetist. Give adrenaline (=epinephrine) 1mg IM every 10min until BP improved; chlorpheniramine (=chlorphenamine) 10–20mg slow IV; salbutamol 2.5mg nebulized.
Non-haemolytic febrile transfusion reaction Shivering and fever usually 30–60min after starting transfusion.	SLOW or STOP the transfusion. Give an antipyretic eg paracetamol 1g Monitor closely. If recurrent, use leucocyte depleted blood or white cell filter.
Allergic reactions Urticaria and itch.	SLOW or STOP the transfusion; give chlorpheniramine (chlorphenamine) 10mg slow IV/IM. Monitor closely.
Fluid overload Dyspnoea, hypoxia tachycardia, ↑JVP, and basal crepitations.	SLOW or STOP the transfusion. Give oxygen and a diuretic eg frusemide 40mg IV initially. Consider CVP line and exchange transfusion.

1 *Drug Ther Bul* 1993 **31** 89 2 *Handb of Transf. Med.* 1996 HMSO, London 3 S Stern 1997 *Lancet* **349** 135

Nutritional support in hospital[1]

▶Almost 50% of hospital in-patients may be malnourished. Hospitals can become so focused on curing disease that they ignore the foundations of good health. Malnourished patients will recover more slowly, and experience more complications, than those well fed.

Why are so many hospital patients malnourished?
1 Increased nutritional requirements (eg sepsis, burns, surgery).
2 Increased nutritional losses (eg malabsorption, output from stoma).
3 Decreased intake (eg dysphagia, sedation, coma).
4 Effect of treatment (eg nausea, diarrhoea).
5 Enforced starvation (eg prolonged periods *nil by mouth*).
6 Missing meals through being whisked off, eg for investigations.
7 Difficulty with feeding and no one available to give enough help.
8 Unappetizing food: "They feed me stuff I wouldn't give my cat".

Identifying the malnourished patient
History: Recent weight change; recent reduced intake; diet change (eg recent change in consistency of food); nausea, vomiting, pain, diarrhoea which might have led to reduced intake.

Examination: Examine for state of hydration (p636): dehydration can go hand in hand with malnutrition, and overhydration can mask the appearance of malnutrition. Evidence of malnutrition: skin hanging off muscles (eg over biceps); no fat between fold of skin; hair rough and wiry; pressure sores; sores at corner of mouth.

Investigations: Generally unhelpful. Low albumin suggestive (but is affected by many things other than nutrition).

Prevention of malnutrition Assess nutritional status, and weight, on admission and regularly (eg weekly) thereafter. Identify those at risk (see above). Ensure that investigations and treatment do not interfere substantially with nourishment. Provide food appetizing to patient.

Calorie needs Most patients are well-nourished with 2000–2500kCal and 7–14g nitrogen/24h. Even catabolic patients rarely need more than 2500kCal. Very high calorie diets (eg 4000kCal/24h) can lead to fatty liver. If patient requires nutritional support seek help from dietician.

Approximate energy contents Glucose 4kCal/g; fat 10kCal/g. To convert kCal to kJ multiply by 4.2.

Enteral nutrition (ie nutrition given into gastrointestinal tract)
If at all possible give nutrition by mouth. An all-fluid diet can meet requirements (but get advice from dietician). If danger of choking (eg after stroke) consider semi-solid diet before abandoning food by mouth.

Tube feeding: This is giving liquid nutrition through an enterally placed tube (eg nasogastric, or nasojejunal, directly into stomach via gastrostomy. Use nutritionally complete, commercially prepared feeds. Standard feeds (eg Nutrison standard®, Osmolite®) normally contain 1kCal/mL and 4–6g protein per 100mL. Most people's requirements are met in 2 litres/24h. Specialist advice from dietician is essential. Nausea and vomiting is less of a problem if feed given continuously with pump, but may have disadvantages compared with intermittent nutrition.

Guidelines for success ●Use fine-bore NG feeding tube when possible.
●Check position of nasogastric tube before starting feeding.
●Build up feeds gradually to avoid diarrhoea and distension.
●Weigh weekly, check blood glucose and plasma electrolytes (including zinc and magnesium if previously malnourished).
●Close liaison with dietician is essential.

1 J Lennard-Jones 1992 *A positive approach to nutrition as treatment*, Kings Fund Report

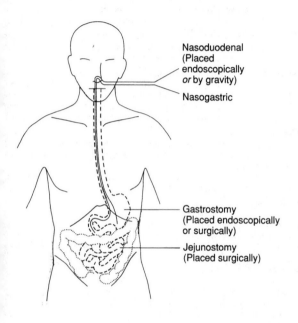

Nasoduodenal
(Placed
endoscopically
or by gravity)

Nasogastric

Gastrostomy
(Placed endoscopically
or surgically)

Jejunostomy
(Placed surgically)

Parenteral (intravenous) feeding

Do not undertake parenteral feeding lightly: it has risks.
Specialist advice is vital.

Only consider parenteral feeding if the patient is likely to become malnourished without it. This normally means that the gastrointestinal tract is not functioning (eg bowel obstruction), and is unlikely to function for at least 7 days. Parenteral feeding may supplement other forms of nutrition (eg in active Crohn's disease when insufficient nutrition can be absorbed in the gut) or be used alone (total parenteral nutrition—TPN).

Administration Nutrition is normally given through a central venous line as this usually lasts longer than if given into a peripheral vein. Insert under strictly sterile conditions and check its position on x-ray.

Requirements There are many different regimens for parenteral feeding. Most provide ~2000kCal and 10–14g nitrogen in 2–3 litres; this amount to be given daily. ~50% of calories are provided by fat and 50% by carbohydrate. Regimens comprise vitamins, minerals, trace elements, and electrolytes; these will normally be included by the pharmacist.

Complications
Sepsis: (Eg *Staph epidermidis* and *aureus*; *Candida*; *Pseudomonas*; infective endocarditis). Look for spiking pyrexia and examine wound at tube insertion point.
Metabolic imbalance: Electrolytes; plasma glucose; deficiency syndromes.
Mechanical: Pneumothorax; embolism of IVI tip.

Guidelines for success
- Liaise closely with nutrition team and pharmacist.
- Meticulous sterility. Do not use central venous lines for uses other than feeding. Remove line if you suspect infection. Culture its tip.
- Review fluid balance at least twice daily, and requirements for energy and electrolytes daily.
- Check weight, fluid balance, and urine glucose daily throughout period of parenteral nutrition. Check plasma glucose, creatinine and electrolytes (including calcium and phosphate), and full blood count daily until stable and then 3 times a week. Check LFTs and lipid clearance 3 times a week until stable and then weekly. Check zinc and magnesium weekly throughout.
- Do not rush. Achieve the maintenance regimen by small steps.

Diabetic patients on surgical wards

Insulin-dependent diabetes mellitus (=type 1 diabetes mellitus)
- Stress of intercurrent illness increases basal insulin needs (see p535).
- Always try to put the patient first on the list (surgery, endoscopy, bronchoscopy, etc.). Inform the surgeon and anaesthetist early.
- Stop all long-acting insulin the night before. Get IV access *before* you need it urgently. If surgery is in the morning, stop *all* SC morning insulin. If surgery is in the afternoon, have the usual short-acting insulin in the morning at breakfast. No medium or long-acting insulin.
- Check U&E on the morning of surgery, and start an IVI of 1 litre of 5% dextrose with 20mmol KCl/8h to continue until the patient is eating normally. Check saline needs, but do not give *only* saline: dextrose may need constant infusion to maintain the blood glucose.
- Add 50u short-acting insulin (eg Actrapid®, Humulin S®, Velosulin®) to 50mL 0.9% saline to give via an infusion pump—give according to a sliding scale below adjusted in the light of blood glucose.
- Check blood glucose hourly. Aim for 7–11mmol/L during surgery.
- Post-op, continue IV insulin and dextrose till the patient eats his 2nd meal. Fingerprick glucose every 2h. Switch to usual SC insulin regimen.

Practical hints:
- If blood glucose persistently <4mmol/L, decrease insulin infusion by 0.5–1.0u/h; if always >11mmol, increase by 0.5–1u/h.
- In Type 1 diabetes mellitus, aim for some insulin to be infused all the time as patients are insulin deficient; eg a patient usually on Mixtard® 40u/35u needs 75u insulin/24h, ie ~3u/h basal requirement. Adjust sliding scales accordingly. •Some prefer to add soluble insulin to 500mL bags of 5% dextrose with 20mmol KCl/4–6h and adjust the amount of insulin added according to the mean glucose level in the previous 4h. This is useful if close monitoring (hourly glucose ward tests) is not possible as there is no risk of giving insulin without dextrose.

Non-insulin-dependent diabetes mellitus (=type 2 diabetes)
These patients are usually controlled on oral hypoglycaemics (see p530). Perform a fasting blood glucose: if >10mmol/L, treat as for type 1 diabetes. Otherwise halve the dose of long-acting sulfonylurea (eg chlorpropamide) the day before surgery and omit the tablet on the day of surgery. Check a fasting glucose on the morning of surgery and at time of premedication: if >15mmol use insulin, either IV as above or SC sliding scale (below). Use half the normal drug dose (and supplement with SC soluble insulin before meals) until a normal diet is established. Convert to IV insulin for major surgery. Fingerprick glucose every 1–2h.

Diet controlled diabetes Usually there is no problem, but the patient may become temporarily insulin-dependent.

IV Insulin Sliding Scale (This is only a guide.)

Fingerprick glucose (mmol/L)	IV soluble insulin*	Alternative SC insulin**
<2 (see p784)	None (50% glucose IV)	None (50% glucose IV)
2–5	No insulin	No insulin
5–10	1u/h	2u
10–15	2u/h	5u
15–20	3u/h	7u
>20 urgent diabetologist review	6u/h	urgent diabetologist review

*Check glucose hourly and adjust insulin accordingly.

**▶Only use SC route if IV route is problematic as it is associated with much variability; check fingerprick glucose every 2–4h if NBM—or premeals if using SC insulin to supplement other hypoglycaemic agents.

Principle source: D Sprigings *et al* 1995 *Acute Medicine*, Blackwell, ISBN 0-632-03625-4

th obstructive jaundice are particularly prone to developing
e after surgery (the hepato-renal syndrome). This may be
oxic effect of bilirubin on the kidney. In practice this means
l urine output must be maintained in such patients around the
gery. The following regimen is one way of ensuring this.

Preoperative preparation Avoid morphine in the premedication.
sert iv line and run in 1 litre of 0.9% saline over 30–60mins following
pre-med (unless the patient has heart failure).
- Insert a urinary catheter.
- Give 500mL of 10% mannitol iv over 20min 1h before surgery.
- A 'renal' dose dopamine (2–5µg/kg/min) iv *may* be indicated: remember
  there may be side-effects from any central line used, and from the drug:
  −Sepsis (immune dysfunction) −Arrhythmias   −Gut and myocardial perfusion↓
  −Diuresis when hypovolaemic −Catabolism↑   −Gastric motility decreased
  −Pulmonary hypertension   −Impaired hypoxic ventilatory responses[1]

During surgery ●Measure urine output hourly.
- Give 100mL of 10% mannitol iv if the urine output <60mL/h.
- Give 0.9% saline iv to match the urine output.

For 48h after surgery ●Measure urine output every 2h.
- Give 100mL 10% mannitol iv over 15min if urine output < 100mL in 2h.
- Give 0.9% saline at rate to match urine output and fluid lost through
  NGT; and give 2 litres of dextrose-saline every 24h.
- Measure urea and electrolytes daily.
- Give 20mmol of potassium per litre of fluid after 24h post-op if urine
  output good.

Surgery in patients taking steroids

Patients taking steroid drugs or those with Addison's disease may need
extra steroid cover to cope with the stress of surgery.

Major surgery Give hydrocortisone 100mg IM with the pre-medica-
tion and then every 6h IV/IM for 3 days. Then return to previous medication.

Minor surgery Prepare as for major surgery except that hydrocortisone is given for 24h only.

The major risk with adrenal insufficiency is hypotension, so if this is
encountered without an obvious cause, it may be worthwhile giving a
dose of 100mg hydrocortisone IV.

Thyroid disease and surgery

Thyroid surgery for hyperthyroidism If severe give carbimazole
until euthyroid (p542). Arrange operation date and 10–14 days before
this, start aqueous iodine oral solution (Lugol's solution), 0.1–0.3mL/8h
PO well diluted with milk or water. Continue until surgery.

Mild hyperthyroidism Start propranolol 80mg/8h PO and Lugol's solution as above at the first consultation. Stop Lugol's solution on the day
of surgery but continue propranolol for 5 days post-op.

1 BH Cuthbertson 1997 *BMJ* i 690

The acute abdomen

Someone who becomes acutely ill and in whom symptoms and signs are chiefly related to the abdomen has an acute abdomen. Prompt laparotomy is sometimes essential: *repeated examination is the key to making the decision.*

Clinical syndromes which usually require laparotomy

1 *Rupture of an organ* (Spleen, aorta, ectopic pregnancy) Shock is the leading sign. Abdominal swelling may be seen. Note any history of trauma. Peritonism may be surprisingly mild. *Delayed* rupture of the spleen may occur some weeks after trauma.

2 *Peritonitis* (Perforation of a peptic ulcer, diverticulum, appendix, bowel, or gall bladder) Signs: prostration, shock, lying still, +ve cough test (p30), tenderness (± rebound, p56), board-like abdominal rigidity and no bowel sounds. An erect CXR may show air under the diaphragm. Note: *acute pancreatitis* (p116) produces this syndrome but does *not* require a laparotomy—so always check the serum amylase.

Syndromes which may not require a laparotomy

1 *Local peritonitis:* Eg diverticulitis, cholecystitis, salpingitis, and appendicitis. (The latter *will* need surgery.) If abscess formation is suspected (swelling, swinging fever, and WCC↑) arrange a diagnostic ultrasound or CT. Drainage can be percutaneous (ultrasound or CT guided), or by laparotomy. Look for 'meteorism' on the plain AXR (p720).

2 *Colic:* This is a regularly waxing and waning pain. It is caused by muscular spasm in a hollow viscus (gall bladder, gut, ureter, uterus). The patient is restless with the pain (unlike in peritonitis).

Obstruction of the bowel See p130.

Tests U&E; FBC; amylase; urinoscopy; laparoscopy may avert unneeded surgery.[1] CT can be helpful *provided it is readily available and causes no delay.*[2]

Pre-op care ►Do not rush to theatre. Anaesthesia compounds shock, so resuscitate properly first (p767) unless blood is being lost faster than it can be replaced in ruptured ectopic pregnancy, OHCS p24, or a leaking abdominal aneurysm, p118. Put to bed, then:

- Nil by mouth for ≥2h pre-op
- IVI (0.9% saline)
- Treat shock (p766)
- Relieve pain (p90) •Consent
- CXR + ECG if >50yrs •Crossmatch eg 2u
- Plain x-rays*
- Blood culture
- IV/PR antibiotics**

Medical causes of acute abdominal symptoms

Myocardial infarction	Pneumonia (p332)	Sickle-cell crisis (p588)
Gastroenteritis or UTI	Tabes (p233)	Phaeochromocytoma (p788)
Diabetes mellitus (p528)	Zoster (p202)	Malaria (p194)
Bornholm disease (p694)	Tuberculosis (p200)	Typhoid fever (p228)
Pneumococcal peritonitis	Porphyria (p656)	Cholera (p228)
Henoch–Schönlein (p700)	Thyroid storm (p786)	*Yersinia enterocolitica* (p225)
Narcotic addiction	PAN (p674)	Lead colic

Computer help Accuracy in diagnosing acute abdomen is ~45%; this is improvable to ~70–80% by using a computer,[2] not because computers are so clever, but because they are so stupid—and rigid: they have no intuition, and they need clear answers to a full set of questions. They allow no escape. You have to take a proper history, and you have to conduct a careful examination. This enforced virtue accounts for most (but not all) of the improved performance when a computer is used.[3]

---

1 *Br J Surg* 1993 **80** 279 2 D Jack & A Malone 1997 *Lancet* **349** 1079 & 1774 3 J Britton 1994 OTS 1377
*Consider erect or decubitus films, but these are rarely helpful. **Give antibiotics for peritonitis, eg cefuroxime 1.5g/8h IV with metronidazole 500mg/8h IV/PR.

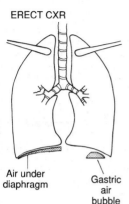

ERECT CXR

Air under diaphragm

Gastric air bubble

Causes of air under the diaphragm

- Perforation of bowel
- Gas-forming infection
- Pleuroperitoneal fistula
  (carcinoma, TB, trauma)
- Crohn's disease
- Iatrogenic (surgery, laparoscopy)
- *Per vaginam*
  (post partum, waterskiiers)
- Interposition of bowel between liver
  and diaphragm

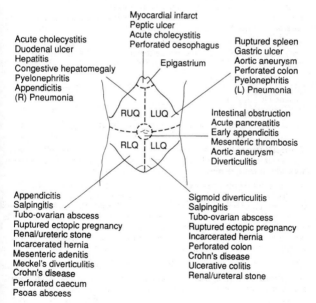

Myocardial infarct
Peptic ulcer
Acute cholecystitis
Perforated oesophagus

Acute cholecystitis
Duodenal ulcer
Hepatitis
Congestive hepatomegaly
Pyelonephritis
Appendicitis
(R) Pneumonia

Epigastrium

Ruptured spleen
Gastric ulcer
Aortic aneurysm
Perforated colon
Pyelonephritis
(L) Pneumonia

RUQ | LUQ

RLQ | LLQ

Intestinal obstruction
Acute pancreatitis
Early appendicitis
Mesenteric thrombosis
Aortic aneurysm
Diverticulitis

Appendicitis
Salpingitis
Tubo-ovarian abscess
Ruptured ectopic pregnancy
Renal/ureteric stone
Incarcerated hernia
Mesenteric adenitis
Meckel's diverticulitis
Crohn's disease
Perforated caecum
Psoas abscess

Sigmoid diverticulitis
Salpingitis
Tubo-ovarian abscess
Ruptured ectopic pregnancy
Incarcerated hernia
Perforated colon
Crohn's disease
Ulcerative colitis
Renal/ureteral stone

Acute appendicitis

The most common surgical emergency (lifetime incidence: 6%).

Pathogenesis Gut organisms invade the appendix wall after lumen obstruction by lymphoid hyperplasia, faecolith, or filarial worms—or there may be impaired ability to prevent invasion, brought about by improved hygiene (so less exposure to gut pathogens). This 'hygiene hypothesis' explains the rise in appendicitis rates in the early 1900s and its later decline (as pathogen exposure dwindles further).

Symptoms As inflammation begins, there is central abdominal colic. Once peritoneum becomes inflamed, the pain shifts to the right iliac fossa and becomes more constant. Anorexia is almost invariable but vomiting rarely prominent. Constipation is usual. Diarrhoea may occur.

Signs		Signs in the right iliac fossa:
Tachycardia	Lying still	Tenderness, guarding (p46)
Fever 37.5–38.5°C	Foetor ± flushed	Rebound tenderness (p56)
Furred tongue	Coughing hurts	PR painful on right
	Shallow breaths	

Special tests: Rovsing's sign (pain more in the RIF than the LIF when the LIF is pressed). In women, do a vaginal examination: does she have salpingitis (+ve cervical excitation, *OHCS* p50)? If rapidly available, consider CT.[1,2]

Variations in the clinical picture ●The schoolboy with vague abdominal pain who will not eat his favourite food.
●The infant with diarrhoea and vomiting.
●The shocked, confused octogenarian who is not in pain.

Hints and pitfalls ●Don't rely on tests (eg WCC; urinoscopy).
●If the child is anxious use his hand to press his belly.
●Do not ignore right-sided tenderness on rectal examination: it may be the only sign of an inflamed retrocaecal appendix.

►Expect your diagnosis (both of 'appendicitis' and 'not appendicitis') to be wrong half the time. This means that those who seem not to have appendicitis should be re-examined often. Laparoscopy may be helpful.

Differential diagnosis

Ectopic pregnancy	Diverticulitis	Perforated ulcer
Mesenteric adenitis	Salpingitis	Cystitis
Food poisoning	Cholecystitis	Crohn's disease

Treatment Prompt appendicectomy. Metronidazole 1g/8h + cefuroxime 1.5g/8h, 3 doses IV starting 1h pre-op, reduces wound infections.

Complications Perforation with peritonitis with later infertility in girls (so have a lower threshold for surgery in girls); appendix mass (inflamed appendix surrounded by omentum); appendix abscess.

Treatment of an appendix mass There are 2 schools of thought: *conservative* and *early surgery*. Try the former initially—NBM and antibiotics (eg cefuroxime 1.5g/8h IV and metronidazole 500mg/8h IV). Mark out the size of the mass and proceed to surgery if it enlarges or the patient gets more toxic (pain↑; temperature↑; pulse↑; WCC↑). If the mass resolves it is usual to do an interval (ie delayed) appendicectomy. Exclude a colonic tumour in the elderly.

Treatment of an appendix abscess Surgical drainage.

Appendicitis in pregnancy (1/2000 pregnancies) Pain and tenderness are higher due to displacement of the appendix by the uterus. Appendicectomy is well tolerated but fetal mortality approaches 30% after perforation—so prompt assessment is vital.

1 DB Jack 1997 *Lancet* 349 1079   2 AJ Malone 1997 *Lancet* 349 1774

Acute pancreatitis

▶This unpredictable disease (mortality 5–10%) is often managed on surgical wards, but because surgery is often not involved it is easy to think that there is no acute problem: *there is*—due to self-perpetuating pancreatic inflammation (and other retroperitoneal tissues). Litres of extracellular fluid are trapped in the gut, peritoneum, and retroperitoneum. There may be rapid progress from a phase of mild oedema to one of necrotizing pancreatitis. In fulminating cases the pancreas is replaced by black fluid. Death may be from shock, renal failure, sepsis, or respiratory failure, with contributory factors being protease-induced activation of complement, kinin, and the fibrinolytic and coagulation cascades.

Causes 'GET SMASHED': Gallstones, Ethanol, Trauma, Steroids, Mumps, Autoimmune (PAN), Scorpion venom[1], Hyperlipidaemia (↑Ca^{2+}, hypothermia), ERCP, (also emboli) Drugs (eg azathioprine, asparaginase, mercaptopurine, pentamidine, didanosine, ?diuretics); also pregnancy. Often none found.

Symptoms Gradual or sudden severe *epigastric* or *central abdominal pain* (radiates to back); vomiting is prominent. Sitting forward may help.

Signs (may be mild in serious disease!) Tachycardia, fever, jaundice, shock, ileus, rigid abdomen ± local/generalized tenderness and periumbilical discolouration (Cullen's sign or, at the flanks, Grey Turner's sign).

Tests Serum amylase >1000u/mL (lesser rises in cholecystitis, mesenteric infarction, perforated peptic ulcer, renal failure; amylase may be ↔ even in severe pancreatitis.) Abdominal films: no psoas shadow (retroperitoneal fluid↑), 'sentinel loop' of proximal jejunum (solitary air-filled dilatation). CT (helps assess severity[2]). Ultrasound (for gallstones; AST↑ too). ERRP. *Differential diagnosis:* Any acute abdomen (p112), myocardial infarct.

Management Obtain expert help. Nil by mouth (may need NGT).
1 Set up IVI and give plasma expanders (eg Haemaccel®) and 0.9% saline until vital signs are satisfactory and urine flows at >30mL/h. If shocked or elderly consider CVP. Check weight daily. Insert a urinary catheter.

2 Analgesia: eg morphine 10mg/4h with prochlorperazine 12.5mg/8h IM.

3 Hourly pulse, BP, and urine flow; daily FBC, U&E, Ca^{2+}, glucose, amylase, blood gas. Repeat ultrasound may show peripancreatic fluid.

4 If deteriorating, take to ITU. In suspected abscess formation or pancreas necrosis (on contrast-enhanced CT), consider parenteral nutrition ± laparotomy and debridement. Antibiotics may have a rôle in severe disease.[2]

5 ERCP + gallstone removal may be needed if there is progressive jaundice.

Prognosis (See table opposite.) C-reactive protein can be a helpful marker. Some patients suffer *recurrent oedematous pancreatitis* so often that near-total pancreatectomy is contemplated. Evidence is accumulating▣ that 'oxidant' stress is important here, and anti-oxidants apparently do work—eg selenium, methionine and β-carotene: seek expert help.

Complications—*Early:* Shock, ARDS (p350), renal failure, DIC, Ca^{2+}↓, (10mL of 10% calcium gluconate IV slowly is, rarely, necessary; albumin replacement has also been tried), glucose↑ (transient; 5% need insulin). *Later* (>1 week): *Pancreatic necrosis*, *pseudocyst* (fluid in lesser sac, eg at ≥6 weeks), with fever, a mass, and persistent ↑amylase/LFTs. It may resolve or need drainage, externally, or into the stomach (may be laparoscopically[3]). *Abscesses* need draining. *Bleeding* is caused by elastase eroding a major vessel. Skilled angiographists can stop bleeding, and allow planned surgery under more favourable circumstances. *Thrombosis* may occur in the splenic and gastro-duodenal arteries, or in the colic branches of the superior mesenteric artery, causing bowel necrosis.

1 Commonest cause in Trinidad (E Lajeunesse) 2 J Baillie BMJ 1998 i 44 3 C Corvera 1997 *Lancet* 350 586

Modified Glasgow criteria for predicting severity of acute pancreatitis

WBC >15 × 10^9/litre
Glucose >10mmol/litre
LDH >600iu/litre
AST >200iu/litre

Serum urea >16mmol/L
Serum Ca^{2+} <2mmol/L
Serum albumin <32g/L
P_aO_2 <8kPa

The greater the number of factors, the poorer the prognosis.
Outcome is also influenced by the cause of the inflammation.
These criteria have been validated for pancreatitis caused by gall-stones and alcohol (Ranson's criteria are valid for alcohol-induced pancreatitis only).

Aneurysms of arteries

These are abnormal dilatations of arteries.[■] They may be fusiform or sac-like (eg Berry aneurysms in the circle of Willis). Common sites: aorta, iliac, femoral, and popliteal arteries. Atheroma is the usual cause; also penetrating injuries and infections (eg endocarditis, or syphilis).

Complications from aneurysms: rupture; thrombosis; embolism; pressure on other structures; infection.

Dissecting thoracic aortic aneurysm Blood splits aortic media, with sudden tearing chest pain (radiates to back). The cause may be cystic medial degeneration in the artery. As dissection unfolds, branches of the aorta occlude leading sequentially to hemiplegia (carotid), unequal arm pulses and BP, paraplegia (anterior spinal artery) and anuria (renal arteries). Aortic incompetence and inferior MI may develop if dissection extends proximally. ▶▶Action: crossmatch blood (10u); do ECG and CXR (expanded mediastinum is rare). Organise urgent CT, MRI or trans-oesophageal echocardiography (TOE). Treatment: take to ITU; hypotensives (keep systolic BP at ~100–110mmHg); ask a cardiologist: 'is surgery appropriate?'.

Ruptured abdominal aortic aneurysm Incidence/yr rises with age: 22/100,000 of those aged 60–64; 177/100,000 if 80–84.

Presentation: Intermittent or continuous abdominal pain (radiating to the back, iliac fossae, or groins), collapse, and an *expansile* abdominal mass (ie the mass expands and contracts: swellings that are simply pulsatile merely transmit the pulse, eg nodes overlying the aorta). It may be possible to aspirate blood from the peritoneum. The main differential diagnosis is pancreatitis. If in doubt, assume a ruptured aneurysm.

If the aneurysm ruptures into the GI tract, there is overwhelming haematemesis and a swift death.

Management: ▶▶Summon the most experienced surgeon and anaesthetist available. Warn theatre. Put up several large IVIs. Treat shock with ORh–ve blood (if desperate), but keep systolic BP ≤100mmHg (but Note: *raised* BP is common early on). Take blood for amylase, Hb, crossmatch (10–40u may eventually be needed). Take the patient straight to theatre. Do not waste time doing x-rays: fatal delay may result. Catheterize the bladder. Give prophylactic ampicillin + flucloxacillin—both 500mg IV. Surgery involves clamping the aorta above the leak, and inserting a Dacron® graft (eg trouser graft, with each 'leg' attached to an iliac artery). Mortality—treated: 21–70%; untreated: 100%.

Unruptured abdominal aortic aneurysm Prevalence: 3% of those >50 yrs. They may be symptomless, or cause abdominal or back pain. They may be discovered incidentally on abdominal examination (this misses ~⅓ of even quite big aneurysms). Ultrasound, plain abdominal films (with a lateral), and CT are good tests, which may be repeated to keep small aneurysms (<6cm across) under review: but small aneurysms *do* rupture. The aim is to operate before the 30% which are destined to rupture actually do so. Elective operative mortality is ~5%—this makes informed consent (the Rees' rules, OHCS p430) the key issue in developing ultrasound-based screening of 'healthy' people.

Diverticular disease

A *diverticulum* is an outpouching of the wall of the gut. The term *diverticulosis* means that diverticula are present, whereas *diverticular disease* implies they are symptomatic. *Diverticulitis* refers to inflammation within a diverticulum. Although diverticula may be congenital or acquired and can occur in any part of the gut, by far the most important type are acquired colonic diverticula, to which this page refers.

Pathology Most occur in the sigmoid colon with 95% of complications at this site but right-sided diverticula do occur. Lack of dietary fibre is thought to lead to high intraluminal pressures which force the mucosa to herniate through the muscle layers of the gut. One-third of the population in the Western world has diverticulosis by the age of 60 years.

Diagnosis PR *examination* (may reveal a pelvic abscess, or colorectal cancer, the chief competing diagnosis), *sigmoidoscopy, barium enema, colonoscopy*.

Complications of diverticulosis

1 *Painful diverticular disease:* There may be altered bowel habit; pain— usually colicky, left-sided, and relieved by defecation; nausea and flatulence. A *high-fibre diet* (wholemeal bread, fruit, and vegetables, see p482) is usually prescribed. *Antispasmodics* such as mebeverine 135mg/8h PO may help. *Surgical resection* is occasionally resorted to.

2 *Diverticulitis*—with features above plus signs of inflammation: pyrexia, WCC↑, and ESR↑. The colon is tender and there may be localized or generalized peritonism. Treatment: bed rest, NBM, IV fluids, and antibiotics—cefuroxime 1.5g/8h IV with metronidazole 500mg/8h IV/PR are suitable until the results of cultures are available. Most settle on this regimen but there may be abscess formation or perforation (below).

3 *Perforation:* There is ileus, peritonitis ± shock. *Mortality:* 40%. Manage as for an acute abdomen (p112). At laparotomy a Hartman's procedure may be used: (temporary colostomy + partial colectomy). It is sometimes possible to do colon lavage via the appendix stump, then immediate anastomosis (so avoiding repeat surgery to close the colostomy).

3 *Haemorrhage* is usually sudden and painless. This is a common cause of big rectal bleeds. Bleeding usually stops with bed rest but transfusion may be needed. Embolization or colonic resection may be necessary after angiography or colonoscopy has located the bleeding point.

4 *Fistulae* may form between the colon and the bladder (so causing pneumaturia and intractible UTIs), vagina, or small bowel. Treatment is surgical, including colonic resection.

5 *Abscesses* eg with swinging fever, leucocytosis, and localizing signs eg boggy rectal mass (pelvic abscess—drain rectally). If no localizing signs, remember the aphorism: *pus somewhere, pus nowhere = pus under the diaphragm*. A subphrenic abscess is a horrible way to die, so do an *urgent* ultrasound. Antibiotics ± ultrasound-guided drainage may be needed.

6 *Post-infective strictures* may form in the sigmoid colon.

Barium enema examination

This should be preceded by rectal and sigmoidoscopic examination. It is useful in the diagnosis of polyps, carcinoma, diverticulosis, and inflammatory bowel disease. Do not do it if you suspect perforation of the colon or toxic megacolon (p514). *Preparation:* Avoid high fibre food (fruit, vegetables, cereals) for 2 days. Give clear fluids only for one day; laxatives for 1–2 days; then an enema ± colonic washout before the examination.

Gallstones

Bile contains cholesterol, bile pigments (from broken-down haemoglobin), and phospholipids. If the concentrations of these vary, different kinds of stones may be formed.[1] *Pigment stones:* small, friable, irregular and radiolucent. Risk factors: haemolysis. *Cholesterol stones:* large, often solitary, radiolucent. Risk factors: female sex, age, obesity, clofibrate. *Mixed stones:* faceted (calcium salts, pigment and cholesterol): 10% radiopaque. *Gallstone prevalence:* 9% of those over 60 years old. Risk factors for stones becoming symptomatic are smoking and parity.

Stones may cause acute or chronic cholecystitis, biliary colic, pancreatitis, or obstructive jaundice (p484).

Acute cholecystitis follows impaction of a stone in the cystic duct, which may cause continuous epigastric or RUQ pain, vomiting, fever, local peritonism, or a gall bladder (GB) mass. The main difference from biliary colic is the inflammatory component (local peritonism, fever, WCC↑). If the stone moves to the common bile duct (CBD) jaundice may occur. *Murphy's sign:* Lay 2 fingers over the RUQ. Ask the patient to breathe in. This causes pain and arrest of inspiration as an inflamed GB impinges on your fingers. It is only +ve if the same test in the LUQ doesn't cause pain.

Tests: WCC, ultrasound (thickened GB wall, pericholecystic fluid, and stones), HIDA cholescintigraphy (to reveal a blocked cystic duct).

Treatment: NBM, pain relief, IVI and an antibiotic such as cefuroxime 1.5g/8h IV. In suitable candidates cholecystectomy is performed within 48h. If it is delayed relapses occur in 18%. Mortality 0–1%. Otherwise perform cholecystectomy after 3 months.

Chronic cholecystitis Stones cause chronic inflammation ± colic. Vague abdominal discomfort, distension, nausea, flatulence and intolerance of fats may also be caused by reflux, ulcers, irritable bowel syndrome, relapsing pancreatitis, or tumour (stomach, pancreas, colon, GB).

Ultrasound is used to image stones, and to assess the diameter of the CBD. IV cholangiograms (IV contrast outlines the CBD) are less often used. *Treatment:* Cholecystectomy (eg laparoscopic). If ultrasound shows a dilated CBD with stones, ERCP with sphincterotomy is used to remove stones, usually prior to surgery. No comparative trials favour lithotripsy.

Biliary colic RUQ pain (radiates to back) ± jaundice. *Treatment:* Pain control (morphine, eg 5–10mg IM/4h + prochlorperazine); cholecystectomy. *Differential diagnosis* can be hard as the above may overlap. Urinoscopy, CXR, and ECG help exclude other diseases. *Other presentations:*

● *Obstructive jaundice with common bile duct stones*—ERCP (p498) then cholecystectomy may be needed, or open surgery with CBD exploration (if there is no obstruction/cholangitis, a stone-trapping basket on the end of a choledochoscope introduced through the cystic duct at laparoscopy can be done as part of laparoscopic cholecystectomy).[1]

● *Cholangitis* (bile duct infection) causing RUQ pain, jaundice and rigors. Treat with eg cefuroxime 1.5g/8h IV and metronidazole 500mg/8h PR.

● *Gallstone ileus:* a stone perforates the GB, ulcerating into the duodenum. It may pass on to obstruct the terminal ileum. X-ray: air in CBD, small bowel fluid levels, and a stone.

● *Pancreatitis.* ● *Empyema:* the obstructed gall bladder fills with pus.

● *Silent stones:* many advise elective surgery. An alternative for small cholesterol-rich radiolucent stones in a functioning GB is medical dissolution, eg ursodeoxycholic acid 8–15mg/kg/24h PO for up to 2yrs (causes less diarrhoea than chenodeoxycholic acid), but high recurrence on lithotripsy.

1 CU Corvera 1997 *BMJ* i 586 (success is possible in 95% of patients; morbidity is as with ERCP)

> ### *Complications of gallstones*
>
> **1 In the gall bladder**
>   a. biliary colic
>   b. acute and chronic cholecystitis
>   c. empyema
>   d. mucocele
>   e. carcinoma
>
> **2 In the bile ducts**
>   a. obstructive jaundice
>   b. pancreatitis
>   c. cholangitis
>
> **3 In the gut**
>   a. gallstone ileus

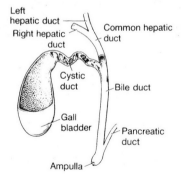

Reproduced from *Cunningham's Manual of Practical Anatomy* 14 ed, OUP 1997, Vol. 2, p138, with kind permission.

Gangrene and necrotizing fasciitis

Gangrene is death of tissue due to damaged vascular supply. Tissues are black and may slough. If tissue death and infection occur together, *wet* gangrene is said to exist. Dry gangrene means death with *no* infection.

Note a line of demarcation between living and dead tissue. Take cultures; look out for group A streptococci (one of the causes of Fournier's- or Meleney's-type gangrene—a rapidly progessive necrotizing fasciitis or myositis[1,2]). ▶*In any atypical cellulitis, get prompt surgical help.* Radical debridement (possibly preserving a skin flap[3]) ± amputation is needed—always covered by antibiotics, including eg 5 days' IV benzylpenicillin 600mg/6h starting 1h pre-op, to prevent gas gangrene (± clindamycin 0.6–1.2g/6h IVI/IM). Enlist the help of a plastic surgeon.

Gas gangrene is a *Clostridium perfringens* myositis. Risk factors: diabetes mellitus, trauma, malignancy. Toxaemia, delirium and haemolytic jaundice occur early. There is surface oedema, crepitus (usually) and bubbly brown pus. *Treatment:* Remove all dead tissue (may involve amputation) and give benzylpenicillin as above (metronidazole if hypersensitive).

1 T Burge 1994 BMJ i 1453   2 I Loudon 1994 *Lancet* 344 1416   3 H Cox 1994 BMJ ii 341

Ischaemia of the gut

►AF with abdominal pain should suggest the idea of bowel ischaemia. This relative rarity is classified into *small bowel* or *colonic* ischaemia. The former may be acute or chronic. Less common causes of ischaemia include vasculitis, trauma, radiotherapy, and strangulation, eg hernias.

Acute small bowel ischaemia This may follow superior mesenteric artery (SMA) embolism or thrombosis, low flow states or venous thrombosis. Embolism is now uncommon and thrombosis is the commonest cause of acute ischaemia. Low flow states usually reflect poor cardiac output but there may be other factors such as DIC. Venous thrombosis is uncommon and tends to affect smaller lengths of bowel.

A classical clinical triad: Acute severe abdominal pain; no abdominal signs; and rapid hypovolaemia (causing shock). Pain tends to be constant and around the right iliac fossa. The degree of illness is often out of proportion to the clinical signs. Pointers to diagnosis are Hb↑ (due to plasma loss), WCC↑, modestly raised plasma amylase, and a persistent metabolic acidosis. Early on the abdominal x-ray shows a 'gasless' abdomen. Arteriography helps but many diagnoses are made at laparotomy.

Treatment: Fluid replacement, antibiotics (eg gentamicin and metronidazole—p181 & p750) and, usually, heparin. At surgery dead bowel must be removed. Revascularization may be attempted but is difficult and often necessitates a second laparotomy.

Prognosis: This is poor with less than 20% survival.

Chronic intestinal ischaemia may present as severe, colicky postprandial abdominal pain ('gut claudication') with PR bleeding. The patient may avoid food and so lose weight. The condition is notoriously difficult to diagnose but, following angiography, surgery may be helpful.

Ischaemia usually follows low flow in the inferior mesenteric artery territory and presents as lower left-sided abdominal pain and bloody diarrhoea. There is often pyrexia, tachycardia, blood per rectum and a leucocytosis. 90% of the time this 'ischaemic colitis' resolves, but it may progress to gangrenous ischaemic colitis. A diagnostic test is a barium enema—may show 'thumb-printing' indentation of the barium due to submucosal swelling. Symptoms may be mild and result in stricture formation.

Treatment: This is usually conservative with fluid replacement and antibiotics. Most recover but strictures are common.

Gangrenous ischaemic colitis This may follow ischaemic colitis and is signalled by more severe pain, peritonitis and hypovolaemic shock. After resuscitation necrotic bowel should be resected and a colostomy formed.

Volvulus (rotation) of the stomach

If the stomach twists, the classical triad of gastro-oesophageal obstruction may occur: vomiting (then non-productive retching), regurgitation of saliva, and failure to pass an NG tube. Dysphagia and noisy gastric peristalsis (relieved by lying down) may occur in chronic volvulus.

Risk factors Pyloric stenosis; congenital bands; paraoesophageal hernia.

Tests Look for gastric dilatation and a double fluid level on erect films.

Treatment If acutely unwell, arrange prompt resuscitation and laparotomy. In organoaxial volvulus, rotation is typically 180° left to right, about a line joining the relatively fixed pylorus and oesophagus. Mesenteroaxial rotation is at right angles to this line (and is from right to left).

✛ Limb embolism and ischaemia

Chronic ischaemia This is almost always due to atherosclerosis.

Symptoms: Intermittent claudication (from the Latin, meaning *to limp*) is pain felt in the leg or buttock on exercise. The calves are the most common site. After walking for a fairly consistent distance (the claudication distance), cramping pain forces the patient to stop. He can resume exercise after rest. *Ulceration, gangrene*, and pain *at rest*, eg burning pain at night relieved by hanging legs over side of bed are the 3 cardinal features of critical ischaemia. Buttock claudication and impotence imply Leriche's syndrome (p702). *Signs:* Absent pulse(s); cold, white leg(s); atrophic skin; punched out ulcers (usually painful); postural colour change.

Tests:[1] FBC (anaemia, infection); U&E (renal disease); ESR/CRP (vasculitis); lipids (hyperlipidaemia); syphilis serology; glucose (DM); ECG (cardiac ischaemia). Do clotting and group-and-save if planning arteriography. *Ankle–brachial pressure index (Doppler):* Normal $\approx$ 1. Claudication $\approx$ 0.9–0.6. Rest pain $\approx$ 0.3–0.6. Impending gangrene $\leq$0.3 or ankle systolic pressure <50mmHg. Do *arteriography* ± digital subtraction arteriography to assess the extent and location of stenoses and the quality of distal vessels ('run off'). If *only* distal obliterative disease is seen, and little proximal atheroma, suspect arteritis, previous embolus, or diabetes mellitus.

Management: Many claudicants improve with *conservative treatment*. Aim to stop smoking, reduce weight, and increase exercise (eg >3 30min walks/week [2]). Treat diabetes, hypertension (avoid β-blockers), and hyperlipidaemia. Vasodilators rarely help. Reduction of atheromatous plaques with chelation therapy (EDTA) has been tried in the USA, but randomized trials are few and give conflicting results.

Percutaneous transluminal angioplasty is particularly good for short stenoses in large proximal arteries and involves inflating a balloon within the narrowed segment. More recently, stents have been used to maintain artery patency after angioplasty. If atheromatous disease is extensive but distal run off is good (ie distal arteries filled by collateral vessels), he may be a candidate for *arterial reconstruction* with a bypass graft. Vein grafts are generally used but prosthetic grafts are an option. *Sympathectomy* (chemical or surgical) is sometimes used for ulceration or rest pain. This redistributes blood, diverting it to the skin rather than increasing the amount entering the limb. *Amputation* may be performed to relieve intractable pain or to prevent sepsis and death from a gangrenous leg. The decision to amputate must be made by the patient, usually against a background of failed alternative strategies. The level of amputation must be high enough to ensure healing of the stump. Rehabilitation should be started early with a view to limb fitting.

Acute ischaemia This may be due to an embolus, thrombosis, or trauma. There is little difference in presentation.

Signs and symptoms: Six Ps—the part is pale, pulseless, painful, paralysed, paraesthetic, and 'perishing with cold'. The onset of fixed mottling of the skin implies irreversible changes. Emboli commonly arise from the heart (infarcts, AF) or an aneurysm (aorta, femoral, or popliteal).

Management: ▶This is an emergency and may require urgent surgery. If diagnosis is in doubt, perform an urgent arteriogram. If the occlusion is embolic the options are surgical embolectomy (Fogarty catheter) or local thrombolysis eg t-PA (p282, 593). Anticoagulate with heparin after either procedure. Later, look for the emboli's source: echocardiogram; USS aorta, popliteal and femoral arteries. Ischaemia following trauma and acute thrombosis may require urgent reconstructive surgery.

1 AM van Rij 1994 *Circulation* 90 1194   [2] AW Gardner 1996 E-BM 1 85

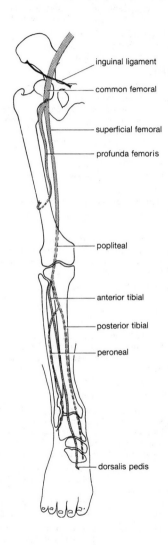

::: Obstruction of the bowel

Features of obstruction Anorexia, nausea, vomiting with relief. Colicky abdominal pain with distension. Constipation need not be absolute (ie no faeces or flatus passed) if obstruction is high. Active, 'tinkling' bowel sounds. For the features of gastric volvulus, see p126.

On AXR (plain abdominal x-ray) look for abnormal gas patterns (gas in the fundus of stomach and throughout the large bowel is normal). On erect AXR look for horizontal fluid levels.

The key decisions

1 *Is the obstruction of the small or large bowel?* In small bowel obstruction vomiting occurs earlier, distension is less, pain is higher in the abdomen. ►*The supine AXR plays a key rôle in diagnosis.* In small bowel obstruction AXR shows central gas shadows and no gas in the large bowel. Small bowel is identified by valvulae conniventes which completely cross the lumen (large bowel haustra do *not* cross all the lumen's width).

In large bowel obstruction pain is more constant and often over a distended caecum; AXR shows gas proximal to the block (eg in caecum) but not in the rectum.

2 *Is there ileus* (functional obstruction due to reduced bowel motility) or *mechanical obstruction?* In ileus there is no pain; bowel sounds are absent.

3 *Is the bowel strangulated?* Signs: the patient is more ill than you would expect. There is a sharper and more constant pain than the central colicky pain of the obstruction and it tends to be localized. Peritonism is the cardinal sign. There may be fever and wcc↑.

Causes *Small bowel:* Adhesions, herniae external/internal, intussusception, Crohn's, gallstone ileus, tumour, swallowed foreign body (eg smuggled cocaine). *Large bowel:* Tumour, sigmoid or caecal volvulus, faeces, diverticulitis.

Management The site, speed of onset, and completeness of obstruction determine therapy. Strangulation and large bowel obstruction require surgery soon. Paralytic ileus and incomplete small bowel obstruction can be managed conservatively, at least initially.

Conservative: Pass NGT and give IV fluids to rehydrate and correct electrolyte imbalance (p100)—ie 'drip and suck'.

Surgery: Strangulation requires urgent surgery (within 1h), as does large bowel obstruction with gross dilatation (>8cm) and tenderness over the caecum—as perforation is close. Usually large volumes of IV fluid must be given. For less urgent large bowel obstruction there is time for an enema to try to clear the obstruction and to correct fluid imbalance.

Sigmoid volvulus occurs when the bowel twists on the mesentery and can produce severe, rapid strangulated obstruction. There is a characteristic AXR with an 'inverted U' loop of bowel. It tends to occur in the elderly, constipated patient and is often managed by sigmoidoscopy and insertion of a flatus tube. For stomach volvulus, see p126.

Pseudo-obstruction resembles mechanical obstruction of the large bowel but no cause for obstruction is found. The condition should be treated conservatively. There is a case for investigating the cause by colonoscopy or water-soluble contrast enema in most instances of suspected mechanical obstruction.

Some paediatric surgical emergencies

Congenital hypertrophic pyloric stenosis ►See *OHCS* p198. This usually presents not at birth but in the first 3–8 weeks as projectile vomiting. ♂:♀≈4:1. The baby is malnourished and always hungry and the diagnosis is made by palpating the pyloric mass in the RUQ during a feed. The baby can be severely depleted of water and electrolytes and this imbalance needs correction before surgery. Pass a nasogastric tube. Treatment is by Ramstedt's pyloromyotomy which involves incision of the muscle down to the mucosa.

Intussusception The small bowel telescopes, as if swallowing itself. The patient may be any age (usually 5–12 months) and presents with intermittent crying associated with vomiting and drawing the legs up, and passing blood PR—classically 'red-currant jelly'. This is less common in older patients who are more likely to have a long history (>3 weeks) and contributing pathology (lymphoma, Henoch–Schönlein purpura, Peutz–Jeghers' syndrome; cystic fibrosis, ascariasis, or nephrosis).

A sausage-shaped abdominal mass may be felt and the patient may quickly become shocked and moribund. ~60% of early intussusceptions (<24h) may be reducible by hydrostatic pressure during a barium enema. If this fails surgery is needed. Absolute CI to barium enema: peritonitis; perforation; severe hypovolaemia.

Torsion of the testis

The aim is to recognize this condition before the cardinal signs and symptoms are fully manifest, as prompt surgery saves testes.
►If in any doubt, surgery is required.

Cardinal symptoms Sudden onset of pain in one testis—which makes walking most uncomfortable. (Pain in the abdomen, nausea, and vomiting are common.)

Cardinal signs Inflammation of one testis—it is tender, hot, and swollen. (The testis tends to lie high and transversely.) Doppler USS may demonstrate blood flow (or lack of) to testis.

Torsion may occur at any age but is most common at 11–30yrs.

Treatment: ►Ask the patient's consent for possible orchidectomy and for *bilateral* fixation (orchidopexy). At surgery expose and untwist the testis. If its colour looks good, return it to the scrotum and fix *both* testes to the scrotum.

Differential diagnosis: The main one is epididymitis but here the patient tends to be older, there may be symptoms of urinary infection, infected urine, and more gradual onset of pain. Also consider tumour, trauma and an acute hydrocoele. Note: *torsion of the hydatid of Morgagni*—remnants of the Müllerian ducts—occurs a little earlier, and causes less pain (the patient can often walk with no pain, unlike in testicular torsion)—and its tiny blue nodule may be discernible under the scrotum. It is thought to be due to the surge in gonadotrophins which signal the onset of puberty.[1] *Idiopathic scrotal oedema* is a benign condition, and is differentiated from torsions by the absence of pain and tenderness.[1]

1 M Davenport 1997 *BMJ* i 435

✜ Urinary retention and catheters

Retention is the inability to empty the bladder completely and follows failure of bladder pressure to overcome urethral resistance. Thus it may be seen in bladder weakness or urethral obstruction. It is subdivided into acute and chronic. (See also *Voiding difficulties*, OHCS p71.)

Acute retention There is pain and complete failure of micturition. The bladder usually contains around 600mL of urine. The cause in men is nearly always prostatic obstruction. For questions to detect obstruction, see p30. Retention may be precipitated by anticholinergic drugs, 'holding on', constipation, alcohol ingestion, or infection (p374).
Examine: Abdomen, PR, perineal sensation (cauda equina compression).
Investigations: MSU, U&E, FBC, prostate specific antigen, and IVU.
Treatment: Catheterization ± an elective prostate procedure (below).

Chronic retention is more insidious. Bladder capacity may be >1.5 litres. Presentations: overflow incontinence, acute on chronic retention, a lower abdominal mass, UTI, or renal failure. Prostatic enlargement is the common cause. Others: pelvic malignancy, CNS disease. ►Only catheterize the patient if there is pain, urinary infection, or renal impairment (eg urea >12mmol/L). Institute definitive treatment promptly.

Catheters *Size* (in French gauge): 12 is small; 16 is large. Usually a 12 or 14 is right. Use the smallest you can. Latex is soft; *simplastic* rather firmer. A *silastic* (silicone) catheter is suitable for long-term use, but costs more. Foley is the typical shape. Coudé catheters have an angled tip to ease around the prostate but are potentially more dangerous. Teeman catheters have tapered ends for a similar reason.
Problems with catheters: 1 Infection (do not use antibiotics unless systemically unwell). Consider bladder irrigation—eg chlorhexidine 1/10,000.
2 *Bladder spasm* may be painful. Try reducing the water in the balloon or using anticholinergic drugs, eg propantheline 15mg/8h PO.

Benign prostatic hypertrophy (BPH) is common (24% if aged 40–64; if older, 40%). ↓Urine flow (eg <15mL/sec) is associated with frequency, urgency (►p52) and voiding difficulty. Exclude cancer and renal failure (rectal exam ± biopsy, prostate specific antigen, U&E); then consider:
1 *Transurethral resection of the prostate* (TURP) is a common operation; ≤14% become impotent. Crossmatch 2u. Consider peri-operative antibiotics, eg cefuroxime 1.5g/8h IV, 3 doses. Beware excessive bleeding post-op and clot retention. ~20% of TURPs need redoing within 10yrs.
2 *Transurethral incision of the prostate* (TUIP) involves less destruction than TURP, and less risk to sexual function. It achieves its effect by relieving pressure on the urethra. It is perhaps the best surgical option for those with glands <30g—ie ~50% of those operated on in some areas.
3 *Retropubic prostatectomy* needs less skill but is an open operation.
4 *Transurethral laser-induced prostatectomy* (TULIP).
5 *Drugs* may be useful in mild disease, and while awaiting TURP, eg:
- α-blockers: terazosin or *indoramin* 20mg/12h PO, ↑dose by 20mg/wk to 50mg/12h. These ↓smooth muscle tone (prostate *and* bladder). SE: depression; dizziness; BP↓; dry mouth; ejaculatory failure; extrapyramidal signs; nasal congestion; weight↑. They are the treatment of choice.[1]
- 5α-reductase inhibitor: *finasteride* (5mg/day PO ↓testosterone's conversion to dihydrotestosterone). It's excreted in semen, so warn to use condoms; ♀: avoid handling crushed pills. SE: impotence; libido↓. Effects on prostate size are limited and slow,[2] so, if α-blockers fail, many try surgery next.[3]
6 'Wait and see' is also an option but inaction in those with moderate symptoms can lead to a bad quality of life (mortality, repeated or intractable retention, residual volumes >350mL, bladder calculi, incontinence and renal failure are used as end-points). ◄4►

1 BMJ 1997 i 1213 2 NEJM 1998 338 557 3 NEJM 1996 335 533+E&M 2 16 ◄4►J Wasson 1995 NEJM 332 75+E&M 1995 1 10

Advice for patients concerning transurethral prostatectomy
- Avoid driving for 2 weeks after the operation.
- Avoid sex for 2 weeks after surgery. Then get back to normal. The amount ejaculated may be reduced (as it flows backwards into the bladder—harmless, but may cloud the urine). It means you may be infertile. Impotence may be a problem after TURP, but do not expect this: in some men erections improve. Rarely, orgasmic sensations are reduced.

- Expect to pass blood in the urine for the first 2 weeks. A small amount of blood colours the urine bright red. Do not be alarmed.
- At first you may need to urinate *more* frequently than before. Do not be despondent. In 6 weeks things should be much better—but the operation cannot be guaranteed to work (8% fail, and lasting incontinence is a problem in 6%; 12% may need repeat TURPs within 8yrs, compared with 1.8% of men undergoing open prostatectomy).
- If feverish, or if urination hurts, take a sample of urine to your doctor.

Catheterizing bladders

1. *Per urethram* This route is used to relieve urinary retention, to monitor urine output in critically ill patients, or to collect urine for diagnosis uncontaminated by urethral flora. It is *contraindicated* in urethral injury (eg pelvic fracture) and acute prostatitis. Catheterization introduces bacteria into the bladder, so aseptic technique is essential. Women are often catheterized by nurses but you should be able to catheterize patients of either sex.
- Lie the patient supine in a well-lit area: women with knees flexed wide and heels together. In women, use a gloved hand to prep urethral meatus in a pubis-to-anus direction, holding the labia apart with the other hand. With uncircumcised men, retract the foreskin to 'prep' the glans; use a gloved hand to hold the penis still and off the scrotum. The hand used to hold the penis or labia should not touch the catheter (use forceps if needed).
- Put sterile lignocaine (lidocaine) 2% gel on the catheter tip and ≤10mL into the urethra (≤5mL if ♀). In men, stretch the penis perpendicular to the body to eliminate any urethral folds that may lead to false passage.
- Use steady *gentle* pressure to advance the catheter. Significant obstructions encountered should prompt withdrawal and re-insertion. With prostatic hypertrophy, a Coudé tip catheter may get past the prostate.
- Insert to the hilt; wait until urine emerges before inflating the balloon. Remember to check the balloon's capacity before inflation. Pull the catheter back so that the balloon comes to rest at the bladder neck.
- Remember to reposition the foreskin in uncircumcised men to prevent massive oedema of the glans after the catheter is inserted.

Self-catheterizations This is a good, safe way of managing chronic retention from a neuropathic bladder (eg in multiple sclerosis, diabetic neuropathy, spinal tumour). Never consider a patient in difficulties from a big residual volume to be too old, young, or disabled to learn. 5-yr-old children can learn the technique, and can have their lives transformed—so motivation may be excellent. There may be *fewer* UTIs as there is no residual urine—and less reflux obstructive uropathy. Assessing suitability entails testing sacral dermatomes: a 'numb bum' implies ↓ sensation of a full bladder; higher sensory loss may mean catheterization will be painless. Get help from your continence adviser who will be in a position to teach the patient or carer that catheterizations must be gentle, particularly if sensation is lacking, and must number >4/day ('always keep your catheter with you; don't wait for an urge before catheterizing').

2. Suprapubic catheterization is sometimes necessary and may be preferred. Ensure the bladder is distended; then clean the skin. Infiltrate with local anaesthetic down to the bladder, nick the skin and then insert the catheter down vertically above the symphysis pubis. After urine is draining advance the catheter over the trocar and tape it down securely.

Bladder tumours

What appear as benign papillomata rarely behave in a purely benign way. They are almost certainly indolent transitional cell (urothelial) malignancies. Adenocarcinomas and squamous cell carcinomas are rare in the West (the latter may follow infestation with *Schistosoma haematobium*).

Incidence 1:5000 in the UK.

Histology is important for prognosis: grade 1—differentiated; grade 2—intermediate; grade 3—poorly differentiated.

Presentation Painless (or painful) haematuria; recurrent UTIs.

Associations Smoking; aromatic amines (rubber industry).

Investigations Urine: culture, microscopy and cytology (bladder papillomas are one cause of 'sterile pyuria'); FBC.
An IVU may show filling defects and ureteric involvement.
EUA is required to assess tumour spread.
Cystoscopy with biopsy is diagnostic.
CT or lymphangiography may show involved pelvic nodes.

TNM staging (EUA = examination under anaesthesia)

T1 Tumour in mucosa or submucosa	Not felt at EUA
T2 Superficial muscle involved	Rubbery thickening at EUA
T3 Deep muscle involved	EUA: mobile mass
T4 Invasion beyond bladder	EUA: fixed mass

Treatment of transitional cell carcinoma

T1: (80% of all patients.) Diathermy via cystoscope. Consider intravesical chemotherapeutic agent for multiple small tumours.

T2: Diathermy via cystoscope. Consider radiotherapy for poorly differentiated tumours.

T3: This is controversial; possibilities are:
- Radical radiotherapy
- Cystectomy
- Combination of radiotherapy and cystectomy.

  Complications of cystectomy include disruption of sexual and urinary function.

T4: Usually palliative radiotherapy. Chronic catheterization and urinary diversions may help to relieve pain.

Chemotherapy is playing an increasingly important rôle and may allow more conservative surgery. One toxic but effective regimen uses methotrexate, vinblastine, doxorubicin and cisplatin.

Follow up History, examination, and cystoscopy every 6 months.

Tumour spread Local—to pelvic structures; lymphatic—to iliac and para-aortic nodes; haematogenous—to liver and lungs.

Survival This depends on age at surgery. For example, the 3-yr survival after cystectomy for T2 and T3 tumours is 60% if 65–75yrs old, falling to 40% if 75–82 years old (in whom the operative mortality is 4%). With unilateral pelvic node involvement only 6% of patients survive 5 years. The 3-year survival with bilateral or para-aortic node involvement is nil.

Massive bladder haemorrhage: This may complicate treatment. Treat by alum solution bladder irrigation (safer than formalin).

Breast lumps and breast carcinoma

All solid lumps need histological or cytological assessment.

History Previous lumps, family history, pain, nipple discharge, change in size related to menstrual cycle, parous state, last period, drugs (eg HRT).

Examination Inspect (arms up and down). Note position, size, consistency, mobility, fixity, and local lymphadenopathy. Any nipple discharge or recent nipple inversion? Is the skin involved (*peau d'orange*)?

Management If cystic, aspirate to dryness. Send the fluid for cytology. If solid and discrete, consider one of: fine-needle aspiration cytology, Tru-cut®, or open biopsy. Consider ultrasound or mammography depending on age and clinical suspicion.

Causes of lumps Fibroadenoma, cyst, cancer, fibroadenosis (diffuse lumpiness, often in upper outer quadrant), periductal mastitis (often secondary to duct ectasia), fat necrosis, galactocoele, abscess, 'non-breast' lumps—eg lipomas, sebaceous cysts.

Causes of discharge Duct ectasia (green/brown/red, often multiple ducts and bilateral), intraduct papilloma/adenoma/carcinoma (red discharge, often single duct), lactation. Management involves diagnosing the underlying cause, for example by mammography, ductogram, microdochectomy or total duct excision, and then treating appropriately.

Breast cancer *Risk factors:* Nulliparity, first pregnancy >30yrs old, early menarche, late menopause, HRT (relative risk↑ × 1.023/yr of use[1]), BRCA genes (p684), not breast feeding, past breast cancer, the Pill (possibly).

Stage by TNM classification: T1 <2cm. T2 2–5cm. T3 >5cm. T4 Fixity to chest wall or *peau d'orange*. N1 Mobile ipsilateral nodes. N2 Fixed nodes. M1 Distant metastases. *Treating early cancer:* Surgery: wide excision + DXT, simple mastectomy, and radical mastectomy give equal survival. Local recurrence may be commoner in smaller procedures. If <50yrs old ovarian ablation improves survival (52% 15yr survival vs 46%).[2] *Discuss all the options with her.* Avoid any delay. Find out if she would like you to talk with her partner. ▶The breast is bound up with what lies deepest—health, beauty, gender, and the nourishing of life. When it is also seen to be harbouring death, complex emotions will be present. Do not presume to confront or reframe these emotions, but by your demeanour your patients will know you, and know if they can trust you to share some of these issues; these issues are discussed on p683).

Consider size of the lump and of the breast, and the lump's exact site. Tamoxifen (oestrogen antagonist, eg 20mg/day PO) improves survival (not just if elderly) whether or not nodes are +ve (saves 12% of patients:[3] it may rarely cause endometrial carcinoma so warn to report vaginal bleeding). Local radiotherapy improves local recurrence rates, but not survival. If >50yrs old, adding chemotherapy to tamoxifen appears not to extend quality-adjusted time without symptoms or toxicity (Q-TWIST).[4]

Distant disease: Assess ESR, LFTs (Alk phos↑), Ca²⁺, CXR, skeletal survey, bone scan, liver ultrasound, or CT. DXT to local, painful bony lesions. For widespread disease tamoxifen 20mg/24h PO is the first choice. If there is initially success but subsequently relapse, consider chemotherapy.

Preventing breast cancer deaths: ●Education ●Self-examination ●Health clinics ●Mammography (using almost negligible radiation)—cancer pick-up rate: 5 per 1000 'healthy' women over 50yrs. Yearly 2-view mammograms could reduce mortality by 40%—but the price is the serious but needless alarm caused: there are ~10 false +ves for each true +ve[5]—but screening every 3 years is probably too lax.[6] Around the menopause breasts are denser and mammograms hard to interpret, and screening appears not to save lives.[3] Cost:☞ ~£5300 per breast cancer detected[7] ▯

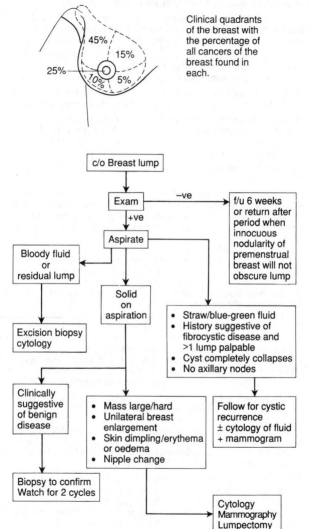

Clinical quadrants of the breast with the percentage of all cancers of the breast found in each.

45% · 15% · 25% · 10% · 5%

c/o Breast lump

Exam

−ve → f/u 6 weeks or return after period when innocuous nodularity of premenstrual breast will not obscure lump

+ve

Aspirate

Bloody fluid or residual lump

↓

Excision biopsy cytology

Solid on aspiration

- Straw/blue-green fluid
- History suggestive of fibrocystic disease and >1 lump palpable
- Cyst completely collapses
- No axillary nodes

Clinically suggestive of benign disease

- Mass large/hard
- Unilateral breast enlargement
- Skin dimpling/erythema or oedema
- Nipple change

Follow for cystic recurrence ± cytology of fluid + mammogram

Biopsy to confirm
Watch for 2 cycles

Cytology
Mammography
Lumpectomy

1 If HRT for ≥5yrs. Risk returns to normal within 5yrs of stopping: *N*=52,705; V Beral 1997 *Lancet* **350** 1047 ◁2▷ Early Breast Cancer Group (EBCG) 1996 *Lancet* **348** 1186 & 1997 E-BM **2** 75 **3** EBCG 1992 *Lancet* **i** 1 & 71 ◁4▷ R Gelber 1996 E-BM **1** 206 **5** C Woodman 1995 BMJ **i** 224 **6** JAMA 1994 **271** 152 **7** N Wald 1995 BMJ **ii** 1189 Breast Cancer Network: http://www.cancer.org/bcn.html

Colorectal adenocarcinoma

The second most common cause of cancer deaths in the UK (20,000 deaths/year). 56% of presentations are in those >70yrs old.

Predisposing factors Neoplastic polyps, ulcerative colitis (and, to a lesser extent, Crohn's disease), family history (p684), familial polyposis, previous cancer, and possibly low-fibre diet. NSAIDs may be protective.

Presentation depends on site: *Left-sided:* Bleeding PR; altered bowel habit; tenesmus; mass PR (60%). *Right:* Weight↓; Hb↓; abdominal pain. *Either:* Abdominal mass; obstruction; perforation; haemorrhage; fistula.

Tests FBC (microcytic anaemia); faecal occult blood; proctoscopy, sigmoidoscopy, barium enema or colonoscopy ± LFTs, CT, liver ultrasound.

Staging is by Dukes' classification:	*Treated survival:*
A Confined to bowel wall	90% 5-year survival
B Extension through bowel wall	65% 5-year survival
C Involvement of regional lymph nodes	30% 5-year survival

Spread This is local, lymphatic, haematogenous (to liver 75%, lung and bone) or transcoelomic.

Treatment Surgery may be performed either to attempt cure (removing the draining lymphatic field) or to relieve symptoms. *Right hemicolectomy* is for tumours in the caecum, ascending or proximal transverse colon. *Left hemicolectomy* is for tumours in the distal transverse colon or descending colon.
Sigmoid colectomy is for tumours of sigmoid colon.
Anterior resection is for low sigmoid or high rectal tumours. Anastomosis is achieved at the first operation. Stapling devices are helpful.
Abdomino-perineal (A-P) resection is for tumours low in the rectum (<~8cm from anal canal): permanent colostomy and removal of rectum and anus (see p97 for total anorectal reconstruction). *Radiotherapy* may be of some value in Ca rectum and decreases local recurrence.
Chemotherapy: Post-op hepatic vein/intraportal IVI of 5-FU improves 5-yr disease-free survival (57% vs 48%) [1]—but metastases >0.5mm are dependent on hepatic artery flow, and may survive this onslaught. There is good but not incontrovertible evidence that 5-FU ± levamisole or folinic acid for 1yr post-op reduces Dukes C cancer deaths by ~12%.[2,3] MRI is more specific than CT in showing liver metastases (99% vs 94%).

Prognosis 60% are amenable to radical surgery, and 75% of these will be alive at 7yrs (or will have died from non-tumour-related causes).[4]
Screening every 2yrs with home tests for faecal occult blood[5] reduces mortality by 18–33%, but false +ve rates are high (10% of those screened) and there are problems with acceptability.[5] The patient has to be on a special diet while 2 out of 3 consecutive stool samples are tested. Best results may occur if the sample is rehydrated.[6]

Polyps are lumps that appear above the mucosa. There are 3 types:
1 *Inflammatory:* Ulcerative colitis, Crohn's, lymphoid hyperplasia.
2 *Hamartomatous:* Juvenile polyps, Peutz–Jeghers' syndrome.
3 *Neoplastic:* Tubular and villous adenomata. These have malignant potential, especially if villous, >2cm, or dysplastic.
Symptoms of polyps: Passage of blood/mucus PR. They should be biopsied and removed if they show malignant change. Most can be reached by the flexible colonoscopy and diathermy can avoid the morbidity of partial colectomy. Check resection margins are clear of tumour.

◁1▷ SAKK 1995 *Lancet* 345 349   2 D Cunningham 1995 BMJ i 247   3 G Mead 1995 BMJ i 246
4 N Gordon 1993 BMJ ii 707   5 J Mandel 1993 NEJM 329 1365   6 R Fletcher 1997 E-BM 2 76

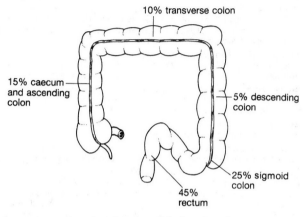

Location of cancers of the large bowel.

Note: these are averages: black females tend to have more proximal neo-plasms, while white men tend to have more distal neoplasms (see p728).

Carcinoma of the stomach

The incidence of gastric carcinoma has shown a sharp decline in Western countries in the last few years but it remains a tumour notable for its gloomy prognosis and nonspecific presentation.

Incidence 33/100,000 in the UK but there are unexplained wide geographical variations, being especially common in Japan. Associations:
●Blood group A ●Atrophic gastritis; pernicious anaemia ●Social class↓
●H pylori[1] (p490) ●Adenomatous polyps ●Smoking

Pathology The adenocarcinoma may be polypoid, ulcerating, or leather bottle type (linitis plastica). Some are confined to mucosa and submucosa—so-called early gastric carcinoma. 50% involve the pylorus, 25% the lesser curve and 10% the cardia.

Symptoms (Often they are nonspecific.) Dyspepsia (p44) lasting longer than a month in patients aged ≥40yrs demands gastrointestinal investigation. Others: weight loss, vomiting, dysphagia, anaemia.

Signs suggesting incurable disease—eg epigastric mass, hepatomegaly, jaundice, ascites (p152), an enlarged left supraclavicular (Virchow's) node (Troissier's sign), acanthosis nigricans (p678).

Spread is local, lymphatic, blood-borne and transcoelomic eg to ovaries (Krukenberg tumour).

Tests Gastroscopy + multiple ulcer edge biopsies. ►Aim to biopsy all gastric ulcers as even malignant ulcers may appear to heal on drug treatment.

Treatment Metastasis is obvious in ≤60% of patients and is a contraindication to curative surgery—which involves wide excision of tumour (5cm margins) and lymph nodes within 3cm of the tumour (D1 resection). For tumours in the distal ²⁄₃, a partial gastrectomy may suffice, but, if more proximal, total gastrectomy may be needed. Removing distant nodes (D2 resection) appears to improve survival in Japanese but not Europeans.[2]

Palliation is often needed for obstruction, pain, or haemorrhage and involves judicious use of drugs, surgery and radiotherapy.

5-year survival < 10% overall, but much better for 'early' gastric carcinoma which is confined to the mucosa and submucosa.

Carcinoma of the oesophagus

Incidence Australia <5 per 1 100,000/yr; UK <9; Brittany >50; China (Linxian) and Iran >100. **Risk factors** Diet (?hot drinks, spicy food), alcohol excess (risk declines quite quickly on abstaining), tobacco, Barrett's oesophagus, achalasia, tylosis, Plummer–Vinson syndrome (p492).

Site 20% occur in the upper part, 50% in the middle, and 30% in the lower part. Most are squamous cell carcinomas but adenocarcinoma can arise from areas of columnar lining (Barrett's oesophagus).

Spread is direct, by extensive submucosal infiltration, and local spread, to lymph nodes and, late, via the bloodstream.

Presentation Poorly localized dysphagia, weight↓, retrosternal chest pain, lymphadenopathy (rare). Signs from upper ¹⁄₃ of oesophagus: hoarseness; cough (may be paroxysmal if aspiration pneumonia).

Differential diagnosis Any cause of dysphagia (p492).

Tests Barium swallow, CXR, oesophagoscopy with biopsy/brushings, CT.

Treatment We do not know how to treat this disease. Radiotherapy and surgery compete for the most dismal statistics (6% vs 4% 5-year survival). Radiotherapy is cheaper and safer. The only prospective comparative trial failed from low recruitment. Palliation: p498.

1 B Walt 1998 Lancet 351 887 (prevention by mass eradication of H pylori is very problematic, and could lead to antibiotic resistance ± lower oesophageal disease) ◀2▶ A Cuschieri 1996 E-BM 1 207 & Lancet 347 995

Lumps

►Examine the regional lymph nodes as well as the lump. If the lump is a node, examine its area of drainage.

History How long has it been there? Does it hurt? Any other lumps? Is it getting bigger? Ever been abroad? Otherwise well?

Physical exam Remember the six Ss: site, size, shape, smoothness, surface, and surroundings. Other questions: does it transilluminate (see below)? Is it fixed to skin or underlying structures? Is it fluctuant? Lumps in certain sites call to mind particular pathologies (see lumps in groin and scrotum p146). Remember to feel if a lump is pulsatile; this may seem to be a minor detail until faced with a surprise on a minor operations list.

Transilluminable lumps Find a dark room and a bright, thin 'pencil' torch, and place it on the lump, from behind, so the light is shining through the lump towards your eye. If the lump glows red it is said to transilluminate. Fluid-filled lumps such as hydrocoeles are good examples of transilluminating swellings.

Lipomas These benign fatty lumps, occurring wherever fat can expand (*not* scalp or palms), have smooth, imprecise margins and a hint of fluctuance. They only cause symptoms due to pressure. Malignant change is very rare (suspect if rapid growth, hardening or vascularization occurs).

Sebaceous cysts These are intradermal, so you cannot draw the skin over them. Look for the characteristic punctum marking blocked sebaceous outflow. Infection is quite common, and foul pus exits through the punctum. *Treatment:* Shelling them out whole can be tricky: learn from an expert. After achieving haemostasis, close with subcuticular catgut.

Causes of lymph node enlargement Infections: glandular fever; brucellosis; TB; HIV; toxoplasmosis; actinomycosis; syphilis. Others: malignancy (carcinoma, lymphoma); sarcoidosis.

Cutaneous abscesses Staphylococci are the most common organisms. Haemolytic streptococci are only common in hand infections. Proteus is a common cause of non-staphylococcal axillary abscesses. Below the waist faecal organisms are common (aerobes and anaerobes). *Treatment:* Incision and drainage alone usually cures. *Boils (furuncles)* are abscesses which involve a hair follicle and its associated glands. *A carbuncle* is an area of subcutaneous necrosis which discharges itself onto the surface through multiple sinuses.

Rheumatoid nodules These are collagenous granulomas which appear on the extensor aspects of joints—especially the elbows. They occur in established cases of rheumatoid arthritis.

Ganglia These are degenerative cysts from an adjacent joint or synovial sheath commonly seen on the dorsum of the wrist or hand and dorsum of the foot. They may transilluminate. 50% will disappear spontaneously. For the rest, the treatment of choice is excision rather than the traditional blow from your bible (the *Oxford Textbook of Surgery*!).

Fibromas These may occur anywhere in the body, but most commonly they are under the skin. These whitish, benign tumours contain collagen, fibroblasts, and fibrocytes.

Dermoid cysts contain dermal structures; often found in the midline.

Malignant tumours of connective tissue These include the fibrosarcoma, liposarcoma, leiomyosarcoma (smooth muscle), and rhabdomyosarcoma (striated muscle). Sarcomas are staged using a modification of the TNM system which includes tumour grade. Incisional biopsies of large tumours precede excision. Any lesion suspected of being a sarcoma should not be simply enucleated in what might erroneously be considered a 'conservative' operation.

Lumps in the groin and scrotum

►Any lump within the tunica vaginalis is cancer until proved otherwise.[1]
►Acute, tender enlargement of the testis is torsion until proved otherwise.

Diagnosing groin lumps Think of nearby structures: femoral/ inguinal herniae, saphena varix (p162—both have cough impulse), nodes, femoral aneurysm, ectopic testis, skin lumps, psoas abscess (may present with back pain, limp, and swinging pyrexia. Diagnose with ultrasound.

Diagnosis of lumps in the scrotum 1 *Can you get above it?* If not, it is an inguinoscrotal hernia (inguinal hernia extending into scrotum, p160).
2 *Is it separate from the testis?*
3 *Is it cystic or solid?* (Does it transilluminate?—see p144.)

Separate and cystic—epididymal cyst.
Separate and solid—epididymitis (may also be orchitis).
Testicular and cystic—hydrocoele.
Testicular and solid—tumour, orchitis, granuloma, gumma.

Ultrasound may help in sorting out testis tumours from other lumps. Do not assume that an injured testis was normal before the injury: this is not a rare mode of tumour presentation; ultrasound may help here.

Epididymal cysts These usually develop in adult life and contain either clear or milky (spermatocoele) fluid. They lie above and behind the testis. Remove if they are symptomatic.

Hydrocoeles (Fluid within the tunica vaginalis) may be *primary* (idiopathic—associated with a patent processus vaginalis, which typically resolves during the first year of life) or *secondary*. Primary hydrocoeles are more common, larger, and usually develop in younger men. If secondary, suspect associated testis tumour, trauma, or infection. These are treated by aspiration (may need repeating) or surgery.

Epididymo-orchitis This may be due to *E coli*, mumps, gonococcal infection, or TB. The area is usually tender. Take a urine sample and look for urethral discharge. Note: a 'first catch' will be more likely to show abnormalities than a midstream sample.

Testis tumours are now the commonest malignancies of young men.

Varieties: Seminoma (30–40yrs); teratoma (20–30yrs); tumours of Sertoli or Leydig cells. ~10% of malignancies occur in undescended testes, even after orchidopexy. A contralateral tumour is found in 1 in 20 instances.[1]

Typical presentation: Painless testis lump, eg noticed after trauma or infection.
Spread: Initially lymphatic to the para-aortic nodes and then to the mediastinum. Haematogenous spread is usually to the lungs.

Staging is essential: 1 No evidence of metastasis. 2 Infradiaphragmatic node involvement. 3 Supradiaphragmatic node↑. 4 Lung involvement.

Tests: Directed towards staging: CXR, IVU, CT or lymphangiogram, excision biopsy. α-fetoprotein (eg >3IU/mL)* and β-human chorionic gonadotrophin (β-HCG) are useful tumour markers and of value in diagnosis and monitoring of treatment. Do levels before and during treatment.

Treatment: Orchidectomy via an inguinal incision, with the spermatic cord occluded before mobilization (less risk of intra-operative spread). Options are constantly being refined (surgery, radiotherapy, chemotherapy). Seminomas are exquisitely radiosensitive. Stage 1 seminomas may be treated by orchidectomy + radiotherapy to give cure rates of ~95%. Do close follow-up to detect relapse. Chemotherapy aims to achieve cure, eg *cisplatin*, *vinblastine* (or *etoposide* in teratomas), and *bleomycin*.[2]

5-year survival: This is good (>~70%—more for early disease).

Prevention of late presentation: Self-examination.

*AFP is **not** raised in pure seminoma (**may also be raised in:** hepatitis; cirrhosis; hepatocellular carcinoma; open neural tube defects). **1** C Dawson 1996 BMJ i 1146 **2** *Drug Ther Bul* 1994 **32** 62

Diagnosis of scrotal masses

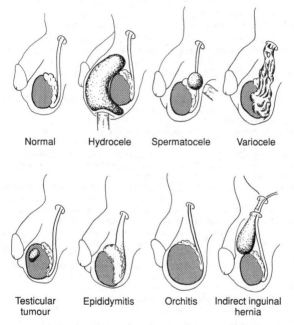

Normal Hydrocele Spermatocele Variocele

Testicular tumour Epididymitis Orchitis Indirect inguinal hernia

After RD Judge, GD Zeidema, FT Fitzgerald 1989 *Clinical Diagmosis* 5 ed, Little Brown, Boston.

Lumps in the neck

▶Don't biopsy lumps until tumours within the head and neck have been excluded by an ENT surgeon. Culture all biopsied lymph nodes for TB.

Diagnosis First of all ask for how long the lump has been present. If <3 weeks, self-limiting infection is the likely cause and extensive investigation is unwise. Next ask yourself where the lump is. Is it intradermal?—(sebaceous cyst with a central punctum, or a lipoma). If the lump is not intradermal, and is not of recent onset, you are about to start a diagnostic hunt over complicated terrain:

Midline lumps: If patient <20yrs old, the likely diagnosis is a dermoid cyst, or, if it moves on protruding the tongue and is below the hyoid, a thyroglossal cyst (fluctuant lump developing in cell rests in thyroid's migration path; treatment: surgery). If >20yrs old, it's probably a thyroid mass, unless it's bony hard, when the diagnosis may be a chondroma.

Submandibular triangle: (Below jaw; above anterior belly of diagastric.) If <20yrs, self-limiting lymphadenopathy is likely. If >20, exclude **malignant lymphadenopathy** (eg firm, and non-tender). ▶Is TB likely? If it's not a node, think of submandibular **salivary stone**, **sialadenitis**, or **tumour**.

Anterior triangle: (Below digastric and in front of sternomastoid.) Nodes are common (see above): examine the areas which they serve (skin, mouth, throat, thyroid; is the spleen enlarged?—this may indicate lymphoma). **Branchial cysts** emerge under the anterior border of sternomastoid where the upper 1/3 meets the middle 1/3; age <20. They are due to non-disappearance of the cervical sinus (where the 2nd branchial arch grows down over the 3rd and 4th). Lined by squamous epithelium, their fluid contains cholesterol crystals. Treat by excision. **Cystic hygromas** arise from the jugular lymph sac; transilluminate brightly. Treat by surgery or hypertonic saline sclerosant. **Carotid body tumours** (chemodectoma) are very rare, move from side to side but not up and down, and splay out the carotid bifurcation. It is usually firm occasionally is soft and pulsatile. It does not usually cause bruits. It may be bilateral, familial, and malignant (5%). This tumour should be suspected in tumours just anterior to the upper third of sternomastoid. Diagnose by digital computerized angiography. Treatment: extirpation by vascular surgeon. If the lump is in the supero-posterior area of the anterior triangle, is it a **parotid tumour** (more likely if >40yrs)? **Laryngocoeles** are uncommon causes of anterior triangle lumps: they are painless, and may be made worse by blowing.

Posterior triangle: (Behind sternomastoid, in front of trapezius, above clavicle.) If there are many small lumps, think of nodes—TB or viruses such as HIV or EBV (infectious mononucleosis) or, if over 20yrs, consider lymphoma or metastases. **Cervical ribs** may intrude into this area.

Posterior triangle nodes are the likely cause, eg from GI or bronchial or head and neck neoplasia—or lymphoma or any chronic infection.

Tests Ultrasound shows lump consistency. CT defines masses in relation to their anatomical neighbours. Do virology and Mantoux test. CXR may show malignancy or reveal bilateral hilar lymphadenopathy; here you should consider sarcoid. Consider fine-needle aspiration (FNA).

Salivary gland pathology

There are 3 pairs of major salivary glands: parotid, submandibular and sublingual (also numerous minor glands).

History: lumps; swelling related to food; pain; taste; dry eyes.

Examination: note external swelling; look for secretions; bimanual palpation for stones. Examine VIIth nerve and regional nodes.

Cytology: This may be ascertained by fine-needle aspiration (FNA).

Recurrent unilateral pain and swelling is likely to be due to a stone. 80% are submandibular. The classical story is of pain and swelling on eating—with a red, tender, swollen but uninfected gland. The stone may be seen on plain x-ray or by sialography. Distal stones are removed via the mouth but deeper stones may require excision of gland.

Chronic bilateral symptoms may co-exist with dry eyes and mouth and autoimmune disease—eg Sjögren's or Mikulicz's syndrome (p704–8).

Fixed swellings may be from tumours or sarcoid—or are idiopathic.

Salivary gland tumours: '80% are in the parotid, 80% of these are pleomorphic adenomas, 80% of these are in the superficial lobe.'

▶Any salivary gland swelling must be removed for assessment if present for >1 month. VIIth nerve palsy signifies malignancy.

Benign or malignant:	Malignant:	Malignant:
Cystadenolymphoma	Mucoepidermoid	Squamous carcinoma
Pleomorphic adenoma	Acinic cell	Adenocarcinoma
		Adenoid cystic carcinoma

Pleomorphic adenomas often present in middle age, and grow slowly. Removed by parotidectomy. Adenolymphomas: usually older men; soft; treat by enucleation. Carcinomas: rapid growth; hard fixed mass; pain; facial palsy. Treatment: surgery+radiotherapy. Surgery complications: 1 Facial palsy—often brief. Have a facial nerve stimulator in theatre to aid identification. 2 Salivary fistula: often close spontaneously. 3 *Frey's syndrome* (gustatory sweating); tympanic neurectomy may help here.

Thyroid lumps

Examination Watch the neck during swallowing water. Stand behind and feel thyroid for size, shape (smooth? one or many nodules?), tenderness, and mobility. Percuss for retrosternal extension. Any nodes? Bruits?

If the thyroid is enlarged (goitre), ask these 3 questions:

1 Is the thyroid smooth or nodular?

2 Is the patient euthyroid, thyrotoxic or hypothyroid (see p542–6)?
   Smooth, non-toxic goitre: Endemic (iodine deficiency); congenital; goitrogens; thyroiditis; physiological; Hashimoto's thyroiditis (an autoimmune disease thought to be due to apoptosis induced by lymphocytes bearing Fas ligands combining with thyrocytes bearing Fas:[1] see p593.)
   Smooth, toxic goitre: Graves' disease.

3 If thyroid is nodular are there many nodules or a single lump?
   Multinodular goitre: Usually euthyroid but hyperthyroidism may develop. Hypothyroidism and malignancy are rare.

The *single thyroid lump* is a common problem; ~10% will be malignant. *Causes:* cyst, adenoma, discrete nodule in multinodular goitre, malignancy. First ask: is he/she thyrotoxic? ●Do T3 & T4. Then ●*Ultrasound*, to see if the lump is solid or cystic. ●*Needle aspiration* and send the fluid for cytology. Unless these tests indicate that the lump is definitely benign, arrange surgery. If it *is* benign: leave it alone.

What should you do if high-resolution ultrasound shows impalpable nodules? Such nodules can usually just be observed[2] provided they are:
●<1.5cm across—most will be (ultrasound can detect lumps <2mm across; such 'incidentalomas' are present in 46% of routine autopsies[3]).
●There is no past history of thyroid cancer or radiation.
●No family history of medullary cancer.[3] (If any present, do ultrasound-guided fine-needle aspiration; excise if cytology is malignant.)

Thyroid neoplasia 5 types:

1 *Papillary:* 60%. Often young; spread to nodes and lung. Treatment: total thyroidectomy (to remove non-obvious tumour) + node excision + radioiodine to ablate residual cells may all be needed. Give T4 to suppress TSH. Prognosis is better if young and female.

2 *Follicular:* ≤ 25%. Middle-aged, spreads early via blood (eg to bone, lungs). Well-differentiated. Treat by total thyroidectomy and T4 suppression or radioiodine (^{131}I) ablation.

3 *Anaplastic:* Rare. ♀:♂≈3:1. Elderly, poor response to any treatment.

4 *Medullary:* 5%. Sporadic (80%) or part of MEN syndrome (p546). May produce calcitonin. They do not concentrate iodine. Do thyroidectomy +node clearance (do phaeochromocytoma screen pre-op). Chemotherapy (eg doxorubicin) ± external beam radiotherapy may save lives.

5 *Lymphoma:* 5%. ♀:♂≈ 3:1. May present with stridor or dysphagia. Do full staging before treatment. Assess histology for MALT (mucosa-associated lymphoid tissue) origin. This is associated with a good prognosis.

Thyroid surgery *Indications:* Pressure symptoms, hyperthyroidism, carcinoma, cosmetic reasons. Render euthyroid pre-op, by antithyroid drugs and/or propranolol. Check vocal cords by indirect laryngoscopy.

Complications *Early:* Recurrent laryngeal nerve palsy, haemorrhage (►if compresses airway, instantly remove clips for evacuation of clot), hypoparathyroidism (check plasma Ca^{2+} daily, usually transient), thyroid storm (symptoms of severe hyperthyroidism—treat by propranolol PO or IV, antithyroid drugs, and iodine, p786). *Late complications:* Hypothyroidism.

1 M Kemeny 1998 *BMJ* i 600   2 G Tan 1997 *Ann Int Med* 126 226   3 *Bandolier* 1997 40 6

Abdominal masses

As with any mass determine size, site, shape, and surface. Find out if it is pulsatile and if it is mobile. Examine supraclavicular and inguinal nodes. Is the lump ballottable (like bobbing an apple up and down in water)?

Right iliac fossa masses

Appendix mass	Crohn's disease	Actinomycosis (p223)
Appendix abscess	Intussusception	Kidney malformation
Caecal carcinoma	TB mass	Tumour in an
Pelvic mass (see below)	Amoebic abscess	undescended testis

Abdominal distension Flatus, fat, fluid, faeces, or fetus? Fluid may be outside the gut (ascites) or sequestered in bowel (obstruction; ileus). To demonstrate ascites elicit signs of a fluid thrill and shifting dullness (p31).

Causes of ascites: (see also PLATE 1)   *Ascites with portal hypertension:*

Malignancy	Cirrhosis
Low albumin (eg nephrosis)	Portal nodes
ccf, pericarditis	Budd–Chiari syndrome (p696)
Infection—especially TB	ivc or portal vein thrombosis

Tests: Aspirate ascitic fluid (paracentesis) for cytology, culture, and protein estimation using an 18G needle in the RIF; ultrasound.

Left upper quadrant mass Is it spleen, stomach, kidney, colon, pancreas, or a rare cause (eg neurofibroma)? Pancreas cysts may be true (congenital; cystadenomas; retention cysts of chronic pancreatitis; cystic fibrosis); or pseudocysts (fluid in lesser sac from acute pancreatitis).

Splenomegaly Causes are often said to be *infective, haematological, neoplastic* etc, but clasification by *associated feature* is more useful at the bedside:

Splenomegaly with fever	*With lymphadenopathy*	*With purpura DIC*
Infection* (eg malaria, hepatitis*, SBE/IE, EBV*, TB, CMV, HIV	Glandular fevers*	Septicaemia; typhus
Sarcoid, malignancies*	Leukaemias; lymphoma	Weil's disease; amyloid
	Sjögren's syndrome	Meningococcaemia

With arthritis Sjögren's	*With ascites*	*With a murmur SBE/IE*
Rheumatoid arthritis; SLE	Carcinoma	Rheumatic fever
Infection, eg Lyme (p232)	Portal hypertension*	Hypereosinophilia
Vasculitis/Behçet's (p674)	(see above)	Amyloid* (p616)

With anaemia Sickle-cell*	*With weight↓+CNS signs*	*Massive splenomegaly*
Thalassaemia*; POEMs (p544)	Cancer, lymphoma, TB	Malaria; myelofibrosis
Leishmaniasis*; leukaemia*	Arsenic poisoning	CML*; leishmaniasis
Pernicious anaemia (p544)	Paraproteinaemia*	Gaucher's syndrome*

(See *Mentor*, p17, for a full list of causes by *any* association; * = causes of hepatosplenomegaly)

Smooth hepatomegaly Hepatitis, ccf, sarcoid, early alcoholic cirrhosis (a small liver is typical later); tricuspid incompetence (pulsatile liver).

Craggy hepatomegaly Secondaries or 1° hepatoma. (Nodular cirrhosis typically causes a small, shrunken liver, not an enlarged craggy one).

Pelvic masses *Is it truly pelvic?*—Yes, if by palpation you cannot 'get below it'. Causes: fibroids, fetus, bladder, ovarian cyst/malignancies.

Investigation of the lump There is much to be said for performing an early CT scan (if available). This will save time and money compared with leaving the test to be the last in a long chain of investigations. If CT is not available, ultrasound should be the first test. Other tests: IVU, liver and spleen isotope scans, Mantoux test (p200). Routine tests: FBC (with film), ESR, U&E, LFTs, proteins, Ca²⁺, CXR, AXR, biopsy tests; a tissue diagnosis may be made using a fine needle guided by ultrasound or CT control.

Around the anus

Pruritus ani Itch occurs if the anus is moist or soiled, eg fissures, incontinence, poor hygiene, tight pants, threadworm, fistula, dermatoses, lichen sclerosis, anxiety, contact dermatitis. *Treatment:*
●Careful hygiene ●Moist wipe post-defecation ●Try anaesthetic cream ●No spicy food ●No steroid/antibiotic creams

Fissure-in-ano This is a midline longitudinal split in the squamous lining of the lower anus—often, if chronic, with a mucosal tag at the external aspect—the 'sentinel pile'. 90% are posterior (anterior ones follow parturition), and are perpetuated by internal sphincter spasm. ♂:♀ >1:1.
●Most are due to hard faeces. They make defecation very painful—and spasm may constrict the rectal artery, making healing difficult.
●*Rare causes:* syphilis, herpes, trauma, Crohn's, anal cancer, psoriasis.
●Examine with a bright light. Do a PR ± sigmoidoscopy. Groin nodes suggest a complicating factor (eg immunosuppression from HIV).
●Try 5% lignocaine (=lidocaine) ointment, extra dietary roughage + good anal toilet. Glyceryl trinitrate ointment (0.2–0.3%) relieves pain and ischaemia caused by chronic fissures and spasm, and can prevent need for surgery, but may cause headache.[1] Otherwise, consider day-case *lateral partial internal sphincterotomy* or, less reliably, *manual anal dilatation* under GA; SE temporary loss of control of faeces/flatus; prolapsing piles.

The perianal haematoma (also called a thrombosed external pile). Both names are wrong because it is a clotted venous saccule.[2] It appears as a 2–4mm 'dark blue berry' under the skin. It may be evacuated via a small incision under local anaesthesia or left alone if >1 day old.

Pilonidal sinus Obstruction of natal cleft hair follicles ~6cm above the anus, with ingrowing of hair, excites a foreign body reaction, and may cause devious secondary tracks which open laterally ± abscesses, with foul-smelling discharge. (Barbers get these sinuses between their fingers.) ♂:♀ ≈ 10:1. *Treatment* is excision of the sinus tract ± primary closure, but is unsatisfactory in 10% of patients. Consider pre-op cefuroxime (eg 1.5g IV + metronidazole 1g IV). Complex tracks can be laid open and packed individually, or skin flaps can be used to cover the defect.

Rectal prolapse The mucosa, or rectum in all its layers, may descend through the anus. This leads to incontinence in 75%. It is due to a lax sphincter and prolonged straining. Treatment: fix rectum to the sacrum (± rectosigmoidectomy with no abdominal wound, as exposure is via amputating the prolapse[3]) or encircle the anus with a Thiersch wire.

Anal ulcers are rare: consider Crohn's disease, TB, syphilis.

Skin tags seldom cause trouble but are easily excised. **Piles** See p156.

Ischiorectal/perianal abscess These are usually caused by bowel organisms (rarely staphylococci or TB). Incision and drainage should be performed. Associations are diabetes, Crohn's disease, and malignancy. Occasionally a fistula results, especially in Crohn's disease, and further surgery may be required. Antibiotics should not be used routinely.

Anal cancer *UK incidence:* 300/yr. *Risk↑:* Syphilis, anal warts, anoreceptive homosexuals (often young). *Histology:* Squamous cell cancers, rarely basaloid or small cell. *The Patient:* may present with bleeding, pain, bowel habit change, pruritus ani, masses (ulcerated or submucosal), stricture formation. *Differential diagnosis:* Condyloma acuminata, leucoplakia, lichen sclerosus, Bowen's or Crohn's disease. *Treatment: Radiotherapy* eg with 45Gy in 20–25 fractions over 4–5 weeks—for squamous or basaloid cancers + *mitomycin* (12mg/m² IV) + *5-FU* (1g/m² IVI for 4 days in the first and final week of radiotherapy) is as effective as *anorectal excision* with colostomy—and 75% of patients retain normal anal function.[3]

1 J Lund 1997 *Lancet* **349** 11 & 573 2 W Thomson 1982 *Lancet* ii 467 3 UKCCCR anal group 1996 *Lancet* **348** 1049

Examination of the rectum and anus

Explain what you are about to do. Make sure curtains are pulled and doors are closed. The patient (and passers-by!) will appreciate it. Have the patient on his left side, his knees brought up towards the chest. Use gloves and lubricant. Part the buttocks and inspect the anus. Press your index finger against the side of the anus. Ask the patient to breathe deeply and insert your finger slowly; press with the pad of the finger first then twist and push in the tip. Feel for masses (haemorrhoids are not palpable) or impacted stool. Twist your arm so that the pad of your finger is feeling anteriorly. Feel for the cervix or prostate. Note consistency and size of prostate. If there is a concern about the spinal cord, ask the patient to squeeze your finger and note the tone. Note stool or blood on the glove and test for occult blood. Wipe anus. Consider proctoscopy (for the anus) or sigmoidoscopy (which mainly inspects the rectum).

Haemorrhoids (piles)

The anus is lined by mainly discontinuous masses of spongy vascular tissue—the anal cushions, which contribute to anal closure. Viewed from the lithotomy position, their positions are at 3, 7, and 11 o'clock. They are attached by smooth muscle and elastic tissue, but are prone to displacement and disruption, either singly or together. The effects of gravity (our erect posture), increased anal tone (?stress), and the effects of straining at stool may make them become both bulky and loose, and so to protrude to form piles (Latin *pila*, meaning a ball). They are vulnerable to trauma and bleed readily from the capillaries of the underlying lamina propria, hence their other name—haemorrhoids (meaning *running blood* in Greek).[1] Because the bleeding is from capillaries, it is bright red. (Piles are *not* varicose veins.)

Classification *First-degree piles* remain in the rectum. If *second-degree,* they prolapse through the anus on defecation but spontaneously reduce. *Third-degree piles:* As for second-degree but require digital reduction. *Fourth-degree piles:* These remain persistently prolapsed.

As there are no sensory fibres above the dentate line (squamomucosal junction), piles are not painful unless they thrombose when they protrude and are gripped by the anal sphincter, blocking venous return.

Differential diagnosis Perianal haematoma, fissures, abscess, tumour, proctalgia fugax (idiopathic, intense, stabbing rectal pain). Never ascribe bleeding to piles without adequate examination or investigation.

Causes Constipation with prolonged straining is the key factor. Congestion from a pelvic tumour, pregnancy, CCF, or portal hypertension are important in only a minority of cases.

Pathogenesis There is a vicious circle: vascular cushions protrude through a tight anus, become more congested, so hypertrophying to protrude again more readily. These protrusions may then strangulate.

The Patient notices bright red rectal bleeding, often coating stools or dripping into the pan after defecation. There may be mucus discharge and *pruritus ani.* Severe anaemia may occur. In all rectal bleeding do:
- An abdominal examination to rule out other diseases.
- A rectal examination: prolapsing piles are obvious. Internal haemorrhoids are not palpable.
- Proctoscopy to see the internal haemorrhoids.
- Sigmoidoscopy to identify rectal pathology higher up (you can get no higher up than the rectosigmoid junction).

The best treatment Unknown, as meta-analyses differ. *Infra-red coagulation* applied for 1.5–2sec, 3–8 times to localized areas of piles works by coagulating vessels, and tethering mucosa to subcutaneous tissue. Doing all the piles may take a few sessions.[1] *Sclerosants* (2mL of 5% phenol in oil injected into the pile above the dentate line; SE: impotence[1]; prostatitis) or *rubber band ligation* (SE: bleeding; infection); do <3 band-treatments per session; a cheap treatment, but needs skill. Banding produces an ulcer to anchor the mucosa (SE: pain, bleeding, infection). Freezing (cryo) is also used.

A high-fibre diet may also help. Soft paraffin soothes. Correct anal spasm (if present) by manual dilatation under general anaesthesia.

In all but grade IV piles, these may obviate need for haemorrhoidectomy (excision of piles ± ligation of vascular pedicles, as day-case surgery, needing ~2 weeks off work, p94). SE: haemorrhage or stenosis.

Treatment of thrombosed piles is with analgesia, and bed rest. Pain usually resolves in 2–3 weeks. Some surgeons advocate early operation.

1 J Pfenninger 1997 BMJ i 1211+ ii 882 2 W Thomson 1975 *Br J Surg* 62 542 & 1995 *personal communication*

157

Hernias

Definition Any structure passing through another so ending up in the wrong place is a *hernia*. Hernias involving bowel are said to be *irreducible* (ie *incarcerated*) if they cannot be pushed back into the right place. This does not mean that they are either necessarily obstructed or strangulated. Gastrointestinal hernias are *obstructed* if bowel contents cannot pass through them—the classical features of intestinal obstruction soon appear. They are *strangulated* if ischaemia occurs—the patient becomes toxic and requires urgent surgery.

Inguinal hernia The commonest kind, described on p160.

Femoral hernia Bowel enters the femoral canal, presenting as a mass in the upper medial thigh or above the inguinal ligament where it points down the leg, unlike an inguinal hernia which points to the groin. They occur more often in women than men and are likely to be irreducible and to strangulate. The *neck* of the hernia is felt below and lateral to the pubic tubercle (inguinal hernias are above and medial to this point).

The boundaries of the femoral canal are *anteriorly* and *medially* the inguinal ligament; *laterally* the femoral vein and *posteriorly* the pectineal ligament. The canal contains fat and Cloquet's node.

Surgical repair is recommended.

Paraumbilical hernias These occur just above or below the umbilicus. Risk factors are obesity and ascites. Omentum or bowel herniates through the defect. Surgery involves repair of the rectus sheath.

Epigastric hernias These pass through linea alba above the umbilicus.

Incisional hernias These follow breakdown of muscle closure after previous surgery. The patient is often obese so repair is not easy, and is often not recommended.

Spieghelian hernias These occur at the lateral edge of the rectus sheath, below and lateral to the umbilicus.

Lumbar hernias These occur through one of the lumbar triangles.

Richter's hernia This involves bowel wall only—not lumen.

Obturator hernias These occur through the obturator canal. Typically there is pain along the medial side of the thigh in a thin woman.

Other examples of hernias
- Of the nucleus pulposus into the spinal canal (slipped disc).
- Of the uncus and hippocampal gyrus through the tentorium (tentorial hernia) in space-occupying lesions.
- Of the brainstem and cerebellum through the foramen magnum (Arnold–Chiari malformation).
- Of the stomach through the diaphragm (hiatus hernia, p491).

Inguinal hernias

Indirect inguinal hernias pass through the internal inguinal ring and, if large enough, out through the external ring. Direct hernias pass through a defect in the abdominal wall into the inguinal canal. Predisposing conditions: chronic cough, constipation, urinary obstruction, heavy lifting, ascites, previous abdominal surgery.

Landmarks *The internal ring* is at the *mid-point* of the inguinal ligament, 1½ cm above the femoral pulse (which crosses the mid-inguinal point). *The external ring* is just above and medial to the pubic tubercle (the bony prominence forming the medial attachment of the inguinal ligament).

The relations of the inguinal canal

Floor: The inguinal ligament.
Roof: Fibres of transversalis and internal oblique.
Front: The aponeurosis of external oblique, with internal oblique for the lateral third.
Back: Laterally, transversalis fascia; medially, the conjoint tendon. The canal contains the spermatic cord (the round ligament in the female) and the ilioinguinal nerve.

Examining the patient Always look for previous scars, feel the other side and examine the external genitalia. Then ask: •Is the lump visible? If so, ask the patient to reduce it—if he cannot, make sure that it is not a scrotal lump. Ask him to cough. Inguinal hernias appear inferomedial to the external ring. •If no lump is visible, feel for a cough impulse. •If there is no lump, ask the patient to stand and repeat the cough.

Distinguishing direct from indirect hernias This is loved by examiners but is of little clinical use. The best way is to reduce the hernia and occlude the internal ring with 2 fingers. Ask the patient to cough—if the hernia is restrained it is indirect, if it pops out it is direct.

Indirect hernias:	Direct hernias:	Femoral hernias:
Common (80%)	Less common (20%)	Often in females
	Reduce easily	Often irreducible
Can strangulate	Rarely strangulate	Often strangulate

Irreducible hernias You may be called because a long-standing hernia is now irreducible and painful. It is always worth trying to reduce these yourself—to prevent strangulation and bowel necrosis (a grave event, demanding prompt laparotomy). Learn how to do this from an expert— ie one of your patients who has been reducing his hernia for years, then you will be well-equipped to act correctly when the incipient emergency presents. You will notice that such patients use the flat of the hand, directing the hernia from below, up towards the contralateral shoulder. Sometimes, as the hernia obstructs, reduction requires perseverance, which may be rewarded by a gurgle from the retreating bowel, and a kiss from the attendant spouse, who feared that surgery was inevitable.

Repairs Advise the patient to diet and stop smoking pre-op. Various methods of repair are used, eg 'Shouldice' with its multi-layered suture involving both anterior and posterior walls of the inguinal canal. Recurrence rate is less than with older methods, eg 'nylon darns' (eg <2% vs 10%).◁1▷ Laparoscopic repair is possible, and *may* be associated with fewer recurrences as tissue disturbance is minimized. Mesh repairs are now increasingly used (the mesh reinforces the posterior wall).

Local anaesthetic techniques and day-case 'ambulatory' surgery may halve the price of surgery. This is important because this is one of the most common operations (70,000 per year in the UK).

Return to work: we used to advise 4 weeks' rest and convalescence over 10 weeks—but with new mesh repairs, if comfortable for patients, return to manual labour after just 1–2 weeks is safe.[2] Explain pre-op.

◁1▷ MP Simons *Br J Surg* **83** 734 & *E-BM* 1996 **1** 209   2 AG Shulman 1994 *BMJ* ii 216

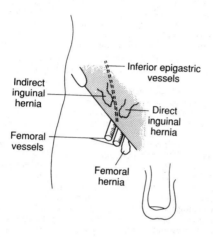

Varicose veins[1]

Varicose veins are common, leading to 50,000 admissions/yr in the NHS.

Essence Blood from superficial veins of the leg passes into the deep veins by means of perforator veins (they perforate the deep fascia) and at the sapheno-femoral junction. Normally, valves prevent blood from passing from deep to superficial veins. If they become incompetent (venous hypertension from prolonged standing, occlusion by fetus, fibroids, ovarian tumour, previous DVT) dilatation (*varicosities*) of the superficial veins occurs. See *Oedema*, p52.

Symptoms "My legs are ugly" ± pain, oedema, eczema, ulceration, skin pigmentation (haemosiderin), haemorrhage, and thrombophlebitis. On their own, even in (non-smoking) takers of the Pill, and even associated with local phlebitis, varicose veins do not cause DVTs (*proximally spreading phlebitis of the long saphenous vein in the thigh may be an exception*).[2]

Method of examination (Start with the patient standing.)
1 Note signs of poor skin nutrition: ulcers usually above the medial malleolus (varicose ulcers, OHCS p596) with deposition of haemosiderin causing brown edges, eczema, and thin skin.
2 Feel for a cough impulse at the sapheno-femoral junction (this signifies incompetence). The percussion test: tap the top of a vein and feel how far down its length you can feel the repercussions, which are normally interrupted by competent valves.
3 The Trendelenburg test determines if the sapheno-femoral junction valve is competent: lie the patient down and raise the leg to empty the vein. Place 2 fingers on the sapheno-femoral junction (5cm below and medial to femoral pulse). Ask her to stand, keeping fingers in place. Do the varicosities fill? If so, there are deep or communicating valve leaks. Then release fingers—if veins fill quickly the sapheno-femoral valve must be incompetent. In the latter, the Trendelenburg operation (disconnection of the saphenous and femoral veins) should help.
4 Doppler ultrasound probes, to listen to flow in incompetent valves, eg the sapheno-femoral junction, or the short saphenous vein behind the knee (the calf is squeezed, and flow on release lasting over ½–1sec indicates significant reflux). If incompetence is not identified and treated at the time of surgery, varicosities will return.[3]
5 Before surgery, ensure that all varicosities are indelibly marked.

Treatment
1 Patient education. Avoid prolonged standing; support stockings; lose weight; regular walking (calf muscle action aids venous return).
2 Injection therapy—especially for varicosities below the knee if there is no gross sapheno-femoral incompetence. Ethanolamine is injected and the vein compressed for a few weeks to avoid clotting (intravascular granulation tissue obliterates the lumen). Unsuitable for perforation sites. Use ≤10–12mL; take care to prevent extravasation.
3 Operative. There are several choices, depending on vein anatomy and surgical preference, eg sapheno-femoral disconnection; multiple avulsions; stripping from groin to upper calf (stripping to the ankle is not needed, and may damage the saphenous nerve). *Post-op:* Bandage legs tightly, and elevate them for 24h. Thereafter encourage walking 3 miles a day—many short walks rather than as one long trek.

Saphena varix This is a dilatation (varicosity) in the saphenous vein at its confluence with the femoral vein. It is one of the many causes of a lump in the groin (p146). Because it transmits a cough impulse, it may be mistaken for an inguinal hernia—but on closer inspection, it may have a bluish tinge to it, and it disappears on lying down.

1 D Tibbs 1992 *Varicose Veins*, Butterworth 2 B Campbell 1996 BMJ i 198 3 W Campbell 1990 BMJ i 763

The mind and the vain: why varicose veins become an illness

When do patients perceive varicose veins as an illness? The obvious answer is that they do so when they hurt. But for *some* patients, this is far too simplistic. Thanks to Albert Camus, we all know that 'certain illnesses are desirable: they provide, in their own way, a compensation for a functional disorder which, in their absence, would express itself in a more serious disturbance'.[1] In one study quoted by the Camus enthusiast, Joseph Herman,[2] ~50% of those undergoing varicose vein surgery had been involved in various family crises or emotional upsets in the period leading up to referral—the implication being that they became interested in their veins as a displacement activity to a less palatable preoccupation with insoluble problems.[3] In short, *we adopt the sickness rôle when we want sympathy*.

But beware of thinking that varicose vein surgery is the middle-aged equivalent of an overdose, and that if the result is less than satisfactory, the patient may be *pleased* as more sympathy is engendered:
► *any surgery done for cosmetic reasons all too easily leads to litigation.*

Somatization (of which this is just one example) is hard to manage: here is one general approach which may be suitable for some people.
● Give time; don't dismiss these patients as "just the 'worried well' ".
● Explore the factors which perpetuate illness behaviour (disordered physiology, misinformation, unfounded fears, misinterpretation of sensations, unhelpful 'coping' behaviour, social stressors).
● Agree a management plan which focuses on each issue and makes sense to the patient's holistic view of him- or herself.
● Treat any underlying depression (*OHCS* p340–p342).
● Offer cognitive therapy (see *OHCS* p370 & R Mayou 1997 *BMJ* ii 562).

1 *The Enigma* in *Selected Essays & Notebooks*, Penguin 2 *BMJ* 1997 ii 589 3 J Holmes 1970 *Practitioner* 207 549

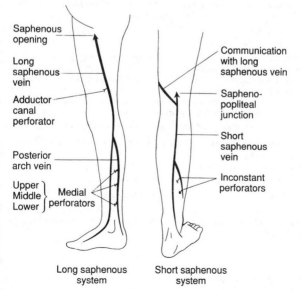

Saphenous opening
Long saphenous vein
Adductor canal perforator
Posterior arch vein
Upper Middle Lower } Medial perforators

Communication with long saphenous vein
Sapheno-popliteal junction
Short saphenous vein
Inconstant perforators

Long saphenous system   Short saphenous system

Gastric surgery and its aftermath

Peptic ulcers and gastric carcinomas are the commonest indications for gastric surgery.

Partial gastrectomy (the Billroth operations)

Billroth I: Partial gastrectomy with simple re-anastomosis (rejoining).
Billroth II (Polya gastrectomy): Partial gastrectomy. The duodenal stump is oversewn (leaving a blind loop), and anastomosis is achieved by a longitudinal incision further down the duodenum.

Operations for duodenal ulceration See p166.

Operations for benign gastric ulceration Those near the pylorus may be considered similarly to duodenal ulceration (p166). Away from the pylorus, elective operation is rarely needed as ulcers respond well to medical treatment, stopping smoking, and avoidance of NSAIDs—but a partial gastrectomy may be needed.

Haemorrhage is usually treated with partial gastrectomy or simple excision of the ulcer. Perforation is treated with excision of the hole for histology, then closure.

Gastric carcinoma See p142. Surgery differs in different parts of the world: in Japan, where gastric cancer is common, and patients are often younger and fitter, the most radical surgery is performed with removal of N_2 and N_1 nodes (pergastric) plus *en-bloc* distal pancreatectomy and splenectomy (known as D_2 surgery). UK surgeons are usually less radical (D_1 surgery). A randomized study ($N=400$) found much greater post-op morbidity with D_2 surgery (46% *vs* 28%), and survival was *worse* (30% 3yr survival *vs* 50%).[1]

Physical complications of peptic ulcer surgery

Recurrent ulceration: Symptoms are similar to those experienced pre-operatively but complications are more common and response to medical treatment is poor. Further surgery is difficult.

Abdominal fullness: Feeling of early satiety (perhaps with discomfort and distension) improving with time. Advise to take small, frequent meals.

Dumping syndrome: Fainting and sweating after eating, possibly due to food of high osmotic potential being dumped in the jejunum, and causing oligaemia because of rapid fluid shifts. 'Late dumping' is due to hypoglycaemia and occurs 1–3 hours after taking food. It is relieved by eating glucose. Both problems tend to improve with time but may be helped by taking more protein and less glucose in meals.

Bilious vomiting: This is difficult to treat—but often improves with time.

Diarrhoea: This can be particularly disabling after a vagotomy. Codeine phosphate may help.

Metabolic complications

Weight loss: This is usually due to poor calorie intake.

Bacterial overgrowth ± *malabsorption* (the blind loop syndrome) may occur.

Anaemia: This is usually due to iron deficiency following hypochlorhydria and stomach resection. B_{12} levels are frequently low but megaloblastic anaemia is rare.

1 A Cuschieri 1996 *Lancet* 347 995

Complications of peptic ulcer surgery			
	Partial gastrectomy	Vagotomy & pyloroplasty	Highly selective vagotomy
Recurrence	2%	7%	>7%
Dumping	20%	14%	6%
Diarrhoea	1%	4%	<1%
Metabolic	++++	++	0
(These are approximate and depend on the skill of the surgeon.)			

STOMACH

Billroth I   DUODENUM   Billroth II (or Polya)

Operations for duodenal ulcer

Peptic ulcers usually present as epigastric pain and dyspepsia (p490). There is no reliable method of distinguishing clinically between gastric and duodenal ulcers. Although management of both is usually medical in the first instance (including *H pylori* eradication[1]), surgery still has a rôle.

Surgery is considered if medical treatment has failed or there are complications: *haemorrhage*, *perforation*, and *pyloric stenosis*.

Several types of operation have been tried but, as whenever considering an operation, one must consider efficacy, side-effects and mortality.

1 **Elective surgery** may be undertaken for symptoms which fail to respond to medical treatment. Operations to consider:

  a. *Gastrectomy* (p164).

  b. *Vagotomy and drainage procedure:* A vagotomy reduces acid production from the stomach body and fundus, and reduces gastrin production from the antrum. However, it interferes with emptying of the pyloric sphincter and so a drainage procedure must be added. The commonest is a pyloroplasty in which the pylorus is cut longitudinally and closed transversely. A gastroenterostomy is an alternative.

  c. *Highly selective vagotomy (HSV).* The vagus supply is denervated only where it supplies the lower oesophagus and stomach. The nerve of Laterget to the pylorus is left intact; thus gastric emptying is unaffected. The results of surgery are greatly dependent on the skill of the surgeon.

2 **a.** **Haemorrhage** may be controlled endoscopically by injection, diathermy, laser coagulation, or heat probe. Operation should be considered for haemorrhage >5 units or rebleeding, especially in the elderly. The ulcer is oversewn to stop the bleeding. The pylorus is opened at operation so it is common to perform a definitive vagotomy and pyloroplasty.

  b. **Perforation** Most often, all that is needed is a limited supra-umbilical laparotomy (or minimal access surgery) to close the hole with an omental plug—with post-op *H pylori* eradication (p490).[1] Consider a vagotomy and pyloroplasty too if there has been a long history of pain or dyspepsia with no response to *Helicobacter* eradication therapy.

  c. **Pyloric stenosis** This is a late complication, presenting with vomiting of large amounts of food some hours after meals. (Adult pyloric stenosis is a complication of duodenal ulcers, and has nothing to do with congenital hypertrophic pyloric stenosis.) Surgery is always required—usually a vagotomy and drainage procedure. Some may attempt highly selective vagotomy with dilatation. The operation should be done on the next available list, after correction of the metabolic defect—hypochloraemic, hypokalaemic metabolic alkalosis.

Fundoplication for gastro-oesophageal reflux

The goal This is to re-establish lower oesophageal sphincter tone.

The procedure This involves wrapping the gastric fundus around the lower oesophagus, closing the hiatus, and securing the wrap in the abdomen. There are various types of procedure: Nissen, Toupet, Hill.

Access Via a *large* laparotomy incision—or use of laparoscopy. The latter, *in the most skilled hands,* achieves similar results to open surgery, with less morbidity, pain, hospital dependency and expense[1]—but see p168.

1 J Danesh 1998 *BMJ* i 746 & CU Corvera 1997 *BMJ* i 586—it may be wise to review patients who have had surgery, eg many years ago, to check if *H pylori* and symptoms are present.

Minimally invasive surgery

The term 'keyhole surgery' or minimal access surgery may be preferred, because these procedures can be as invasive as any laparotomy, having just the same set of side-effects—plus some new ones.[1] It is the size of the incision and the use of laparoscopes which marks out this branch of surgery. As a rule of thumb, whatever can be done by laparotomy can also be done with the laparoscope. This does not mean that it *should* be done, but if the patient feels better sooner, has less post-operative pain, and can return to work earlier, then these specific techniques will gain ascendency—provided hospitals can afford the equipment.[2] Established uses for this type of surgery are for oesophageal, gastric, duodenal, and colonic procedures—including the removal of cancers—as well as hernia repairs, appendicectomies and cholecystectomies.

It is worth noting that advantages do not include time. In upper GI procedures, laparoscopic procedures take longer than open procedures. Also, the patient needs to spend a night in hospital, usually. This has economic implications when comparing laparoscopic hernia repair with its open alternative done under local anaesthesia (after which the patient can go home the same day). The other side of the economic equation for hernia repair is that post-operative discomfort is much less after laparoscopic procedures, and the patient can return to full employment after a week.[1]

Problems with minimal access surgery: for the surgeon
Inspection: Anatomy looks different—eg in hernia repairs which are approached differently in open procedures. (In cholecystectomy, visualization may be facilitated by the laparoscope which can gain access to areas which require difficult traction to reveal in open surgery.)
Palpation is impossible during laparoscopic procedures. This may make it hard to locate colon lesions prior to cutting them out. This means that pre-operative tests may need to be more extensive (eg colonoscopy *and* barium enema). Alternatively, colonoscopy can take place during the procedure, or methylene blue can be injected at the first colonoscopy.
Skill: Here the problem is not just that a new skill has to be learned and taught. Old skills may become attenuated if most cholecystectomies are performed via the laparoscope, and new practitioners may not achieve quite the level of skill in either sphere if they try to do both.

Problems for the patient and his general practitioner
Post-operative complications: What may be quite easily managed on a well-run surgical ward (eg haemorrhage) may prove a challenge for a GP and be terrifying for the patient, who may be all alone after early discharge.
Loss of tell-tale scars: After laparoscopy there may only be a few abdominal stab wounds, so the GP or the patient's future carers have to guess at what has been done. The answer here is not to tattoo the abdomen with arrows and instructions, but to communicate carefully and thoroughly with the patient, so that he or she knows what has been done.

Problems for the hospital
Just because minimal access surgery is often cost-effective, it does not follow that hospitals can afford the procedures. Instruments are continuously being refined, and quickly become obsolete—so that many are now produced in disposable single-use form. Because of budgeting boundaries, hospitals cannot use the cash saved by early return to work or by freeing-up bed use to pay for capital equipment and extra theatre time which may be required.

1 JR Monson 1993 *BMJ* ii 1346   2 K Lawrence 1994 *Lancet* 343 308

6. Infectious diseases

Relevant pages in other chapters:
Prophylactic antibiotics in gut surgery (p84); infective endocarditis and its prevention (p312 & p314); pneumonia (p332); unusual pneumonia (p334); management of pneumonia (p336); lung abscess (p334); bronchiectasis (p338); fungi and the lung (p340); urinary tract infection (p374); encephalitis (p441); ►►meningitis (p442, p444); septic arthritis (p662).

In OHCS: Endometritis (*OHCS* p36); pelvic infection (*OHCS* p50); prenatal & perinatal infection (*OHCS* p98–p101); measles, mumps, and rubella (*OHCS* p214); parvoviruses (*OHCS* p215); overwhelming neonatal infection (*OHCS* p238); the ill and feverish child (*OHCS* p248); TB meningitis (*OHCS* p260); orbital cellulitis (*OHCS* p484); ophthalmic shingles (*OHCS* p484); mastoiditis (*OHCS* p534); sinusitis (*OHCS* p554); tonsillitis (*OHCS* p556); skin infections/infestations (*OHCS* p590 & p600); osteomyelitis (*OHCS* p44).

Notifiable diseases in the UK (Marked ND on relevant pages.) Inform the Consultant in Communicable Disease Control (CCDC).

Anthrax	Malaria	Rubella
Cholera	Measles	Scarlet fever
Diphtheria	Meningitis (acute)	Tetanus
Dysentery (amoebic,	Meningococcal sepsis	Tuberculosis
typhoid/paratyphoid)	Mumps	Typhus
Ebola virus disease	Ophthalmia neonatorum	Viral haemorrhagic fevers
Encephalitis	Plague	including Lassa fever
Food poisoning (any)	Poliomyelitis	Viral hepatitis
Leprosy	Rabies	Whooping cough
Leptospirosis	Relapsing fever	Yellow fever

Note: In the UK, reporting AIDS is voluntary—and in strict confidence—to the Director, Communicable Disease Surveillance Control, 61 Colindale Ave, London NW9 5EQ. UK telephone advice: 0181 200 6868 or 0181 965 1118. Report only if the patient gives consent.

The essence of infectious diseases First of all define a clinical syndrome. Look for a possible causative organism. Then entertain Koch's (1843–1910) postulates—ie 1 Show that you can find the organism in all instances of the disease; 2 Culture the organism; 3 Show that the culture can reproduce the disease when inoculated into an animal; 4 Recover the organism from the experimental animal.

The next step is to clone the organism's genome; then design a molecule to kill it, or, better still, a vaccine to prevent its effects, and so to raise the possibility of extinguishing the organism's life on earth for ever. But before this happy state of affairs exists, there is the hardest hurdle of all for a great discovery: you must make its application available and desired by all members of our species.▫ In no other area is the gap so great between how much we *know* and how much of this knowledge we have *applied*. Millions of children are dying because they are unimmunized against preventable infectious diseases; 1,000,000,000 people have no ready access to a safe water supply.[1] The rest of this chapter might be thought of as being almost an inconsequential footnote to these appalling facts.

---

*Junior doctors working in the developed world are unlikely to have much experience with many of these diseases (which may be common abroad). ►The importance of consulting early with experts cannot be overemphasized. Specific treatments are given here principally to enable the reader to have intelligent discussion with the relevant expert.

Sources: OTM 3e; J Sanford 1997 *Guide to Antimicrobial Therapy*, Antimicrobial Therapy Inc, Dallas, ISBN 0-933775-10-5 (available via Visa payment from USA, tel 703-847-4441; fax 703 847 4447 (~$9) 1 J Ciment 1998 BMJ i 571 & J Mackay 1993 *The State of Health Atlas*, Simon & Schuster ISBN 0-671-71151-2. For 1000s of CD-ROM pictures with interactive tutorials, see the Wellcome *Tropical Medicine Resource* 210 Euston Rd, London NW1 2BE. tel. 0171 611 8888.

The classification of pathogens

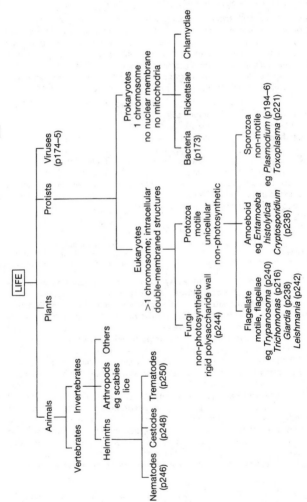

Classification of some pathogenic bacteria

GRAM +VE COCCI
Staphylococci (p222)
  Staph aureus
  Staph epidermidis (coagulase −ve)
Streptococci* (p222)
β-haemolytic Streptococci
  Strep pyogenes (group A)
α-haemolytic Streptococci (viridans)
  Strep mitior
  Strep pneumoniae
  Strep sanguis
Non-haemolytic Streptococci
  Strep bovis
  E faecalis (enterococcus)
  E mutans
Anaerobic Streptococci

GRAM +VE BACILLI (rods)
Aerobic
  Bacillus anthracis
  (anthrax: p222)
  Corynebacterium diphtheriae
  (diphtheria: p222)
  Listeria monocytogenes (p223)
  Nocardia

Anaerobic
  Clostridia
    Clostridium botulinum (botulism: p794)
    Clostridium perfringens
    (gas gangrene: p223)
    Clostridium tetani
    (tetanus: p226)
    Clostridium difficile
    (pseudomembranous colitis: p486)
  Actinomyces israelii
  (actinomycosis: p223)

**ORGANISMS ON THE BORDERLINE
BETWEEN VIRUSES AND BACTERIA**
Mycoplasma (atypical pneumonia: p334)
Rickettsia (typhus: p237; Coxiella
  burnetii: p236-7)
Ehrlichia (p236); Bartonella (p236)
Chlamydia (p220 & p334 & OHCS p50)

GRAM −ve COCCI
Neisseria meningitidis
(= the meningococcus)—meningitis
and septicaemia: p444
Neisseria gonorrhoeae
(= the gonococcus)—gonorrhoea:
p221 Chlamydia.

GRAM−ve BACILLI (rods)
Enterobacteriaceae (p190, p244)
  Escherichia coli
  Proteus mirabilis
  Serratia marcescens
  Klebsiella aerogenes
  Salmonella
  Shigella
  Enterobacter species
  Yersinia enterocolitica
  Yersinia pestis (plague: p224)
Haemophilus influenzae (p224)
Brucella species
  (brucellosis: p224)
Bordetella pertussis
  (whooping cough: p224)
Pasteurella multocida (p225)
Pseudomonas aeruginosa (p224)
Vibrio cholerae
  (Cholera: p228)
Legionella pneumophila
  (atypical pneumonia: p334)
Campylobacter jejuni (food
  poisoning: p190)
Anaerobes
  Bacteroides (wound infections: p84)
  Helicobacter pylori (p490)
Mycobacteria
  Mycobacterium tuberculosis
  (TB, p198–p200)
  Mycobacterium leprae: leprosy (p230)
  'Atypical' mycobacteria, eg M simiae;
  Mycobacterium avium intracellulare (p214)
  M bovis; M scrofulaceum; M ulcerans;
  M zenopi; M maninum; M kansasii
Spirochaetes (p232–p233)
  Treponema—Syphilis; yaws; bejel; pinta
  Leptospira—Weil's disease; canicola fever
  Borrelia—Relapsing fever; Lyme disease

This table is not intended to be comprehensive nor to follow closely bacteriological taxonomy. It is simply a guide for the forthcoming pages.
*The classification of streptococci is as β-, α-, or non-haemolytic, or by Lancefield antigen (mainly β-haemolytic streptococci express Lancefield antigens), or by clinical species (eg Strep pyogenes—see also p222). There is much crossover among these groups; the above is a generalization for the most important organisms.

Viruses (various)

DNA viruses

A) Double-stranded DNA
- Papovavirus—papilloma virus—human warts
  —progressive multifocal leukoencephalopathy
- Adenovirus—10% viral respiratory disease
  —7% viral meningitis
  —there are >30 serotypes
- Herpes viruses 1) Herpes simplex virus 1 (p202)
  2) Herpes simplex virus 2
  3) Herpes (varicella) zoster virus (p202)
  4) Epstein–Barr virus—infectious mononucleosis (p204)
   —Burkitt's lymphoma
   —some nasopharyngeal carcinoma
  5) Cytomegalovirus (p208)
  6) Herpes virus 6 (HHV-6)
   —roseola infantum (Exanthem subitum)—a
   mild, self-limiting infection of infants (OHCS p214)
  7) HHV-8: Kaposi's sarcoma (p702)
- Pox virus 1) Variola—smallpox (now offically eradicated)
  2) Vaccinia—cowpox
  3) Orf: cutaneous pustules in man, contracted from sheep
  4) Molluscum contagiosum: groups of pearly umbilicated
   papules, typically seen in children or with HIV.
- Hepatitis B virus (see p210)

B) Single-stranded DNA: Parvovirus (only group with single-stranded DNA)
  —Erythema infectiosum (known as fifth disease, OHCS p214)
  'slapped cheek appearance' ± aplastic crises

RNA viruses A) Double-stranded RNA—Reovirus
  B) Positive single-stranded RNA   • Picornavirus
     • Togavirus
  C) Negative double-stranded RNA   • Orthomyxovirus
     • Paramyxovirus
     • Arenavirus
     • Rhabdovirus
     • Bunyavirus

A) Reovirus—eg Rotavirus—infantile gastroenteritis
B) • Picornavirus:
  —Rhinovirus—common cold with >90 serotypes infectious
   from 2 days before symptoms for up to 3 weeks.
  —Enterovirus: i) Coxsackie: Group A: meningitis; gastroenteritis
   Group B: pericarditis; Bornholm disease
   ii) Poliovirus (p234)
   iii) Echovirus: 30% viral meningitis
   iv) Hepatitis A (atypical)
  • Togavirus: i) Rubella ii) Alphavirus iii) Flavivirus—yellow fever
   —dengue
C) • Orthomyxovirus—Influenza A, B, C
  • Paramyxovirus—Parainfluenza, Mumps, Measles
   Respiratory syncytial virus: 20% serious
   respiratory disease in children
  • Arenavirus—Lassa fever
   —some viral haemorrhagic fevers
   —lymphocytic-choriomeningitis (LCM) virus
  • Rhabdovirus—Rabies
  • Bunyavirus—certain viral haemorrhagic fevers
D) Retrovirus—Retrovirus HIV I & II (p212 & p214), HTLV I, HTLV II

Travel advice[1]

Most problems are due to ignorance, indiscretions (sex ± alcohol), and lack of immunity: all are partly amenable to forward planning. Accidents (± alcohol abuse) are the commonest problems with travel. ►Take time to advise travellers on the risks of HIV and the benefits of safer sex—or, more reliably, *no sex*. *Malaria* is another big killer: see p194 for prevention. For *cholera* and *traveller's diarrhoea*, see p228 & p190. *Vaccinations*:

[L = live vaccine]	Doses needed	Gap between doses: 1st & 2nd	2nd & 3rd	Booster interval
Yellow fever[L]	1			10 yrs
Typhoid sc (Typhim VI®)	1			3 yrs
Typhoid oral[L*]	4	2 days	2 days	3–5 days
(don't give with mefloquine)				
Tetanus	3	4 weeks	4 weeks	5–10 yrs
Polio[L]	3	>6 weeks	>6 weeks	5–10 yrs
Rabies pre-exposure	3	7–28 days	6–12 months	10 yrs
Meningococci	1			3 yrs
Japanese encephalitis	3	1–2 weeks	2–4 weeks	1–4 yrs
Tick encephalitis	3	1–3 months	9–12 months	5–10 yrs
Hepatitis A (Havrix®)	3	2–4 months	6–12 months	5–10 yrs
Hepatitis B	3	1 month	5 months	2–5 yrs
if travelling soon:	3	1 month	1 month	1 yr

If only one attendance is possible, all is not lost (?make up *en route*): Give *malaria prophylaxis and advice*—p196. *Africa:* Meningitis, typhoid, tetanus, polio, Hepatitis A vaccine ± yellow fever. *Asia:* Meningitis (some areas), typhoid, tetanus, polio, Hepatitis A vaccine. *S America:* Typhoid, tetanus, polio, Hepatitis A vaccine ± yellow fever.[1] *Travel if substantially immunocompromised:* See p215; avoid live[L] vaccines.

Preventing traveller's diarrhoea—*Water:* ►If in doubt, boil all water. Chlorination is an alternative but does not kill amoebae. Tablets are available from pharmacies. In emergency, one drop of laundry bleach (4–6%), or 4 drops of tincture of iodine may be added to 1 litre of water. Filter water before purifying. It is important to distinguish between simple gravity filters and water purifiers (which also attempt to sterilize chemically). Choose a unit which is verified by bodies such as the London School of Hygiene and Tropical Medicine (eg the MASTA[2] *Travel Well Personal Water Purifier*). Make sure that all containers are disinfected. Always try to avoid surface water and intermittent tap supplies. Avoid ice. In Africa assume that all unbottled water is unsafe. With bottled water, ensure the rim is clean and dry.

Other water-borne diseases include schistosomiasis (p250). *Food:* Hot, well-cooked food is safest (prawns need ≥8 mins boiling). In China, for example, a piping hot rat kebab might be a safer bet than a salad. Peel your own fruit. If you cannot wash your hands, discard the part of the food which you are holding (with bananas, careful unzipping obviates this precaution).[1] In those in whom traveller's diarrhoea might be most serious, consider a stand-by course of ciprofloxacin.

*If live oral form used, give 3 doses (1 cap on alternate days, 1h ac, with a cool drink).**1** R Dawood 1992 *Travellers' Health*, OUP **2** Medical Advis. Service for (UK) Travellers Abroad (0171 631 4408) provides detailed written travel advice for ~£5. Also try Healthline (01898 345 081), the Liverpool School of Tropical Medicine (0151 708 9393), and the Royal Geographical Society Expedition Advisory Centre, 1 Kensington Gore, London SW7 2AR; see also DoH 1995 *Health Information for Overseas Travel.* http://www.cdc.gov/epo/mmwr/preview/rr4612.html.

Susceptibility of some bacteria to certain antibiotics.   I=susceptible, first choice.   2=2nd choice.   R=Resistance likely.   0=Usually inappropriate.
R*=resistance is rare in most areas.

	Penicillin V & G	Flucloxacillin	Ampicillin & Amoxycillin	Ticarcillin, Piperacillin, Azlocillin	Cefradine & Cefazolin	Cefuroxime & Cefoxitin	Ceftriaxone & Cefotaxime	Ceftazidime	Imipenem	Erythromycin	Clindamycin	Tetracyclines	Chloramphenicol	Trimethoprim	Aminoglycosides eg Gentamicin	Vancomycin	Metronidazole	Ciprofloxacin	Co-amoxiclav
Staph aureus (penicillin sensitive)	1	2	2	2	0	0	0	0	0	2R	2R	2R	0	2	2	2	0	2	2
Staph aureus (penicillin resistant)	R	1	R	R	0	0	0	0	0	2R	2R	2R	R	2R	R	2	0	2	2
Strep (group A)	1	0	0	0	0	0	0	0	0	2	2	2	0	R	R	2	0	2	2
Strep pneumoniae	1	1	0	0	0	0	0	0	0	2R	2R	2R	0	R	R	2	0	2	2
Enterococcus faecalis	R	R	2	2	R	R	R	R	0	R	R	R	R	R	R	2	0	2	2
N meningitidis	1	0	2	0	0	0	2	0	0	0	0	0	2	R	R	R	0	0	2
Listeria monocytogenes	1	0	2	0	R	R	R	R	2	0	0	0	0	2	2	R	0	0	2
H influenzae	0	R	2	2	IR	R	1	0	2	R	R	R	IR	R	R	R	0	0	2
E coli	R	R	2	2	IR	R	IR	R	2	R	R	R	IR	IR*	2	R	0	2	2
Klebsiella species	R	R	R	2	2R	R	IR	R	2	R	R	R	IR	IR*	2	R	0	2	2
Serratia/Enterobacter species	R	R	R	2	2R	R	IR	R	2	R	R	R	IR	IR*	2	R	0	2	2
Proteus species	R	R	2	2	IR	R	IR	R	2	R	R	R	IR	IR*	2	R	0	2	2R
Pseudomonas aeruginosa	R	R	R	R	R	R	R	2	2	R	R	R	R	R	2	R	0	R	R
Bacteroides fragilis	R	R	R	R	R	2R	R	R	2	2R	2R	2R	R	R	R	–	2	R	2
Other Bacteroides species	2	R	R	R	R	2R	R	R	2	2R	2R	2R	R	R	R	–	2	R	2
Clostridium difficile	0	0	0	0	0	0	0	0	0	0	0	0	R	R	R	0	0	0	0

NB: this table is a guide only, and different populations will exhibit their own (changing) patterns of resistance—so, in many ways, these sorts of tables are often unsatisfactory. ▲ In practice, the best thing is often to talk to a microbiologist.

Antibiotics: penicillins

General advice Our most common error is to give antibiotics with no clear idea of the organism involved, and then to stop them before the infection is controlled. This may promote spread of antibiotic resistance (see p222). In general, avoid antibiotics unless the lab has cultured the organism, or the patient is very ill and/or in need of immediate treatment (see *blind treatment of infections* p182). In which case, culture blood, MSU, sputum and any other relevant samples before treating.

Antibiotic (and its uses):	Usual **adult** dose:	In renal failure:
Amoxycillin As ampicillin but better absorbed PO. For IV therapy, use ampicillin.	250–500mg/8h PO 3g/12h in recurrent or severe pneumonia	↓Dose if cc <10 (cc=creatinine clearance, mL/min)
Ampicillin Broader spectrum than penicillin; more active against Gram −ve rods, but β-lactamase sensitive. Amoxycillin is better absorbed PO. Well excreted in bile.	500mg/4–6h IM/IV	↓Dose dose if cc <10
Azlocillin Antipseudomonal agent.	2–5g/8h IV	If cc <30 give /12h
Benzylpenicillin = penicillin G Most Streps, syphilis, *Neisseria*, tetanus, actinomycosis, gas gangrene, anthrax, many anaerobes	300–600mg/6h IV, more in meningitis. 1 megaunit = 600mg. If dose >1.2g, inject at rate <300mg/min	If cc <10 max dose is 6g/24h
Cloxacillin For Gram +ve β-lactamase producers (*Staph aureus*) only. Less absorbed PO than fluclox.	250mg/4–6h IM 500mg/4–6h IV	Dose unaltered
Co-amoxiclav Augmentin® = clavulanic acid 125mg + amoxicillin 250mg; uses as for ampicillin, but β-lactamase resistance confers a much broader spectrum, but it is hepatotoxic.	1–2* tab/8h; 1.2g/6–8h IV *Avoid clavulanic acid toxicity (LFT↑) by giving 2nd tab as plain amoxicillin	cc: 10–30 <10 — Dose/12h: 1–2 tab or 600mg IV 1 tab or 300mg IV
Flucloxacillin (= **Nafcillin** in USA) As for cloxacillin. Take ½h pre-food.	250mg/6h PO, 250 mg/6h IM; max 1g/6h IV	Dose unaltered if cc >10
Phenoxymethyl-penicillin = penicillin V As for Pen G but less active. Used as prophylaxis or to complete an IV course.	250–500mg/6h PO ½h before food	In severe renal failure, give doses every 12h
Piperacillin Very broad spectrum, with anaerobes and *Pseudomonas*. Keep for severe infections. Combine with aminoglycoside. Antagonized by cefoxitin. It isn't active against *Staphs*.	4g/6h slowly IV	CC: 40–80 20–40 <20 dialysis: — Max dose: 16g/24h 12g/24h 8g/24h 6g/24h
Procaine penicillin (=procaine benzylpenicillin) Depot; good in syphilis (**S**) and gonorrhoea (**G**).	**S**: 0.6–1.2g/24h IM for 10 days; **G**: if female, 3.6g stat (if male, 2.5g stat)	Dose unaltered
Ticarcillin Wide spectrum, eg *Pseudomonas*, *Proteus*. Use with aminoglycoside. More active than azlocillin or piperacillin.	5g/6–8h IV	Reduce dose if cc <20 to 2g/8–12h

Side-effects ●Hypersensitivity: rash (ampicillin rashes do not necessarily indicate penicillin allergy but 'penicillin allergic' implies allergy to *all* penicillins); serum sickness (2%); anaphylaxis (<1:100,000). ●In huge overdose or intrathecal injection: seizures and coma. ●Diarrhoea (pseudomembranous colitis is rare). ●U&E imbalance given IV.

Antibiotics: cefalosporins

Spectrum Most cefalosporins are active against *Staphs* (including those producing β-lactamase), streptococci (except group D, *Enterococcus faecalis* & *faecium*), pneumococci, *E coli*, some *Proteus*, *Klebsiella*, *Haemophilus*, *Salmonella*, and *Shigella*. 2nd generation drugs (cefuroxime, cefamandole) are active against *Neisseria* and *Haemophilus*. 3rd generation (∗) drugs (cefotaxime, ceftazidime, ceftizoxime, ceftriaxone) have better activity against Gram −ve organisms, but less Gram +ve activity, especially against *Staph aureus*. *Pseudomonas* is often susceptible to ceftazidime: reserve for this.

Uses Indications are controversial, and vary from place to place. Oral cefalosporins (cefaclor, cefadroxil, cefradine, cefalexin, cefuroxime axetil) may be used in pneumonias, otitis media, skin and soft tissue lesions, and UTIs, but they are not first line agents. (The effect on *Haemophilus influenzae* varies.) They may be used as second-line agents or to complete a course that was started with an IV cefalosporin. The major use of cefalosporins is parenteral, eg as prophylaxis in surgery (p84) and in post-op infection. Suspected life-threatening infections due to Gram −ve bacteria may be treated blindly with a third generation drug. In neutropenic patients, if the organism has been identified, third generation drugs are very useful, but their place in 'blind' treatment is unclear. Cefalosporins may also become the drugs of first choice in other special circumstances, such as penicillin sensitivity or where aminoglycosides are better avoided—but they have no unique rôle here. *Klebsiella* pneumonia is best treated with two agents, or a third generation cefalosporin.

The principal **adverse effect** of the cefalosporins is hypersensitivity. This is seen in <10% of penicillin-sensitive patients. There may be GI upsets, reversible rises in transaminases or alk phos, eosinophilia, rarely neutropenia, nephrotoxicity, and colitis. There are some reports of clotting abnormalities, and there may be false +ve reactions for glycosuria, and false +ve Coombs' test. There is increased risk of nephrotoxicity when first generation cefalosporins are co-administered with frusemide (=furosemide), gentamicin, and vancomycin, but 2nd and 3rd generation drugs are probably safe. Cefamandole may potentiate warfarin.

ANTIBIOTIC:	USUAL ADULT DOSE:	NOTES: cc=creatinine clearance /mL/min. RF=renal failure. cc^M=cc/1.73 m² body area
Cefaclor	250mg/8h PO Max: 4g/24h	Oral route. No dose change in RF
Cefadroxil	½–1g/12h PO	RF load with 1g, then: cc^M 26–50: 1g/12h;11–25: 1g/24h; 0–10: 1g/36h
Cefalexin	Minor infection: ½g/8h PO Max: 4g/24h PO	An oral cefalosporin. ↓dose proportionately in RF if cc<60. If cc<10: ½g/24h
Cefamandole	½–2g/4–8h IM or IV	Similar to cefuroxime. In RF load with 1–2g; then cc 50–80: ¾–2g/6h cc 25–50: ¾–2g/8h; 10–25: ½–1g/8h 2–10: ½–1g/12h; <2: ¼–¾g/12h
Cefazolin	Minor infection ½g/8–12h IM/IV	Less stable to β-lactamase than cefuroxime. In RF, load with ½–1g; then: cc 40–70: 250–1250mg/12h cc 20–40: 125–600mg/12h cc 5–20: 75–400mg/24h cc <5: 37.5–200mg/24h

*Our usage, and international nomenclature, uses an *f* not *ph* here. ③=3rd generation

Cefixime
Syrup=100mg/5mL
½–1yr 3.75mL/day
1–4yrs 5mL/day
5–10yrs 10mL/day
Adult dose:
200mg/12–24h PO

Active against streps, coliforms, *Proteus*, *Haemophilus* (eg β-lactam +ve), anaerobes, staphylococci, *E faecalis*, and *Pseudomonas* are resistant. Renal failure: normal dose if cc >20mL/min

Cefotaxime[Ⓡ]
1g/12h
IV/IM; max 4g/8h
(Gonorrhoea:
1g stat)

If cc <5, halve dose. Wide spectrum. Variable activity against *Pseudomonas*; not for *E faecalis*, *Bacteroides* or *Listeria*. For serious infections only (eg meningitis or pneumonia).

Cefoxitin
1–2g/6–8h
IV/IM
Max dose:
12g/24h

Active against *Bacteroides*, so useful in bowel surgery and pre-op. RF—cc: cc 30–50: 1–2g/8–12h; cc 5–9: ½–1g/12–24h; cc 10–29: 1–2g/12–24h; cc <5: ½–1g/24–48h

Cefradine
¼–½g/6h PO or
½–1g/12h PO or
½–2g/6h IM/IV

Less active than cefuroxime. In RF load with 750mg; then 500mg at frequency dictated by cc[M]: >20: 6–12h; 15–19: 12–24h; 10–14: 24–40h; 5–9: 40–50h; <5: 50–7

Ceftazidime[Ⓡ]
UTI: ½–1g/12h
Other: 1–2g/8h
Max: 2g/8h
Route: IV/IM

Wide spectrum, incl. most *Pseudomonas*, but not *E faecalis* or *Bacteroides*. For serious infections only. Also used in blind treatment of PUO in neutropenia. In RF: cc 31–50: 1g/12h; cc 6–15: 0.5g/24h; cc 16–30: 1g/24h; cc ≤5: 0.5g/48h

Ceftizoxime[Ⓡ]
UTI: ½–1g/12h
Other: 1–2g/8h
Max: 2.7g/8h
Route: IV/IM

Wide spectrum, poor against *Pseudomonas*, *E faecalis*, *Bacteroides*. For serious infections only. Used in hospital-acquired infections and aspiration pneumonia. In RF: cc 50–79: ½–1½g/8h; 5–49: ¼–1g/12h; ≤5: ½–1g/48h

Ceftriaxone[Ⓡ]
Many Gram –ve & +ve infections. Long t½
1–4g once daily IM/IVI
(give ≤1g at 1 IM site,
dilute with lignocaine
(=lidocaine) 1% 3.5mL
per g of ceftriaxone).
Gonorrhoea: ¼g stat IM.
Pre-colon surgery: 2g IM
+ agent against anaerobes.
Children: OHCS p248.

Can use in renal failure unless cc <10mL/min. Limit dose to 2g/day or less here; do levels, also do levels if on dialysis Used extensively in meningitis, p444 Activity is poorer against listeria, entero-cocci and *Pseudomonas aeruginosa*

Cefuroxime
¼–½g/12h PO
¾g/8h IM/IV
Severe: 1½g/8h
Max IV: 3g/8h
Max IM: ¾g/8h

Wide spectrum & good Gram –ve activity. Very useful in surgery for prophylaxis and post-op infections. In RF: cc 10–20: 750mg/12h; <10: 750mg/24h.

Neomycin: Some Gram +ve and many Gram ⊖ve.

Antibiotics: others

Antibiotic (and uses)	Adult dose	Notes (CC=creatinine clearance, mL/min)

Amikacin*
See gentamicin.

7.5mg/kg/12h IV; lower dose in renal failure)

Resistance is less common than with gentamicin.

Chloramphenicol Rarely used now as a first-line drug. May be used in typhoid fever and *Haemophilus* infection. Also in blind treatment of meningitis if *Haemophilus* could be cause. Avoid late in pregnancy and when breast feeding. Toxicity is overstated.

500mg/6h PO; 12.5mg/kg/6h IV (PO is the best route)

SE: marrow aplasia, neuritis; GI upset (all rare). ↓Dose in hepatic failure. Avoid if CC <10mL/min. Avoid long or repeated courses. Do FBC often. Interactions: warfarin, phenobarbitone, phenytoin, rifampicin, sulfonylureas.

Ciprofloxacin Used in adult cystic fibrosis, typhoid, and other enteric infections; *Campylobacter*, prostatitis, and serious multiple or resistant infections. Avoid overuse.

200–400mg/12h IVI over ½h or 250–750mg/12h PO; UTI: 250–500mg/12h PO

The only good oral anti-pseudomonal agent. Not good for S pneumoniae. ↓Dose by 50% if CC <20. β-lactamase resistant. It potentiates theophylline. SE: rashes, D&V, LFTs↑.

Clarithromycin A macrolide like erythromycin used for: *Staph aureus*, streps, *Myco-plasma, H pylori, chlamydia, Mycobacterium avium* (MAC in HIV p214).

250–500mg/12h PO for 7 days. MAC: may need 12 weeks (p214); *H pylori*: 500mg/12h PO for 2 weeks—see p490

½ dose if CC <30; interacts with ergot, warfarin, astemi-zole, terfenadine, carbemaze-pine, theophyllines, zido-udine, protease inhibitors. SE: D&V, glossitis; phlebitis.

Clindamycin Active against Gram +ve cocci including penicillin resist-ant Staph, and anaerobes.

150–300mg/6h PO or 0.2–0.9g/8h IV or IM

May cause pseudomembra-nous colitis (p486). Used in Staphylococcal bone and joint infections/peritonitis.

Co-trimoxazole Sulfameth-oxazole 400mg + trimetho-prim 80mg, ∴=480mg. Only first choice in pneumocystis (p334), toxoplasmosis and nocardia. ?2nd/3rd choice in some *Haemophilus* infections (eg in COPD, otitis media) and travellers' diarrhoea—only if 2 agents are *really* needed.NB: can act against *S aureus*. Use trimethoprim alone in UTI.

960mg/12h PO 960mg/12h IM/IV; higher in Pneumocystis see—p334).

SE: (elderly at ↑risk) jaundice; Stevens–Johnson sy; marrow depression; folate↓; Reduce dose in renal failure: if CC 15–25: halve the dose after 3 days. Avoid if CC <15, unless haemodialysis is available. CI: G6PD↓. Interactions: warfarin, phenytoin, sulfonylureas, methotrexate. Most SEs are due to sulfonamide.

Doxycycline Useful in travellers' diarrhoea, leptospirosis, and (with rifampicin) brucellosis.

200mg PO first day then 100mg/24h

As for tetracycline, but may be used in renal failure if necessary.

Erythromycin Similar to penicillin but spec-trum wider, so used in penicillin allergy. Good in pneumonia (esp. *Leg-ionella*); *Campylobacter* enteritis; mycoplasma; chlamydia—so a good drug in pelvic inflammatory disease. (OHCS p50).

250–500mg/6h PO (≤4g/day in Legionella). IVI dose: 6.25–12.5 mg/kg/6h (adult and child)

SE: D&V; painful phlebitis (IV route). Potentiates warfarin, theophylline, terfenadine, ergotamine, carbamazepine, cyclosporine (=ciclosporin). NB: estolate form is obso-lete; use lactobionate form IV and the stearate or 'phEur' enteric-coated pellets (Ery-max® 250mg capsules).

Fusidic acid Narrow-spec-rum anti-staph agent (inc. e MRSA, p222); helpful (in actice) in osteomyelitis.

500mg/8h PO; 500mg/8h IVI over 6h; avoid intravenous route if possible

Combine with another anti-Staph drug. SE: GI upset, reversible changes in LFTs.

Antibiotic (and uses):	Adult dose:	Notes
Gentamicin* Spectrum wide but <u>poor against strep-tococci and anaerobes</u>, so use with a penicillin and/or metronidazole. Synergy with ampicillin against Entero-coccus. For potentially seri-ous Gram −ve infections or prophylaxis in endocarditis.	0.7–1.7mg/kg/8h IV Load with 2mg/kg CC Dose example: 70 80mg/8h IV 50 80mg/12h IV 20 80mg/24h IV 10 80mg/48h IV <5 80mg/4 days after dialysis	▶See nomogram, p750. In ur-aemia, give usual loading dose then ↓frequency. Avoid: ●pro-longed use ●Concurrent frusem-ide/furosemide ●In pregnancy/ myasthenia gravis. SE: oto- and nephrotoxicity. Typical once-daily dose: 160mg/day (p750) in uncomplicated infection. Single stat dose for 'simple' infections: 5mg/kg then no more or review.
Imipenem (+cilastatin) Very broad spectrum: Gram +ve and −ve, anaerobes (incl-uding B fragilis) + aerobes. β-lactamase stable.	250mg/6h–1g/8h IVI CC Dose example: 31–70 500mg/6–8h 21–30 500mg/8–12h 5–20 250–500mg/12h	Avoid in pregnancy and lactation. SE: fits; D&V; myoclonus, eosinophilia, WCC↓, Coombs' +ve; LFTs abnormal.
Metronidazole Drug of choice against <u>anaerobes</u>, Gardnerella, Entamoeba histolytica, and Giardia. Also in pseudomembranous colitis—by PO route p486.	400mg/8h PO. PR dose: 1g/8h for 3 days then 1g/12h. IVI dose: 500mg/8h for ≤7 days	Disulfiram reaction with alcohol, interacts warfarin, phenytoin, cimetidine. CI: liver failure. Pregnancy and breast feeding: avoid high-dose regimens.
Minocycline Spectrum > tetracycline. 2nd line meningococcal prophylaxis.	100mg/12h PO	As for tetracycline, but more SE: vertigo, chronic active hep-atitis/eosinophilic pneumonitis.
Nalidixic acid Used only for UTIs. It is a non-fluorinated quinolone. Resistance rapidly develops.	1g/6h PO for 7 days, reducing to 500mg/6h PO If CC <20, avoid	SE: allergy; D&V; myalgia; weakness; phototoxicity; jaundice; fits; disturbed vision. Avoid if G6PD↓ and lactation; care in liver dis-ease; potentiates warfarin.
Netilmicin* Spectrum sim-ilar to gentamicin but less active against Pseudo-monas. Route: IM or IV.	2–3mg/kg/12h; max 7.5mg/kg/day (<48h) CC Max dose (IV): 80 2.0mg/kg/8h 50 1.37mg/kg/8h	SE: as for gentamicin, but less toxic; complete deafness unreported. Typical once a day UTI dose: 150mg/day.
Nitrofurantoin Used only for urinary tract infections.	50–100mg/6h PO with food	CI: CC <50; G6PD↓. SE: D&V, neuropathy, fibrosis.
Oxytetracycline	250–500mg/6h PO ac	See tetracycline.
RifampicinUK=**Rifampin**USA <u>Mycobacteria</u>, some Staphs (don't use alone), prophylaxis in some <u>meningitis</u> contacts.	450–600mg/24h PO ac	↓Dose in liver disease. Interferes with contra-ceptive pill. SE: p200.
Tetracycline Used in chronic bronchitis; first line in <u>Chlamydia, Lyme disease,</u> mycoplasma, brucellosis (in combination), rickettsia.	250–500mg/6h PO ac 500–1000mg/12h IVI (not if liver disease)	Avoid if <12 years old, in pregnancy, and if CC <50. Absorption↓ by iron, milk, and antacids. SE: photosensitivity, D&V.
Tobramycin* As gentamicin; <u>better against Pseudomonas</u>.	1–1.6mg/kg/8h IV Dose↓ in renal failure	?Less toxic than gentamicin. Once-daily dose: 2mg/kg/day.
Trimethoprim Use in UTI and in some COPD. Dose in prophylaxis: 100mg/24h PO.	200mg/12h PO 150–250mg/12h IV	SE: folate, marrow, depres-sion, D&V. Lower dose if CC <20.
Vancomycin* PO: pseudo-membranous colitis only if metronidazole is contraindi-cated; IV: <u>resistant Staph</u> and other <u>Gram +ve organisms</u> (not erysipelothrix species).	125mg/6h PO 500mg/6h IVI over 60mins or 1g/12h IVI over 100mins	CC dose/day CC dose/day 100 21mg/kg 10 2mg/kg 50 11mg/kg 5 1mg/kg SE: rashes and ototoxicity. Do not over use (↑risk of multi-ple resistance, p222).

⚕ 'Blind' treatment of infection

Follow hospital guidelines, if available, based on local microbiology and resistance patterns; change to the most appropriate agent once sensitivities are known. If in doubt, ask a microbiologist. For doses, see p176–81.

Infection	Likely cause	Blind treatment*
PUO See p186. (Only after very exhaustive investigation, it may be necessary to resort to a theraputic trial, guided by a detailed travel history	Tuberculosis	see p200
	Malaria, p196	quinine or chloroquine
	Enteric fever	ciprofloxacin
	Brucellosis	see p224
	Kala-azar	see p242
	Endocarditis	see below
	??	anti-TB drugs
Septicaemia (no clues)	??	cefuroxime+gentamicin
Septicaemia (abdomen or pelvis)	Gram −ve or anaerobes, + enterococcus	ampicillin + metronidazole + gentamicin
Septicaemia if immunocompromised eg neutropenic/post-transplant ►See *neutropenic regimen*, p598	*Pseudomonas*	ceftazidime ± metronidazole +gentamicin OR piperacillin+gentamicin
Septicaemia from a UTI	Coliforms	cefuroxime+gentamicin
Septicaemia with a purpuric rash	*Meningococcus* rarely *Pneumococcus** or other bacteria	benzylpenicillin (high-dose)+ cefotaxime
Septicaemia from skin or bone	Gram +ve organisms	benzylpenicillin + flucloxacillin
Meningitis (p444)	*Meningococcus* *Pneumococcus** *Haemophilus* *Listeria* (cover for this if old or immunosuppressed)	high-dose benzyl-penicillin+ceftriaxone or cefotaxime ampicillin
Pneumonia	See p332–7	
Osteomyelitis/ Septic arthritis	*Staph aureus* *Pseudomonas*	flucloxacillin ciprofloxacin
Endocarditis (p312)	Streptococci	high-dose benzylpen-icillin or ampicillin + gentamicin
Endocarditis (on prosthetic valves, get expert help)	*Staph epidermis* Streptococci	vancomycin + gentamicin ± rifampicin
Cellulitis (PLATE 6)	Streptococci	flucloxacillin ± benzylpenicillin
UTI	Coliforms	trimethoprim

Tests: ►Microscope urine yourself (p370). If possible, culture before treating. 3 sets of blood cultures, swabs, MSU, faeces pathogens, sputum culture, and immediate Gram stain, CXR, serum for virology. FBC, ESR, U&E, ͚ood gases, coagulation studies.

͚ *sis:* Bad if: very old or young, BP↓, WCC↓, P_aO_2↓, DIC, hypothermia.

͚ ocation where pneumococcal resistance to penicillin is a problem, include vancomycin.

Using a side-room laboratory

Any side room with a sink and power point may be suitable to convert into your lab. Your repertoire of techniques will grow as your patients present you with material. This enables you to have intelligent conversations with lab staff, and, with experience, may obviate the need to call them at night. It gives you a feel for the limitations of a given technique, and keeps you in touch with fluids and tissues.

Blood Adhere to local policies for specimens that could be HBsAg or HIV +ve. Watch a technician make a good blood film, then try yourself. First allow the film to dry, then stain as follows. Cover with 10 drops of Leishman's stain. (Leishman's stain is most beautiful—almost however tired you are, its bright and subtle shades will lift your spirits.) After 30sec add 20 drops of water. Leave for 15mins. Pick up the slide with forceps (to avoid purple fingers) and rinse in fast-flowing tap water—for 1 sec only. Allow to dry. Now examine under oil immersion. Note red cell morphology. Do a differential white count. Polymorphs have lobed nuclei. Lymphocytes are small (just larger than red cells) and round, having little cytoplasm. Monocytes are larger than lymphocytes, but similar, with kidney-shaped nuclei. Eosinophils are like polymorphs, but have prominent pink-red cytoplasmic granules. Basophils are rare, and have blue granules. Learn to use a white cell counting chamber—don't expect this to be as accurate as electronic methods.

Malaria: See p194. Many clinicians working in the UK are unlikely to gain enough experience, but, for those using this book in the tropics, with ready access to enough material to 'get their eye in' with regular practice with this capricious protazoon, Field's stain is easy to use and gives the best results. It also will allow detection of trypanosomiasis and filaria. Dip a thick film in solution A for 5sec and B for 3sec. Dip in tap water for 5sec after each staining. Stand to dry. Examine the film for at least 5mins before saying that it is negative.

Pus (Gram stain) Make a smear and fix by gentle heat. Flood the slide with cresyl violet for 30 sec. Wash in running water. Flood with Lugol's iodine for 30sec. Wash again with running water. Decolorize with acetone for 1–3sec until no blue colour runs out. Over-zealous decolorization may mislead. Counterstain for 30sec with neutral red or safranin. Wash again, and dry. Gram +ve organisms appear blue-black, and Gram –ve ones look red, but are easier to miss.

Aspirates (eg ascites) and CSF require too much skill for the amateur.

Urine should be examined under the microscope as described on p370. Dipstick analysis should also be performed.

Near-patient biochemistry[1] In one sense this is less taxing than the above tests—all the skill has been concentrated in making the reagents and test-strips easy to use. But a very real problem is quality control and the black box effect: when you put a strip into a machine, eg to measure cardiac enzymes, you cannot observe the workings of the black box—it simply produces a deceptively accurate-looking figure. With haematology, you can see that your stain is poor, and should be discarded. Frequent calibration of biochemical equipment is only a partial answer to this, and it is only after you have spent a long time trying to get good results from near-patient analysers, and comparing paired samples with the lab, that one really appreciates the reproducability, and almost 100% reliability of the formal laboratory. ►Speed of reporting is useless if you cannot trust the results.[2]

1 Assoc^n Clin. Biochem. (London WIV OBN) & Roy Col Path 1993 *Guidelines for Implementation of Near-Patient Testing (NPT)* 2 F Hobbs 1997 *Review of NPT in Primary Care*, Health Technology Assessment 1 5

Drug abuse and infectious diseases See PLATE 2

►Always consider this when there are unexplained findings, especially in younger patients. Ask direct questions: 'Do you use any drugs? Have you ever injected any drug? Does your partner use any drugs? Do you share needles? Have you ever had a HIV test? How do you finance your drugs (eg male or female prostitution)? Ever in prison?' List drugs used, and prescribed drugs, with names of prescriber. Behavioural clues:
- 'Just passing through your area . . . I just need some pethidine for my renal colic.' Evasive answers. Temporary resident seen by GP.
- Erratic behaviour on the ward; unexplained absences; mood swings.
- Unrousable in the mornings; agitation from day 2; petty theft.
- Demands analgesia/anti-emetics (cyclizine). Knows pharmacopoeia well.
- Heavy smoking; strange smoke smells (cannabis, cocaine, heroin).

Physical clues: • Acetone or glue smell on breath (solvent abuse).
- Small pupils (opiates) enlarging on day 2 if no narcotics supplied.
- Needle tracks on arms, groin, legs, between toes (PLATE 2); IV access hard.
- Abscesses and lymphadenopathy in nodes draining injection sites.
- Signs of drug associated illnesses (eg endocarditis, p312; AIDS, p214).
- Odd tattoos: eg over veins; dots around the neck; self-harm signs (eg cigarette burns, wrist lacerations); scars from accidents or violence.

Common and possible presentations in drug abusers

Unconscious (see p762)	Narcotics (naloxone, p794), barbiturates, solvents, benzodiazepines (if in ITU consider flumazenil 0.2mg IV over 15sec then 0.1mg/min as needed, to 2mg).
Psychosis or agitation	Ecstasy (p795), LSD, amphetamine, anabolic steroids, benzodiazepines. Haloperidol may help (p13).
Asthma/dyspnoea	Is there opiate-induced pulmonary oedema? Note: asthma may follow the smoking of heroin.
Lung abscess	Right-sided endocarditis (Staph) until proved other.
Fever/PUO	Is it endocarditis, eg with no cardinal signs (p312)?
Shivering & headache	After a 'bad hit' (chemical/organism contamination). Do blood cultures; start eg gentamicin (p180 & 750).
Hyperpyrexia	Ecstasy (p795). Beware myoglobinuria, DIC, renal failure.
Abscesses	If over injection site, then often of mixed organisms.
DVT (p92)	Eg on injecting suspended tablets into groin. Is there compression damage (compartment syndrome)? Do CK.
Pneumonia	Pneumococcus, haemophilus, TB, pneumocystis.
Tachyarrhythmia	(If young); cocaine, amphetamines, endocarditis.
Jaundice	Hepatitis B, C, or D; anabolic steroids (cholestasis).
'Glandular fever'	May be presentation of HIV seroconversion illness.
Osteomyelitis	Including spinal. Staph aureus/Gram −ve organisms.
Constipation	If severe, opiate abuse may be the cause.
Blindness	Consider fungal ophthalmitis ± endocarditis.
Runny nose	Opiate withdrawal (+colic/diarrhoea, yawns, lacrimation, dilated pupils, insomnia, piloerection, myalgia, mood↓); cocaine use.
Neuropathies	(And any odd CNS signs) Consider solvent abuse.
Infarctions	(eg of spinal cord, brain, heart): suspect cocaine use.

General management A non-judgmental approach will produce better co-operation and may avoid self-discharge. Establish firm rules of acceptable ward behaviour. NSAIDs are useful for pain relief. Do not prescribe benzodiazepines or chlormethiazole (=clormethiazole).

Commercial sex workers need STD screen, speculum exam (OHCS p2), ~d cervical cytology as carcinoma *in situ* is common (OHCS p35). Screen ~epatitis B (vaccination, p513, use gloves); safe sex and safe injection . HIV testing (p212). ►Liaise with community teams. See OHCS p362.

The vocabulary of drug abusers[1]

The first step in helping a drug abuser is to communicate. To understand what he or she is telling you, the following may be helpful.

Amphetamines	Speed; whiz; Billy; pink champagne
Amyl-nitrate	Goldrush; poppers; snappers
Barbiturates	Barbs; idiot pills
Cocaine	Coke; Charlie; uncle; the white; the nice; snow
(free base)	Rock; crack; nuggets; wash; gravel
Dihydrocodeine	Dfs
Drug-induced sleep	Gauching; nodding; going on the nod
Drug intoxication	Stoned; off it; bladdered; ripped; wiped out
Heroin (± cocaine)	Smack; the nasty; gear; brown; scag; hit; Harry
Ecstasy (MMDA)	E; X; echo; disco biscuit; love drug; XTC
Febrile reaction	Bad hit
Filter	A bud (usually a cigarette tip, through which drugs are drawn before being injected).
Injecting	Hitting up; jacking up; cranking; having a dig
subcutaneous	Skin popping
IM	Muscle popping
subclavian	Pocket shot
failed	Miss
LSD	Acid; trips; cardboard; tabs
Marijuana	Weed; pot; draw; ganja; grass; resin; Mary; hash
Methadone	Mud
Needles	Spikes; nails
Obtaining drugs	Score (selling drugs=deal)
PCP	Angel dust; KJ; ozone; missile
Physeptone ampoules	Amps
Prostitution	Working the block/square; doing business; on the game; on the batter; flogging ones golly.
Prostitute's client	Mush; punter
Shoplifting	Grafting
Smoking cocaine	Bonging
Smoking heroin	Chasing the dragon
Syringes	Works; tools (barrel of a syringe=gun)
Temazepam	Temazies; eggs; jellies (fluid-filled capsules)
Tourniquet	Key
Wanted by police	'On me toes'; keeping head down
White heroin	China white
Withdrawing from opiates	Turkeying, clucking
Zopiclone	zim-zims

1 D Stockley 1992 *Drug Warning*, Optima Books, London

Pyrexia of unknown origin (PUO)

Contrary to Gustave Flaubert, most fevers are not caused by plums, melons, April sunshine, etc,[1] but by self-limiting viral infections; here fever may be quite helpful, enhancing neutrophil migration and secretion of antibacterials and cytokines, increasing production and activity of interferon, and T-cell proliferation. Prolonged fever (>3 weeks) which has resisted diagnosis after a week in hospital constitutes a PUO, and requires thorough investigation in order to 'resolve the enigma of the fever chart'. Predictors of bacteraemia include confusion, renal failure, neutrophilia, ↓plasma albumin[1] and ↑CRP (acute phase response, p650).

Causes[2] Infection (23%); multisystem diseases, eg connective tissue diseases (22%); tumours (7%); drug fever (3%); miscellaneous diseases (14%); it is often impossible to reach a diagnosis (25% in this series).

- ●**Infections** Abscesses (subphrenic, perinephric, pelvic); TB (CXR may be normal—take any opportunity to culture any body fluid for AFBs); other granulomata (eg actinomycosis, toxoplasmosis); parasites (eg amoebic liver abscess, malaria—including 'baggage' malaria, p188); bacteria (brucella, salmonella); rheumatic fever; endocarditis (p312, may be culture –ve, eg Q fever); *Chlamydia psittaci*; fungi; HIV;and other viruses.

- ●**Neoplasms** Especially *lymphomas* (any temperature pattern: the Pel–Ebstein fever, p606, is rare). Occasionally *solid tumours* (especially GI and renal cell carcinoma). Frequently, the patient does not feel hot during fevers. The fever associated with *leukaemia* is usually infective.

- ●**Connective tissue disease** SLE, PAN, cranial arteritis, polymyalgia rheumatica, rheumatoid arthritis, Still's disease.

- ●**Others** Drugs (may be months after starting drug, but fever drops within days of stopping; look for eosinophilia); rheumatic fever; sarcoid; pulmonary emboli; Crohn's/UC; intracranial pathology; familial Mediterranean fever (genetic recurrent polyserositis with intermittent fever, abdominal pain, pleurisy and arthritis; treat with colchicine); factitious.

Examples of intermittent fevers SBE; TB; filarial fever; amyloid; brucella. *Daily fever spikes:* Abscess; malaria; schistosomiasis; *Saddleback fever (eg fever for 7d, then ↔ for 3d):* Colorado tick fever; *borrelia; leptospira;* dengue; ehrlichia[3] (p236). *Longer periodicity:* Pel–Ebstein (p606). *Remitting (diurnal variation, not dipping to normal):* Amoebiasis; malaria; salmonella; Kawasaki disease; CMV.

History Note especially sexual history, IV drug abuse, immunosuppressive illness, foreign or distant travel (►see p188), animal (or people) contacts, bites, cuts, surgery, rashes, mild diarrhoea, drugs (including non-prescription), immunization, sweats, weight↓, lumps, and itching.

Examination Remember teeth, rectal/vaginal exams, skin lesions, lymphadenopathy, hepatosplenomegaly (p152), nails, joints, temporal arteries.

Tests *Stage 1 (the first days):* FBC, ESR, U&E, LFTs, CRP, WBC differential, blood cultures (several, from different veins, at different times of day—prolonged culture may be needed for *brucella*); baseline serum for virology, sputum microscopy and culture (specifying also for TB); urine dipstick, microscopy and culture stool for microscopy (ova, cysts, and parasites); CXR. If very ill, consider blind treatment as in septicaemia (p182).
Stage 2: Repeat history and examination every day. Protein electrophoresis, CT (chest, abdomen). Rheumatoid factor, ANA, anti-streptolysin titre, Mantoux, ECG, bone marrow, lumbar puncture. Consider PSA, carcionembryonic antigen, and withholding drugs, one at a time for 48h each. Consider temporal artery biopsy (p674). HIV test cousnselling.
Stage 3: Follow any leads uncovered. Consider echocardiography. Further isvestigate the abdomen (eg indium-labelled white cell scan) CT, arium studies, IVU, liver biopsy, exploratory laparotomy. ?Bronchoscopy.
Stage 4: ?Treat for TB, endocarditis, vasculitis, or trial of aspirin/steroids.

ert 1913 *Dictionary of Received Ideas* ISBN 014-03-8904-0   2 PH Chandrasekar 1994 *Arch Int* 1–9 3 H Horowitz 1998 *Lancet* **351** 650. *See also* D Knockaert 1992 *Arch Int Med* **152** 51–5

⁝⁝⁝ Diagnosing the tropical traveller

Tropical medicine centres *UK phone numbers:* Glasgow 0141 946 7120, Liverpool 0151 708 9393, London 0171 636 8636. *USA:* 770-488-4086.

188

In every ill traveller consider:

1 *Malaria* (p194–p196): The best way to exclude this is for an expert to examine thick films (p183). Very prolonged microscopy may be needed with thin films. Note: the tropical traveller can sometimes be mosquitoes, not the patient—they may stowaway in luggage causing malaria in non-tropical destinations.[1]

2 *Typhoid* (p228): Fever, relative bradycardia, abdominal pains, dry cough, and constipation are suggestive; an enlarged spleen and rose spots more so. Diagnose by blood or bone marrow culture.

3 *Amoebic liver abscess* (p238). 4 *Dengue fever* (p234).

Jaundice Think of malaria, viral hepatitis, leptospirosis, yellow fever, typhoid, liver abscess, thalassaemia, sickle-cell disease, dengue fever, alcohol, G6PD deficiency. Look for anaemia.

Hepatosplenomegaly See p152. Malaria, brucella, schistosomiasis, typhoid.

Gross splenomegaly Malaria, kala-azar, also chronic myeloid leukaemia.

Diarrhoea & vomiting (p190 & p486) Examine fresh stool. *E coli* commonest (toxin-producing). Consider *Salmonella, Shigella, Campylobacter, Cholera, Giardia* and *E histolytica*. Also *Vibrio parahaemolyticus, Staph aureus, Clostridium perfringens, Plesiomonas*. Remember pathogens which need special stains for identification: cyclospora and cryptosporidia.

Erythema nodosum TB, leprosy, fungi, sulfonamides, sarcoid. Also UC, Crohn's, post-streptococcal, the Pill and other drugs, pregnancy.▣

Anaemia Malaria, hookworm, kala-azar, malabsorption.

Skin lesions Onchocerciasis (itchy nodules), scabies (itchy allergic rash + burrows, eg in finger web-spaces; it's a common disease *anywhere*, see p220 & *OHCS* p600), leprosy (ulcers, depigmented areas, insensitive areas), tropical ulcers, typhus ('eschar' = scab), leishmaniasis (ulcers/nodules).

Acute abdomen Sickle-cell crisis, ruptured spleen, perforation of a typhoid ulcer, toxic megacolon in amoebic or bacillary dysentery.

Rarities to consider ►Use local emergency isolation policy.
- *Yellow fever* (p234) Antibodies appear in the second week.
- *Lassa fever:* Suspect in rural travellers from Nigeria, Sierra Leone, or Liberia, presenting with fever, sore throat (exudative), facial oedema, and prostration. Diagnosis: EM, serology. Isolate and refer. ▣
- *Marburg and Ebola virus:* Fever, myalgia, D&V, knife-like pleuritic pain, hepatitis, shock, and bleeding tendency. (Sudan, Zaire, Kenya). On white skins, a maculopapular rash appears on day 5–7 (lasts <5 days before desquamation). Patients may bleed from all orifices and gums.[2] From known incubation periods it is possible to exclude Ebola, Marburg and Lassa fever if the patient fell ill >3 weeks after leaving Africa.
- *Viruses causing haemorrhage:* Eg haemorrhagic fever with renal syndrome (HFRS, eg with oliguria), Crimea-Congo haemorrhagic fever.
- *Rabies* (p234). • *Viral encephalitis.*

The world is big: ultimately only experts have the geographical knowledge necessary to construct a differential diagnosis, and to know local drug resistances. Even within one region risks vary. The urban visitor is less risk than the intrepid hiker. The details of the travel history are important, even if you cannot interpret them yourself.

1993 *Tr Roy Soc Trop Med Hyg* **87** 394   2 DI Simpson 1995 *Lancet* **345** 1252

Gastroenteritis

The ingestion of certain bacteria, viruses and toxins (bacterial and chemical) is a common cause of diarrhoea and vomiting (p60, p486). Contaminated food and water are common sources, but often the specific origin is never identified. The history should include details of food and water taken, how it was cooked, time until onset of symptoms, and whether fellow-diners were affected. The food eaten, incubation period, and clinical picture give clues as to the causative organism. Note: food poisoning is a notifiable disease in the UK (p171).

Organism/Source	Incubation	Symptoms	Food
Staph aureus	1–6h	D&V, P, hypotension	Meat
B cereus (emetic)	1–5h	D&V	Rice
Red beans	1–3h	D&V	
Heavy metals, eg zinc	5 mins–2h	V, P; with zinc, (delayed fever ±flu-like features after a weekend away from exposure at work: 'Monday morning fever', OTM 2e p1114)	
Scombrotoxin (from fish)	10–60 mins	D, flushing, sweating erythema, hot mouth	Fish
Mushrooms	15min–24h	D&V, P, fits, coma, renal and liver failure	
Salmonella	12–48h	D&V, P, T°↑, septi-caemia+local infections	Meat, eggs, poultry
Clostridium perfringens	8–24h	D, P, no fever	Meat
Clostridium botulinum	12–36h	V, paralysis	Processed food
V parahaemolyticus	12–24h	Profuse D; P, V	Seafood
Campylobacter	2–5 days	bloody D, P, T°↑	Milk, water*
Listeria		Meningoencephalitis, 'flu-like symptoms, miscarriages	Soft cheese pâtés
Small round structured viruses	36–72h	D&V, T°↑, malaise—	Any food
E coli	12–72h	like cholera or dysentery;*	Some bred in
type *0157*, has toxins causing haemolytic–uraemic syndrome, p397			abattoirs
Y enterocolitica	24–36h	D, P, T°↑	Milk*
Cryptosporidium	4–12 days		Cattle→water→man
Giardia lamblia	1–4 weeks	See p238	Water*
Entamoeba histolytica	1–4 weeks	See p238	*
Rotavirus	1–7 days	D&V, T°↑, malaise	*
Shigella	2–3 days	bloody D, P, T°↑	Any food

v=vomiting; D=diarrhoea; P=abdominal pain; T°↑ =fever; *May be food- or water-borne.

Tests *Stool microscopy and culture (p487) if:* patient has been abroad, is from an institution or at day care, or an outbreak is suspected. In these circumstances, culture of the food source is also useful, hence the value of early notification of the local Public Health doctor.

Prevention Basic hygiene; longer cooking and rewarming times (to a core T° ≥70°C for ≥2mins) with prompt consumption.

Management None is usually needed. Give fluids PO (Rehidrat® oral rehydration sachets help replace salt and water). Give *anti-emetic* (eg prochlorperazine 12.5mg/6h IM) and antidiarrhoeal (codeine 30mg PO/IM) only for *severe* symptoms (but not in dysentery). Give antibiotics in:
- Cholera: tetracycline reduces transmission.
- Salmonella bacteraemia: ciprofloxacin 200–400mg/12h IV.
- Severe shigella infection: ciprofloxacin 500mg/12h PO.
- Severe campylobacter: ciprofloxacin or erythromycin ¼–½g/6h PO.
- Traveller's diarrhoea: use ciprofloxacin (500mg/12h PO × 3–5d; one tablet be adequate) + loperamide, eg 4mg stat then 2mg after each stool. other antibiotics may be more appropriate; check sensitivities.

✝ Immunization

Active immunization usually stimulates antibody production. BCG stimulates native cell-mediated immunity. *Passive immunization* provides preformed antibody (nonspecific or antigen-specific). ▣

Immunizations The new UK DoH schedule[1] (L=live vaccine)

3 days	BCG[L] (if TB in family in last 6 months). See below.
	Hepatitis B vaccine if mother is HBsAg +ve. See *OHCS* p208.
2 months	**'Triple'** (pertussis, tetanus, diphtheria) 0.5mL SC;
	HiB=*Haemophilus influenzae type b, OHCS* p209; oral **polio**[L].
	Note: If premature still give at 2 postnatal months.
3 months	Repeat **'triple'**, HiB and **polio**[L].
4 months	Repeat **'triple'**, HiB and **polio**[L].
12–18 months	**Measles/Mumps/Rubella**[L] (MMR$_{II}$® vaccine): 0.5mL SC.
4–5 years	**Tetanus, diphtheria & polio**[L] booster. MMR$_{II}$® dose 2.
10–14 years	BCG[L]. (Also Rubella[L] for girls who have missed MMR$_{II}$®)
15–18 years	**Polio**[L]+Tetanus+low-dose **Diphtheria 'Td'** booster. ▣
~65 years	? a last one-off **Tetanus** booster[1] ± Pneumovax II if indicated (p332; consider yearly **'flu vaccine** (p206).

▶*An acute febrile illness is a contraindication to any vaccine.* Give live vaccines either together, or separated by ≥3 weeks. Do not give live vaccines if there is a *primary* immunodeficiency disorder, or if taking steroids (>60mg/day prednisolone, >2mg/kg/day if a child), or from 3 weeks before to 3 months after injection of human normal immunoglobulin. *HIV infection and AIDS:* (*OHCS* p217; avoid BCG in areas where TB prevalence is low). ▶*Contraindications to vaccines are given in OHCS p208.*

BCG (bacille Calmette–Guérin) Live attenuated anti-TB vaccine (effective in up to 80% subjects for ~10yrs). If TB is rife, or if past TB in family in the last 6 months, give BCG (*intradermally*—0.05mL for neonates; 0.1mL if older). Make a 7mm blanched wheal (for volumes of ~0.1mL) between the top and middle thirds of the arm (deltoid's insertion) or, for cosmetic reasons, the upper, outer thigh. Use a short needle with a short bevel. Expect to feel marked resistance as the injection is given. If, during the injection, propagation of the wheal stops, the vaccine is going too deep: re-insert. A swelling appears after 2–6 weeks, developing into a papule or small ulcer. Avoid air-occluding dressings (air access helps). SE: pain, local abscess. CI: pyrexia, oral steroids (not inhaled), sepsis or eczema at vaccination site, immune pareses (eg HIV, malignancy).

Mantoux test (p200) Offered (in UK) to those at risk of TB (eg TB contacts, health workers) and those 10–13yrs, to find those needing BCG.

Travel immunization ▶See p175. Take expert advice (Liverpool School of Tropical Medicine, UK tel. 0151 708 9393).[2] Agents available: *Yellow fever* (single dose) gives immunity after 10 days for 10yrs. *Monovalent (whole cell) typhoid*, or oral form (p175). *Cholera* vaccine (p228). *Polio* booster or course if not previously vaccinated. Consider also *tetanus, diphtheria, rabies, human immunoglobulin/Hepatitis A vaccine*.

Advice to travellers is more important than vaccination: eg malaria prophylaxis, simple hygiene, and protective techniques (eg avoiding insect bites). Remember to advise about safe sex.

Other vaccines Hepatitis B, p513; anthrax; botulism; influenza; pneumococcal (p332); meningococcal (group A & C); rabies; Japanese encephalitis.

~ization *Against Infectious Disease,* DoH, 1996; note: the 65-yr tetanus booster is *not*
~e, but is reckoned to be cost-effective ($4527/life saved *vs* $8000/life saved for
~n screening—see C Bowman 1996 *Lancet* 348 1664) 2 *Drug Ther Bul* 1993 31 11

Plasmodium protozoa, injected by anopheles mosquitoes (~20 sporo-zoites/bite), multiply in RBCs (>10^{11} trophozoite ring forms per infection) so causing haemolysis, RBC stasis, and cytokine release. *Protective factors:*[1]

Sickle-cell trait; HLA-B53 +ve, found in many non-Europeans, enabling killing of parasite-infected hepatocytes by cytotoxic T lymphocytes.

P falciparum malaria Incubation: ~7–14 days (up to 1yr if semi-immune or after prophylaxis). Most travellers present within 2 months. After a prodrome of headache, malaise, myalgia, and anorexia, there may be paroxysms lasting 8–12h: sudden coldness, a severe rigor for up to 1h, then high fever, flushing, vomiting, and drenching sweats. ►Classical tertian and subtertian periodicity (paroxysms separated by 48 and 36h) are quite rare; daily (quotidian) or irregular paroxysms are commoner. Signs: anaemia, jaundice, and hepatosplenomegaly without lymph-adenopathy or rash. There are no relapses after successful cure.

Complications: Cerebral malaria (Mortality: 20%; 80% of deaths.) Signs: psychosis; fits; apnoea/hyperventilation; coma; tone & reflexes↑; extensor posture; upgoing plantars; nystagmus; dysconjugate gaze; teeth-grinding; papilloedema; flaccidity. ►Exclude hypoglycaemia/meningitis.

Hypoglycaemia occurs especially in severe malaria, pregnancy, or with quinine therapy. There may be extensor posturing and oculogyric crises.

Acute renal failure from BP↓ or haemoglobinuria ('blackwater fever').

Pulmonary oedema from over-rehydration, uraemia or, ARDS (see p350).

'Algid' malaria is the complex of shock complicating a serious manifestation of malarial infection, eg pulmonary oedema, acidosis, or bacterial infection. ►Also consider splenic rupture.

In pregnancy: Risk of death (mother or fetus) is high: ►see *OHCS* p159. Use chemoprophylaxis in pregnant women in areas of transmission.

Other severe signs: Anaemia, DIC, T°≥42°C, jaundice, parasitaemia >2%.

Benign malaria has a very low mortality although the acute illness is very similar to that of *falciparum* malaria. Incubation periods are longer: *P ovale,* 15–18 days; *P vivax,* 12–17 days; *P malariae,* 18–40 days; 5–10% of *malariae* malaria presents over 1 year after infection. Benign tertian malaria is caused by *P vivax* or *P ovale:* fever occurs every 3rd day (ie days 1, 3, 5, etc). Benign quartan malaria is caused by *P malariae:* fever recurs every 4th day (ie days 1, 4, 7, etc), but fever regularity is often not seen early in the infection. Relapse occurs as parasites lie dormant in the liver (*P vivax* and *ovale*) or blood (*P malariae*). *Complications:* Nephrotic syndrome (glomerulonephritis) occurs in chronic *P malariae* infection.

Diagnosis Repeated thin & thick film microscopy. In partially treated patients, examine bone marrow smears if blood smears are –ve. Serology is only helpful epidemiologically. *Other tests:* FBC (anaemia, WCC often normal), platelets (usually low), glucose, U&E (hyponatraemia, uraemia), urinalysis, blood culture. Always ask yourself: Have I excluded *falciparum?* If it is falciparum, what is the level of parasitaemia?

Poor prognostic signs (*falciparum*) Age <3yrs or pregnant; deep coma, fits, no corneal reflex, decerebrate rigidity, retinal haemorrhage, lung oedema, blood glucose <2.2mmol/L, hyperparasitaemia (>5% of RBCs or 250,000/µl), WCC >12 × 10^9/L, Hb <7g/dL, DIC, creatinine >265µmol/L, lactic acid↑ (>6mmol/L CSF or plasma), plasma 5'-NT↑, antithrombin III↓.[2] >20% (or >10^4/µL) of parasites are mature trophozoites or schizonts, prognosis is bad, even if few parasites seen (reflects critical mass of ...ered RBCs[3]); also finding malaria pigment in >5% of neutrophils.[4]

5 *Lancet* 345 1003 2 H Gilles 1991 *Management of Severe & Complicated Malaria,* WHO 93 *Tr Roy Soc Trop Med Hyg* 87 436 & 1996 335 800 4 N Phu 1995 *Tr R Soc Trop M Hy* 89 200

⋔ Malaria: pitfalls, treatment, and prophylaxis[1]

Treatment ▶If species unknown or mixed infection treat as *P falciparum*. ▶Nearly all *P falciparum* are now resistant to chloroquine—treat with quinine unless chloroquine-sensitive for sure. ●Chloroquine is the drug of choice for benign malarias (p194) in most parts of the world—but chloroquine-resistant *P vivax* occurs in Papua New Guinea, Indonesia, Brazil, Colombia and Guyana.[1] ●Never rely on chloroquine if used as prophylaxis.

Falciparum malaria: If can swallow and no complications (p194) give 600mg quinine salt/8h po for 7 days; then Fansidar® (pyrimethamine + sulfadoxine) 3 tabs stat, or if Fansidar®-resistance could be a problem, give tetracycline 250mg/6h for 7 days with quinine. *Alternative:* Malarone® (atovaquone + proguanil; 4 tabs once daily for 3 days with food⬛). If seriously ill, take to ITU, give quinine salt 20mg/kg (max 1.4g) IV over 4h, then after 8–12h give 10mg/kg (max 700mg) over 4h every 8–12h.   Give IV until can swallow and complete oral course. Use Fansidar®/tetracycline as above. Correct for hydrochloride/dihydrochloride/sulfate, but bisulfate has less quinine.[2]

Benign malarias: Give chloroquine po as 600mg base, 300mg 8h, later then 300mg/24h for 2 days.[2] Primaquine 15mg/24h for 14 days (21 days if Chesson strain from SE Asia/west Pacific) after chloroquine if *vivax/ovale* to destroy liver phase and prevent relapse (screen for G6PD deficiency first).

Other treatment: Tepid sponging + paracetamol for fever. Transfuse if severe anaemia. Consider exchange transfusion if parasitaemia >10% and patient deteriorating. If cerebral malaria give prophylactic phenobarbitone (=phenobarbital) 3.5mg/kg IM: avoid steroids and osmotic diuretics. Treat 'algid' malaria as malaria + bacterial shock (p766).

Monitor TPR, BP, urine output, blood glucose frequently. Daily parasite count, platelets, U&E, plasma creatinine, and bilirubin.

Prophylaxis[3] ●Prophylaxis doesn't give full protection. Try to reduce bites (nets; repellents; long-sleeved clothes in evening—the mosquito biting time). ●Take drugs from 3 weeks before travel (to reveal any SE) to 4 weeks after return. ●None required if just visiting cities of Hong Kong, Thailand or Singapore. ●There is no good protection for parts of SE Asia.[2]

Drug examples: Low-risk areas (eg N Africa, Middle East, Central and parts of S America): chloroquine base 300mg/week po + proguanil 200mg/24h po. Folate supplements with proguanil if pregnant.

High-risk: Sub-Saharan Africa, Indonesia (not Bali), Laos, Vietnam, rural China, Myanmar (Burma), rural Philippines, Cambodia: mefloquine (1 tab/wk for adults *with no risk of pregnancy*; or in W Cambodia, Thailand, Papua New Guinea, and Solomons, doxycycline 100mg/24h po). If poor medical care and not pregnant, also carry treatment course: eg Fansidar® 3 tab stat (or mefloquine 15mg/kg, max 2 tab of 250mg each repeated at 6h).[3]

Side-effects: Chloroquine: Headache, D&V, psychosis, retinopathy (chronic use). *Fansidar®:* Stevens–Johnson syndrome, haemopoiesis↓.

Primaquine: Haemolysis if G6PD (test blood first), methaemoglobinaemia.

Mefloquine: D&V, dizziness, fits, neuropsychiatric signs (can be terrible), long t½; avoid if: ●Low risk of highly-chloroquine-resistant malaria, eg 2 week trip to East African coast resorts[2] ●Past or family history of epilepsy, psychosis ●Delicate tasks need performing (eg pilots) ●Risk of pregnancy within 3mths of last dose. Consider a pre-travel test-dose. Interaction: quinidine.

Children: Chloroquine & proguanil: to 5 weeks old, ⅛ adult dose; 6–52 weeks, ¼; 1–5yrs old, ½; 6–11yrs, ¾; then full dose. *Fansidar®:* avoid below 6 weeks; to 4yrs, ¼ adult dose; to 8yrs, ½ to 14yrs, ¾; then full dose. NB: due to resistance patterns, proguanil + atovaquone may have a rôle.[4]

Mefloquine—weekly dose: If under 15kg, not recommended. 15–19kg: ▪ a tablet. 20–30kg: ½ a tablet. 31–45kg: ¾ of a tablet. >45kg: 1 tablet. ⟂t dose to 3 months; see warnings above.

⟂ help: *tel* 0151 7089393 2 150mg chloroquine base = 250mg chloroquine phosphate (PO) ⟂hloroquine sulfate (IV). 3 PHLS 1997 *Com Dis Rep Rev* 7:R 137 4 B Lell 1998 *Lancet* 351 709

Pitfalls in managing malaria patients

- Belief that drugs will work, whereas the parasite is often one step ahead.
- Failing to take a full travel history, including stop-overs in transit.
- Relying on regular fever or splenomegaly to make the diagnosis.
- Not examining enough thick & thin films before saying 'it's not malaria'.
- Delay while seeking lab confirmation. ►►Prompt action saves lives.
- Giving an inappropriate quinine loading dose, if he's already had quinine.
- Not having ıv quinine immediately available (here quinidine gluconate is an alternative, eg a loading dose of 10mg/kg over 1–4h then 0.02mg/kg/min ıvı by pump for 72h or until the patient can swallow).
- Not observing falciparum patients closely for the first few days.

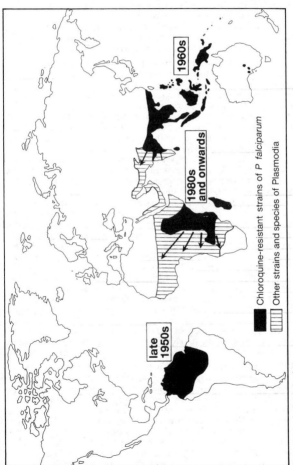

After GC Cook 1988 *Lancet* i 32

Mycobacterium tuberculosis: clinical features

▶No other pathogen kills more adults. Worldwide prevalence: 1½ billion people; UK incidence: 5700/year. 10% are drug-resistant; more in USA.

Primary TB The initial infection with *Mycobacterium tuberculosis*, often in childhood, is usually pulmonary (by droplet spread). A peripheral lesion forms, and its draining nodes are infected. There is an early spread of the bacilli throughout the body, but immunity rapidly develops, and the infection becomes quiescent at all sites. The commonest non-pulmonary *primary* infection is GI, most commonly affecting the ileocaecal junction and associated lymph nodes.

Post-primary TB Any form of immunocompromise may allow reactivation, eg malignancy; diabetes mellitus; steroids; debilitation, especially HIV or old age. The lung lesions progress and fibrose (usually upper lobe). Any other site may become the main clinical problem. In the elderly or Third World children, dissemination of multiple tiny foci throughout the body (including back to the lungs) results in miliary TB. Dissemination also occurs in the immunocompromised.

Primary TB is usually asymptomatic, but there may be fever, lassitude, sweats, anorexia, erythema nodosum, cough, sputum, or phlyctenular conjunctivitis (small, multiple, yellow-grey nodules near the limbus). AFBs (acid-fast bacilli) may be found in sputum. CXR may help.
- *Pulmonary TB:* This may be silent or cause cough, sputum, haemoptysis (may be massive), pneumonia, pleural effusion, and chest pain. Again CXR and sputum are important. When a pleural effusion is tapped parietal pleural biopsy is taken at the same time as biopsy has a higher yield. A mycetoma (p340) may form in the cavities.
- *Miliary TB:* This causes a characteristic CXR. Clinical features may be nonspecific. Look for retinal TB (*OHCS* p500). Biopsy of liver, marrow, lymph nodes, or lung parenchyma may yield AFBs or granulomata.
- *Meningeal TB:* See p442. Treatment of TB meningitis: *OHCS* p260.
- *Genitourinary TB:* This causes dysuria, loin or back pain, haematuria, and frequency, with, classically, sterile pyuria (ie white cells but no growth). Take 3 early morning urine samples (EMUs) for AFBs. Renal ultrasound and IVU are helpful. Renal TB may spread to bladder, seminal vesicles, epididymis, or the Fallopian tubes. For endometrial TB, see *OHCS* p36.
- *Bone TB:* Look for vertebral collapse adjacent to a paravertebral abscess (Pott's vertebra). Do x-rays and biopsy culture (*OHCS* p644).
- *Skin TB (lupus vulgaris):* Look for jelly-like nodules, eg on face or neck.
- *Peritoneal TB:* This causes abdominal pain and GI upset. Look for AFBs in ascites (send a *large* volume to lab); laparotomy may be needed.
- *Acute TB pericarditis:* Think of this as a primary exudative allergic lesion.
- *Chronic pericardial effusion* and *constrictive pericarditis:* These reflect chronic granulomata. Fibrosis and calcification may be prominent, with spread to myocardium. (Giving steroids to these patients for 11 weeks with their anti-TB drugs reduces need for pericardiectomy.▪)

Additional points in all those with TB ▶Consider HIV.
- ▶Ensure regular checking for drug concordance (p3) and drug toxicity.
- ▶Notify CCDC (consultant in communicable disease control) to arrange contact tracing, and screening (preferably by a chest physician).
- ▶Explain that prolonged treatment will be necessary, and explain that taking the tablets as prescribed is important. Monitoring of blood tests will be needed (LFTs). Explain *why* directly observed therapy (DOT) may needed—to reduce the risk of inducing drug-resistance.
- ular clinical monitoring during treatment is used. "*If you get problith treatment, come and see us: don't just stop taking the tablets.*"
- the need for respiratory isolation procedures while infectious.

TB with AIDS—and multi-drug-resistant (MDR) TB

TB is a common, serious, but treatable complication of HIV infection (p214). It is estimated that 30–50% of those with AIDS in the developing world also have TB.[1] Interactions of HIV and TB are as follows:[2]

- Mantoux tests may be falsely negative.
- There is increased reactivation of latent TB.
- Presentation may be atypical.
- Previous BCG vaccination may not stop those with HIV from getting TB.[3]
- Smears may be negative for acid-fast bacilli. This makes culture all the more important—and is vital to characterize drug resistance.
- Those smears which are positive tend to contain less AFBs.
- Atypical CXR: lobar or bibasilar pneumonia, hilar lymphadenopathy.
- Extra-pulmonary and disseminated disease much more common.
- There is good response to drugs, but they tend to be more toxic.
- Get expert help on need for isoniazid prophylaxis in HIV+ve individuals; lifelong prophylaxis with isoniazid is probably *not* helpful (controversial),[3] but everyone agrees that regular clinical monitoring is vital.

▶Remember to use full respiratory isolation when TB patients are near HIV +ve patients. Nosocomial (hospital-acquired) and multi-drug-resistant TB are now big problems, not only in the USA, affecting both HIV +ve and HIV −ve people. Mortality is ~80% in patient-to-patient spread. Test TB cultures against 1st and 2nd-line chemotherapeutic agents:[4]

First-line antitubercular agents:		*Second-line agents:*
Isoniazid	Streptomycin	Ofloxacin, ciprofloxacin
Rifampicin	Amikacin	Cycloserine
Pyrazinamide	Kanamycin	Ethionamide
Ethambutol	Capreomycin	Aminosalicylic acid

Stopping spread of multi-drug resistant TB (MDR-TB) Chief goals: *Early identification*; *full treatment*; *isolation*. Control may be linked to:[5]

- Directly *observing and confirming* that patients take all prescribed drugs.
- Not waiting to *prove* TB before using an isolation room. A suspicious x-ray or a past history of MDR-TB is enough.
- Wearing of special masks (discard when wet) by staff and the patient when s/he leaves the isolation room (only when absolutely required).
- The ability to do ZN stains day and night (a 2-hour turnaround time).
- Sputum induction/expectoration being confined to isolation rooms.
- The doors to these rooms should have automatic closing devices.
- Providing −ve air pressure in isolation rooms (frequently monitored).
- Only stop isolation after >2 sputa are AFB −ve *on culture for MDR-TB*, or if there is a good response to therapy, which must include 4 anti-TB drugs.
- Frequent tuberculin skin surveillance tests for workers and contacts.

Exact guidelines on dealing with MDR-TB are continually under review. Discuss these issues with a microbiologist, and refer early to a consultant in infectious diseases. Specific advice is available from the British Thoracic Society and the USA National Institutes of Health.

1 M Merson 1992 *BMJ* i 209 2 British Thoracic Society advice 1992 *BMJ* i 1231 3 E Ong 1992 *BMJ* i 1567
4 M Iseman 1993 *NEJM* 329 784. See also: British Thoracic Society Guidelines for TB Treatment:
L Oimerod 1990 *Thorax* 45 403–8 5 A Catanzaro and P Wenger 1995 *Lancet* 345 204 & 235

✚ TuberculosisND: diagnosis and treatment

Diagnosis *Microbiology:* Auramine-stained *Mycobacterium tuberculosis* resists acid-alcohol decolourization ('acid [–alcohol] fast bacilli', A[A]FBs). The clinical picture dictates the most useful specimens. *Histological* or *radiological* diagnosis may come from finding characteristic pathology—granulomata (caseating, ie like soft cheese), calcification, and cavitation (forming cavities). *Immunological evidence of TB* are also helpful:

●In the tuberculin test TB antigen is injected intradermally and the cell-mediated response at 48–72h is recorded.

●In the Mantoux test, 0.1mL of 1 in 10,000, 1 in 1000, and 1 in 100 dilutions provide 1, 10, and 100 tuberculin units (TU) respectively. The test is +ve if it produces ≥10mm induration, and –ve if <5. Always state tuberculin concentration and mm of induration.

●The Heaf and Tine tests are for screening and consist of a circle of primed needles which inject the tuberculin.[1]

●A +ve tuberculin test proves only that the patient has immunity not active infection. It may indicate previous exposure or BCG. A strong positive more probably means active infection. *False –ve tuberculin tests* occur in immunosuppression, including miliary TB, sarcoid, AIDS, lymphoma.

●If active TB is strongly suspected, use 1 TU. If it is +ve, infection is likely. Otherwise, interpret in the clinical context.

Treatment of pulmonary TB *Before treatment:* Stress importance of adhering to regimens (helps the patient, *and* stops spread of resistance; check with urine sample: rifampicin turns it orange-red). Assess liver and kidney function. Test colour vision before and during treatment as ethambutol may cause ocular toxicity which is reversible if stopped quickly.

▶If you think he will forget to take his pills, use directly observed therapy.

●*Initial phase* (8 weeks on 3–4 drugs):
  1 Rifampicin 600–900mg (child 15mg/kg) PO ac 3 times/wk.
  2 Isoniazid 15mg/kg PO 3 times/wk.
  3 Pyrazinamide—child: 50mg/kg; adult: 2.5g PO (2g if <50kg) 3 times/wk.
  4 If resistance possible, add ethambutol 25mg/kg/24h PO (not children) or streptomycin 0.75–1g/24h IM (child 15mg/kg/24h). Do LFTs weekly.

●*Continuation phase* (4 months on 2 drugs) rifampicin and isoniazid at same doses. (2 Rifinah 300® tablets = rifampicin 600mg + isoniazid 300mg.) If too poor to buy much rifampicin (it is the best anti-TB drug), twice weekly rifampicin (600mg) + isoniazid (900mg) works well.[2] If resistance is a problem, use ethambutol 15mg/kg/24h PO.

●Give pyridoxine (maximum dose: 10mg/24h) throughout treatment.

Steroids, normally anathema to TB microbiologists (immunosuppression, ∴ ↑risk of TB) *may* be indicated in meningeal and pericardial disease, p198.

Main side-effects ▶Seek help in renal or hepatic failure, or pregnancy. *Rifampicin:* Hepatitis (stop if bilirubin rises; a small rise of AST is not significant), orange urine, contact lens staining, contraceptive steroid inactivation, flu-like syndrome with intermittent use.

Isoniazid: Neuropathy, hepatitis, pyridoxine deficit, agranulocytosis.

Ethambutol: Optic neuritis (colour vision is the first to deteriorate).

Pyrazinamide: Arthralgia (gout is a contraindication), hepatitis.

Preventing TB in HIV +ve people Consider isoniazid 300mg/day PO (children 5mg/kg, max 300mg) for 1 year—if the patient has not had BCG and the Mantoux test is >5mm (Heaf 1–4). If BCG vaccinated (>10yrs ago), only use prophylaxis if Mantoux >10mm (Heaf 3–4). If prophylaxis is not used, monitor clinical state and CXR.[3]

1 GAT 1997 75 2 A Castelo 1989 *Lancet* ii 1173 3 Brit Thoracic Soc recommendation 1992 *BMJ* i 1231

Herpes infections

Varicella zoster Chickenpox (*OHCS* p216) is the primary infection; after infection virus remains dormant in dorsal root ganglia. Reactivation causes shingles. Shingles affects 20% at some time. High-risk groups: elderly or immunosuppressed. *Features of shingles:* Pain in a dermatomal distribution precedes malaise and fever by a few days. Some days later macule-papules+vesicles develop in the same dermatome. Thoracic dermatomes and the ophthalmic division of trigeminal nerve (ophthalmic shingles, *OHCS* p484) are most vulnerable. If the sacral nerves are affected, urinary retention may occur. Motor nerves are rarely affected. *Ramsay Hunt syndrome* (zoster of the ear + VII-nerve palsy, *OHCS* p756). Recurrence suggests HIV. *Tests (if needed):* Rising antibody titres; culture; electron microscopy of vesicle fluid.

Treatment: It is not clear if everyone with shingles needs aciclovir (to reduce viral replication▣)—but if it is going to be used, use it as early as possible: 800mg 5 times a day PO for 5 days (if immunocompromised: 10mg/kg/8h by slow IVI for 10 days and monitor renal function). Famciclovir offers an alternative twice-daily regimen. Control pain with oral analgesic or low-dose amitriptyline. There is evidence to support a 4-week course of prednisolone to reduce post-herpetic neuralgia. If the conjunctiva is affected, apply 3% aciclovir ointment 5 times a day. Beware iritis. Measure acuity often. Tell to report *any* visual loss at once (*OHCS* p484). SE of aciclovir: vomiting, urticaria, encephalopathy.

Complication: Post-herpetic neuralgia, in the affected dermatome, can persist for years, and be life-ruining, and very difficult to treat. Try carbamazepine, then phenytoin, or capsaicin cream (counter-irritant). As a final step, ablation of the appropriate ganglion may be tried (often with no success) and it leaves the patient with an anaesthetic dermatome.

Herpes simplex virus (HSV) Manifestations of primary infection:

1 *Systemic infection*, eg with fever, sore throat, and lymphadenopathy may pass unnoticed. If immunocompromised it may be life-threatening with fever, lymphadenopathy, pneumonitis, and hepatitis.

2 *Gingivostomatitis:* Ulcers filled with yellow slough appear in the mouth.

3 *Herpetic whitlow:* The virus gains access to the digit through a breach in the skin and local irritating vesicles form.

4 *Traumatic herpes (herpes gladiatorum):* Vesicles develop at any site where HSV is ground into the skin by brute force.

5 *Eczema herpeticum:* HSV erupts on eczematous skin; may be extensive.

6 *Herpes simplex meningitis:* This is uncommon and is self-limiting (typically HSV II in women during a primary attack).

7 *Genital herpes:* ♂: Anus or penis (shaft or glans) develop small, grouped vesicles and papules (± palm, feet, or throat sites too). Also pain, fever, dysuria. ♀: *OHCS* p30. Give analgesia + famciclovir 125mg/12h PO for 5 days.▣ Advise condoms. If frequent (eg ≥6/year) or severe recurrences, try continuous aciclovir ≤400mg/12h PO.

8 *HSV keratitis:* These are corneal dendritic ulcers. See *OHCS* p480.

9 *Herpes simplex encephalitis:* (Usually HSV I, spread centripetally, eg from cranial nerve ganglia, to frontal and temporal lobes) ►*Suspect if* fever, fits, headaches, odd behaviour, dysphasia, hemiparesis, or coma—or subacute brainstem encephalitis, meningitis, or myelitis. *Diagnosis:* PCR on CSF sample (± brain biopsy; CT/MRI and EEG are nonspecific and unreliable[1]). High mortality. Seek expert help: admit to ITU; careful fluid balance to minimize cerebral oedema (consider mannitol, p780); ►►*prompt* aciclovir 10mg/kg/8h (if U&E↔) IV for 10 days saves lives.[1]

Tests: Rising antibody titres in 1° infection; culture; PCR for fast diagnosis.

Recurrent HSV may lie dormant in ganglion cells and be reactivated by eg any intercurrent illness, immunosuppression, menstruation, or even sunlight. Cold sores (perioral vesicles) are one manifestation—and the response to aciclovir cream is often disappointing.

Infectious mononucleosis (glandular fever)

This is a common disease of young adults (although patients may be of any age) which may pass unnoticed or cause acute illness—rarely followed by months of lethargy. It is caused by the Epstein–Barr virus (EBV), which preferentially infects B lymphocytes. There follows a proliferation of T-cells (the 'atypical' mononuclear cells—see below) which are cytotoxic to EBV-infected cells. The latter are 'immortalized' by EBV infection, and, very rarely, proliferate to form a picture indistinguishable from immunoblastic lymphoma in immunodeficient individuals whose supressor T-cells fail to check multiplication of these B-cells.

The incubation period is uncertain, but may be 4–5 weeks, or less. Spread is thought to be by saliva or droplet.

Symptoms and signs Sore throat, fever, anorexia, malaise, lymphadenopathy, petechiae on palate, splenomegaly, hepatitis, and haemolytic anaemia. Occasionally encephalitis, myocarditis, pericarditis, neuropathy. Rashes may occur—particularly if the patient is given ampicillin (this does not indicate lifelong ampicillin allergy).

Investigations Blood film shows a lymphocytosis with many atypical lymphocytes (eg 20% of all WBCs). Such cells may be seen (usually in fewer numbers) in many viral infections (especially CMV), toxoplasmosis, drug hypersensitivity, leukaemias, lymphomas, and lead intoxication.

Heterophil antibody tests (eg Monospot® or Paul–Bunnell): Heterophil antibodies develop early and disappear after ~3 months. These antibodies agglutinate sheep red blood cells. They can be absorbed (and thus agglutination is prevented) by ox red cells, but not guinea-pig kidney cells. This pattern distinguishes them from other heterophil antibodies. These antibodies do not react with EBV or its antigens. *False +ve* Monospot® tests occur (rarely) in hepatitis, parvovirus infections, lymphoma, leukaemia, rubella, malaria, carcinoma of pancreas, and SLE.

Immunology: EBV-specific IgM implies current infection, IgG shows that the patient has been previously infected.

Differential diagnosis Cytomegalovirus, viral hepatitis, HIV seroconversion illness, toxoplasmosis, leukaemia, streptococcal sore throat (may co-exist), diphtheria.

Treatment Bed rest. Avoid alcohol. Rarely, experts recommend prednisolone PO for severe symptoms or complications (80mg, 45mg, 30mg, 15mg, and 5mg on successive days, then stop). Its use is non-standard.

Complications Low spirits, depression, and lethargy which may persist for months. Also thrombocytopenia, ruptured spleen, upper airways obstruction (may need observation on ITU), secondary infection, pneumonitis, aseptic meningitis, Guillain–Barré syndrome, renal failure, lymphoma, and autoimmune haemolytic anaemia. All are rare.

Other EBV-associated diseases EBV (augmented by malaria and HIV infection) is a cause of Burkitt's lymphoma (p608). EBV+ve large cell (B-cell) lymphomas occasionally appear in the immunocompromised. The EBV genome has been found in the Reed–Sternberg cell of Hodgkin's lymphoma, and EBV is also associated with nasopharyngeal carcinoma. There are some pointers to its presence in SLE.

Influenza

This is the most important viral respiratory infection[1] because of its frequency and complication rate, particularly in the elderly. In pandemics, millions die, particularly when new strains are involved.

The virus (RNA orthomyxovirus) has 3 types (A, B, C). Subtyping (for type A) is by haemagglutinin (H) and neuraminidase (N) characteristics.

Frequent mutations give strains with new antigenic properties. Minor changes (antigenic drift) and especially major changes (antigenic shift) place whole areas at risk. WHO specifies: *type; host origin; geographic origin; strain number; year of isolation; and subtype,* eg A/Swine/Taiwan/2/87/ (H3,N2).

Spread is by droplets. **Incubation period** 1–4 days. **Infectivity** 1 day before to 7 days after symptoms start. **Immunity** Those attacked by one strain are immune to that strain only.

Pathology An acute necrotizing (and even haemorrhagic) inflammatory process involves the upper and lower respiratory tract.

The Patient Abrupt fever, malaise, headache, and myalgia—also prostration, vomiting, and depression. Convalescence may be slow.

Diagnosis is easy in epidemics (a fatal pitfall is not asking about travel, so missing malaria). Serology may help (↑titres over 2 weeks) if firm diagnosis is essential. Culture is possible.

Complications Bronchitis (in 20%[1]), viral or bacterial pneumonia (especially *Staph aureus*), sinusitis, otitis media, encephalitis, pericarditis.

Treatment Bed rest ± aspirin. Amantadine 100mg/24h PO for 5d markedly reduces symptoms in some outbreaks (H2,N2; H3,N2; H1,N1).[1] In those few who develop severe pneumonia (± secondary infection), most authorities recommend rapid transfer to ITU as dyspnoea and anoxia frequently progress very fast to circulatory collapse and death.

Prevention[2] ●Use whole *trivalent vaccine* (from inactivated viruses), reserving split (fragmented virus) for those <13yrs old. It is prepared from current serotypes; it takes <2 weeks to work. *Indications:* Diabetes; chronic lung, heart or renal disease; immunosuppression; haemoglobinopathies; medical staff (in epidemics); those ≥60yrs old. *Dose:* 0.5mL SC (deltoid) once; children repeat after 5–6 weeks (½ dose if <3yrs old and use anterolateral thigh). SE: Mild pain or swelling (17%). Guillain–Barré and pericarditis are rare. Fever, headaches and malaise are often reported (10%), but no more so than in those given a placebo injection.[3] ●6 weeks of *amantadine* 100mg/24h PO can give good cover (eg 91% for H2,N3 and H1,N2 subtypes of A virus). SE: Insomnia, nervousness. Uraemia and immunosuppression are reasons for vaccine failure—so consider this oral prophylaxis.

The logistics of vaccinating all those in the at-risk groups (above) poses a challenge, particularly in ageing populations.

The common cold (coryza)

Rhinoviruses are the chief cause (>80 strains), producing self-limiting nasal discharge (gets mucopurulent over a few days). *Incubation:* 1–4d. *Complications:* (6% in children) Otitis media, pneumonia, febrile fits. *Treatment:* None is usually needed. ▢ If nasal obstruction in infants hampers feeding, 0.9% saline nose drops may help. In adults, a careful study has shown that zinc gluconate trihydrate 13.3mg in a candy lozenge, 5 × daily, reduced duration by ~50%; SE: nausea, metallic taste. ◁3▷

---

1 A Connolly 1993 *BMJ* ii 1452 2 L Van Voris 1981 *JAMA* 245 1128–31 ◁3▷ S Mossad 1996 *E-BM* 1 204
Further information on current outbreaks is available on http://www.open.gov.uk/cdsc/flufact.htm

Toxoplasmosis

The protozoan *Toxoplasma gondii* infects via gut, lung, or broken skin. Cats (the definitive host) excrete oocysts, but eating poorly cooked infected meat may be as important as contact with cat faeces. In humans, the oocysts release trophozoites, which migrate widely, with a predelection for eye, brain and muscle. Toxoplasmosis occurs worldwide, but is common in the tropics. Infection is lifelong. HIV may reactivate it.

The Patient ►*In any granulomatous uveitis or necrotizing retinitis think of toxoplasmosis, especially in the immunosuppressed.* Most infections are asymptomatic: in the UK 50% have been infected by 70yrs. Symptomatic acquired toxoplasmosis resembles infectious mononucleosis, and is usually self-limiting lasting a few months. Eye infection, usually congenital, presents with posterior uveitis causing blurring and ache, often in the 2nd decade of life; it may cause cataract. In the immunocompromised (eg AIDS), encephalitis and myocarditis can occur (may be fatal).

Tests 4-fold antibody titre rise over 4 weeks or specific IgM implies acute infection (unreliable if HIV +ve). The 'dye test' was the first serological test used. Parasite isolation is hard, but lymph node or CNS biopsy may be diagnostic. CNS CT may show lesions (enhanced by contrast).

Treatment is controversial;[1] often none is needed; get expert help. If the eye is involved, or in the immunocompromised (but non-pregnant), pyrimethamine 25–50mg/8h PO for 5 days then 25–50mg/24h PO for 4 weeks, + sulfadiazine 4–6g/24h PO *may* be recommended. ►If pregnant, get expert help; consider spiramycin ± sampling of fetal cord blood, eg at 21 weeks for IgM (may indicate serious fetal infection). Toxoplasmosis in HIV, see p214.

Congenital transplacental toxoplasmosis (*OHCS* p98) May induce abortion—or neonatal fits, chorioretinitis, hydrocephalus, microcephaly, or cerebral calcification may occur; worse prognosis if early infection.

Cytomegalovirus (CMV)

CMV may be acquired eg by kissing, sexual intercourse, blood transfusion, or organ transplants. Like other herpes viruses, it lies latent after acute infection for the rest of the patient's life, and may reactivate at time of stress or immunocompromise.

The Patient Most infections are unnoticed. 50% of women of childbearing age have been infected. Symptoms may resemble infectious mononucleosis. It is more serious if immunocompromised (eg transplant recipients or AIDS), when it may cause: pneumonia; CNS infection; chorioretinitis; colitis; hepatitis (RUQ pain, jaundice); WCC↓; platelets↓.

Diagnosis Isolation and growth of the virus is slow. Also there may be prolonged CMV excretion following distant infection, making diagnosis of acute CMV infection difficult. Serology is much more helpful. Specific IgM implies acute infection (unreliable if HIV +ve).

Treat only if serious infection (eg if immunocompromised), with ganciclovir 5mg/kg/12h IVI over 1h. Immunization is being explored. Alternative: foscarnet; see CMV in HIV, p214.

Prevention post-transplantation[1] If seropositive pre-op, ganciclovir eg 2.5mg/kg/day IV for the first 2 post-op weeks. Reduce dose frequency if creatinine↑ (see *Ann Int Med* 1995 123 18). Use CMV-free blood or filtered blood when transfusing transplant recipients, leukaemia or HIV patients.

Congenital CMV (*OHCS* p98) Look for: jaundice, hepatosplenomegaly, and purpura. Chronic defects include mental retardation, cerebral palsy, epilepsy, deafness, and eye problems. Treatment: none is established.

1 J Sanford 1997 *Guide to Antimicrobial Therapy* pages 86 & 95

Viral hepatitis

Hepatitis A *Spread:* Faecal–oral, often in institutions or travellers. Most infections pass unnoticed in childhood. *The Patient:* After 2–6 weeks' incubation and a prodrome (anorexia, nausea, joint pain, fever) comes jaundice ± tender hepatomegaly, splenomegaly, and adenopathy. *Tests:* Serum transaminases rise 22–40 days after exposure. Specific antibodies rise from 25 days: IgM signifies recent infection, and IgG remains detectable for life. *Treatment:* Supportive. Avoid alcohol until LFTs ↔. *Prevention:* After infection immunity is *probably* lifelong. Normal human immunoglobulin (0.02mL/kg IM) gives <3 months' passive immunity to those at risk (travellers; *all* household contacts) and during incubation. Havrix® is an inactivated protein from hepatitis A virus, grown in human diploid cells); *dose:* 2 IM doses (into deltoid), 2–4 wks apart, if >16yrs old—lasts 1yr (10yrs if further booster is given at 6 months). Use Havrix Junior® if 1–15yrs old. *Prognosis:* Usually self-limiting; rarely fulminant. There is no carrier state; chronic liver disease does not occur.

Hepatitis B virus (HBV) *Spread:* Blood products, secretions, and sexual intercourse. Risk groups: homosexuals, haemophiliacs, health workers, heroin (or other IV drug) users, haemodialysis, and those in 'homes'/institutions—eg prison. Endemic in tropics and Mediterranean area.
Clinical features resemble those of hepatitis A, but with 1–6 months' incubation. Urticaria and arthralgia are more common with hepatitis B. *Tests:* HBsAg (surface antigen) is present from 1–6 months after exposure. The presence of HBeAg (e-antigen) *implies high infectivity*; it is usually present for 1½–3 months after the acute illness. The persistence of HBsAg for >6 months defines carrier status. This follows 5–10% of infections. Antibodies to HBcAg (core antigen, ie anti-HBc) imply past infection; to HBsAg (ie anti-HBs) alone implies vaccination.
Vaccination may be universal in childhood or just for high-risk groups (UK policy, p513). Passive immunization (specific antihepatitis B immunoglobulin) may be given to non-immune contacts after high-risk exposure.
Treatment: Supportive. Use local infection-control rules. No alcohol. Chronic hepatitis B may respond to IFN-α. Immunize sexual contacts.
Complications: Fulminant hepatic failure (rare, p504); relapse; prolonged cholestasis; chronic hepatitis (5–10%, p512, ± cirrhosis ± liver carcinoma). Others: glomerulonephritis; cryoglobulinaemia.

Hepatitis C (a flavivirus spread like HBV.) It is a major cause of post-transfusion hepatitis. ~50% develop chronic infection; 5% develop cirrhosis (15% of these risk hepatoma).[1] Newer antibody tests are +ve at ≤4mths (eg c200 and c22-3 antigens, ± 5-1-1, c-100-3, c33c). Transfused blood is screened for HCV (offer HCV+ve donors expert advice about need for liver biopsy). Interferon (IFN-α$_{2b}$, eg 3,000,000u, 3 doses/week SC for 1 year) slows infection and progress to hepatoma.[2] Tribavirin (ribovirin) improves virus clearance and response to INF. Monitor with ALT ± PCR. Retreatment may help the 50% who relapse[1] (£1300/course). *Gamma-globulin* gives *some* protection pre-unscreened transfusion. As HCV is often subclinical, screening is suggested:[3] *spouses are at particular risk.*

Hepatitis D—delta agent (an incomplete RNA virus only existing with HBV) Spread: same routes as HBV. It increases the incidence of both acute hepatic failure and cirrhosis. A serological test is available. Interferon (IFN-α) has limited success in treatment of delta infection.

Hepatitis E (an RNA virus) is similar to hepatitis A in transmission and clinical features with no apparent risk of chronic liver disease. In some areas it is the commonest viral cause of hepatitis in adults and older children and mortality if pregnant may be up to 20%. Incubation: 2–9 weeks. Diagnosis: serology. Gammaglobulin is ineffective; there is no vaccine.[4]

Hepatitis GB (Named after its first victim) One type of this flavivirus (HGB-C) can cause fulminant liver failure.

Differential diagnosis *Acute hepatitis:* Drugs, toxins, alcohol, infectious mononucleosis, Q fever, leptospirosis, syphilis, malaria, yellow fever, obstructive jaundice. *Chronic hepatitis:* Alcohol, drugs, chronic autoimmune hepatitis (p512), Wilson's disease (p712).

Markers of **infection**	HBV Acute infection *[marker peak, mths from infection]*	..............Carriers:.......... Infectivity high	Infectivity low	Past infection
HBeAg	Present early then absent [4½]	Present*	Present*	Absent
HBsAg	Present [5]	Present	Present	Absent
anti-HBc IgM	High titre [7]	Absent/low	Absent	Absent
anti-HBc IgG	Moderate titre	High titre	Moderate	Moderate
anti-HBe	Absent early [9]	Absent	Present	Present
anti-HBs	Absent [>10]	Absent	Absent	Present
DNA polymerase	Present	Present	Absent	Absent
LFTs	↑↑↑	↑	Normal	Normal

Most patients recover from HBV infection completely; this is mirrored by disappearance of HBsAg and development of antibodies to HBsAg. Anti-HBs appears late (implying immunity).

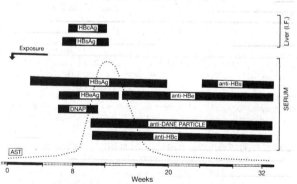

Virological events in acute hepatits B in relation to serum amino-transferase (AST) peak. I.F.=immunofluorescence; Ag=antigen; HBs=hepatitis B surface; HBe=hepatitis B e; DNAP=DNA polymerase.

1 *Drug ther Bul* 1993 **31** 61 2 BMJ 1997 i 1070 3 C Seymour 1994 BMJ i 211 4 *Lancet* 1995 **346** 519

Human immunodeficiency virus (HIV)

AIDS (defined below) represents the end of a spectrum associated with HIV infection and immunodeficiency. The US Center for Disease Control (CDC) asserts that HIV positivity with low CD4 lymphocyte count ($<200 \times 10^6$/L) is sufficient for diagnosis of AIDS. HIV-1 (a retrovirus) is responsible for most cases worldwide, with the related HIV-2 producing a similar illness, perhaps with a longer latent period. ~30 million people are HIV+ve, and ~3 million have AIDS; most are women and children in sub-Saharan Africa.[1] In the UK, incidence appears now *not* to be rising (~30/10^6/year).

Transmission is by sexual intercourse (vaginal or anal: 75% of cases worldwide), infected blood or blood products and from mother to fetus. (Screening of blood donors and sterilization of blood products reduce risks from these to minimal levels in developed countries). In the developing world, heterosexual spread is commonest with equal numbers of men and women affected, and increasing numbers of infected children born to seropositive mothers (vertical transmission, OHCS p98).

4 stages of HIV infection HIV binds to CD4 receptors on helper T-lymphocytes (CD4 cells), monocytes and neural cells. During seroconversion (p216) there is dissemination of virus with seeding of lymphoid organs.[2] A day or so after its infection, the CD4 cell dies and releases large numbers of new virions which exist free in plasma for ~6h. They then enter new susceptible CD4 cells typically in lymphoid tissue. Billions of virions are produced and destroyed each day during the phase of *clinical latency* (which may last 7 or more years). Daily turnover of infected CD4 cells is also in the billions. When host ability to replenish CD4 cells wanes, immunodeficiency manifests as ↑risk of opportunistic infection (p214).

Before developing an AIDS-defining illness, there may be systemic symptoms such as weight loss, seborrhoeic dermatitis ± *persistent generalized lymphadenopathy:* This is defined as nodes >1cm diameter at ≥2 extra-inguinal sites and persisting for 3 months or longer (biopsy if there are symptoms or obvious asymmetry). *Acquired immunodeficiency syndrome (AIDS)* is defined as the development of one or more AIDS-indicating conditions in the presence of evidence of HIV infection. CD4 counts are usually $<200 \times 10^6$/L. These illnesses (described on p214) are:

Pneumocystis pneumonia	Kaposi's sarcoma	CNS toxoplasmosis
Non-Hodgkin's lymphoma	Oesophageal candidiasis	Tuberculosis
Primary CNS lymphoma	Cancer of the cervix	Wasting syndrome
Progressive multifocal	Mycobacterium avium	CMV retinitis; Dementia
leukoencephalopathy	intracellulare	Cryptococcal meningitis

Diagnosis is based on detecting anti-HIV antibodies in serum. Most will develop antibodies within 3 months of exposure. Before seroconversion, detection of the virus by PCR may make the diagnosis.

Direct HIV effects •*Seroconversion illness* (p216). •*Small bowel enteropathy* ± partial villous atrophy (weight↓; diarrhoea; malabsorption), CNS illness (dementia; myelopathy; neuropathy, often sensory and asymmetrical). *Renal effects:* Fibrosis, glomerulosclerosis, mesangial proliferation, tubule dilatation. •*HIV-induced lymphomas:* Usually non-Hodgkin's of B-cell type, at any site, eg small bowel and CNS). Often aggressive, but may respond well to chemotherapy with highly active anti-retroviral therapy (HAART).

Because of immunosuppression, HIV patients should not receive BCG vaccination, yellow fever, oral typhoid or live oral polio immunizations.

AIDS prognosis Untreated, death in ~20 months; longer if treated, p218.

---

1 K Morris 1997 *Lancet* 350 1683   2 A Fanci & G Pantaleo 1996 *Ann Int Med* 124 654-63

HIV biology and drug engineering

HIV virus enters lymphocytes: here its RNA is reverse-transcribed, making double-stranded viral DNA which integrates with the cell's DNA. Expression of this DNA produces large polyproteins on the cell surface. These produce immature virions which are later released. The number of viral nucleic acid molecules ('viral load') predicts progression. If >100,000 molecules/mL, progression to AIDS is likely in 3 years (if no antivirals are given). If >300,000/mL, progression is likely in 1 year. At ~10,000 molecules, time to progression is 3–19 years.

Virion maturation involves polyprotein cleavage by HIV proteases. Computers have found chemicals to match and block the cleavage site (we know its 3D structure). These *protease inhibitors* are now being used (p218) and they ↓viral load (as do other anti-retroviral agents). In those in whom they produce a fall in viral load within 8 weeks of starting, the risk of disease progression is halved. If viral load subsequently rises, progression to AIDS is likely.[1] They also cause ↑CD4+ counts (eg by 100–250 cells/μL).[2]

1 *Bandolier* 1997 4 5 2 USPHS/IDSA CDC MMWR 1997 RR-12

Opportunistic diseases after HIV infection

- **TB** p199 ● **Leishmaniasis** p242 ● **HHV-8** (Kaposi's sarcoma) p702.

- **Oropharynx** *Candida* affects 80% at some time in HIV infection, with sore mouth, angular cheilitis, <u>dysphagia</u> (if oesophagus involved). <u>If no oesophageal involvement</u>, try <u>nystatin pastilles</u> or <u>amphotericin lozenges</u>. Systemic treatment: eg fluconazole 50–200mg/24h PO for 2 weeks (resistance can occur). It is likely to relapse so give standby courses.

- **Pulmonary**—*Pneumocystis carinii* pneumonia: ►p334. If CD4 <200 × 10⁹/L give <u>co-trimoxazole prophylaxis</u>, 960mg <u>3 times a week</u>, dapsone or <u>pentamidine</u>. *M tuberculosis*: Drug resistance (p199). Late problems: fungi (*Aspergillus* or *Cryptococcus*); nocardia. CMV pneumonitis (rare)—use <u>ganciclovir</u> 5mg/kg/12h IV. In ganciclovir resistance use <u>foscarnet</u> IV (see 'eye', below); SE: rash, vomiting, headache, urea↑, fits, Ca²⁺↓, glucose↓.

- **CNS** *Toxoplasma gondii* is the chief focal CNS pathogen in AIDS, producing abscesses visible as <u>ring-enhancing lesions</u> on CT/MRI. Treat with <u>pyrimethamine</u>: get expert help. Loading dose, eg 200mg then 50–70mg/day (give <u>folinic acid</u> 10mg/24h with it) + <u>sulfadiazine</u> 100mg/kg/24h PO for 6 months. (<u>Clindamycin</u> is an alternative.) Follow by <u>lifelong secondary prophylaxis</u>. *Cryptococcus neoformans* (p244) causes an insidious <u>meningitis</u> in up to 8%. Beware a high opening CSF pressure (associated with blindness and ↑mortality). Fluconazole IV/PO may be an alternative to <u>amphotericin/flucytosine</u> in less severe disease. Lifelong secondary prevention with fluconazole ~200mg/day PO is needed (discuss dose with expert). <u>Therapeutic LP</u> may be needed to lower pressures.

- **Eye** *CMV* causes retinitis (acuity↓ ± blindness) may affect <u>45%</u> of those with AIDS. Early diagnosis and anti-CMV drugs may somewhat diminish progression. Dose example: <u>ganciclovir 5mg/kg/12h IV</u> or <u>foscarnet</u> (eg 60mg/kg/8h IVI for <u>2 weeks</u>' induction), then eg 60mg/kg/24h indefinitely: <u>renal failure is a problem</u>—*see datasheet for dose-reduction*). This treatment is difficult, expensive, and carries all the <u>hazards of indwelling catheters</u>. Oral ganciclovir is a partial answer—but is less effective. Once-weekly infusions of cidofovir are under trial (probenecid may ↓ <u>nephrotoxicity</u>). Another option is ganciclovir-containing intraocular implants. These show a <u>median time to progression of 216 days</u> compared with 104 days for IV ganciclovir. The problem here is post-op retinal detachment (5% in one study, 18% in another). One implant cannot prevent CMV infecting the other eye—or taking root elsewhere.[1]

    Once retinitis is established, IV cidofovir or IV ganciclovir <u>with</u> foscarnet may be tried. Prevention with ganciclovir is unreliable and costly.

- **Gut** <u>Chronic diarrhoea</u> from *Cryptosporidium parvum* can be debilitating: p486. There is limited success with <u>paromomycin</u> (not on UK market; available *via* IDIS, tel. 0181 410 0700). Other causes include *Isospora belli* (use <u>co-trimoxazole</u>), *Microsporidium*, CMV colitis (abdominal pain suggestive), HIV enteropathy and *Mycobacterium avium* complex (MAC) infection (fevers, sweats, weight↓, abdominal pain, wasting, hepatosplenomegaly, Hb↓, alk phos↑). It may be grown from sputum or blood. MAC may infect up to 50% of those with AIDS, and prophylaxis, which may fail, is recommended if CD4 lymphocytes fall to <75 × 10⁶ cells/L.[1] Azithromycin, clarithromycin, or <u>rifabutin</u> can prevent most infections, but there may be problems with interaction with protease inhibitors. Treatment is problematic, with multi-drug regimens, eg clarithromycin ½–1g/12h PO + ethambutol 15–25mg/kg/day or rifabutin 300mg/day PO (SE: uveitis).[2] Allow 2–12 weeks for a response. Discuss with a microbiologist.

- **PUO** Important, treatable PUOs in HIV having no clinical focus may be from mycobacteria, <u>pneumococci</u>, <u>salmonellae</u>, fungi, or toxoplasma.

1 C Beiser 1997 BMJ i 579 + J Bartlett 1996 *Med. Care of Pat. with HIV*, Williams & Williams 2 GAT Sanford 1997 p86

When to suspect Pneumocystis carinii pneumonia

- Any respiratory symptom, particularly tachycardia, tachypnoea, cyanosis, or fever combined with known risk factors for HIV (but note that chest pain, wheeze, and orthopnoea are *not* typical).
- Chronic cough, eg non-productive, and slowly worsening (ask yourself: *Does this patient also have tuberculosis?*).
- Breathlessness in any adult, particularly if exertional, and with no known reason for dyspnoea. A useful clue, especially if CXR is −ve, is to check O_2 saturation pre- and post-exertion.
- Nodular, reticular, or granular change on CXR ± pneumothorax.

Do not give oral co-trimoxazole 'just in case'. Doing so will make diagnosis harder. Admit to hospital or recognized HIV treatment centre: diagnosis may depend on analysis of saline lavage at bronchoscopy ± DNA amplification. Do send off a sputum sample.

▶Pneumocystosis is the leading cause of HIV-associated morbidity: remember that co-trimoxazole prophylaxis has a very significant impact on reducing mortality, so start it in good time.

Self-help to avoid opportunistic infections in immunodeficiency

Infections may be prevented by 'safe' sexual practices, and avoiding dietary risks. Risk depends on degree of immunosuppression (CDC recommends acting on the patient's worst CD4 count, not the most recent), and on local prevalence of disease. Eg during outbreaks of cryptosporidiosis, or if CD4-count $<100 \times 10^6$/L, water should be boiled for >1min (pasteurized drinks, beers and commercially-packaged drinks which do not require refrigeration are probably safe; treating water with iodine or chlorine ± home-based filters may be less safe).[1]

Travellers may be recommended to take ciprofloxacin (500mg/day), and should favour piping hot food, and bottled water. They should have all the usual vaccinations, but not live ones (except possibly measles if non-immune). Use inactivated polio vaccine. If travel to a yellow fever area, this live vaccine may be offered, but it has uncertain safety and efficacy if HIV +ve. If not given, provide a letter of exemption. In any case, take all measures to avoid mosquito bites. Cholera vaccine is not recommended for ordinary tourist activities, even in cholera areas. It may be sensible to avoid travel to areas where TB and leishmaniasis are prevalent. 1 USPHS/IDSA CDC MMWR 1997 RR-12

What every doctor should know about HIV

Preventing HIV spread ●Promote *lifelong* safer sex, barrier contraception, and reduction in the number of partners. Videos, followed by interactive discussions, is one way to double the use of condoms.[■] Another way is the *100% condom programme* involving distribution of condoms to brothels, with enforcement programme enabling monitoring and encouragement of condom use at any sex establishment. Such programmes are estimated to have prevented 2 million HIV infections in Thailand.
●Warn heterosexuals about the dangers of sexual tourism/promiscuity.
●Tell drug users not to share needles. Use needle exchange schemes.
●Vigorous control of other STDs can reduce HIV incidence by 40%.[■]
●Strengthen awareness of clinics for sexually transmitted diseases.
●Reduce unnecessary blood transfusions.
●Encourage pregnant women to have HIV tests. (Caesarean sections and zidovudine during birth can prevent vertical transmission, OHCS p98.)

Occupational exposure and needle-stick (?HIV+ve) injury[1]
(Seroconversion rate: ~0.4% for HIV; 30% for Hepatitis B—if HBeAg +ve)
●Wash well; encourage bleeding; do not suck or immerse in bleach.
●Note name, address, and clinical details of 'donor'; been on any anti-HIV drugs?
●Report incident to Occupational Health. Fill in an accident form.
●Store blood from both parties. If possible, ascertain HIV and HBsAg of both. Immunize (active and passive) against hepatitis B at once, if needed. Counsel (HIV risk <0.5% if 'donor' is HIV +ve) and test recipient at 3, 6, and 8 months (seroconversion may take this long).
●Weigh risks by questioning 'donor'; if HIV+ve, what is the CD4 and viral load count? Before prophylaxis, do a pregnancy test. Get informed consent. Was there a large inoculum? Was injury deep? (Mucous membrane exposure carries very low risk; if conjunctival, somewhat higher.) Give 4 weeks of drugs, if possible within 1 hour of exposure: **Low-risk exposure:** No antiviral medication. **Higher-risk:** Zidovudine 300mg/12h + lamivudine 150mg/12h, and, particularly for worst episodes, indinavir 800mg/8h, all PO. Drug choice may change as evidence accrues.

HIV test counselling If in doubt, get help from a genitourinary clinic.
●Determine level of risk (eg unprotected sex; sex overseas).
●Explore benefits of the test (eg anxiety↓; protection of partner; planning the future; avoiding vertical transmission; getting treatment).
●What are the difficulties? Will you tell family and friends? How? Explain possible effects on: job, mortgage, insurance (in the UK there is no obligation for doctors to disclose HIV status: just leave the box blank).
●Do post-test counselling (eg to re-emphasize ways to ↓ risk exposure).
●*Counselling throughout HIV illness:* A key issue when a couple is dying from HIV is making a will, and guardianship of any children; a lawyer's help may be needed, and also with housing and employment. Drawing up advance directives also needs special skill. Later in the illness, hospices and domiciliary teams from departments of sexual health (genitourinary medicine) help with terminal care. The GP also has a central rôle.

Acute seroconversion As HIV gets more treatable, so recognizing this early phase becomes more desirable. With fever, myalgia, a maculopapular rash and lymphadenopathy, it is unfortunately like infectious mononucleosis. It is a moot point whether all those with these signs should be offered HIV tests (antibody tests may be ↔ but viral 'p24' and HIV RNA levels are ↑↑). Do think of these tests if there are unusual signs (oral ulcers, oral candidiasis, leucopenia, or CNS signs). As ever, the first, best 'test' is to take a good history—and to know your patient, and the community he comes from. If you do identify acute seroconversion illness, get expert help promptly: vigorous anti-HIV combination treatment may be indicated.

1 Internat. AIDS SOC & UK 1997 Guidelines—*see* P Easterbrook 1997 *BMJ* ii 557

Monitoring HIV—and when to treat

There is more to monitoring HIV than periodic measurements of the CD4 count. HIV RNA levels in plasma strongly predict progression to AIDS and death, whatever the CD4 count. This test typically involves quantitative reverse transcriptase PCR to amplify DNA copies of the target RNA—or branched-chain DNA manipulation (DNAb) to amplify target RNA. HIV patients in the lowest quartile of HIV load (HIV RNA ≤4530 RNA copies/mL) had an 8% chance of progressing to AIDS in 5yrs *vs* 62% in those in the top quartile (>36,270 RNA copies/mL).

Clinical benefit from anti-HIV agents depends not just on improving the CD4 count; further benefit comes from decreasing HIV RNA by at least 70%—which is now possible with combination therapy (p218).

In deciding when to recommend anti-HIV treatment, no recent long-term studies involving clinical end-points such as death are available. Short-term studies have led to the recommendation that treatment be started when plasma HIV RNA values exceed 5000–30,000copies/mL or when the CD4 count is <500 cells × 10^6/L.[1]

Use CD4 and HIV RNA quantification to monitor treatment, eg every 3 months.[2] There is an argument for changing treatment when and if plasma HIV RNA returns to within 70% of its pretreatment level[2]—or if there is a consistent fall in the CD4 count, or if new symptoms supervene: see p218. The new regimen should include at least 2 drugs new to the patient. Note that triple-drug therapy imposes logistic constraints, some needing to be taken with food, and others on an empty stomach. Always check *Datasheets* for interactions: a serious problem.

1 CC Carpenter 1996 *JAMA* **276** 146 2 JA Cohn 1997 *BMJ* **i** 487 See also http://www.cdcnac.org

Using anti-HIV agents

This is an expensive, if complicated, luxury for most of the world's HIV patients. Even in wealthy countries, resources may not be forthcoming.
▶In many ways *all* anti-HIV treatment is experimental—so perhaps the
best question to ask is not *What is the best treatment for HIV?* but *Which is the most appropriate trial to enter my patient into?* Discuss these issues with your patient and consultants in infectious diseases.

Combinations eg of two nucleoside analogue reverse transcriptase inhibitors (NRTI) with a protease inhibitor give best results.[1] NRTIs are:
- *Zidovudine (AZT)* eg 250–300mg/12h PO or 1–2mg/kg/4h IVI. SE: marrow suppression, headache, nausea, myalgia, insomnia.
- *ddi (didanosine)* dose example: if body weight <60kg, 125mg/12h PO; if ≥60kg: 200mg (tablets) every 12h. Chew thoroughly—or crush and disperse in water (± clear apple juice for flavour). *Cautions:* Be alert to:
  1 Pancreatitis (possible great danger here). Stop if plasma amylase rises. It may be safe to restart very cautiously once pancreatitis has been excluded, and the amylase is normal, and beware concurrent treatment with pentamidine isetionate and other pancreatoxic agents. Triglycerides are also pancreatoxic, so check these too.
  2 Liver failure (monitor LFTs, stop if significant elevation).
  3 Renal failure. 4 Peripheral neuropathy. 5 Hyperuricaemia.
  Avoid ddi if: Breastfeeding; also on tetracycline (at same time of dose). Other SE of ddi: hyperuricaemia (suspend treatment if measures to reduce urate concentration fail); diarrhoea; vomiting; confusion; insomnia; fever; headache; pain; rash; pruritus; seizures.
- *Zalcitabine (ddC)* eg 0.75mg/8h. SE: neuropathy (in 20%); pancreatitis (1%).
- *Lamivudine*[1] *(3TC)* eg 150mg/8h PO, take without food. SE: neuropathy is rare.
- *Stavudine (D4T)*, eg 40mg/12h PO if weight >60kg; if less, 30mg/12h PO; stop if LFT↑ or neuropathy. Other SE: neutropenia; platelets↓; pancreatitis. Zidovudine co-therapy may inhibit stavudine's intracellular activation.

Selective protease inhibitors such as *ritonavir* (600mg/12h PO with food) and *indinavir*, 800mg at 'strictly 8h intervals, 1h before or 2h after a meal, or with a low-fat light meal' (SE: nausea, D&V, abdominal pain, lethargy, rashes, LFT↑, visceral fat↑; as it contains 43% ethanol, co-therapy with disulfiram or metronidazole is ill-advised).[2] An alternative is *saquinavir* 600mg/8h PO. SE: diarrhoea, abdominal discomfort, nausea, and mouth ulcers.

HIV protease mediates the final development of HIV, and inhibiting it slows cell-to-cell spread, and lengthens time to the first clinical event. All protease inhibitors inhibit the cytochrome P450 enzyme system, and so may increase concentrations of benzodiazepines, astemizole, cisapride, terfenadine, and rifabutin (ritonavir dangerously so). If taking ketoconazole, the dose of indinavir may need reducing to 600mg/8h PO.

Non-nucleoside reverse transcriptase inhibitors include nevirapine (200mg /day for 2 weeks, then 200mg/12h PO). This is a powerful anti-HIV agent, but resistant mutants emerge readily. SE: Stevens–Johnsone syndrome.[3]
Integrase inhibitors may also have a rôle in the future.[4]

Relapse and drug resistance When anti-HIV treatment fails to control symptoms, or CD4 counts are falling, or plasma HIV RNA returns to within 70% of its pretreatment level, use a new anti-HIV agent—trying to avoid cross-resistance. (There is not much point in substituting indinavir for ritonavir, as resistance to one generally implies resistance to the other.)

1 http://www.hivatis.org & J Montaner 1997 *Lancet* 349 1042 & *BMJ* 1997 i 699 & Delta committee 1996 *Lancet* 348 283 & E-BM 1997 2 17 2 D Cameron 1998 *Lancet* 351 543+867 3 *Lancet* 1998 351 567 4 *Drug Ther Bul* 1997 34 25 & *Lancet Review* 1995 346 s12 & B Larder 1995 *Science* 269 696

Golden rules in anti-HIV treatment
- Aim to stop viral replication permanently.
- Monitor plasma viral load and CD4 count (see p217).
- Start antiretroviral treatment early *before* immunodeficiency sets in.[1]
- Use 3 antiviral drugs (minimizes replication and cross resistance).
- Change to a new combination if plasma viral load rebounds.
- Explain to patients that regimens are complex: take time to harmonize pharmacodynamics with the patient's expectations and lifestyle.

Sexually transmitted infection (STI)

►Refer early to Genitourinary Medicine Clinic (GUM) for full microbiology and partner notification. Some clinics give an on-call service for out-of-hours advice and most see patients immediately during the working day. Avoid giving antibiotics until seen in GUM clinic or at least discussed.

Presentation—Discharge (opposite) or HIV (p212) or genital lesions:
Herpes, p202;   Syphilis, p233;   Genital warts, OHCS p592;
Salpingitis, OHCS p50   Crab lice OHCS p600 (*Phthirias pubis*; R$_x$: malathion)

Scabies mites are arachnids (8 legs). Spread is common in families. *Presentation:* A papular rash (on abdomen or medial thigh; itchy at night) + burrows (look *and feel* web spaces and flexor wrist surfaces). *Incubation:* ~6 weeks (during which time sensitization to the mite's faeces and/or saliva occurs). Lesions on the penis produce red nodules. *Diagnosis:* Trying to tease a mite out of her burrow with a needle for microscopical examination (× 10) often fails—but if a drop of oil is placed on the lesion, a few firm scrapes with a scalpel will provide microscopically recognizable faeces and eggs. *Treatment:* ►Treat all the household. Give written advice (OHCS p600). Apply malathion 0.5% liquid (Derbac-M®), or, if pregnant or <6 months old, monosulfiram (=sulfiram) 25% in methylated spirit (diluted in 3 parts water to 1 part of the liquid), from the neck down (include the head in those <2 years old—and if elderly or immunocompromised). Remember to paint *all* parts, including the soles. ►Avoid the eyes. Wash off after 24 hours.

Lymphogranuloma Rarely, STI presents as inguinal lymphadenopathy ulceration, eg from *Lymphogranuloma venereum*, chancroid*, or granuloma inguinale (Donovanosis, caused by *Calymmatobacterium granulomatis* giving extensive, painless, red genital or other ulcers and pseudobuboes, ie abscesses *nearby* inguinal nodes, with possible elephantiasis ± malignant change. Diagnosis: find 'closed safety-pin' inclusion bodies in histiocytes' cytoplasm. Treatment: >14 days of tetracycline).

History Sexual contacts; timing of last intercourse; duration of relationship; sexual practices and orientation; contraceptive method; contact history; past STIs, menstrual and medical history; antimicrobial therapy.

Examination Detailed examination of genitalia including inguinal nodes and pubic hair for lice/nits. Scrotum, subpreputial space, and male urethra. PR and proctoscopy (if indicated); PV and speculum examination.

Tests Refer to GUM clinic. Urine: dipstix analysis and send MSU. Ulcers: HSV cultures (viral transport medium) and dark ground microscopy of smears for *T pallidum*. *Men:* Urethral smear for Gram stain and culture for *N gonorrhoeae* (send quickly to lab in Stuart's medium); urethral swab for chlamydia. *Women:* High vaginal swab in Stuart's for microscopy and culture (*Candida, Gardnerella vaginalis*, anaerobes, *Trichomonas vaginalis*—may need specific culture medium depending on local facilities); take endocervical swab for *Chlamydia trachomatis* (this obligate intracellular bacteria is the trickiest STI to diagnose; unfortunately it is also the most common. Special medium is needed, or direct immunofluorescence: serology is difficult (cross-reacts with *C pneumoniae*[1])—and we cannot rely on urine tests based on plasmid probes and ligase chain reactions[2]). *Blood tests:* Syphilis, hepatitis, and HIV serology after full counselling.

Follow-up Arrange to see patients at 1 week and 3 months, with repeat smears, cultures, and syphilis serology.

1 G Scott 1995 *Lancet* 345 207   2 H Lee 1995 *Lancet* 345 213 *In the Tropics, chancroid is a common cause of sexually acquired genital ulcers—typically with a granular, yellow base, and ragged edges (± inguinal buboes, which may need draining through a wide-bore needle; see TMR image 980/16991); the cause is *Haemophilus ducreyi*. The WHO recommends erythromycin 500mg/8h PO for 7 days, ceftriaxone 250mg IM (1 dose), or ciprofloxacin 500mg (1 dose). Chancroid facilitates spread of HIV.

Vaginal discharge and urethritis

Non-offensive vaginal discharge may be physiological. Most are smelly and itchy and are due to infection. A very foul discharge may be due to a foreign body (eg forgotten tampons, or beads in children).

►Discharges rarely resemble their classical descriptions.

►Untreated GU inflammation ↑ viral shedding of HIV-1 in semen 3-fold.

Thrush (*Candida albicans*) Thrush is the commonest cause of discharge, which is classically white curds. Vulva and vagina may be red, fissured, and sore. Her partner may be asymptomatic. *Risk factors:* Pregnancy, the Pill, immunodeficiencies, antibiotics, diabetes (check for glycosuria). *Diagnosis:* Microscopy reveals strings of mycelium or typical oval spores. Culture on Sabouraud's medium. *Treatment:* A single imidazole pessary, eg clotrimazole 500mg, plus cream for the vulva (and partner) is convenient. She may need reassurance that thrush is not necessarily sexually transmitted. Recurrent thrush: see *OHCS* p48.

Trichomonas vaginalis (TV) Produces vaginitis and a thin, bubbly, fishy smelling discharge. It is sexually transmitted. Exclude gonorrhoea (may co-exist). The motile flagellate may be seen on wet film microscopy, or cultured. *Treatment:* Metronidazole 200mg/8h PO for 7 days or 2g PO stat; treat the partner; if pregnant, use the 7-day regimen.

Bacterial vaginosis presents with fishy-smelling discharge (cadaverine and putrescine). Vaginal pH is >5.5. The vagina is not inflamed and itch is uncommon. Mixed with 10% potassium hydroxide on a slide under the nose, a whiff of ammonia may be emitted. Stippled vaginal epithelial 'clue cells' may be seen on wet microscopy. There is altered bacterial flora ± overgrowth eg of *Gardnerella vaginalis*, *Mycoplasma hominis*, peptostreptococci, *Mobiluncus* and anaerobes, eg *Bacteroides* species—with too few lactobacillae. There is ↑risk of preterm labour and amniotic infection if pregnant. *Diagnosis:* Culture. *Treatment:* OHCS p48.

Gonorrhoea *Neisseria gonorrhoea* (gonococcus; GC) can infect any columnar epithelium—urethra, cervix, rectum, pharynx, conjunctiva, but not vagina (which is squamous). Incubation: 2–10 days. *The Patient:* ♂: Purulent urethral discharge & dysuria; or proctitis, tenesmus, and discharge PR if homosexual. ♀: Usually asymptomatic, but may have vaginal discharge, dysuria, proctitis. Pharyngeal disease is often asymptomatic. *Complications—Local:* Prostatitis, cystitis, epididymitis, salpingitis, Bartholinitis. *Systemic:* Septicaemia, eg with petechiae, hand/foot pustules, arthritis (metastatic or sterile), endocarditis (rare). *Obstetric:* Ophthalmia^ND (*OHCS* p100). *Long-term:* Urethral stricture, infertility.
Treatment: 1 dose of *amoxicillin* 3g PO + *probenecid* 1g PO, or *procaine penicillin* (*procaine benzylpenicillin*) 2.4g (4.8g for ♀) IM + *probenecid* 1g PO. Trace contacts. No intercourse or alcohol till cured. If penicillin resistance/allergy, use *ofloxacin* 400mg PO stat or *ciprofloxacin* eg 500mg stat PO. β-lactamase producing strains: *cefuroxime* 1.5g IV + *probenecid* 1g PO.

Non-gonococcal urethritis is commoner than GC. Discharge is thinner and signs less acute, but this does not help diagnosis. Women (typically asymptomatic) may have cervicitis, urethritis, or salpingitis (pain, fever, infertility). Rectum and pharynx are not infected. *Organisms:* *Chlamydia trachomatis*; *Ureaplasma urealyticum*, a kind of Mycoplasma; *Mycoplasma genitalium*; *Trichomonas vaginalis*; *Gardnerella*; Gram −ve and anaerobic bacteria; *Candida*. *Complications:* The local but not the systemic complications of GC. *Chlamydia* cause Reiter's syndrome and neonatal conjunctivitis. *Treatment:* 1 week of oxytetracycline 250mg/6h PO 1h ac, or doxycycline 100mg/12h PO for 1 week. Trace contacts. Avoid intercourse during treatment and alcohol for 4 weeks. Treatment failures: erythromycin 500mg/12h PO (1 week).

Non-infective urethritis Traumatic; chemicals; cancer; foreign body.

Miscellaneous Gram positive bacteria

Staphylococci When pathogenic these are usually *Staph aureus*. Most commonly, they cause localized infection of skin, lids, or wounds—or septicaemia. Deep infections with *Staph aureus*: cavitating pneumonia, osteomyelitis, septic arthritis, endocarditis. These infections are usually acute and severe. Production of β-lactamase which destroys many antibiotics (p176–p182) is the main problem. *Staph aureus* toxins may cause food poisoning (p190) or the toxic shock syndrome toxin (TSST-1): shock, confusion, fever, a rash with desquamation, diarrhoea, myalgia, CPK↑, platelets↓—eg associated with the use of hyperabsorbent tampons, which provide an ideal milieu for toxin-producing *Staph aureus*. *Staph epidermidis (albus)* is increasingly recognized as a pathogen in the immunocompromised, particularly in connection with IV lines or any prosthesis. It is often enough to remove the infected line, and it is often multiply resistant to antibiotics. In other circumstances, when isolated from a culture, *Staph epidermidis* can usually be assumed to be a contaminant (unless seen in several blood cultures, or in neonates). Deep staph infections need ≥4 weeks of flucloxacillin 500mg/6h IV ± removal of foreign bodies such as arthroplasties. Check sensitivities with the lab. *Methicillin-resistant Staphylococcus aureus (MRSA)* is the big issue in hospital-acquired infection, causing pneumonia, septicaemia, wound infections, and deaths. In the USA 29% of hospitals have MRSA problems (a problem in smaller community units, as well as tertiary hospitals).◫ Carriage rates (eg nosal): 1–10%. Risk factors: HIV, dialysis, being on ITU. MRSA may also be community-acquired. *Management:* Talk with a microbiologist. Only some types are sensitive to vancomycin.[1] Preventive measures:

- Now wash your hands—and your stethoscope!
- Ask about need for eradication (with *mupirocin*) in those likely to need ITU.
- Be meticulous in looking after intravascular catheters when on ITU.
- Surveillance culture of patients during outbreaks.
- Ask about need for gowns/gloves if dealing with infected or colonized patients. Masks may be needed during contact with MRSA pneumonia.
- Ask about grouping all MRSA patients together on one ward.
- Patients simply colonized with MRSA *may* not need isolation.◂

Streptococci Group A streps (eg *Strep pyogenes*) are common pathogens, causing wound and skin infections (eg impetigo, erysipelas, *OHCS* p590), tonsillitis, scarlet fever[ND], necrotizing fasciitis (p124), toxic shock (above), or septicaemia. Late complications are rheumatic fever and glomerulonephritis. *Strep pneumoniae* (the pneumococcus—a diplococcus) causes pneumonia, otitis media, meningitis, septicaemia, peritonitis (rare). Resistance to penicillin is becoming a problem. *Strep sanguis, mutans* and *mitior* (of the 'viridans' group), *bovis*, and *Enterococcus faecalis* all cause endocarditis. *Enterococcus faecalis* also causes UTI, wound infections, and septicaemia. *Strep mutans* is a very common cause of caries. *Strep milleri* forms abscesses eg in CNS, lungs, and liver. Most streptococci are sensitive to the penicillins, but *Ent faecalis* and *Ent faecium* may present some difficulties. They usually respond to a combination of ampicillin and an aminoglycoside, eg gentamicin, p181 & p750.

Anthrax[ND] (*Bacillus anthracis*, eg in Africa, China, Asia, East Europe, Haiti) is spread by handling infected carcasses. Well-cooked meat poses no risk.◫ Common form: local cutaneous 'malignant pustule'. Sometimes oedema is a striking sign, eg with fever ± hepatosplenomegaly. Inhaled or swallowed spores may cause pulmonary or GI anthrax respectively—with massive GI haemorrhage and breathlessness (± meningoencephalitis). Gram stain is characteristic (Gram +ve rod). Treatment: benzylpenicillin.

6. Infectious diseases

Diphtheria[ND] is caused by the toxin of *Corynebacterium diphtheriae*. It usually starts with tonsillitis ± a false membrane over the fauces. The toxin may cause neuritis, often starting with cranial nerves. Shock may occur (myocarditis, toxaemia, conducting system disease). Treat with antitoxin (*OHCS* p276) and erythromycin IV. Vaccination has been very effective in the UK. Consider diphtheria in the differential diagnosis of skin lesions in recent visitors to the Tropics or Eastern Europe. Those born before 1942 visiting Russia (or Ukraine) who have *close contact* with locals need a primary *low-dose* course: 0.1mL IM of the single antigen paediatric vaccine (Evans Medical—3 doses, at monthly intervals). Give a booster, eg 0.5mL of Diftavax® (contains tetanus toxoid too) to *close* diphtheria contacts if primary immunization was >5yrs ago. Explain that it may not work. Schick tests are no longer available. All close contacts should also get prophylactic antibiotics, eg 10 days of erythromycin 250mg/6h PO *before* swab results are known.

Listeriosis is caused by *Listeria monocytogenes*. It is a Gram +ve bacillus with an unusual ability to multiply at low temperatures. Possible sources of gastroenteritis outbreaks are pâtés, milk, raw vegetables, and soft cheeses (brie, camembert, and blue-vein types). Person-to-person spread is not reported. It may cause a nonspecific 'flu-like illness, pneumonia, meningoencephalitis, ataxia, rash, or PUO, especially if immunocompromised (eg pregnancy, where it may cause miscarriage or stillbirth) and neonates.[1] *Diagnosis:* Culture blood, placenta, amniotic fluid, CSF, and any expelled products of conception. ▶Do blood cultures in any pregnant *patient with unexplained fever for ≥48h.* Serology, vaginal and rectal swabs don't help (it may be a commensal here). *Treatment:* Ampicillin IV (erythromycin if allergic) + co-trimoxazole. *Prevention in pregnancy:* ●Avoid soft cheeses, pâtés, and under-cooked meat. ●Observe 'use by . . .' date. ●Ensure reheated food is piping hot all through; observe standing times when using microwaves; throw away any left-over.

Nocardia species cause subcutaneous infection (eg Madura foot) in warm climes. If immunocompromised, it may cause chest, cerebral, or liver abscesses. *Microscopy:* Branching chains of cocci. *Treatment:* eg 3g sulfamethoxazole/12h PO for 6 wks;[2] check blood levels if renal failure.

Clostridia cause wound infections and gas gangrene (± shock or renal failure) after surgery or trauma (*C perfringens*). Debridement is essential; benzylpenicillin 1.2–2.4g/6h IV, antitoxin and hyperbaric oxygen may also be used. Amputations may be needed, particularly in theatres of war. *Clostridia* food poisoning: p190. *C difficile:* p486. Botulism, p794.

Actinomycosis Cause: *Actinomyces israelii*. *Presentation:* Usually a subcutaneous infection which forms chronic sinuses with sulfur granule-containing pus. It most commonly affects the area of the jaw (or IUCDs, *OHCS* p62). It may cause abdominal masses. *Treatment:* Benzylpenicillin (p177) for ≥2 weeks post clinical cure. Remove IUCD. Liaise with surgeons.

1 S Tabaqchali 1997 *Lancet* 350 1644   2 Dose not in *BNF*, see N Beeching *Infectious Diseases* 1994 Wolfe

Miscellaneous Gram negative bacteria

Enterobacteria Some are normal gut commensals, others environmental organisms. However, they may be pathogenic. They are the commonest cause of UTI and intra-abdominal sepsis, especially post-operatively and in the acute abdomen. They are also a common cause of septicaemia. Unusually, they may cause chest infections (especially *Klebsiella*), meningitis, or endocarditis. These organisms are often sensitive to ampicillin and trimethoprim, but in serious infections, cefuroxime ± an aminoglycoside should be used. *Salmonella* and *Shigella* are discussed on p190 and p228.

Pseudomonas aeruginosa is a serious pathogen, especially in the immunocompromised and cystic fibrosis. As well as pneumonia and septicaemia, it may cause UTI, wound infection, osteomyelitis, and cutaneous infections. The principal problem is its increasing resistance. Each isolate should have sensitivities assessed, but a good combination is piperacillin or azlocillin plus an aminoglycoside. Ciprofloxacin, ceftazidime and imipenem (p181) are newer agents useful against *Pseudomonas*.

Haemophilus influenzae typically affects unvaccinated children usually <4yrs old, causing otitis media, pneumonia, meningitis, osteomyelitis, septicaemia, and acute epiglottitis. Adults: exacerbations of chronic bronchitis. It is unreliably sensitive to ampicillin; cefotaxime is more reliable. Capsulated types tend to be much more pathogenic than non-capsulated types. Immunization (p192) has lead to markedly falling incidence.

Plague[ND] Cause: *Yersinia pestis*; spread by fleas of rodents or (rarer) cats. Bubonic plague presents with lymphadenopathy (buboes). Pneumonic plague may also be spread by droplets from other infected humans. *Incubation:* 1–7 days. It may present with lymphadenopathy or a 'flu-like illness leading to dyspnoea, cough, copious, bloody sputum, septicaemia and a haemorrhagic fatal illness. *Diagnosis:* Phage typing of bacterial culture, or a 4-fold rise in antibodies to F antigen of *Y pestis*.[1] *Treatment:* Isolate suspects. 1 week's oxytetracycline (250mg/6h PO 1h ac) or streptomycin (used prophylactically too, but no trials have shown efficacy)—if in first trimester, amoxicillin 250–500mg/8h PO; if later in pregnancy, co-trimoxazole 480mg/12h PO; children: co-trimoxazole.[2] Staying at home, quarantine (inspect daily for 1 week), insect sprays to legs and bedding, and avoiding dead animals helps stop spread. Vaccines give no *immediate* protection (multiple doses may be needed).

Brucellosis This zoonosis (domestic animals) is common in the Middle East. Symptoms may last years; the main problem is thinking of it. Cause: a Gram –ve coccobacillus—*Brucella melitensis* (the most virulent), *B abortus*, *B suis*, or *B canis*. *The Patient:* Typically a vet or farmer, eg with:

Fever (PUO); sweats	Anorexia; weight loss	Complications—eg:
Myalgia; backache	Rash; bursitis; orchitis	Osteomyelitis; SBE/IE
Vomiting; malaise	Hepatosplenomegaly	Liver abscess
Depression; lassitude	Arthritis; sacroiliitis	Spleen/lung abscess
Constipation; diarrhoea	Pancytopenia	Meningoencephalitis

Tests: Blood culture (≥6 weeks, contact lab); serology: if titres equivocal (eg >1:40 in non-endemic zones) do ELISA ± immunoradiometric assays. *Treatment:* Doxycycline 100mg/12h PO + streptomycin 1g/day IM for 2–3 weeks (↓ relapse rate from 2–10% vs >20%).[3] If a child, get expert help.

Bordetella pertussis[ND] causes whooping cough. This begins with a nonspecific catarrhal phase of fever and cough. Only after a week or so, does the child develop the characteristic paroxysms of coughing and inspiratory whoops. Most children recover without complication, although the illness may last some months, but some, especially the very young, may develop pneumonia and consequent bronchiectasis, or convulsions and brain damage. Erythromycin should be given early, if only to limit spread. See immunization, p192 and OHCS p208.

Pasteurella multocida is acquired via domestic animals, especially cat or dog bites. It can cause cutaneous infections, septicaemia, pneumonia, UTI, or meningitis. Treat with co-amoxiclav 625mg/8h PO.

Yersinia enterocolitica *Presentation:* In Scandinavia, this is a common cause of reactive, asymmetrical polyarthritis of weight-bearing joints, and, in America, of enteritis. It also causes uveitis, appendicitis, mesenteric lymphadenitis, pyomyositis, glomerulonephritis, thyroiditis, colonic dilatation, terminal ileitis and perforation, and septicaemia. *Tests:* Serology is often more helpful than culture, as there may be quite a time-lag between infection and the clinical manifestations. Agglutination titres >1:160 indicate recent infection. *Treatment:* None may be needed—or ciprofloxacin 500mg/12h PO for 3–5 days.

Moraxella catarrhalis (a diplococcus) is an increasingly recognized cause of pneumonia, exacerbations of COPD, otitis media, sinusitis, septicaemia, endocarditis, and meningitis. It is usually sensitive to amoxicillin.

Tularaemia is caused by *Francisella tularensis* (Gram −ve bacillus), which may be acquired by handling infected animal carcasses. It causes rashes, fevers, tonsillitis, headaches, malaise, hepatosplenomegaly, and lymphadenopathy. There may be papules at sites of inoculation (eg fingers). *Complications:* Meningitis, osteomyelitis, SBE/IE, pericarditis, septicaemia. *Diagnosis:* Telephone your local microbiologist. Only use laboratories with safety cabinets suitable for dangerous pathogens. Swabs and aspirates must be transported in approved containers.
Treatment: Streptomycin 7.5–10mg/kg/12h IM for 2 weeks. Oral tetracycline may be suitable for chemoprophylaxis.
Prevention: Find the particular animal vector; reduce human contact with it as far as possible. Vaccination may be possible for high-risk groups.

Cat scratch disease *Cause:* Mostly due to *Bartonella henselae*, a small, curved, pleomorphic, Gram −ve rod (once classified in the genus Rickettsiales). *Diagnosis:* Think of this disease when any 3 of the following co-exist: an inoculating cat scratch; regional lymphadenopathy with −ve results on lab tests looking for other causes of lymphadenopathy (p50); +ve cat scratch skin test antigen response—or microabscesses found in lymph nodes. *Treatment:* Uncertain as usually unresponsive *in vivo* despite susceptibility *in vitro*. Agents to consider: rifampicin, ciprofloxacin, co-trimoxazole, gentamicin (p178–p181).

See also **spirochaetes** p232; *Neisseria*, p444, and *Legionella* p334.

1 F Charlton 1994 *BMJ* i 1060 2 D Dennis 1994 *BMJ* ii 893 3 G Luzzi 1993 *Tr Roy Soc Trop Med Hy* 87 138

TetanusND

Essence Tetanospasmin, *Clostridium tetani*'s *exotoxin*, causes muscle spasms and rigidity, cardinal features of tetanus (='to stretch').

Incidence ~50 people/yr in the UK. Mortality: 40% (80% in neonates).

Pathogenesis Spores of *Clostridium tetani* live in faeces, soil, dust, and on instruments. A tiny breach in skin or mucosa, eg cuts, burns, ear piercing, banding of piles, may admit the spores. (Diabetics are at especial risk.) Spores may then germinate and make the exotoxin. This then travels up peripheral nerves and interferes with inhibitory synapses.

The Patient Signs appear from 1 day to several months from the (often forgotten) injury. There is a prodrome of fever, malaise, and headache before classical features develop: *trismus* (=lockjaw; Greek trismos = grinding, hence difficulty in opening the mouth); *risus sardonicus* (a grin-like posture of hypertonic facial muscles); *opisthotonus* (arched body with hyperextended neck); *spasms* (which at first may be induced by movement, injections, noise, etc, but later are spontaneous; they may cause dysphagia and respiratory arrest); autonomic dysfunction (arrhythmias and wide fluctuations in BP).

Differential diagnosis is dental abscess, rabies, phenothiazine toxicity, and strychnine poisoning. Phenothiazine toxicity usually only affects facial and tongue muscles; if suspected, give benztropine 1–2mg IV.

Bad prognostic signs are short incubation, rapid progression from trismus to spasms (<48h), development post-partum or post-infection, and tetanus in neonates and old age.

Treatment Get expert help; use ITU. Monitor ECG+BP. Careful fluid balance.
- Clean/debride wounds, IV penicillin or metronidazole 1g/8h PR for 1wk.
- Give human tetanus immune globulin (HTIGS) 500u IM to neutralize free toxin. (If only horse antitetanus serum (ATS) is available, give a small SC test dose before giving 10,000u IV and 750u/d to the cut for 3 days.) Some advocate the intrathecal administration of antitoxin.
- Early ventilation and sedation if symptoms progress.
- Control spasms with diazepam 0.05–0.2mg/kg/h IVI or phenobarbitone 1.0mg/kg/h IM or IV with chlorpromazine 0.5mg/kg/6h IM (IV bolus is dangerous) starting 3h after the phenobarbitone. If this fails to control the spasms, paralyse (tubocurarine 15mg IV) and ventilate.

Prevention Active immunization with tetanus toxoid is given as part of the 3-stage 'triple' vaccine during the first year of life (p192). Boosters are given on starting school and in early adulthood. Once 5 injections have been given, revaccinate only at the time of significant injury, and consider a final one-off booster at ~65yrs.[1,2] *Primary immunization of adults:* 0.5mL tetanus toxoid IM repeated twice at monthly intervals.
Wounds: Any cut merits an extra dose of 0.5mL toxoid IM, unless already fully immune (a full course of toxoid or a booster in last 10 years). The non-immune will need 2 further injections (0.5mL IM) at monthly intervals. If partially immune (ie has had a toxoid booster or a full course >10 years previously), a single booster is all the toxoid that is needed.[2]
Human tetanus immunoglobulin: This is required for the partially or non-immune patient (defined above) with dirty, old (>6h), infected, devitalized, or soil-contaminated wounds. Give 250–500 units IM, using a separate syringe and site to the toxoid injection.
▸If immune status is unknown, assume that the patient is non-immune. Routine infant immunization started in 1961, so many adults are at risk.
▸Hygiene education and wound debridement are of vital importance.

1 C Bowie 1996 *Lancet* 348 1195 2 DoH 1996; the 65-yr booster is *not* DoH advice, but is reckoned cost-effective ($4527/life saved vs $8000/life saved for hypertension screening—C Bowman 1996 *Lancet* 348 1664; this regimen may still be inadequate for some—R Sehgal 1997 *Lancet* 349 573)

Enteric feverND

Typhoid and paratyphoid are caused by *Salmonella typhi* and *S paratyphi* (types A, B, and C) respectively. (Other salmonellae cause diarrhoea and vomiting, but rarely typhoid-like illness; see p190, p486.)

Incubation: 3–21 days. Spread: Faecal–oral. 1% become chronic carriers.
Presentation: Usually malaise, headache, high fever with relative bradycardia, cough, and constipation (or diarrhoea). CNS signs (coma, delirium, meningism) are serious. Diarrhoea is more common after the first week. Rose spots occur on the trunk of 40%, but may be very difficult to see. Epistaxis, bruising, abdominal pain, and splenomegaly may occur.
Diagnosis: Blood culture in first 10 days; faecal/urine culture in 2nd 10 days. Marrow culture has the highest yield. The Widal test is unreliable.
Treat with fluid replacement and good nutrition. Chloramphenicol is still used in many areas: 1g/8h PO until pyrexia diminishes, then 500mg/8h for a week and 250mg/6h to make up 14 days (can be shorter). Ciprofloxacin 500mg/12h PO for 14 days, amoxicillin 1g/6h PO for 14 days are alternatives (IV therapy may be needed, and resistance is likely). In encephalopathy ± shock, give dexamethasone 3mg/kg IV stat, then 1mg/kg/6h for 2 days. Antibiotic resistance is a problem (even with ciprofloxacin).
Complications: Osteomyelitis (eg in sickle-cell disease); DVT; GI bleed or perforation; cholecystitis; myocarditis; pyelonephritis; meningitis; abscess. Infection is said to have cleared when 6 consecutive cultures of urine and faeces are −ve. Chronic carriage is a problem; treat if at risk of spreading disease (eg food handlers). Amoxicillin 4–6g/day + probenecid 2g/day for 6 weeks may work, but cholecystectomy may be needed.
Prognosis: If untreated, 10% die; if treated, 0.1% die. *Vaccine:* p192.

Bacillary dysenteryND

Shigella causes abdominal pain and bloody diarrhoea ± sudden fever, headache, and occasionally neck stiffness. CSF is sterile. Its incubation period is 1–7 days. School epidemics in Britain are usually mild (often *S sonnei*), but imported dysentery may be severe (often *S flexneri* or *S dysenteriae*). Spread is by the faecal–oral route. The organism should be cultured from the faeces. Treatment is supportive with fluids. Avoid antidiarrhoeal agents. Drugs: ciprofloxacin 500mg/12h PO for 3–5 days. Imported shigellosis is often resistant to several antimicrobials: sensitivity testing is important. There may be associated spondyloarthritis (p669).

CholeraND

Vibrio cholerae (Gram −ve comma-shaped rod)
Incubation: A few hours–5 days. *Spread:* Faecal–oral. Pandemics may occur. It produces profuse watery ('rice water') stools (eg 1 litre/h), fever, vomiting, and rapid dehydration, which is the cause of death.
Diagnosis: Direct stool microscopy; culture. *Epidemics:* eg 1990s epidemic in S America, Zaire, and Bangladesh (Bengal *Vibrio cholerae 0139*).
Treatment: Strict barrier nursing. Replace fluid and salt losses meticulously, by 0.9% saline IVI only if desperate (eg shocked); add 20mmol/L K⁺ until U&E known (avoid plain Ringer's lactate◻). Oral rehydration using WHO formula (20g glucose/L) is not nearly so effective as cooked rice powder solution (50–80g/L) in reducing stool volume, perhaps because WHO fluid does not contain enough glucose to enable absorption of all the sodium and water in the rehydration fluid. Its high osmolarity (310mmol/L vs 200mmol/L) is also unfavourable to water absorption.[1] Tetracycline 10mg/kg/6h PO for 2 days reduces fluid losses.
Prevention: Only drink treated water. Cook all food well; eat it hot. Avoid shellfish. Peel all vegetables. Oral vaccines (live and killed) are becoming available (CVD 103-HgR can give near-complete protection within 8 days).[2]

---

1 Cholera Working Group 1993 *Lancet* **342** 387 & S Gore 1992 BMJ i 287 2 M Levine 1997 *Lancet* **349** 220, 231

Historical note on the enteric fevers

Typhoid means *like typhus*, τυφος (*tuphos = smoke*) denoting *stupor*, or *darkening of the intellect as if wrapped in smoke* (seen in severe typhoid).

The provision of clean drinking water and other hygienic measures have lessened the impact of the enteric fevers. But over the centuries, and, even now, in many places such as India and South America, typhoid and typhoid-like illnesses cause significant mortality. Perhaps the most significant such death occurred at noon on April 23 1851 in Malvern—that of a little-known girl whose death is securely, though circuitously, woven into our twentieth-century consciousness. Her name was Annie Darwin, her father's, Charles. Annie was Charles's favourite fun-loving daughter, and with her lingering enteric death Darwin gave up all belief in a just and moral universe. Thus unimpeded, his mind was able to frame and compellingly justify the most devastating answer to the oldest question: that we are here by accident, thanks to natural selection, the survival of the fittest, and the 'wasteful, blundering low & horridly cruel works of nature'.[1]

A remark of Darwin's in 1856, before starting his *Origin of Species*, and quoted in *Darwin* by Adrian Desmond and James Moore, 1989, Penguin

Leprosy[ND]

►The diagnosis of leprosy must be considered in all who have visited endemic areas who present with painless disorders of skin and nerves. It is not just a tropical disease, and may occur in the USA, eg in Texas, Louisiana, and California, as well as Hawaii and Puerto Rico.

Mycobacterium leprae affects some millions of people in the Tropics and subtropics. Since the widespread use of dapsone prevalence has fallen (from 0.5% to 2/1000 in Uganda; from 11% to 4/1000 in parts of India).[1]

The Patient The incubation period is months to years, and the subsequent course depends on the patient's immune response. If the immune response is ineffective, 'lepromatous' disease develops, dominated by foamy histiocytes full of bacilli, but few lymphocytes. If there is a vigorous immune response, the disease is 'tuberculoid', with granulomata containing epithelioid cells and lymphocytes, but few or no demonstrable bacilli. Between these poles lie those with 'borderline' disease.

Skin lesions: Hypopigmented anaesthetic macules, papules, or annular lesions (with raised erythematous rims). Erythema nodosum occurs in 'lepromatous' disease, especially during the first year of treatment.▪

Nerve lesions: Major peripheral nerves may be involved, leading to much disability. Sometimes a thickened sensory nerve may be felt running into the skin lesion (eg ulnar nerve above the elbow, median nerve at the wrist, or the great auricular nerve running up below the ear).

Eye lesions: ►*Refer promptly to an ophthalmologist.* The lower temperature of the anterior chamber favours corneal invasion (so secondary infection and cataract). Inflammatory signs: chronic iritis, scleritis, episcleritis. There may be reduced corneal sensation (V nerve palsy), and reduced blinking (VII nerve palsy) and lagophthalmos (difficulty in closing the eyes; *lagos* is Greek for hare), ± ingrowing eyelashes (trichiasis).

Diagnosis Biopsy a thickened nerve; *in vitro* culture is not possible. As an incidental curio, armadillo (or mouse) foot-pad culture works, but do not taunt your lab by requesting this test! Skin or nose-blow smears for AFB are +ve in borderline or lepromatous disease. Classification matters as it reflects the biomass of bacilli, influencing treatment: the more organisms, the greater the chance that some will be drug-resistant. Other tests: neutrophilia, ESR↑, IgG↑, false +ve rheumatoid test.▪

Treatment[2] Ask a local expert about: ●Resistantce patterns, eg to dapsone, when ethionamide may (rarely) be needed ●Using prednisolone for severe complications ●Is surgery ± physiotherapy needed as well as chemotherapy? In the UK, advice from the panel of Leprosy Opinion is essential. In other areas, the administration of some drugs should be supervised (s) whereas others need no supervision (NS). For lepromatous and borderline disease, WHO advises rifampicin 600mg PO monthly (s), dapsone 100mg/24h PO (NS), and clofazimine 300mg monthly (s) + 50mg/24h (NS) for 2yrs. In tuberculoid leprosy, rifampicin 600mg monthly (s) and dapsone 100mg/24h (NS) for 6 months. Dapsone may cause haemolysis. ►Beware sudden permanent *paralysis* from nerve inflammation caused by dying bacilli (± *orchitis*, *prostration*, or *death*); this 'lepra reaction' may be mollified by thalidomide (*NOT* if pregnant). Liaise urgently with a leprologist.

WHO regimens are problematic as many find it hard to attend for supervised therapy (nomads, jungle-dwellers, those living in remote mountains). Shorter courses of treatment may be practical and effective.[2]

1 K Meeran 1989 *BMJ* i 364   2 MF Waters 1993 *Tr Roy Soc Trop Med Hyg* 87 500

✝✝ Spirochaetes

Lyme disease (*Borrelia burgdorferi[et al]*) is tick-borne. *Don't make the mistake of thinking it's confined to Lyme (Connecticut): it's a global(izing) disease.* ►Ask: "Do you remember being bitten by an insect?" Not all will remember. It may begin with *erythema chronicum migrans* (p678), ± malaise, cognition↓, stiff neck; lymph nodes↑; arthralgia (later erosive arthropathy); myocarditis; heart block; meningitis; ataxia; amnesia; cranial nerve palsies; neuropathy; lymphocytic meningoradiculitis (Bannwarth's syndrome). *Diagnosis:* Clinical ± serology (if −ve, PCR may help.)▪ *Treat* skin condition with doxycycline 100mg/12h PO (amoxicillin or penicillin V if <12yrs) for 10–21 days, and later complications with high-dose IV benzylpenicillin, cefotaxime or ceftriaxone. *Prevention:* Keep limbs covered; use insect repellent; tick collars for pets; check skin often when in risky areas. Advice differs on prophylaxis after a tick bites. In highly endemic areas this may be worthwhile (eg if risk is >1%). *Removing ticks:* Suffocate tick with eg petroleum jelly, then gently remove by grasping close to mouth parts and twisting off; then clean skin. (See http://www.lymenet.org/)

Endemic treponematoses *Yaws* is caused by *Treponema pertenue*, serologically indistinguishable from *T pallidum*. It is a chronic granulomatous disease prevalent in children in the rural Tropics. Spread is person-to-person, via skin abrasions, and is promoted by poor hygiene. The primary lesion (an ulcerating papule) appears ~4 weeks after exposure. Scattered secondary lesions then appear, eg in moist skin, but can be anywhere. These may become exuberant. Tertiary lesions are subcutaneous gummatous ulcerating granulomata, affecting skin and bone. Cardiovascular and CNS complications do not occur. *Pinta* (*T carateum*) affects only skin; seen in Central and South America. *Endemic non-venereal syphilis (bejel; T pallidum)* is seen in Third World children, when it resembles yaws. In the developed world, *T pallidum* causes venereal syphilis (p233). *Diagnosis:* clinical. *Treatment:* procaine penicillin (p177).

Weil's disease[ND] *Cause:* Leptospira interrogans (eg serogroup *L icterohaemorrhagiae*). Spread is by contact with infected rat urine, eg while swimming. *Signs:* Fever, jaundice, headache, red conjunctivae, tender legs (myositis), purpura, haemoptysis, haematemesis, or any bleeding. Meningitis, myocarditis, and particularly renal failure may develop. AST rise may be small.
Diagnosis: Complement fixation test, the Schuffner agglutination test, and blood, urine and CSF culture.
Treat symptomatically and give benzylpenicillin 600mg/6h for 7 days, or doxycycline 100mg/12h PO. Doxycycline is useful prophylaxis for high-risk groups. The Jarisch–Herxheimer reaction is rare in leptospirosis. This is a systemic reaction several hours after the first dose of antibiotic is given. There is fever, tachycardia, and vasodilatation; death is rare. It is thought to be due to the sudden release of endotoxin.

Canicola fever is an aseptic meningitis caused by *Leptospira canicola*.

Relapsing fever[ND] This is caused by *Borrelia recurrentis* (louse-borne) or *B duttoni* (tick-borne). It typically occurs in pandemics following war or disaster, and may kill millions. *Presentation:* After 2–10 days' incubation there is abrupt fever, rigors, and headache. A petechial rash (which may be faint or absent), jaundice, and hepatosplenomegaly may develop. Crises of very high fever and tachycardia occur. When the fever abates, hypotension due to vasodilation may develop. It may be fatal. Relapses occur, but are milder. *Tests:* Organisms are seen on Leishman-stained thin or thick films. *Treatment:* Tetracycline 500mg PO or 250mg IV as a single dose (but for 10 days for *B duttoni*). The Jarisch–Herxheimer reaction (above) is fatal in 5%: meptazinol 100mg IV slowly is given as prophylaxis with the tetracycline, repeated 30mins later (with the chill phase) and during the flush phase (if systolic BP <75mmHg). Delouse the patient. Doxycycline (p180) is useful prophylaxis in high-risk groups.

Syphilis—the archetypal spirochaetal (treponemal) disease

Treponema pallidum enters via an abrasion, during sex. All features are from endarteritis obliterans (reduction in lumen of small arteries by proliferation of intima). It is commonest in homosexuals—but by trying to avoid AIDS their risk is lessening. *Incubation:* 9–90 days. 4 stages:

- *Primary:* A macule at site of sexual contact becomes a very infectious, painless hard ulcer (*primary chancre*).
- *Secondary:* Occurs 4–8wks after chancre. Fever, malaise, lymphadenopathy, rash (trunk, palms, soles), alopecia, condylomata lata (anal papules), buccal snail-track ulcers; rarely hepatitis, meningism, nephrosis, uveitis.
- *Tertiary syphilis* follows 2–20yrs latency (when patients are non-infectious): there are *gummas* (granulomas occurring in skin, mucosa, bone, joints, rarely viscera eg lung, testis).
- *Quaternary syphilis—Cardiovascular:* Ascending aortic aneurysm ± aortic regurgitation. *Neurosyphilis: a Meningovascular:* Cranial nerve palsies, stroke; *b General paresis of insane (GPI):* Dementia, psychoses (fatal untreated; treatment *may* reverse it); *c Tabes dorsalis:* Sensory ataxia, numb legs, chest, and bridge of nose, lightning pains, gastric crises, reflex loss, flexor plantars, Charcot's joints (p476). *Argyll Robertson pupil* (p56).

Pitfalls: Always ask yourself: *Is there HIV complicating this illness?* ►Any genital sore is syphilis until proven otherwise—but there *are* other causes: trauma, herpes, scabies, Behçet's disease, cancer, chancroid, lymphogranuloma venereum, granuloma inguinale. *Serology* (2 types):

1 Cardiolipin antibody: detectable in primary disease but wanes in late syphilis. It indicates active disease and becomes negative after treatment. *False +ves* (with negative treponemal antibody): pregnancy, immunization, pneumonia, malaria, SLE, TB, leprosy.
Examples: VDRL (venereal disease research laboratory slide test), RPR (rapid plasma reagin), WR (Wassermann reaction).

2 Treponeme-specific antibody: +ve in **1°** disease, remaining so despite treatment. *Examples:* TPHA (*T pallidum* haemagglutination test), FTA (fluorescent treponemal antibody), TPI (*T pallidum* immobilization test); none distinguish syphilis from nonvenereal yaws, bejel, or pinta.

Other tests In **1°** syphilis, treponemes are demonstrated by dark ground microscopy of chancre fluid; serology at this stage is often –ve. In **2°** syphilis, treponemes are seen in the lesions and both types of antibody tests are positive. In late syphilis, organisms may no longer be seen, but both types of antibody test usually remain +ve (cardiolipin antibody tests may wane). In neurosyphilis, CSF antibody tests are +ve. If HIV+ve, serology may be –ve during syphilis reactivation.

Treatment: Procaine penicillin (=procaine benzylpenicillin) 600mg/24h IM for 10 days (tertiary or CVS disease: 14 days; CNS: 14 days). Beware *Jarisch–Herxheimer reaction* (p232), commonest in 2° disease; most dangerous in 3°. Consider steroids. Trace contacts. If HIV+ve, penicillin may not stop neurosyphilis; consult microbiologist. *Congenital syphilis:* OHCS p98.

PoliomyelitisND

Polio is a highly contagious picornavirus. *Spread:* Droplet or faeco–oral.
The Patient: 7 days' incubation, then 2 days' 'flu-like prodrome, leading to a 'pre-paralytic' stage, consisting of fever (eg 39°C), tachycardia, headache, vomiting, neck stiffness, and unilateral tremor. This proceeds in 65% of those reaching the pre-paralytic stage to the paralytic stage with myalgia and lower motor neurone signs and respiratory failure.
Tests: CSF: WCC↑, polymorphs then lymphocytes, otherwise normal; paired sera (14 days apart); throat swab and stool culture identify virus.
Natural history: < 10% of those with paralysis die; anterior horn cell loss is permanent,so appropriate support will be needed. There may be *delayed progression* of paralysis. *Risk factors for severe paralysis:* Adulthood; pregnancy; post-tonsillectomy; muscle fatigue/trauma during incubation period.
Prophylaxis: Live vaccine by oral route (p192). In the Tropics the killed parenteral vaccine is needed to induce adequate immunity. Adults should be revaccinated when their children are vaccinated.

RabiesND

Rabies is a rhabdovirus spread by bites from any infected mammal, eg bats (bites may go unnoticed[1]), dogs, cats, foxes, or raccoons. *The Patient:* Usually 9–90 days' incubation, so give prophylaxis even several months after exposure. Prodromal symptoms of headache, malaise, abnormal behaviour, agitation, fever, and itching at the site of the bite proceeds to 'furious rabies', eg with water provoking muscle spasms often accompanied by profound terror (hydrophobia). In 20%, 'dumb rabies' starts with flaccid paralysis in the bitten limb and spreads. *Pre-exposure prophylaxis* (eg vets, zoo-keepers, customs officials, bat handlers, remote expeditions): Give human diploid cell strain vaccine (1mL IM, deltoid) on days 0, 7, & 28, and again at 2–3 yrs if still at risk. *Treatment if bitten in a country where rabies is endemic* (if unvaccinated or possibly not): ►Seek expert help (UK *virus reference lab*, tel.: 0181 200 4400). Observe the biting animal if possible, to see if the animal dies (but it is possible that it may not die of rabies before the patient does);[2] asymptomatic carriage occurs but has not (yet) produced rabies in man. Clean the wound. Give the vaccine on days 0, 3, 7, 14, 30, and 90 (1mL IM) and human rabies immunoglobulin (20u/kg on day 0; half given IM and half locally infiltrated around wound). Rabies is usually fatal once symptoms begin, but survival has occurred, if there is optimum CNS and cardiorespiratory support. Staff in attendance should be offered vaccination.

Viral haemorrhagic feversND

Yellow fever: An epidemic arbovirus disease spread by *Aedes* mosquitoes (Bolivia, Peru, and moist central/w African savannas). Immunization: p192.
The Patient: 2–14-day incubation, then in mild forms, fever, headache, nausea, albuminuria, myalgia, and relative bradycardia. If severe: 3 days of headache, myalgia, anorexia ± nausea—then abrupt fever; after brief remission, prostration, dramatic jaundice (± fatty liver), haematemesis and other bleeding, oliguria. *Mortality:* < 10% (day 5–10). *Diagnosis:* ELISA. *Treatment:* Symptomatic.

*Lassa fever*ND, *Ebola virus*^{ND,} *Marburg virus*ND, and *dengue haemorrhagic fever* (dengue is the most prevalent arbovirus disease)[3] These diseases may start with sudden-onset headache, pleuritic pain, backache, myalgia, conjunctivitis, prostration, dehydration, facial flushing (dengue), and fever. Soon bleeding supervenes. There may be spontaneous resolution, or renal failure, encephalitis, coma, and death. *Treatment:* Symptomatic. ►*Use special infection control measures (Lassa, Ebola, Marburg); get expert help at once.*

1 *Morbid & Mortal Weekly Rec* 1998 **47** 1 2 T Hemachudha 1991 *NEJM* **324** 1890 3 T Monath 1997 reports that dengue is very unlikely to become haemorrhagic if AST ↔; other signs: haemostasis↓, +ve tourniquet test (>10 petechiae/2.5cm² skin), platelets↓, PCV↑, WCC <5, pleural effusion (do decubitus CXR)—*Lancet* **350** 1719.

> ### Polio: an exercise in prevention
>
> - Pre-1950 distribution was worldwide.
> - April 12 1955: vaccination starts.
> - 1991: transmission interrupted in the western hemisphere.
> - 1993: China institutes national immunization days (>80,000,000 children vaccinated in 2 days; 1 year later only 5 cases of virus-confirmed wild polio, so on target for global eradication by 2000, except perhaps for parts of Africa and India).
> - 1997: 1 case of 'wild' polio confirmed in the entire European Region.
> - Any polio seen in the West will be the very rare kind that may follow vaccination. Half these people will be adult contacts of child vaccinees.

Rickettsia and arthropod-borne bacteria

Rickettsia are intracellular bacteria spending at least part of their time in specific host arthropods before invading human mononucuclear cells, neutrophils or blood vessels (vasculotropic types). All the cataclysmic events of the 20th century have favoured infestation with lice—war, revolution, flood, famine, overcrowding, and the disintegration of empires: as a result, Rickettsia (notably typhus, opposite) have killed uncounted millions.

Q fever *Coxiella burnetii* causes about 100 cases of Q fever per year in the UK. It is so named because it was first labelled 'query' fever in workers in an Australian abattoir. *Epidemiology:* It occurs worldwide, and is usually rural with its reservoir in cattle and sheep. The organism is very resistant to drying and is usually inhaled from infected dust. It can be contracted from unpasteurized milk, directly from carcasses in abattoirs, sometimes by droplet spread, and occasionally from tick bites.

The Patient: Q fever should be suspected in anyone with prolonged PUO or atypical pneumonia. It may present with fever, myalgia, sweats, headache, cough, and hepatitis. If the disease becomes chronic, suspect endocarditis ('culture-negative'). This usually affects the aortic valve, but clinical signs may be absent for many years. It also causes miscarriages.

Tests: CXR (consolidation, eg lower lobe, or 1 or more masses, persisting for months during resolution). Liver biopsy may show granulomata. The diagnosis is made serologically. The presence of phase I antigens indicates chronic infection; phase II antigens indicate acute infection.

Treatment: Tetracycline is effective *in vitro* (rickettsiostatic), but has not been shown to speed recovery. It is given in the hope of preventing chronicity. Drugs for chronic disease include rifampicin and tetracycline.

Bartonellosis is a non-contagious, infectious disease caused by a Gram –ve, motile, bacillus-like organism *Bartonella bacilliformis* which parasitizes RBCS. Spread is by dawn- or dusk-biting sandflies—in the Andes, Peru, Equador, Colombia, Thailand, and Niger. Transient immunosuppression leads to associated infections (eg salmonella). *The Patient:* Fever, rashes, lymphadenopathy, hepatosplenomegaly, cerebellar syndromes,[1] dermal nodules (verrugas), retinal haemorrhages, pericardial effusion, oedema, CSF pleocytosis, haemolysis (Coombs' –ve, ± dyspnoea and jaundice), and hypochromic, macrocytic red cells with a megaloblastic marrow.

Tests: Organisms are cultured, or seen on Giemsa-stained thin or thick films.

Treatment: It responds to penicillin, but chloramphenicol (50mg/kg/day for 7d) is often used because of its frequent association with salmonelloses.

Trench fever is caused by *Bartonella quintana* inoculated from infected louse faeces, not only in soldiers, but also in the homeless, and in alcoholics.

The Patient may exhibit fever, headache, myalgia, dizziness, back pain, a rash (macules 2–4mm across), eye pain, leg pain, splenomegaly, and, rarely, endocarditis. It is not fatal; it may relapse. *Treatment:* Tetracycline.

Ehrlichiosis *Ehrlichia chaffeensis* is an obligate intracytoplasmic Gram –ve organism related to Rickettsia and is spread by ticks (*Dermacentor variabili*). It causes fever, headache, anorexia, malaise, abdominal pain, epigastric pain, conjunctivitis, lymphadenopathy, jaundice, rash, confusion, and cervical lymphadenopathy.

Test results: Leukopenia, thrombocytopenia, AST↑.[2]

Treatment: It may respond to doxycycline.

---

1 JE Gonzalez-Mendoza 1993 *Tr Roy Soc Trop Med Hyg* **87** 367   2 D Pierard 1995 *Lancet* **346** 1233

Typhus: the archetypal rickettsial disease

Typhus rickettsia are conveyed between hosts by arthropods. The incubation period is 2–23 days. There follows an acute illness of sudden onset which may be associated with severe headache, vomiting, photophobia, deafness, and toxaemia. With some species, an *eschar* may be present. This is a single skin lesion at the site of the initial inoculation, which goes on to ulcerate and form a black scar. Later in the acute illness (5th–6th day) a more generalized skin rash occurs (see below). It may be of a maculopapular nature, resembling measles or rubella, or be haemorrhagic. Asymptomatic or mild illness is common.

Pathology: Widespread vasculitis and endothelial proliferation may affect any or all organs, and thrombotic occlusion may lead to gangrene. Patients die of shock, renal failure, DIC, or stroke.

Diagnosis: This is difficult as often the picture is nonspecific, the organisms are difficult to grow, and the traditional heterophil antibody Weil–Felix test has low specificity and sensitivity. Immunofluorescence and ELISA tests on paired sera are a great help, and skin biopsy can be diagnostic in Rocky Mountain spotted fever.

The two chief types of typhus are:
- *Louse-borne epidemic typhus: R prowazeki* is carried by the human louse *Pediculus humanus*, faeces of which are inhaled or pass through skin. It may become latent and recrudesce later (Brill–Zinsser disease).
- *Rocky Mountain spotted fever* is tick-borne (*R rickettsi*) and is the other major killer in this group. There are marked asynchronous geographic flutuations in incidence. The typical locality is the south-eastern states of the USA, where the incidence is ~600 people/year.

Risk factors for fatal disease: Older, male, black, or G6PD deficiency.

The Patient with typhus: A characteristic rash *may or may not* appear, typically by the 4th day of fever (pink macules, starting on palms, soles and wrists)—in a few days, lesions become purpuric and slightly papular. Haemolysis may occur, with thrombocytopenia in up to 50%. Later there may be oedema of hands and feet, and bleeding from orifices from DIC.

Complications: Respiratory failure (12%); renal failure (14%). ▶A history of tick exposure only occurs in 60% of patients.

Tests: Latex agglutination, indirect immunofluorescence, and enzyme immunoassays are available.

Treatment: ▶▶Do not wait for serology. All types are treated with tetracycline 500mg/6h for 7 days (or chloramphenicol 500mg/6h for 7 days). Resistance problems are reported in northern Thailand.

Other forms of typhus include *murine (endemic) typhus*, *tick typhus (fièvre boutonneuse)*, *rickettsialpox* (*R akari*—its rash is papular, and may become vesicular), and *scrub typhus* (which is most common in SE Asia).

Giardiasis

Giardia lamblia is a common flagellate protozoon which lives in the duodenum and jejunum. It is transmitted by faeces. Risk factors: travel, immunosuppression, homosexuality, achlorhydria, and playgroups where nappies/diapers are changed. Drinking water may become contaminated.

Presentation: Often asymptomatic. Lassitude, bloating, flatulence, loose stools, and abdominal discomfort ± explosive diarrhoea are typical features. Malabsorption (weight↓) and disaccharide intolerance may occur.

Diagnosis: Repeated stool microscopy for cysts or trophozoites may be –ve, and duodenal fluid analysis (by aspiration or absorption on to a piece of swallowed string (Enterotest® ▣)) may be tried. An ELISA test is available. Finally, a blind therapeutic trial may be needed.

Differential: Any cause of diarrhoea (p188, p190, p486), tropical sprue (p522), coeliac disease (p522). See http://vm.cfsan.fda.gov/~mow/intro.html.

Treatment: Scrupulous hygiene. Give metronidazole 400mg/8h PO for 5 days or 2g/24h for 3 days, or tinidazole 2g PO once (advise to avoid driving and alcohol) or mepacrine hydrochloride 100mg/8h PO for 5–7 days (cheap, but SEs common). If treatment fails, check for concordance (p3) and consider treating the whole family. If diarrhoea persists, avoid milk as lactose intolerance may persist for 6 weeks.

Other GI protozoa *Cryptosporidium* (p486) and *Isospora* (particularly common in AIDS), *Balantidium coli*, and *Sarcocystis*.

Amoebiasis

Entamoeba histolytica distribution is worldwide. Spread is faecal–oral. It is necessary to boil infected food to destroy cysts. Trophozoites may remain in the bowel or invade extra-intestinal tissues, leaving 'flask-shaped' GI ulcers. Infection may be asymptomatic, or cause only mild diarrhoea. Dysentery lies at the other extreme of the spectrum.

Amoebic dysentery[ND] may begin years after infection. Diarrhoea begins slowly, becoming profuse and bloody. High fever, colic and tenesmus are rare, but an acute febrile prostrating illness does occur, as do remissions and exacerbations. Diagnose by microscopy of fresh stool. Serology indicates whether the patient has at some time been infected.

Differential diagnosis: Amoebic dysentery has a gradual onset with pus, red cells, and trophozoites in the stool. Bacillary dysentery often has a sudden onset and may cause dehydration. Its stools may be more watery and have no trophozoites. Acute ulcerative colitis also has a more gradual onset. Dehydration is rare, and the stools are very bloody with relatively few pus cells. Other causes of bloody diarrhoea: p486.

Amoebic colonic abscesses may perforate causing peritonitis.

Amoeboma is an inflammatory mass most often found at the caecum, where it must be distinguished from other RIF masses.

Hepatic abscesses are usually single masses in the right lobe, and contain anchovy-sauce-like fluid. There is usually a high swinging fever, sweats, RUQ pain, tenderness, and WCC↑. LFTs may be normal but mechanical obstruction may occur. Diagnosis is suggested by ultrasound and CT appearances, and positive serology. Aspiration may be required.

Treatment Metronidazole 800mg/8h PO for 5 days (SE: neuropathy; fits; WCC↓) for acute amoebic dysentery (very active against vegetative amoebae), then diloxanide furoate 500mg/8h PO for 10 days to destroy gut cysts (SEs rare). Diloxanide is also best for chronic disease when *Entamoeba* cysts, not vegetative forms, are in stools. Amoebic liver abscess: metronidazole 400mg/8h PO for 10 days; repeat at 2 weeks as needed; aspirate if no improvement after 72h giving diloxanide course post-metronidazole.

Trypanosomiasis

African trypanosomiasis (sleeping sickness) *T gambiense* causes a slow, wasting illness with a long prepatent (latent) period (West African variety). *T rhodesiense* causes a more rapidly progressive illness (rural East Africa). The organism enters the skin following a bite from an infected tsetse fly, and spreads to nodes, blood, spleen, heart, and brain.

The Patient: Signs include a subcutaneous chancre at the site of infection, with fevers, lymphadenopathy (posterior cervical nodes are particularly enlarged with *T gambiense* infection: Winterbottom's sign), headache, rashes, joint pains, weight loss, amenorrhoea/impotence, peripheral and pulmonary oedema, ascites, pericardial effusions, and nephritis. Later in the natural history, patients develop CNS features (apathy, depression, ataxia, dyskinesias, dementia, hypersomnolence, and coma).

Diagnosis is by demonstration of the organisms in the blood or lymph nodes. CSF should be examined.

Treatment: Seek expert help. ●Treat the anaemia and other infections first.
●Early (haemolymphatic) phase: suramin 20mg/kg IV on days 1, 3, 7, 14, 21. Give 200mg test dose IV first.
●CNS disease: see opposite.

Suramin predictably causes proteinuria and often increased serum urea and creatinine; therefore check renal function frequently.
Melarsoprol causes lethal encephalopathy in up to 10% of patients, characterized by abnormal behaviour, fits, and coma. This is partly preventable with prednisolone 1mg/kg/24h PO (max 40mg) starting the day before the first injection.[1] Seek expert help.

Arseno-resistant trypanosomiasis was uniformly fatal until the introduction of difluoromethylornithine (DFMO) in 1984. Dose example: 100mg/kg/6h IVI over 1h for 14 days, followed by 75mg/kg/6h PO for 3–4 weeks. SE: anaemia; diarrhoea; seizures; leucopenia; hair loss. It is also being assessed in Chagas' disease.

American trypanosomiasis (Chagas' disease) is caused by *Trypanosoma cruzi*. It is spread by Reduviid bugs or blood transfusion. After implantation, a nodule (Chagoma) forms which may then scar.
Presentation: Fever; unilateral bipalpebral oedema (Romañas' sign); ophthalmia (=eye inflammation); lymphadenopathy; hepatosplenomegaly—or there may be a long latent period (eg 20yrs) followed by signs of multi-organ invasion and damage, affecting especially heart and GI smooth muscle. GI: Megaoesophagus, dilated stomach, megacolon.
Heart: Dilated cardiomyopathy, bundle branch blocks, syncope, emboli, LVF, ST elevation, T-wave inversion, left ventricular aneurysm; sudden death.
CNS: With Chagas' disease in those with HIV, there may be cerebral lesions.
Diagnosis: Acute disease: protozoa may be seen in or grown from blood, CSF, or node aspirate. Chronic disease: serology (Chagas' IgG ELISA).
Treatment: This is unsatisfactory. Nifurtimox 2mg/kg/6h PO or benzidazole (3.7mg/kg/12h PO for 60 days) are used in acute disease (toxic agents which only eliminate the parasite in 50% of patients[2]). Chronic disease can only be treated symptomatically. Allopurinol can reduce parasitaemia.

---

1 J Pepin 1989 *Lancet* **i** 1246   2 L Kirchhoff 1993 *NEJM* **329** 389

Melarsoprol in late sleeping sickness

One regimen involves 12 doses as follows

Day	
1	0.4mg/kg IV slowly
2	0.8
3	1.0
10	2.0
11	2.0
12	2.0
19	2.0
20	2.5
21	3.0
28	3.5
29	3.5
30	3.5

In debilitated patients, start with 2 stat IV doses of suramin 0.2g separated by 24h.

►Seek expert help.

See J Sanford 1997 *Guide to Antimicrobial Therapy,* 87

Leishmaniasis

This intracellular infection, caused by *Leishmania* protozoa, is spread by sandflies, and occurs widely in Africa, India, Latin America, the Middle East, and Mediterranean. It gives rise to sometimes lethal granulomata.

Cutaneous leishmaniasis (oriental sore) A major disease affecting >300,000 people. It may be mild and localized, or diffuse and severe. Lesions develop at the site of the bite, beginning as an itchy papule, from which the crust may fall off to leave an ulcer. Most heal spontaneously with scarring, which may be disfiguring if the lesions are extensive. Cause: *L tropica* or *L mexicana* (which tends to cause destruction of the pinna). Diagnosis is by microscopy of material aspirated from the edge of the ulcer. *Treatment:* If no spontaneous healing, use sodium stibogluconate (Sb^V, ie pentavalent antimony) 10mg/kg/12h IV (max 850mg per day) for 10 days. This is only sometimes effective. Local infiltration may be used. Seek expert advice—aminosidine may be indicated: dose example: 14mg/kg/day IM for 60 days with 10mg Sb^V/kg/day IM.[1] An ointment form is also used.

Mucocutaneous leishmaniasis (espundia) is caused by *L brasiliensis* and occurs in S America. Often primary skin lesions are complicated by spread to mucosae of the nose, pharynx, palate, larynx, and upper lip (in that order). This results in serious scarring and death from pneumonia. *Diagnosis:* As the parasites may be scanty, a Leishmanin skin test is often necessary to distinguish the condition from leprosy, TB, syphilis, yaws, and carcinoma. Indirect fluorescent antibody tests are available. *Treatment:* This is unsatisfactory once mucosae have become involved, so all cutaneous lesions in areas where *L brasiliensis* occurs should be treated with pentavalent antimony as above.

Kala-azar (visceral leishmaniasis) *Kala-azar* means black sickness, denoting hyperpigmentation (face, hands, feet, abdomen, as seen in India). Cause: *L donovani*, *L chagasi* or *L infantum* (or, rarely, 'visceralizing' of *L tropica* eg in Iran, Israel, and NE India).[2] Protozoa spread via lymphatics from minor skin lesions. In the reticuloendothelial system, organisms multiply in macrophages (Leishman–Donovan bodies). ♂:♀>3:1. It is HIV-associated.

Presentation:[3]

●Fevers 100%	●Splenomegaly 96%	●Weight↓ 95%	
●Sweats 90%	●Fatigue 88%	●Appetite↓ 87%	●Rigors 83%
●Cough 69%	●Liver↑ 63%	●Burning feet 52%	●Insomnia 42%
●Abdo pain 42%	●Arthralgia 36%	●Epistaxis 19%	●Lymph nodes↑

Tests: Hypersplenism (anaemia, platelets and WCC↓), albumin↓, IgG↑; –ve Leishmanin skin test. Diagnosis depends on finding organisms in marrow (80%), lymph nodes, or splenic aspirate (95%). Solid-state serology is being developed for field use (K39 antigen).[3] Serology may be –ve if HIV+ve.
Treatment: Request expert help. WHO regimen: pentavalent antimony (sodium stibogluconate, Sb^V) 20mg/kg/24h IV or IM, up to 850mg/day, for 30 days. SE: malaise (patient curls up under the bed clothes all day, not eating), cough, substernal pain, long Q–T interval, arrhythmias, anaemia, uraemia, hepatitis. Regimens are changing—eg 10mg Sb^V/8h for 10 days,[1] without the 850mg limit—as 25% fail to respond or relapse. Here pentamidine may be used: deep IM 3–4mg on alternate days, up to 10 doses: SEs may be fatal (BP↓, arrhythmias, glucose↓, permanent diabetes in 4%[1]). Other anti-leishmanials: aminosidine (paromomycin), liposomal amphotericin B (AmBisome®).[4]
Post kala-azar dermal leishmaniasis, with lesions resembling those of leprosy, may occur months or years following successful treatment.

1 S Teklemariam 1994 *Tr Roy Soc Trop Med Hyg* 88 334 2 D Sacks 1995 *Lancet* 345 959 3 S Sundar 1998 *BMJ* i 563 (sensitivity: >98%; specificity: >95%) 4 F Hashim 1994 *Tr Roy Soc Trop Med Hyg* 88 431

Fungi

Fungi may cause disease by acting as airborne allergens, by deploying toxins, or by direct infection. Fungal infection may be superficial or deep, and both are much commoner in the immunocompromised.

Superficial mycoses Dermatophyte infection (*Trichophyton, Microsporum, Dermatophyton*) causes tinea (ringworm). Diagnose by microscopy of skin scrapings and treat with topical clotrimazole 1% 12-hourly. Continue for 14 days after healing. In intractable lesions, griseofulvin 0.5–1g/24h PO for up to 18 months was previously required, but itraconazole and terbinafine have emerged as promising alternatives.

Candida albicans causes oral (p500) and vaginal (p221) thrush.

Malassezia furfur causes pityriasis versicolor: a macular rash, brown on pale skin and pale on tanned skin. Treat with clotrimazole cream or ketoconazole 400mg PO as a single dose. Some superficial mycoses penetrate the epidermis and cause chronic subcutaneous infections such as Madura foot or sporotrichosis. Treatment is complex and sometimes even requires amputation of the affected limb.

Systemic mycoses *Aspergillus fumigatus* may colonize the lung or cause allergic damage. Invasive systemic aspergillosis occurs in the immunosuppressed. Aspergillosis is discussed fully on p340. Systemic candidiasis also only occurs in the immunocompromised: consider this *whenever* they get a PUO. *Candida* UTI occurs in DM and *Candida* is a rare cause of endocarditis on prosthetic valves. Take repeated blood cultures and do serology. If it does not resolve when the predisposing factor (eg IV line) is removed, the treatment is amphotericin B IV (use the regimen given on p340) or fluconazole 400mg stat then 200mg/day PO.

Cryptococcus neoformans may cause meningitis, or pneumonia in the immunocompromised. It is especially common in AIDS, but also occurs in sarcoid, Hodgkin's, and those on steroids. The history may be long and there may be features suggestive of raised intracranial pressure, eg confusion, papilloedema, and cranial nerve lesions. This may delay CSF examination which is the key investigation. If this diagnosis is suspected, specifically request Indian-ink staining of the CSF. The organism may also be successfully cultured and the antigen detected by the latex test in CSF and blood. HIV –ve cryptococcus meningitis is treated with amphotericin B IV 0.5–0.8mg/kg/day + flucytosine 37.5mg/kg/8h PO until afebrile and culture –ve (eg 6 weeks). Adjust flucytosine to give a peak level of 70–80mg/L; trough 30–40. When culture –ve, start fluconazole 400mg daily PO for 8–10 weeks. Response may be monitored clinically and by serum. If HIV+ve, see opposite. Cryptococcal pneumonia is the other major manifestation (commonest in USA). Treatment is similar.

There are other fungi, most commonly found in the Americas and Africa, which may cause deep infection. *Histoplasma capsulatum, Coccidioides immitis, Paracoccidioides brasiliensis,* and *Blastomyces dermatitidis* may cause asymptomatic infections, acute or chronic pulmonary disease, or disseminated infection. Acute histoplasma pneumonitis may be associated with arthralgia, erythema nodosum, and erythema multiforme. Chronic disease, which is commoner with the other 3 fungi, may cause upper-zone fibrosis or radiographic 'coin lesions'. Diagnosis is by serology, culture, and biopsy. These diseases are treated with amphotericin B (p340), except *Paracoccidioides*, which responds to itraconazole 50–100mg/day PO.

Preventing fungal infections This is a goal in the immunocompromised, and may be achievable with oral fluconazole: eg 50–400mg daily after an episode of (treated) cryptococcal meningitis in HIV patients, or after cytotoxics or radiotherapy (400mg if systemic infection likely, eg after bone marrow transplant)—preferably started before the onset of neutropenia, and continued for 1 week after WCC returns to normal.

Candida on ITU: colonization → invasion → dissemination

Not everyone with a positive yeast culture needs treatment: candida is a common commensal (eg on skin, pharynx, or vagina)—but if many sites (urine, sputum, or surgical drains) are colonized, risk of invasion rises, particularly when on ITU with known risk factors:[1]

- Prolonged ventilation
- Urinary catheters
- Intravascular lines
- Broad spectrum antibiotics
- Immunosuppression
- IV nutrition

Invasion implies fungus in normally sterile tissues.

Dissemination entails invasion of non-contiguous organs via the blood (eg endophthalmitis + fungi in lung or kidney). Consider IV amphotericin (p340) or fluconazole (itraconazole if unresponsive) in these unequivocal circumstances (especially if your patient is deteriorating):[2]

- A single well-taken +ve blood culture—if risk factors present (above).
- Isolation of candida from any sterile site except urine.
- Yeasts on microscopy on a sterile-site specimen, before culture known.
- Positive histology from normally sterile tissues in those at risk (above).

▶ *Before starting systemic antifungals, get help from a microbiologist.*

1 J Lipman 1997 BMJ i 266 2 British Soc for Antimicrobial Chemo 1994 *Intensive Care Med* **20** 522

Cryptococcal meningitis in HIV patients

- It may be necessary to lower CSF pressure by ~50% by removing CSF.
- Amphotericin B 0.5–0.8mg/kg/day IV until response, then. . .
- Fluconazole 400mg PO daily for 2 months, then. . .
- Maintenence fluconazole 200mg daily PO indefinitely.

Note: studies have shown no benefit in adding flucytosine to amphotericin in this context (but it may have a rôle with fluconazole). Confer with experts.

Nematodes (roundworms)

Worldwide, ~1,000,000,000 people are hosts to nematodes (give or take a few hundred million[1]). Many live with us quite peacefully—but note that ascariasis can cause fatal GI obstruction, hookworms can stunt growth, necatoriasis can cause debilitating anaemia, and trichuriasis causes dysentery (ie bloody diarrhoea) and rectal prolapse—so mass population treatment (eg albendazole 400mg/24h PO for 3 days to all school-children) in areas of high prevalence *may* be beneficial.

Necator americanus and ***Ancylostoma duodenale* (Hookworms)** Both occur in the Indian subcontinent, SE Asia, Central and N Africa, and parts of Europe. Necator is also found in the Americas and sub-Saharan Africa. Numerous small worms attach to upper GI mucosa, causing bleeding (a major cause of iron-deficiency anaemia). Eggs are passed in faeces and hatch in soil. Larvae penetrate feet, so starting new infections. Oral transmission of *Anclostoma* may occur. *Diagnose* by stool microscopy. *Treat* with mebendazole 100mg/12h PO for 3 days, and iron.

Strongyloides stercoralis is endemic in (sub)tropics. Transmitted percutaneously, it causes rapidly migrating uriçaria over thighs and trunk (cutaneous larva migrans). Pneumonitis, enteritis, and malabsorption occur, as do acute exacerbations. Chronic signs: diarrhoea, abdominal pain, and urticaria. The worms may take bacteria into the bloodstream, causing septicaemia ± meningitis if they gain access to the CSF. *Diagnose* from stool microscopy and culture, serology, or duodenal aspiration. *Treat* with albendazole 5mg/kg/12h PO for ~3 days (recommended doses may not be enough,[2] and 800mg/day PO has been advised for some adults). Open studies have obtained good results with ivermectin, which may become the treatment of choice.[3] Hyperinfestation is problem if immunocompromised (eg on steroids, or, more rarely, in AIDS). Alternative: thiabendazole (=tiabendazole) (22mg/kg/12h PO, max 3g/d, eg for 2d).

Ascaris lumbricoides occurs worldwide. It looks like (and is named after) the garden worm (*Lumbricus*). An unusual characteristic is that it has 3 finely-toothed lips. Transmission is faecal–oral. It migrates through liver and lungs, and settles in the small bowel. It is usually asymptomatic, but death may occur from GI obstruction or perforation. It may grow very long (eg 25cm). Look for: ●Faecal ova (stained orange by bile; 60–45μm across; the rate of egg production being ~200,000/day). ●Worms on barium x-rays. ●An eosinophilia (may be absent if immunosuppressed). *Treat* with mebendazole as in hookworm (above).

Trichinella spiralis is transmitted by uncooked pork worldwide. It migrates to muscle, and causes myalgia, myocarditis, periorbital oedema, fever and swellings. *Treat* with prednisolone 40mg/day for 5 days, then mebendazole 300mg/8h PO for 3 days, then 500mg/8h for 10 days.

***Trichuris trichiura* (whipworm)** may cause nonspecific abdominal symptoms. Diagnose by faecal microscopy. *Treat* as for hookworm.

***Enterobius vermicularis* (threadworm)** is common in temperate climes. It causes anal itch as it leaves bowel to lay eggs on the perineum. Apply sticky tape to the perineum and identify eggs microscopically. *Treat* with mebendazole 100mg PO (1 dose); repeat at 2 wks if ≥2yrs; if aged 6 months–2yrs: pyrantel 10mg/kg PO (1 dose; tabs are 125mg). Treat whole family. *Hygiene is more important than drugs*—adult worms die after 6 wks and do not multiply in colon. Continued symptoms means *reinfection*.

Toxocara canis Commonest cause of *visceral larva migrans*; any other invasive helminth may be causative; presents with eye granulomas (squint, blindness) or gross visceral involvement (fever, myalgia, hepatomegaly, asthma, cough). *Diagnosis* may require histology. *Treatment* with thiabendazole (=tiabendazole) or diethylcarbamazine is often unsatisfactory. Toxocara is commonly acquired by ingesting soil contaminated with animal faeces—so deworm pets regularly, and exclude them from play areas.

Filariasis

This is very common: Prevalence: 18 million worldwide.

1 **Onchocerca volvulus** causes blindness (river blindness) in 72% of some communities in tropical Africa and America—causing abandonment of large areas of fertile land (eg with 40% of those >50yrs being blind). A nodule forms at the bite; it sheds microfilariae to distant skin sites which develop altered pigmentation, lichenification, loss of elasticity and poor healing. Eyes may develop keratitis, uveitis, cataract, fixed pupil, fundal degeneration, or optic neuritis/atrophy. Lymphadenopathy and elephantiasis also occur. *Diagnosis* is by visualizing microfilaria in eye or skin snips. Remove a fine shaving of clean, unanaesthetized skin with a scalpel. Put on slide with a drop of normal saline (0.9%) and look for swimming larvae after 30 minutes.

2 Lymphatic filaria (eg *Wuchereria bancrofti*) cause lymphadenitis, leg lymphoedema (elephantiasis), hydrocoeles, and tropical pulmonary eosinophilia—mainly in tropical Asia. *Tests:* Thick films; serology. *Complications:* Immune hyperreactivity may cause tropical pulmonary eosinophilia (cough, wheeze, lung fibrosis, very high blood eosinophil counts + IgE and IgG↑↑). It is a major public health problem (prevalence 120 million), and is targeted by WHO for elimination, eg with mass treatment with ivermectin ± diethylcarbamazine.[4]

3 **Loa loa** causes transient, cellulitis-like 'Calabar' swellings, and may migrate across the conjunctiva. Occurs in West & Central Africa.

Treatment: This needs expert help as dying filaria may provoke a severe allergic reaction (Mazzotti reaction: pretreating with prednisolone 1mg/kg/24h for 2 days may prevent this cause of blindness). Ivermectin, a semisynthetic macrocyclic lactone, does not precipitate the allergic reaction and is now the drug of choice (1 dose of 150µg/kg PO repeated, eg each year for onchocerca—see *OHCS* p512, 20µg/kg PO as a single dose for wuchereia[4]). It does not kill adult worms, so repeat treatment may be needed in 6–12 months. This replaces diethylcarbamazine. Give every 6–12 months until adult worms die. Mass treatment campaigns may prevent blindness in some communities, but side-effects may pose problems.[5] The drug company has made ivermectin freely available to these communities. Lymphoedema responds to compression garments (hard to use)—or benzopyrone (coumarin) 400mg/24h PO.[6]

1 D Bundy 1994 *Tr Roy Soc Tr Med Hyg* **88** 259 2 N Beeching 1995 Ibid **89** 342 3 A Datri 1994 Ibid **88** 344
4 M Bockarie 1998 *Lancet* **351** 162 & J Sanford 1997 *Guide to Antimicrobial Therapy, Dallas,*
ISBN 0-933775-30-X   5 D Mabey 1993 *Lancet* i 154   6 JR Casley-Smith 1993 *BMJ* ii 1037

⊹ Cestodes (tapeworms)

These worms adhere to small bowel mucosa, but do not suck blood.

Taenia solium infection occurs by eating 'measly' pork, or from contaminated water, and *T saginata* is contracted from uncooked, infected beef. They cause vague abdominal symptoms and malabsorption. Contaminated food and water contain cysticerci which develop into adult worms within the gut. However, if a human swallows eggs of *T solium* (faecal–oral route), they may enter the circulation and disseminate throughout his body, becoming cysticerci within the human host (cysticercosis). This tapeworm encysts in muscle; skin; heart; eye; and CNS, causing focal signs. Examine the arms and legs for palpable subcutaneous lesions.

Neurocysticercosis: Signs depend on *how many* and *where* cysticerci are located, usually in *cerebrum* (with seizures, focal CNS signs ± dementia, or no symptoms at all), *ventricles*—here cysticerci may cluster (='racemose form') like bunches of grapes, with hydrocephalus if intraventricular foramina are blocked, and *basal cysterns* (may cause a basal meningitis, cranial nerve lesions, and, if arachnoiditis blocks CSF flow, ICP rises). *Spinal cysticerci* may cause radicular or compressive symptoms (p426).

Signs vary with degree of vasculitis and inflammatory reaction cysticerci incite, and whether the parasite is alive and producing granulomata. In the 'inactive' phase there is calcification and fibrosis. Lesions show on MRI/CT; here cysts may be so numerous as to give the scan a starry sky appearance.

Treat with niclosamide 2g in 2 doses, separated by 1h PO followed 2h later with a purge. It may be helpful to use an anti-emetic on waking. In neurocysticercosis, try albendazole 5mg/kg/8h PO or praziquantel 20mg/kg/8h PO for 14 days. An allergic response to the dying larvae should be covered by dexamethasone 12mg/day PO for 21 days. The rôle of steroids in the routine treatment of neurocysticercosis is controversial. Obtain expert help (*tel:* 0151 708 9393[UK]). Note: if CSF ventricles are involved, you may need to shunt before starting drugs, and drugs may worsen the acute phase of cysticercotic encephalitis.

Diphyllobothrium latum It is acquired from uncooked fish, causing similar symptoms to *T solium*, and is treated similarly with niclosamide. It may cause a vitamin B_{12} deficiency as the worm consumes it.

Hymenolepis nana and **H diminuta** (dwarf tapeworms) are rarely symptomatic. Treat with niclosamide 2g first day, then 1g/24h for 6 days. *H nana* may be treated with a single dose of praziquantel (25mg/kg PO).

Hydatid disease Cystic hydatid disease is a zoonosis—by ingesting eggs of the dog parasite *Echinococcus granulosus* (a cestode—ie a tapeworm), by contact with dog faeces, eg in rural sheep-farming regions. Hydatid is an increasing public health problem in parts of China, Russia, Alaska, Wales, and Japan. *Presentation* is usually due to a large cyst forming in the lungs (causing eg dyspnoea, pain, or haemoptysis, or anaphylaxis on its discharge through the large airways) or liver (causing hepatomegaly, obstructive jaundice, cholangitis, or PUO). But it may migrate almost anywhere. It may be an incidental finding (eg it is on the differential diagnosis of solitary, or even multiple shadows, on chest x-rays). It may occasionally occur in other organs (eg CNS). *Diagnosis* is aided by plain x-ray, ultrasound and CT of the cyst. A reliable serological test has replaced the variably sensitive Casoni intradermal test. *Treatment:* Excise symptomatic cysts. Beware spilling cyst contents, as this may provoke an anaphylactic reaction. The drug of choice is albendazole, eg 5mg/kg/12h for ~28 days pre-excision (± repeat × 1, after a 14-day gap): get expert help. The PAIR approach: puncture→aspirate cyst→inject hypertonic saline→reaspirate. (Alveolar hydatid is caused by *E multilocularis*.)

Diagnosis of cysticercosis

This is by faecal microscopy and examination of perianal swabs.

- Differentiate *Taenia solium* from *T saginata* by examining the scolex or a mature proglottid; the eggs are indistinguishable.
- A less technical means of species identification is to ask your patient about *movement* of the worm. If he describes worms vigorously wriggling out of the rectum, they will be *T saginata*.
- An indirect haemagglutination test is available.
- The CSF may show eosinophils in neurocysticercosis, and a CSF antigen test is available.
- CT or MRI scan may locate cysts. SXR and x-rays of soft tissues of the thigh may show calcified cysts.

✂ Trematodes (flukes)

Schistosomiasis (bilharzia) is the most prevalent disease caused by flukes, affecting 200 million people worldwide. The snail vectors release cercariae which can penetrate the skin, eg during paddling—may cause itchy papular rash ('swimmer's itch'). The cercariae shed their tails to become schistosomules and migrate via lungs to liver where they grow. ~2 weeks after initial infestation there may be fever, urticaria, diarrhoea, cough, wheeze, and hepatosplenomegaly ('Katayama fever', a self-limiting, ?immune complex phenomenon). In ~8 weeks mature flukes couple and migrate to resting habitats, ie vesical veins (*haematobium*) or mesenteric veins (*mansoni* and *japonicum*). Eggs released from these sites cause granulomata and scarring. Clinical schistosomiasis is an immunological process on the part of the human host which is known to be due to a type IV hypersensitivity (at least for *S mansoni*) to schistosomal eggs.

The Patient: He is likely to have visited or be from Africa, the Middle East, or Brazil (*S mansoni*), and present with abdominal pain and bowel upset, and, later, hepatic fibrosis, granulomatous inflammation, and portal hypertension (transformation into true cirrhosis has not been well-documented). *S japonicum*, often the most serious, occurs in South-east Asia, tends to affect the bowel and liver, and may migrate to lung and CNS—'travellers myelitis'. Urinary schistosomiasis (*S haematobium*) occurs in Africa, the Middle East, Spain, Portugal, Greece, and the Indian Ocean. Signs: frequency, dysuria, haematuria (± haematospemia), incontinence. It may progress to hydronephrosis and renal failure. *Diagnosis* is based on finding eggs in the urine (*haematobium*—collect at midday as diurnal variation in egg output; egg has terminal spine) or faeces (*mansoni*—egg has lateral spine, or *japonicum*) or rectal biopsy (all types). Ultrasound is a good screening test for GU morbidity in *S haematobium* infections as it identifies renal congestion, hydronephrosis, thickened bladder wall (but not calcification).

Treatment is with praziquantel: 40mg/kg PO with food divided into 2 doses separated by 4–6h for *S mansoni* and *S haematobium*, and 20mg/kg/8h for 1 day in *S japonicum*. Sudden transitory abdominal pain and bloody diarrhoea may occur shortly after treatment.

Fasciola hepatica is spread by sheep, water, and snails. It causes liver enlargement followed by fibrosis. It causes fever, abdominal pain, diarrhoea, weight loss, and mild jaundice with eosinophilia. *Tests:* Stool microscopy; serology. *Treatment:* Triclabendazole 10mg/kg PO, one dose (may be repeated once), or bithionol 25mg/kg/8h PO for one day.

Opisthorchis and **Clonorchis** are liver flukes common in the Far East, where they cause cholangitis, cholecystitis, and cholangiocarcinoma. *Tests:* Stool microscopy. *Treatment:* Praziquantel 25mg/kg/8h PO for 1 day.

Fasciolopsis buski is a big intestinal fluke ~7cm long causing ulcers or abscesses at the site of attachment. It is treated with praziquantel.

Paragonimus westermani (a fluke) is contracted by eating raw freshwater crabs or crayfish. The parasite migrates through gut and diaphragm to invade the lungs, where it causes cough, dyspnoea, and haemoptysis. Secondary complications: lung abscess and bronchiectasis. It occurs in the Far East, South America, and the Congo, where it is commonly mistaken for TB (similar clinical and CXR appearances). *Tests:* The sputum contains ova—will be missed if you do not consider diagnosis and only look for AFB. *Treatment:* Praziquantel (25mg/kg/8h PO for 2 days) or bithionol (20mg/kg/12h PO days for 14 doses[1]).

1 J Sanford 1997 *Guide to Antimicrobial Therapy*, Antimic.Ther.Inc, Dallas, ISBN 0-933775-30-X

Exotic infections[1]

Exotic infections may be *community-acquired*. Ask:

- Any foreign trips?
- Any foreign bodies, eg hip?
- What pets does he keep?
- Any exposure at work?
- Where else has he visited in the past?
- Any immunosuppression or risk factors for HIV?
- Any necrotic tissues to entice pathogens?
- What or who has bitten the patient?

Alternatively, infections may be from hospitals—ie *nosocomial*. With the arrival of transplantation and immunosuppression, along with HIV, and selection of multi-drug-resistant strains by the omnipresence of antibiotics, exotic infections are an increasing problem. New techniques such as PCR are enabling more putative infective agents to be characterized.

When you suspect an infection (fever, sweats, inflammation, D&V, WCC↑, or *any* unexplained symptom), liaise with a microbiologist. Treatments offered opposite are drug-only; perform debridement ± surgical drainage as appropriate. Remember that for many new organisms Koch's postulates (p171) will not all have been met—so the list opposite is suspect; it is certainly incomplete, and the drugs referred to are a guide only. The importance of trying to culture the organism cannot be over-stated—notwithstanding the frequent pragmatic fact of having to start treatment before the organism is known because the patient is ill.

Do not give up if you cannot culture an organism. Keep talking to the microbiologist. Perhaps the organism is 'fastidious' in its nutritional requirement? If culture *is* achieved, your problems are not over. It may be that the organism is pathogenic, or it could be a commensal (ie part of the normal flora for that patient). If culture is not possible, looking for antibodies or antigen in serum or other body fluids is an option. Tests may need repeating, and it is generally agreed that a 4-fold increase in antibody titres in convalescence (compared with the acute sera) is indicative of recent infection—but it is not proof, and neither is the absence of such a rise proof that the organism in question is innocent. PCR is increasingly being used to make identifications: but, be warned—PCR is far from fallible, and contamination with DNA from the lab or elsewhere is a frequent problem, and a risk which is very difficult to eliminate entirely.

The following table is for reference purposes only: no one can remember *all* the details about even the common infectious diseases for very long—let alone the rare ones. Check with a microbiologist for antibiotic sensitivities.

Antibiotic doses: Cefalosporins, see p178; penicillins, p177; others, p180.

Sources: J Paul 1996 *OTM* 3e 778 & R Mitchell 1987 *OTM* 2e 5.378, OUP; Moorfield's Eye Hospital

ORGANISM	SITE OR TYPE OF INFECTION	TREATMENT EXAM
Acanthamoeba	Corneal ulcers	Propamidine+neomycin, OHCS p
Acinetobacter calcoaceticus	UTI; CSF; lung; bone; conjunctiva	Gentamicin
Actinobacillus actinomycetemcomitans	IE; CNS; UTI; bone; thyroid; lung periodontitis; abscesses	Penicillin ± gentamicin
Actinobacillus lignieresii	CSF; IE; wounds; bone; lymph nodes	Ampicillin±gentamicin
Actinobacillus ureae	Bronchus; CSF post-trauma; hepatitis	Ampicillin±gentamicin
Aerococcus viridans	Empyema; UTI; CSF; bone	Penicillin±gentamicin
Aeromonas hydrophila	IE; CSF; cornea; bone; D&V; liver abscess	Gentamicin or
Agrobacterium radiobacter	Dialysis peritonitis; IE	Co-trimoxazole
Alcaligenes species	Dialysis peritonitis; ear; lung	Ceftazidime
Afipia broomeae	Marrow; synovium	Imipenem or ceftriaxone
Arachnia propionica	Actinomycosis; tear ducts; CNS	Penicillin
Arcanobacterium	Throat; cellulitis; leg ulcer	Penicillin
Bacillus cereus	Wounds; eye; ear; lung; UTI; IE	Gentamicin
Bifidobacterium	Vagina; UTI; IE; peritonitis; lung	Penicillin
Bordetella bronchiseptica	URTI; CSF (after animal contact)	Co-trimoxazole?
Burkholderia cepacia etc (formerly *Pseudomonas*)	Wounds; feet; lungs; IE; CAPD; UTI ecthyma gangrenosa; peritonitis	Ceftazidime Gentamicin
Burkholderia pickettii	CSF (formerly a *pseudomonas*)	Cefalosporin
Burkholderia pseudomallei (formerly *Pseudomonas pseudomallei*)	Meloidosis: self-reactivating septicaemia with multi-organ, protean symptoms eg in rice-farmers, via water or soil in Thailand, Papua, Vietnam, Torres Straits etc: capricious, stealthy, deadly	Ceftazidime or Chloramphenicol
Capnocytophaga ochracea and C sputagena	Oral ulcer; stomatitis; arthritis Blood; cervical abscess	Penicillin or Minocycline
Cardiobacterium hominis	IE (=infective endocarditis)	Penicillin+gentamicin
Chromobacterium violaceum	Nodes; eye; bone; liver; pustules	Erythromycin, chloramphenicol
Citrobacter koseri/diversus	CSF; UTI; blood; cholecystitis	Cefuroxime+gentamicin
Corynebacterium bovis/equi	IE; CSF; otitis; leg ulcer; lung	Erythromycin+rifampicin
Corynebacterium ovis	Joints; liver; muscle; granulomata	Penicillin
Corynebacterium ulcerans	Diphtheria-like ± CNS signs	Penicillin+Diphtheria antitoxin
Cyclospora cayetanensis	Diarrhoea (via raspberries)	Co-trimoxazole
Edwardsiella tarda	Cellulitis; abscesses; BP↓; dysentery via penetrating fish injuries	Cefuroxime+gentamicin
Eikenella corrodens	Sinus; ears; PE post jugular vein phlebitis (postanginal sepsis) via bites	Penicillin+gentamicin
Erysipelothrix rhusiopathiae	Erysipelas-like (OHCS p590); IE	Penicillin
Eubacterium	Wounds; gynaecology sepsis; IE	Penicillin
Flavobacterium meningosepticum	Lungs; epidemic neonatal meningitis; post-op bacteraemia	Penicillin
Flavobacterium multivorum	Peritonitis (spontaneous)	Cefuroxime
Gemella haemolysans	IE; meningitis postneurosurgery	Penicillin+gentamicin
Helicobacter cinaedia	Proctitis in homosexual men	Ampicillin or gentamicin
Kingella denitrificans kingae	Throat; larynx; eyelid; joint; skin	Penicillin
Kurthia bibsonii/sibirica/zipfii	IE (infective endocarditis)	Penicillin
Lactobacillus	Teeth; chorioamnionitis; pyelitis	Cefalosporins, penicillin
Megasphaera elsdenii	IE (infective endocarditis)	Metronidazole
Mobiluncus curtisii/mulieris	Vagina; uterus; septicaemia in cirrhosis	Penicillin
Moraxella osloensis and M nonliquefaciens	Conjunctiva; wound; vagina; UTI; CSF CNS; bone; haemorrhagic stomatitis	Penicillin
Neisseria cani	Wounds from cat bites	Amoxicillin
Neisseria cinerea/mucosa + N subflava; N flavescens	IE; CNS; bone; post human bites or from peritoneal dialysis	Penicillin, cepalosporin
Pasteurella multocida	Bone; lung; CSF; UTI; pericarditis epiglottitis. Post cat/dog bite	Penicillin
Pasteurella pneumotrophica	Wounds; joints; bone; CSF	Penicillin or ciprofloxacin
Peptostreptococcus magnans	Bone; joint; wound; teeth; face	Penicillin or ciprofloxacin
Plesiomonas shigelloides	D&V; eye; sepsis post fishbone injury	Ciprofloxacin
Propionibacterium acnes	Face; wounds; CSF shunts; bone; IE liver granuloma (botyromycosis)	Tetracycline or Penicillin
Prototheca wickerhamii/ zopfii=achlorophyllous algae	Subcutaneous granuloma; bursitis Lymphadenitis; nodules; granuloma	Amphotericin or Ketoconazole
Providencia stuartii	UTI; burn or lung infections	Gentamicin
Pseudomonas maltophilia	Wounds; ear; eye; lung; UTI; IE	Co-trimoxazole
Pseudomonas putrefaciens	CSF post CNS surgery/head trauma	Cefotaxime
Rothia dentocariosa	Appendix abscess	Penicillin+gentamicin
Serratia marcescens	Wound; burns; lung; UTI; liver; CSF; bone; IE; red diaper syndrome	Imipenem, ceftazidime,cip- rofloxacin (multiple resistance)
Sphingomonas paucimobilis	Leg ulcer; CSF; UTI	Ceftazidime
Streptococcus bovis	IE if colon neoplasm; do colonoscopy	Penicillin+gentamicin
Vibrio vulnificus	Wounds; muscle; uterus; fasciitis	Tetracycline, penicillin

7. Cardiovascular medicine

Other relevant pages: Cardiac shock (p768); cardiac arrest (p770); cardiovascular exam (p26); carotid bruit (p40); cough (p42); cyanosis (p42); dyspnoea (p44); haemoptysis (p46); nodules (p52); oedema (p52); oliguria (p52); palpitations (p52); aneurysms (p118); hyperlipidaemia (p654); risk factor analysis (p740); pulmonary oedema (p772); thrombolysis at home (*OHCS* p803).

Cardiovascular health

Ischaemic heart disease causes 30% of male and 22% of female deaths in England (higher in Scotland); its incidence has fallen in the developed world by 2–30% over the last decade or so; but cardiovascular health is not *only* about preventing ischaemic heart disease: health entails the ability to *exercise*, and enjoying vigorous activity (within reason!) is one of the best ways of achieving health, not just because the heart likes it (BP↓, 'good' HDL↑, atheroma regression)—it also may prevent osteoporosis, keep depression at bay, improve glucose tolerance, and augment immune function (eg in cancer and if HIV+ve).[*] People who improve *and maintain* their fitness live longer: ►*age-adjusted mortality from all causes is reduced by >40%.*[1,2] Trying to reduce obesity by dietary means (p482) brings less certain benefit than advice about exercise and smoking (below). This is partly because diets rarely achieve their aims. Also, it is a fallacy to suppose that, because it is healthier to be slim rather than obese, fat people should slim. If they do, the evidence is that they will not live any longer.[3]

Moderate drinking of alcohol (p482) also reduces cardiovascular risk. We also note that alcohol ↓gastric infection with *H pylori*, a known risk marker for cardiovascular disease.[4]

Smoking is another major risk factor for cardiovascular mortality. You *can* help people give up, and giving up *does* undo much of the harm of smoking. *Simple advice works.* Most smokers want to give up, unlike unhealthy diets, to which most people are wedded, p482. Because advice does not *always* work, do not stop giving it. Ask about smoking in consultations—especially those concerned with smoking-related diseases.

- Ensure advice is congruent with the patient's beliefs about smoking.
- Concentrate on the benefits of giving up.
- Invite the patient to choose a date (when there will be few stresses) on which he or she will become a non-smoker.
- Suggest throwing away all smoking accessories (cigarettes, pipes, ash trays, lighters, matches) in advance; informing friends of the new change; practise saying 'no' to their offers of 'just one little cigarette'.
- Consider offering nicotine chewing gum, chewed intermittently (to limit release of nicotine). ≥Ten 2mg sticks may be needed/day. Results have been rather inconsistent, and transdermal nicotine patches may be more reliable (easier to use, with minimal instruction required), ~doubling the give-up rate (eg from 11.7% to 19.4%, compared with placebo). A dose increase at 1 week is helpful for some who are in difficulties.[5] Gum may be preferable to patches in those most addicted (eg craving on waking).[5] Detailed written advice offers no added benefit to simple advice from nurses. Always offer follow-up.

Lipids and BP (p654 & p300–p302) are the other major modifiable risk factors (few can change their sex or genes). The graph of BP against mortality is J-shaped (low-point at 75–79mmHg diastolic).

To calculate how risk factors interact, see the risk equation on p740.

►Apply preventive measures *early* in life to maximize impact, when there are most years of life to save, and before 'bad' habits become ingrained.

◁1▷ I Lee 1995 *JAMA* 273 1179 27   ◁2▷ SN Blair 1995 *JAMA* 272 1092 & *E-BM* 1995 1 26 & 27   3 1995 Oxcheck *BMJ* i 1099   4 DJ Jenkins 1997 *BMJ* ii 1481   5 M Russell 1993 *BMJ* i 1308

✛ Chest pain

▶Cardiac-like pain may have no serious cause—but always think "*Could this ischaemic-type pain really mean a dissecting aneurysm, pericarditis, or pulmonary embolism*". Do BP in both arms; look at the legs: is there a DVT?

Central pain *Nature: Constricting* suggests angina, oesophagitis or anxiety; a *sharp* pain may be from pleura or pericardium (both may be exacerbated by deep inspiration, ie pleuritic). A prolonged (>½h), intense, dull, crushing pain suggests myocardial infarction (MI): "I thought I was going to die"—particularly if said with a clenched fist placed over the sternum (Levine sign +ve). Features which make cardiac pain unlikely are: ●Stabbing or shooting pains ●Pains lasting <30sec, however intense ●Well-localized, left submammary pain ('In my heart, doctor') ●Pains of continually varying location ●Youth.

Radiation: To shoulder, either or both arms, or neck and jaw suggests a lesion of heart, aorta, or oesophagus. The pain of aortic dissection may be interscapular, but is often retrosternal. Epigastric pain may be cardiac.

In pains coming on with exercise, emotion, or palpitations, think of cardiac pain or anxiety; if brought on by food, lying flat, hot drinks, or alcohol, consider oesophagitis—but meals *can* precipitate angina.

If it is *made better* by stopping exercise, suspect a cardiac lesion. If it is alleviated by antacids, suspect oesophagitis. Glyceryl trinitrate helps cardiac and oesophageal pain, but acts much more rapidly in cardiac pain. In pains improving on leaning forward, think of pericarditis.

Associations: In pains associated with dyspnoea, consider cardiac pain, pulmonary embolism, pleurisy or anxiety (ask about the peripheral and perioral paraesthesiae of hyperventilation). Myocardial infarction can occur with nausea, vomiting, or sweating, but so can upper GI lesions.

Angina may not mean coronary artery disease: left ventricular outflow obstructions (aortic stenosis; HOCM—hypertrophic obstructive cardiomyopathy) also give classical angina. Beware attributing angina solely to anaemia: there is usually underlying coronary artery disease too.

In aortic dissection, pain is often tearing and midscapular: see p118.

Pain that is not central This still may very well be cardiac, but other conditions enter the differential diagnosis.
Pleuritic pain: This is worse on inspiration, causing a restriction of breathing. The patient may 'catch his breath'. It implies inflammation of the pleura and localizes the pathology well. While peripheral pulmonary embolism leads to pulmonary infarction and, some days later, pleuritic pain, massive emboli may cause central chest pain resembling myocardial infarction, often with accompanying cardiovascular collapse.
Fractured rib: Gentle pressure on the sternum makes the pain worse.
Ankylosing spondylitis: Note the limited back movement.
Tietze's syndrome (costochondritis): See p708.
Tabes dorsalis: The pain may be 'like a bolt from the blue'.
Gall bladder and *pancreatic disease* may also mimic cardiac pain.

Whenever patients are acutely ill ●Admit unless you're sure the cause is benign. ●Monitor ECG (and do 12-lead ECG) ●Place an IV line ●Give O₂ by mask ●Relieve pain (eg morphine 5–15mg IV slowly with an antiemetic) ●CXR. **Famous traps** Zoster (p202); endoscopy yesterday = ruptured oesophagus today; shock but JVP↑ = cardiac tamponade; ideal textbook 'case' of crushing central chest pain = heroin addiction.

Chest pain with 'no cause' Even after extensive tests, including coronary angiography, and assessment for depression, the pain may be undiagnosed. Do not reject these patients: explain your findings to them carefully. Up to 50% have a 'chronic pain syndrome' which responds to a low-dose tricyclic, eg imipramine 50mg PO at night▯—rather like those with post-herpetic neuralgia (a better-known chronic pain syndrome).

The jugular venous pressure

The internal jugular vein acts as a rather capricious manometer of right atrial pressure. Observe two features: the height (jugular venous pressure—JVP) and the wave form of the pulse. JVP observations are difficult. Do not be downhearted if the skill seems to elude you. Keep on watching necks, and the patterns you see may slowly start to make sense.

Features helping to distinguish venous from arterial pulses: The venous pulse is not usually palpable. It is obliterated by finger pressure on the vein. The venous pressure rises transiently following pressure on the abdomen below the right costal margin (hepatojugular reflux). The JVP alters with changes in posture. Usually there is a double venous pulse for every arterial pulse.

The height Observe the patient at 45°, with his head turned slightly to the left. Look for the right internal jugular vein, which passes just medial to the clavicular head of the sternocleidomastoid up behind the angle of the jaw to the ear lobes. Do not rely on the external jugular vein.

The JVP is the vertical height of the pulse in cm above the sternal angle. It is raised if >4cm.

The waveform There is a double impulse:

1 *a* wave (atrial contraction)

2 *v* wave—seen at the end of ventricular systole, as tricuspid valve is about to open. It represents maximum venous filling of the right atrium.

Between them lie the *x* and *y* descents. The *c wave* represents ballooning back of the tricuspid valve as it closes.

Abnormalities *Raised JVP with normal waveform:* Fluid overload; right heart failure, (eg from fluid overload, reflex ↑in venous tone, impaired right ventricular function and tricuspid regurgitation).

Raised JVP with absent pulsation: SVC obstruction (oedema of the head and neck, collateral veins, and absent venous pulsation).

Large a wave: Tricuspid stenosis, pulmonary hypertension, pulmonary stenosis, some cases of LVH (Bernheim effect).

Cannon wave (Large *a* wave with rapid fall due to atrium contracting against closed tricuspid valve): atria and ventricles contracting simultaneously, eg in complete heart block, atrial flutter, single chamber ventricular pacing, nodal rhythm, ventricular extrasystole/tachycardia.

Absent a wave: Atrial fibrillation.

Systolic (cv) waves: Tricuspid regurgitation (ie occurring during ventricular systole, combining *c* and *v* waves)—look for earlobe movement.

Slow y descent: Tricuspid stenosis.

Constrictive pericarditis and pericardial tamponade: High plateau of JVP (which rises on inspiration) with deep *x* and *y* descents.

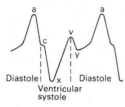

The venous plus wave. After *Clinical Examination* 4 ed, ed J Macleod 1976, Churchill Livingstone

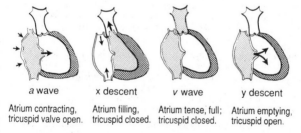

a wave	x descent	*v* wave	y descent
Atrium contracting, tricuspid valve open.	Atrium filling, tricuspid closed.	Atrium tense, full; tricuspid closed.	Atrium emptying, tricuspid open.

Venous pulse. Events occurring in the right atrium are reflected in the jugular waveform.

The heart sounds

▶Listen systematically: sounds then murmurs. While listening, palpate the carotid artery: S_1 is synchronous with the upstroke.

The heart sounds The first and second sounds are usually clear. Confident pronouncements about other sounds and soft murmurs may be difficult. Even senior colleagues disagree with one another about the more difficult murmurs.

The first heart sound (S_1) represents the closure of mitral and tricuspid valves (the exact cause is probably the vibrations occurring immediately after closure). It is therefore best heard in mitral and tricuspid areas. It is loud in mitral stenosis (so loud it may be palpable: the 'tapping' apex, p40), if the PR interval, is short and in tachycardia. It is soft in mitral regurgitation and if PR interval is long. Its intensity is variable in AV block and atrial fibrillation. Splitting in inspiration may be heard and is normal.

The second heart sound (S_2) represents the closure of the aortic and pulmonary valves, producing the A_2 and P_2 components. As with the first heart sound, the exact cause is probably vibrations occurring immediately after closure of the respective valves. Splitting in inspiration (ie A_2 and P_2 heard at very slightly different times) is normal and is due mainly to the variation with respiration of right heart venous return; so it is mainly the pulmonary component which moves, and it is in the pulmonary area that splitting is best heard. Wide splitting occurs in right bundle branch block, pulmonary stenosis, and atrial septal defects (wide and *fixed* splitting, ie not varying with respiration). Reversed splitting (ie splitting increasing on *expiration*) occurs in systemic hypertension, left bundle branch block, and aortic stenosis (but with aortic stenosis A_2 is often very soft or absent: the single component second sound). A_2 is loud in systemic hypertension. P_2 is loud in pulmonary hypertension, and soft in pulmonary stenosis.

A *third heart sound* (S_3) may occur just after S_2. Normal in young people (<35yrs), it is low pitched and best heard with the bell of the stethoscope. It occurs also in left and right heart failure (heard best in the mitral and tricuspid areas respectively), mitral regurgitation, and constrictive pericarditis (when it is early and more high pitched: the 'pericardial knock'). It signifies rapid ventricular filling.

Fourth heart sounds (S_4) occurs just before S_1. Always abnormal, it represents atrial contraction against a ventricle made stiff by any cause, eg aortic stenosis, hypertensive heart disease.

An *ejection systolic click* is heard early in systole with bicuspid aortic valves, and systemic hypertension. The right heart equivalent lesions may also cause clicks. Mid-systolic clicks occur in mitral valve prolapse (p306).

An *opening snap* (noncalcified valves) precedes the mid-diastolic murmur of mitral stenosis; listen with diaphragm between apex and lower sternal edge.

Triple and gallop rhythms A third or fourth heart sound occurring with a sinus tachycardia may give the impression of galloping hooves. When S_3 and S_4 occur in a tachycardia, eg with pulmonary embolism, then they summate and appear as a single sound—a summation gallop.

Note: Added sounds do not occur in atrial fibrillation.

Prosthetic sounds are heard from nonbiological valves on opening and closing.

Heart sound cadence

To help differentiate between S_3 and S_4, listen to the cadence of the heart sounds.

S3 sounds like 'Kentucky':
　　S1——S2—S3
　　KEN——TU—KY

S4 sounds like 'Tennessee':
　　S4—S1——S2
　　TE—NNE——SSEE

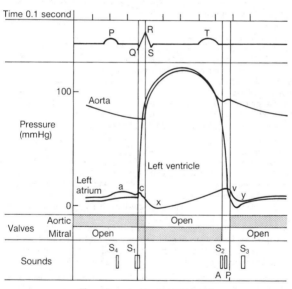

The cardiac cycle. After *Med Intl* **1** (17) 759.

Murmurs

▶Always consider the other physical signs before listening and answer the question: what do I expect to hear? But do not let your expectations determine what you hear. So while listening, ask yourself: can I hear anything unexpected?

▶When in doubt, rely on echocardiography rather than disputed sounds.

Stenotic murmurs occur when a valve is meant to be fully open, and is not; regurgitant murmurs occur when a valve is meant to be closed, and is not. Think about the cardiac cycle while listening. Traditionally, cardiologists grade systolic murmur intensity on a scale out of 6, where 6/6 means loud enough to hear from the end of the bed. Diastolic murmurs, being less loud, are scored out of 4.

Maximize the chance of hearing a murmur by using the stethoscope correctly. The bell should be applied very gently to the skin and is particularly good for hearing low-pitched sounds (eg mitral stenotic murmur). The diaphragm filters out low pitches and makes higher-pitched murmurs easier to detect (eg aortic regurgitant murmur). A bell tightly applied to the skin becomes a diaphragm.

Left heart murmurs are accentuated in expiration and right heart murmurs in inspiration. Other manoeuvres which alter the haemodynamics may be useful. Exercise brings out the murmur of mitral stenosis. The Valsalva manoeuvre makes the murmur softer in mitral regurgitation and aortic stenosis but louder in mitral valve prolapse and hypertrophic obstructive cardiomyopathy; prompt squatting has exactly the opposite effects.

Some murmurs will be better heard by bringing the relevant part of the heart closer to the stethoscope, eg mitral stenosis in the left lateral position, aortic regurgitation by leaning forward.

Systolic murmurs An *ejection systolic murmur* (ESM; crescendo–decrescendo; diamond-shaped [ ] on phonocardiogram) usually originates from the outflow tract and waxes and wanes with the intraventricular pressures. The louder it is, the more likely it is to be significant. Flow murmurs are common in children and high output states (eg tachycardia, pregnancy) and do not have an associated thrill. Organic causes include aortic stenosis and sclerosis, hypertrophic obstructive cardiomyopathy, and pulmonary stenosis.

A *pansystolic murmur* (PSM) is of uniform intensity and merges with the second sound. It is usually organic and may represent mitral or tricuspid regurgitation (S_1 may also be soft in these), or a ventricular septal defect (p320). Mitral valve prolapse may produce a late systolic murmur.

Diastolic murmurs An *early diastolic murmur* (EDM) is high pitched and easily missed: if you suspect it clinically, then listen in early diastole for 'the absence of silence'. An EDM occurs in aortic (and rarely pulmonary) regurgitation. If the pulmonary regurgitation is secondary to pulmonary hypertension which is itself due to mitral stenosis, then the early diastolic murmur is called a Graham Steell murmur.

Mid diastolic murmurs (MDM) are low pitched and rumbling. They occur in mitral stenosis, rheumatic fever (Carey Coombs' murmur: due to thickening of the mitral valve leaflets), and aortic regurgitation (Austin Flint murmur: due to fluttering of the anterior mitral valve cusp caused by the regurgitant stream).

⚕ ECG—a methodical approach

▶When you go for a walk with your eyes over the heart's mountains, expose each hill, valley, precipice, and summit in turn.[1] Learn about each individually, and in due course you will take them all in your stride. First confirm the <u>patient's age and name,</u> and the ECG's date. Then:

- *Rate:* p266 (summary: 300/RR measured in <u>big squares; each is 0.2 sec</u>).

- *Axis:* p266–p267 (summary: if I and II are both 'positive', axis is normal).

- *Rhythm:* If the cycles are not clearly regular, use the 'card method': lay a card along ECG, marking positions of 3 successive R-waves. Slide the card to and fro to check all intervals are equal. If not, note if different rates are multiples of each other (ie varying block), if changes are abrupt (if so, concentrate on that first complex), or if it is totally irregular (eg AF or VF).

- *Initiation of depolarization:* <u>Sinus rhythm</u> means initiation from the sino-atrial node, and is characterized by one normally shaped and timed P-wave preceding each QRS complex. *Atrial fibrillation* (AF) has an <u>irregular baseline</u> and <u>no discernible P-waves</u>; the QRS complexes are irregularly irregular (but can be deceptively regular when the patient is controlled on digoxin). *Atrial flutter* has a 'sawtooth' baseline of atrial depolarization and regular QRS complexes. <u>Nodal rhythm</u> has a normal QRS complex but <u>P-waves which are absent or occur just before (ie very short PR) or within the QRS complex.</u> *Ventricular rhythm* has QRS complexes which are >0.12sec with P-waves following them (paced rhythm p295).

- *P-wave shape* 'P mitrale' (large LA): bifid P-wave, >0.11sec in II and negative deflection in VI. 'P <u>pulmonale</u>' (large RA): <u>tall (>2.5mm) P-wave in II;</u> dominant initial positive vector in <u>P-wave in VI.</u>

- *PR interval:* From start of <u>P-wave to start of the QRS</u> (few people know this arcane fact, and those that do might say that to rename it the 'PQ interval' would be to make medicine too easy). Normal range: <u>0.12–0.21sec.</u> >0.21sec means delay in atrioventricular conduction (heart block, p265).[2] *1st, 2nd, and 3rd degree block* are described on p287. A <u>consistently short PR</u> interval implies unusually fast AV conduction down an accessory pathway (eg Wolff–Parkinson–White or Lown–Ganong–Levine syndromes, p288, p291, p704) or nodal rhythm.

- *QRS width:* <u>If >0.12sec suggests conduction defects</u> (p266, p287).

- *QRS height:* Ventricular hypertrophy (p266). Look for <u>Pathological Q-waves: >25% of succeeding R-waves;</u> >0.04sec wide.

- *QT interval:* From QRS start to end of T. Varies with rate. Estimate interval for 60/min (QT[60] or QT^c) by dividing measured QT interval by the square root of the cycle length, ie QT^c = (Q–T)/($\sqrt{R\text{–}R}$). Normal QT^c is 0.35–0.43sec.

- *ST segment:* <u>Planar elevation (>1mm)</u> or <u>depression (>0.5mm)</u> implies infarction (p287) and ischaemia (p271) respectively. <u>W</u>idespread saddle-shaped elevation occurs in pericarditis (p319).

- *T-wave* is usually <u>abnormal if negative in I, II, V4–6.</u> It is peaked in hyperkalaemia (p269), and flattened in hypokalaemia.

- *U-waves* may be prominent in hypokalaemia but may be normal.

---

1 See RM Rilke, *Exposed on the Heart's Mountains,* Penguin Modern European Poets  2 N Balasuriya 1994 *ABC of ECG,* North Colombo Medical College, Ragama, Sri Lanka

ECG nomenclature

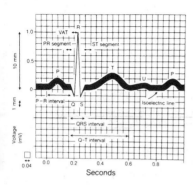

VAT = ventricular activation time

Heart block

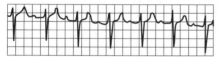

First degree AV block. <u>P–R interval=0.28s</u>

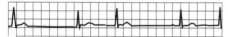

Mobitz type I (Wenkebach) AV block

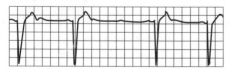

Mobitz type II AV block. Ratio of AV conduction varies from 2:1 to 3:1

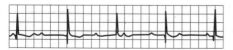

Complete AV block with narrow ventricular complexes. There is no relation between atrial and the slower ventricular activity

⚕ ECG—additional points

Where to place the chest leads

V1: right sternal edge, 4th intercostal space
V2: left sternal edge, 4th space
V3: half-way between V2 and V4
V4: the patient's apex beat (p40)
    All subsequent leads are in the
    same horizontal plane as V4
V5: anterior axillary line
V6: mid-axillary line
(V7: posterior axillary line)

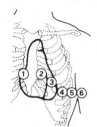

The precordial ECG leads (V1-V6)

Finish a 12-lead ECG with a long rhythm strip in lead II

Rate At usual speed (25mm/sec) each 'big square' is 0.2sec; each 'small square' is 0.04sec. To calculate the rate divide 300 by the R–R interval (in big squares).

The mean frontal axis is the sum of all the ventricular forces during ventricular depolarization. (See p267.)
The 6-limb leads are positioned in the coronal plane (p267).
Normal axis is between −30° and +120° (some say +90°).
Left axis deviation is more negative than −30°.
Right axis deviation is more positive than +120° (some say +90°).

Disorders of the ventricular conduction—*Bundle branch block* (ECGs p285) The evidence of delayed conduction is QRS >0.12sec. Abnormal conduction patterns lasting <0.12sec are incomplete blocks. The area that would have been reached by the blocked bundle depolarizes slowly and late. Take V1 as an example. In V1, right ventricular depolarization is +ve and left ventricular depolarization is −ve. Hence, if the last peak in the QRS complex in V1 is above the isoelectric line (ie positive secondary wave), it is the right ventricle which is depolarizing late. This is *right bundle branch block* (RBBB, ECG on p285). Isolated RBBB may be a variant of normal; with other abnormalities it may indicate ischaemic heart disease, fibrosis, pulmonary hypertension, or congenital heart disease.

If the last peak is below the isoelectric line, it is *left bundle branch block* (LBBB, ECG on p285). In V6 the converse is true. ▶If there is left bundle branch block, no comment can be made on the ST segment or T-wave.

Bifascicular block is the combination of right bundle branch block and left bundle hemiblock (manifest as an axis deviation, eg LAD=left anterior hemiblock).

Trifascicular block is the combination of bifascicular block and first degree heart (atrioventricular) block.

Ventricular hypertrophy can be suggested by unusually large QRS complexes, but there is a great overlap between normals and hypertrophy. The co-existence of a strain pattern of ST depression and inverted T-waves in the chest leads (in V1–3 for right ventricular hypertrophy, V4–6 for left) is strong supportive evidence of hypertrophy. The strain may represent ischaemia of the bulky ventricle.
Examples of cited voltage criteria for hypertrophy are:
    Left: the sum of S in V1 and R in V5 or V6 >35mm.
    Right: dominant R in V1 where there is a narrow QRS excluding RBBB.
Differential diagnosis: true posterior infarction (T-wave is upright), or Wolff–Parkinson–White syndrome type A (delta-wave).

Conduction problems and their effects on ECG axis

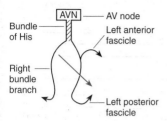

1. Normal conduction → normal axis

2. RBBB → normal axis
   (as left ventricle depolarizes normally)

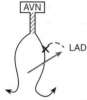

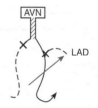

3. Left anterior hemiblock → left axis deviation

4. RBBB and left anterior hemiblock → left axis deviation

After J Hampton *ECG Made Easy* Churchill Livingstone.

Some rules of thumb to determine the ECG axis
- If the complexes in I and II are both predominantly positive, the axis is normal.
- The axis lies at 90° to an isoelectric complex (ie positive and negative deflections are equal in size).

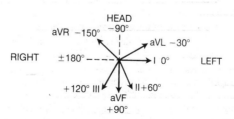

ECG—abnormalities

Myocardial infarction: (For ECG examples, see p281.)

- Within hours, the T-wave *may* become abnormally tall, and the ST segment *may* begin to rise. (ECG signs are at their most capricious when you most want them to be certain: just before you start thrombolysis.)
- Within 24h, the T-wave inverts, as ST elevation begins to resolve.
- Pathological Q-waves also begin to form within a few days.
- Q-waves usually persist, but may resolve completely in 10%.
- T-wave inversion may or may not persist.
- ST elevation rarely persists, except with a ventricular aneurysm.

The leads affected reflect the site of the infarct: inferior (II, III, aVF), anteroseptal (V1–4), anterolateral (V4–6, I, aVL), true posterior (mirror image changes in V1–2: tall R and ST↓). Certain infarcts have ST and T changes without Q-waves ('non-Q-wave infarct').

Pulmonary embolism: Sinus tachycardia with an otherwise normal ECG is commonest; there may be deep S-waves in I, pathological Q-waves in III, inverted T-waves in III ('$S_I Q_{III} T_{III}$'), strain pattern V1–3 (p266), right axis deviation, RBBB (ECG on p285) atrial fibrillation.

Digoxin effect: ST depression and inverted T-wave in V5–6 (reversed tick). Changes are more extensive in digoxin *toxicity* (any arrhythmia, but ventricular ectopics and nodal bradycardia are common).

Hyperkalaemia: (p640) Tall, tented T-wave, ST segment↓, P–R interval↑, wide QRS, absent Ps. (ECG p269.)

Hypokalaemia: Small T-waves, prominent U-waves, ventricular bigemini (a premature extrasystole coupled to each sinus beat).

Hypercalcaemia: Shortens Q–T interval.

Hypocalcaemia: Prolongs Q–T interval.

Acute pericarditis: p318.

Causes of some ECG abnormalities

Right axis deviation: Right ventricular hypertrophy or strain (eg pulmonary embolism), cor pulmonale, pulmonary stenosis, but not right bundle branch block (see p267). Occurring alone with normal QRS, it represents left posterior hemiblock.

Left axis deviation: Left ventricular hypertrophy or strain (eg hypertension, aortic stenosis, HOCM), but not left bundle branch block. Occurring alone, with a normal QRS, it represents left anterior hemiblock.

ST elevation: Infarction, variant (Prinzmetal's, p706) angina, pericarditis, ventricular aneurysm.

ST depression: Ischaemia, hypertrophy with strain, digoxin.

Heart block: Ischaemic heart disease, drugs (digoxin, verapamil), myocarditis, cardiomyopathy, fibrosis, Lyme disease.

Sinus tachycardia: Exercise, emotion, anxiety, pain, fever, MI, shock, heart failure, drugs (eg atropine, nitrates, adrenaline/epinephrine), constrictive pericarditis, myocarditis, endocarditis, hyperthyroidism, smoking, coffee.

Sinus bradycardia: Athletes, vasovagal attack, drugs (eg β-blockers, verapamil, digoxin), infarction (especially inferior), sick sinus syndrome, hypothyroidism, hypothermia, raised intracranial pressure, jaundice.

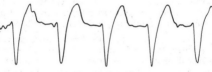

Hyperkalaemia

Exercise ECG testing

This test is used for the diagnosis of ischaemic heart disease, assessment of exercise tolerance, response to treatment, (including surgical revascularization), and prognosis. It is also of value in the assessment of exercise-related arrhythmias.

The patient undergoes a standardized (eg Bruce) protocol of increasing exercise, with continuous 12–lead ECG and blood pressure monitoring. Watch for ST depression, but do not be fooled by J-point depression with steeply upward sloping ST segments: this is associated with a very low incidence of ischaemic heart disease. (The J-point is the junction of QRS complex and ST segment—see p271.)

Stop the test if:
- ST segment depression >2mm.
- The patient is exhausted or in danger of falling.
- There is a ventricular arrhythmia (not just ectopics).
- The blood pressure falls.
- The patient has chest pain (but if it is a diagnostic test, you will have to continue looking for ECG changes—be careful).

Contraindications: Electrolyte disturbance, unstable angina, recent (<7 days) infarction, severe aortic stenosis, pulmonary hypertension, LBBB (p266, you cannot interpret ECG changes—do a thallium scan to assess ischaemia), HOCM, acute myopericarditis, severe hypertension.

Interpreting the test: A positive test only allows one to assess the *probability* that the patient has ischaemic heart disease. 75% with significant coronary artery disease have a positive test, but so do 5% of people with normal arteries. The more positive the result, the higher the predictive accuracy. Down-sloping ST depression is much more significant than up-sloping, eg 1mm J-point depression with down-sloping ST segment is 99% predictive of 2–3 vessel disease.

Mortality: 10 in 100,000; *Morbidity:* 24 in 100,000.

Ambulatory ECG monitoring

Continuous ECG monitoring for 24h (extended to 72h in HOCM) may be used to try and pick up paroxysmal arrhythmias. About one-fifth will have a normal ECG during symptoms: investigate other systems, if appropriate. About 10% will have an arrhythmia coinciding with symptoms.

However, 70% of patients will not have symptoms during the period of monitoring, so little is gained. Give these patients a recorder they can activate themselves during an episode (eg 'Cardiac memo'—least cumbersome, greater monitoring time, and may be able to download information to cardiology departments via telephones; in some centres these devices are the first and preferred specific form of investigation).◁1▷

Recorders may be programmed to detect ST segment depression, either symptomatic (to prove angina), or to reveal 'silent' ischaemia (predictive of reinfarction or death early after MI).

◁1▷S Kinley 1996 E-BM 1 159

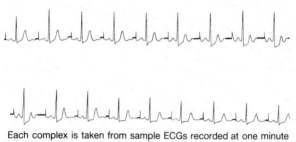

Each complex is taken from sample ECGs recorded at one minute intervals during exercise (top line) and recovery (bottom line). At maximum ST depression, the ST segment is almost horizontal. This is a positive exercise test.

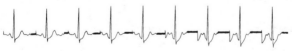

This is an exercise ECG in the same format. It is negative because although the J point is depressed, the ensuing ST segment is steeply upsloping.

Cardiac catheterization

This involves the insertion of a catheter into an artery (to examine the left heart and perform a coronary arteriogram) or vein (for right heart imaging). The catheter is manipulated within the heart and great vessels to measure pressures, sample blood to assess oxygen saturation, and for the injection of radio-opaque contrast medium in conjunction with digital film recording to look at blood flow and the anatomy of the heart and vessels. Using the catheter, it is now possible to insert angioplasty and valvuloplasty balloons, and to perform cardiac biopsy. ECG and arterial pressure are monitored continuously. The opportunity may be taken to perform intravascular ultrasound (using a tiny 1mm probe with a rotating echo transmitter receiver on its end) which helps quantify arterial narrowing.▣

40% are day-case procedures in the UK (this is OK if the patient can rest lying down at home for 4h).

Indications: ●Coronary artery disease: diagnostic (including assessment of bypass graft patency); therapeutic (angioplasty—balloon or laser).
●Valve disease: assessment of severity, and to do therapeutic valvuloplasty. Aortic valvuloplasty (if too ill or declines valve surgery) may be attempted using a retrograde (from the aorta) or a transseptal approach. Mitral and pulmonary valvuloplasty is also performed.
●Other: Congenital heart disease; cardiomyopathy; pericardial disease; endomyocardial biopsy.

Morbidity: Arrhythmias, thrombo-embolism (coronary and systemic), infection, trauma to heart and vessels (eg dissection). Risk of MI, stroke, or death is ~1 per 1000 procedures. If there is much bruising over the site of arterial puncture, consider ultrasound to diagnose a false aneurysm.

Pre-op tests: Check peripheral pulses and general fitness. ECG, CXR, FBC, platelets, U&E, clotting screen, group & save blood. *Post-op:* Frequently check peripheral pulses beyond catheter site; check site for bleeding.

Normal values of pressures and saturations

Location	Pressure (mmHg)		Saturation (%)
Inferior vena cava			76
Superior vena cava			70
Right atrium:	a	2–10	
	v	2–10	
	mean	0–8	
Right ventricle:	systolic	15–30	74
	end-diastolic	0–8	
Pulmonary artery:	systolic	15–30	
	end-diastolic	3–12	
	mean	9–16	
Pulmonary capillary wedge:	a	3–15	
	v	3–12	
	mean	1–10	
Left ventricle:	systolic	100–140	98
	end-diastolic	3–12	
Aorta:	systolic	100–140	
	end-diastolic	60–90	

Gradients (mmHg) across stenotic valves

Valve	Normal gradient	Stenotic gradient		
		Mild	Moderate	Severe
Aortic	0	<30	30–50	>50
Mitral	0	<5	5–15	>15
Prosthetic	5–10			

Intracardiac electrophysiology via a cardiac catheter can determine types and origins of arrhythmias, and locate aberrant pathways. Arrhythmias may be induced, and the effectiveness of control by drugs assessed. Aberrant pathways can be electrically ablated with good success.

Coronary artery anatomy

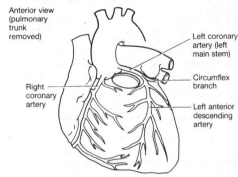

Anterior view (pulmonary trunk removed)

Right coronary artery

Left coronary artery (left main stem)

Circumflex branch

Left anterior descending artery

Angiographic views

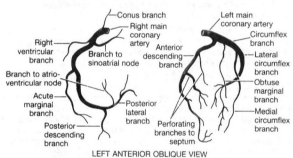

1 RIGHT CORONARY SYSTEM   LEFT CORONARY SYSTEM

Conus branch
Right main coronary artery
Right ventricular branch
Branch to sinoatrial node
Branch to atrioventricular node
Acute marginal branch
Posterior descending branch
Posterior lateral branch

Left main coronary artery
Circumflex branch
Anterior descending branch
Lateral circumflex branch
Obtuse marginal branch
Medial circumflex branch
Perforating branches to septum

LEFT ANTERIOR OBLIQUE VIEW

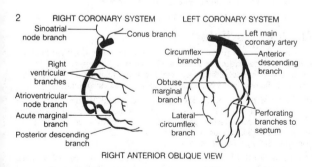

2 RIGHT CORONARY SYSTEM   LEFT CORONARY SYSTEM

Sinoatrial node branch
Conus branch
Right ventricular branches
Atrioventricular node branch
Acute marginal branch
Posterior descending branch

Left main coronary artery
Circumflex branch
Anterior descending branch
Obtuse marginal branch
Lateral circumflex branch
Perforating branches to septum

RIGHT ANTERIOR OBLIQUE VIEW

1. Reproduced with permission from 'Understanding Angina'. ©American Heart ssociation.
2. From M. Sokolow, Clinical Cardiology, Lange, p170, with kind permission

Echocardiography

This non-invasive technique uses the differing ability of various structures within the heart to reflect ultrasound waves. It not only demonstrates anatomy but provides a continuous display of the functioning heart throughout its cycle.

2D echocardiography produces pictures of a 2-dimensional, fan-shaped plane. In this way one sees eg all four chambers in a view from the apex (p40) or a cross-section of the aortic valve from the parasternal region.

M-mode echocardiography offers a picture of the structures in a single narrow beam beneath the transducer. By holding the transducer still, one can record fine movements of the valves which can be timed and measured more easily than in the 2D mode.

Doppler and colour-flow echocardiography will illustrate flow and gradients across valves and septal defects (p320).

Transoesophageal echocardiography (TOE) is more sensitive than conventional transthoracic echocardiography (TTE). TTE is technically limited in 10–25% of patients due to eg obesity and COPD. Placing the ultrasound probe in the oesophagus allows for high-quality images given the proximity of the transducer to the heart without the intervening lung.

Uses of echocardiography *Heart failure:* Diagnosing both its presence and its cause. With colour Doppler, it may find the cause (eg valve pathology or pericardial disease). Comparing LV systolic and end-diastolic size is a good way of measuring LV function; the difference forms the basis of the echo diagnosis of heart failure.

Valve disease: Mitral stenosis is characteristic on M-mode, but aortic stenosis is better demonstrated by 2D. Neither technique is diagnostic in regurgitant lesions which are best evaluated by Doppler. Doppler can also quantify the gradient across a stenosis.

Cardiomegaly: Focal and global hypokinesia, aneurysms, and pericardial effusions show up well on 2D. *Left ventricular hypertrophy:* Echo is 5–10 times more sensitive than the ECG in detecting this. It may be important to detect and follow LVH as, independently of blood pressure, it is a risk factor for sudden cardiac death (relative risk is 1.7 per 50g/m—indexed to height).[1] LVH is related to age, obesity, and blood viscosity, as well as to BP, so echo may play a part in *coronary risk assessment.* Defining LVH is complex, but >134g/m² may be taken as abnormal (>110g/m² if ♀).

Vegetations and *mural thrombi* are less reliably shown.

Pericardial effusion is best diagnosed by echo, using either technique.

Nuclear cardiology

Radionuclide ventriculography is a less invasive investigation than cardiac catheterization, and is very effective at assessing gross ventricular anatomy (eg global and focal dyskinesias) and function (eg ejection fraction). Technetium-99 is used to label red cells or albumin.

Myocardial perfusion is assessed using thallium-201 (its distribution mirrors that of K⁺) injected just before maximum exercise on a treadmill. Exercise scans are compared with resting views taken 2½–3h later: fixed defects (infarct) or reperfusion (ischaemia) can be seen and the coronary artery involved is reliably predicted.

Myocardial infarction can be labelled by technetium pyrophosphate as it is not taken up by normal tissue. This is valuable if the patient presents when it is too late for enzymes to be of value (but within 10 days of infarction), and/or if the ECG is unhelpful (eg LBBB). See PET, p738.

1 J Chambers 1995 *BMJ* ii 273

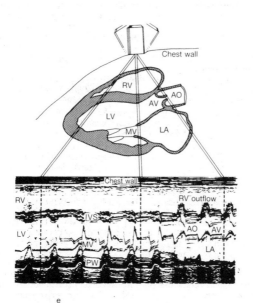

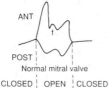

e

ANT

f

POST

Normal mitral valve

CLOSED ¦ OPEN ¦ CLOSED

2. Mitral stenosis
• reduced e-f slope

3. Aortic regurgitation
• fluttering of ant. leaflet

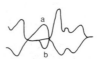

a

b

4. (a) Systolic anterior leaflet movement (SAM) in HOCM
(b) Mitral valve prolapse (late systole)

Normal M-mode echocardiogram. (RV=right ventricle; LV=left ventricle; AO=aorta; AV=aortic valve; LA=left atrium; MV=mitral valve; PW=posterior wall of LV; IVS=interventricular septum. After R Hall *Med Inrl* (17) 774.

Some cardiovascular drugs

Low-dose aspirin Vital antiplatelet rôle in unstable angina/MI (+TIA/stroke); it may have a rôle in primary prevention.[1] It helps keep CABG grafts open (p311).

Beta-blockers decrease sympathetic effects. Blockade of β_1 receptors is negatively inotropic and chronotropic (pulse↓ by delaying AV conduction). Blocking β_2 receptors causes coronary and peripheral vasoconstriction but also bronchoconstriction, so agents which are *relatively* specific for β_1 receptors (cardioselective) are often used (eg bisoprolol 10mg/day PO).

Use β-blockers in angina to decrease myocardial O_2 demand, and to control BP and some arrhythmias, eg post MI (here they ↓mortality). CI: Asthma/COPD, peripheral vascular disease (β_2 effect), heart failure/heart block (unhelpful β_1 effects, but see carvedilol, p298). SE: Lethargy, impotence, *joi de vivre*↓, nightmares, ↓glucose tolerance, headache.

Diuretics are used in hypertension (thiazides) and heart failure. SE: Dehydration. *Frusemide* (=furosemide): ↓K^+, ↓Ca^{2+}, ototoxic; *thiazides*: ↓K^+, ↑Ca^{2+}, ↓Mg^{2+}, ↑urate (± gout), ↑glucose, ↓platelets; *amiloride*: ↑K^+, GI upset.

Vasodilators are used in heart failure, ischaemic heart disease, and hypertension. They may predominantly venodilate (eg nitrates) thus decreasing filling pressure (pre-load), or be arterial dilators (eg hydralazine) which primarily decrease systemic blood pressure (after-load), or do both (eg prazosin). For ACE inhibitors, eg captopril, see p299.

Calcium antagonists These ↓cell entry of Ca^{2+} via voltage-sensitive channels on smooth muscle cells, thereby promoting coronary and peripheral vasodilatation and reducing myocardial oxygen consumption. *Pharmacology:* Effects of specific Ca^{2+} antagonists vary because there are different types of Ca^{2+} channels in different tissues. Verapamil and diltiazem slow conduction at the atrioventricular and sinoatrial nodes and cause coronary vasodilatation. Diltiazem allows normal pulse increase at peak exercise. Don't give verapamil with β-blockers (risk of bradycardia ± LVF). Nifedipine is good if there is coronary artery spasm but can cause a reflex tachycardia, so often used with a β-blocker. Prolonged use of short-acting preparations is implicated (inconclusively) in ↑mortality.[2] *Uses:* Angina (=[A], below), dysrhythmias[D], and hypertension[H]. *Typical doses: Phenylalkylamines:* Verapamil[AHD] 40–120mg/8h PO. *Benzithiazepines:* Diltiazem[AH] eg 60mg/8h PO, max 160mg/8h—less if elderly; (SR tabs are 90, 120, 180, 300mg). *Dihydropyridines:* Nifedipine[AH] 20mg/12h PO pc (as slow-release); amlodipine[AH] 5mg/24h. SE: Flushes, headache, oedema (diuretic unresponsive), LV function↓, gingival hypertrophy. CI: Nifedipine: fertile ♀. Diltiazem: fertile ♀, pulse↓, heart block.

Digoxin[3,4] is used to slow the pulse in fast AF (aim for < 100). As it is a weak +ve inotrope, its rôle in heart failure in sinus rhythm may be best reserved if symptomatic despite optimum ACE therapy (p299);[3] here there is little benefit *vis à vis* mortality (but admissions for worsening CCF are ↓by ~25%).[4] Old people are at ↑risk of toxicity: use lower doses. Do plasma levels >6h post-dose (p751). Typical dose: 500µg stat PO, then 125µg (if elderly) to 375µg/day PO (62.5µg/day is almost never enough).[3] Toxicity risk↑ if: K^+↓, Mg^{2+}↓, or Ca^{2+}↑. $t_{1/2} \approx$ 36h. If on digoxin, use less energy in cardioversion (start with 5J). SE: Any arrhythmia (SVT with AV block is suggestive), nausea, appetite↓, yellow vision, confusion, gynaecomastia. In toxicity, stop digoxin; check K^+; treat arrhythmias; consider Digibind® (p794). CI: HOCM; Wolff–Parkinson–White syndrome (p288 & p316).

Anti-arrhythmics classified by main site of action: 1 *AV node:* Adenosine, verapamil, β-blockers, digoxin. 2 *Ventricles only:* Lignocaine (=lidocaine), mexiletine, phenytoin, flecainide. 3 *Atria, ventricles, and bundle of Kent:* Quinidine, procainamide, disopyramide, amiodarone.

ACE inhibitors p299; **Nitrates** p278; **Antihypertensives** p302.

1 (75mg/day) MRC 1998 Lancet 251 233 2 E&M 1997 2 29 3 Lancet 1997 349 833 & 1994 343 128 4 NEJM 1997 336 525

Atheroma and the mechanism of action of statin drugs

The arrival of statin drugs in the management of atheroma and hyper-lipidaemia is one of the key advances in cardiology in recent times. To understand their rôle, some background is needed. Think of atheroma as the slow accretion of snow on a mountain. Nothing much happens until one day an avalanche devastates the community below. The snow is lipid and lipid-laden macrophages; the mountain is an arterial wall; the avalanche is plaque rupture; and the community below is, all too often, myocardium or CNS neurones. The devastation is infarction (Latin *farcire*, to stuff or obstruct). In assessing risk of thrombi, remember Rudolph Virchow's (1821–1902) triad of *changes in the vessel wall*, *changes in blood flow*, and *changes to the blood constituents*.

Plaque biology Atheroma is the result of cycles of injury and repair to the vascular wall, leading to the accretion of T lymphocytes, which produce growth factors, cytokines, and chemoattractants. LDL gains access by a process called transcytosis, where it undergoes modification by macrophage-derived oxidative free radicals—a process enhanced by smoking tobacco and hypertension. It is rupture of an atheromatous plaque which triggers most acute coronary events.▪ These plaques have a core of lipid-laden macrophages—and a fibrous cap is all that separates them from endothelium. Many factors predispose to plaque formation, eg genetics, sex (♂), blood pressure, smoking, diabetes mellitus. But do not think of plaques as static, dead things. They can regress or accumulate, or become inflamed (eg in unstable angina[2]). The balance between low-density lipoprotein (LDL) efflux and influx is alterable—for example by diet or antilipid drugs. Neither is the vessel wall a non-participatory audience to these great events. A sclerotic arterial wall comprises areas of chronic inflammation, with monocytes, macrophages, and T lymphocytes—with smooth muscle proliferation, and elaboration of extracellular matrix. These macrophages make cholesterol, and also produce enzymes (eg interstitial collagenase, gelatinase, and stromelysin) which have been implicated in digesting the plaque cap. The thinner the cap, and the fewer smooth muscle cells involved, the more unstable the plaque.

After plaque rupture, what happens to fibrinogen and passing platelets partly determines the extent of the impending catastrophe. Hypercholesterolaemia (if present) is associated with hypercoagulable blood and enhanced platelet reactivity at sites of vascular damage.

Plaque pacification What can we do about plaques? First, try to prevent them: eat a healthy diet (p482, ?with vit. E, p529), encourage *some* exercise, discourage smoking; treat high BP and diabetes. Once a plaque is there, it can be bypassed, ablated (physically removed or compressed) or stented (with a metal conduit). Angioplasty splits the plaque, causing an injury response: elastic recoil → thrombus formation → inflammation → smooth muscle proliferation → arterial remodelling. An alternative to this drastic change is to give a 'statin' drug—if there is hypercholesterolaemia—but note that the whole process described above is favourably influenced by statins. These statin drugs are HMG-CoA reductase inhibitors (simvastatin, pravastatin, p654); inhibiting this enzyme has effects which may go far beyond reducing LDL, eg:▪

- ↓Prothrombotic states: serum fibrinogen↓ (not with atorvastatin) platelet aggregation↓, ?*via* ↓platelet thromboxane production.
- Reduction of inflammation around plaques prone to fissuring and rupture (statins inhibit antibody-dependent cellular cytotoxicity).
- Reduction in cholesterol synthesis by within-vessel macrophages.
- Reduction of within-vessel macrophage proliferation and migration.

╫ Angina pectoris

This is central, crushing chest pain which may radiate to the jaw, neck, or one or both arms. It may only be felt in the jaw or arm. It represents myocardial ischaemia. It is precipitated by exertion (often predictably), emotion, cold weather, and heavy meals, and may be associated with dyspnoea and faintness. It is relieved by rest and nitrates. There are usually no physical signs. Angina remits spontaneously in ⅓ of patients.

Causes Usually coronary artery disease. Rarely: valve disease, eg aortic stenosis; HOCM; hypoperfusion from arrhythmias; arteritis; anaemia.

Incidence 5 per 1000 per year in males over 40 years old.

Tests ECG: ST depression; flat or inverted T-waves; Q-waves from old MIs. If resting ECG normal (it usually is), consider exercise ECG (p270), or thalium scan (p274). Angiography indications: uncontrolled angina; diagnostic uncertainty. Exclude anaemia, polycythaemia, giant cell arteritis (FBC & ESR).

Management Screen for modifiable risk factors: smoking; BP; DM; lipids (give a statin if cholesterol ≥5mmol/L, p654); weight; fitness (p255).

Drugs: Unless contraindicated, *all* should have 75–150mg aspirin daily (mortality↓ 34%[1]). For symptoms, give glyceryl trinitrate spray (GTN, 0.4mg/intra-oral puff; sublingual tablets deteriorate after 8 weeks), up to every ½h. Work up to maximum tolerated doses of 'triple' therapy—eg:
- β-blockers: atenolol 50–100mg/24h PO. CI: asthma, LVF, bradycardia.
- Calcium antagonists, eg diltiazem 60mg/8h PO (p276).
- Nitrates, eg isosorbide mononitrate slow-release, 60mg/24h PO (more frequent doses easily cause tolerance), or try adhesive nitrate skin patches (5–10mg/24h, remove for 4–8h in each 24h) or buccal absorption (eg 1mg, 2mg or 3mg Suscard Buccal® pills). SE: headaches.

Finally, consider adding a K⁺-channel activator, eg nicorandil 10–30mg/12h PO.

Coronary revascularization—percutaneous transluminal coronary angioplasty (PTCA) and coronary artery bypass grafting (CABG—p311) are used if drugs fail to control angina or are not tolerated. Choice is determined by the number and distribution of stenoses, clinical setting, eg unstable or stable angina, previous PTCA or CABG etc. In PTCA, a balloon catheter is inflated within a stenosis, but the risk of complete occlusion demands full surgical back-up. 33% relapse *vs* 11% post-CABG at 6 months, and 30% go on to need CABG.[2] Mortality and MI rates in low-risk patients are similar, making angioplasty an attractive option, especially as repeat procedures are possible (repeat CABG is often problematic). Mortality is <2% (but operator variable). 70% get total relief and 20% improvement of symptoms—but pain returns to 50% in 5yrs. Aspirin 75–300mg/24h PO reduces risk of graft closure. *Note:* prognosis is better with CABG if there is left main coronary artery stenosis, many severe stenoses, severely impaired LV function, or concurrent need for valve or LV aneurysm repair.

Unstable angina is angina which is rapidly worsening, eg on minimal or no exertion. Treatment: diltiazem[3] ± β-blockers as above; isosorbide dinitrate 2–20mg/h IVI; aspirin ≥75mg/24h PO; heparin 5000u IV bolus then IV infusion to maintain APTT 1.5–2.5 of control. Low molecular weight heparin is an alterative, eg enoxaparin 1mg/kg/12h SC.[4] Monitor closely on CCU and exclude (and prevent impending) MI. ~15% die in 1yr if untreated (do prompt angiography). If pain is uncontrolled, emergency angiography and CABG or angioplasty is needed. Prinzmetal angina p706.

Mortality 0.5–4% per year (sudden death, MI, LVF), depending on number of affected vessels. It is doubled if there is left ventricular dysfunction.

1 *Lancet* 1992 **340** 1421 2 RITA 1993 *Lancet* **341** 573 3 *Lancet* 1995 **345** 1201 4 ESSENCE 1997 NEJM **337** 447

✝✝✝ Myocardial infarction (MI)

▶*The ECG may be normal: don't discount the diagnosis of MI if the history is clear. Any new ECG changes may imply MI.*

MI implies death of heart muscle. **Incidence** 5/1000 per year (UK).

Causes/associations Male sex, genetic influence, BP↑, smoking, lipids↑, stress (rates may double with severe stress, eg the day after an earthquake). 90% of acute transmural MIs (ECG Q-waves heralded by ST elevation in several leads) are caused by thrombosis, eg following rupture of an atheromatous coronary artery plaque (p277) and so are amenable to thrombolysis. Non-Q-wave MIs and pre-infarction states may be due to intermittent platelet plugs (amenable to heparin and aspirin); ECGs may be normal.

Mortality 50% of deaths occur within 2 hours of symptom onset.

Symptoms Pain is like angina, but often worse and lasts >30 minutes, and may cause vomiting, sweating, and extreme distress. Painless ('silent') infarcts are quite common (eg in diabetics and the elderly).

Signs Often none, but may be distressed, cold, clammy, pulse↑ or↓, BP↑ or↓. May be cyanosed, and sometimes have a mild pyrexia (but look for other causes). Signs of complications, eg LVF: dyspnoea, crepitations.

Tests—*ECG* (p268): ST elevation* (see p282), T inversion, and Q-waves are typical in the leads adjacent to the infarction. Hyperacute peaked T waves may be an early sign, preceding ST elevation. Leads II, III, and aVF look at the inferior aspect of the heart, V1–3, the anterior aspect and V4–6, the lateral aspect (the septum is seen in V3–4). Other leads may show 'reciprocal' ST depression. The absence of Q-waves in a proven infarct is associated with higher risk of subsequent MI. *CXR:* Any evidence of aortic dissection or failure or cardiomegaly? *U&E. FBC.* Also plasma *glucose* may rise (do not ignore this: *vigorous pursuit of normoglycaemia saves lives* ◁1▷). *Lipids* may be lowered from the first 24h post-MI for up to 3 months.

Cardiac enzymes:

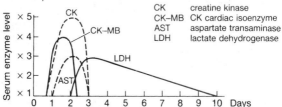

CK	creatine kinase
CK–MB	CK cardiac isoenzyme
AST	aspartate transaminase
LDH	lactate dehydrogenase

Diagnosis Look for 2 or 3 out of the history, ECG changes, and enzyme changes. CK is found in myocardial and skeletal muscle and can be raised after:[1] MI, a fall/trauma, IM injection, prolonged running, or in myositis (eg use of statin drugs), Afro-Caribbeans, hypothermia, and hypothyroidism. Request CK-MB isoenzyme levels if there is doubt as to the source (normal CK-MB/CK ratio <5%). Cardiac troponin T is another marker of myocardial damage; it remains elevated for at least 1 week.[2]

Differential diagnosis: See p256—Angina, pericarditis, myocarditis, aortic dissection (p118), pulmonary embolism and oesophageal reflux/spasm.

◁1▷ *E-BM* 1996 **1** 41 *JK French 1996 *BMJ* **i** 1637—other criteria stipulate ≥2mm in V4-V6 too, but note that other cardiologists state that *one* affected chest lead is enough if ≥1.5mm; also recent onset of left bundle branch block, with appropriate symptoms, is suggestive. **2** R Donelly 1998 *Lancet* **351** 537

Sequential ECG changes following acute MI

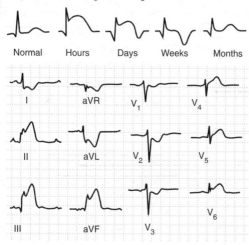

Acute inferolateral infarction with minimal 'reciprocal' ST changes in I, aVL and V_2–V_3.

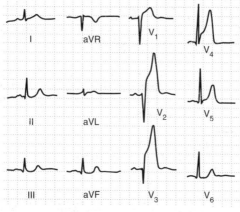

Acute anteroseptal infarction with minimal 'reciprocal' ST changes in III and aVF.

✚ Immediate management of MI

The greatest risk of death is in the first hour; correcting arrhythmias and giving thrombolysis *at home*[1] can cut deaths by half, compared with waiting until hospital admission. See *Thrombolysis at home?*, OHCS p804. The top priority is to decide whether to thrombolyse. ►'Time is muscle.'

A patient presenting to his GP days after his MI is at lower risk; manage at home, unless pain relief or complications are problems.

In the coronary care unit ►Your patient may be terrified; reassure him. Explain that survival is the rule (>90% if in low-risk group, ie typical MI symptoms, <60yrs old, no diabetes, no past history, pulse <100).

- Attach an ECG monitor and ensure a defibrillator trolley is on hand.
- High-flow O_2 (unless CO_2 retaining, eg COPD). • Site an IV cannula.
- Morphine 5–15mg IV at ≤1mg/min, if none before (+ anti-emetic, eg metoclopramide 5–10mg IV). It is: *analgesic; anxiolytic; anti-arrhythmic; venodilatory.*
- Aspirin 300mg (if not already given by GP) for antiplatelet activity.
- Glyceryl trinitrate (0.5mg sublingually) for coronary vasodilatation.
- Could this be *aortic dissection/aneurysm, pericarditis, PE,* or *peptic ulcer*? Do bilateral BPs; any murmur or rub? Check calves; palpate abdomen.
- Thrombolysis—indications:
  Presentation within 12h of typical cardiac chest pain with
  - ST elevation >2mm in 2 or more chest leads, or
      >1mm in 2 or more limb leads, or
  Tall - R waves and ST depression in V1–V3 (posterior infarction), or
  - new onset bundle branch block.
  Presentation 12–24h after onset of cardiac chest pain with continuing pain ± ECG evidence of evolving infarction.

Contraindications to thrombolysis: see opposite (trying to distinguish relative and absolute contraindications may be oversimplistic). Warn patient of the 1% risk of stroke. Streptokinase (SK) is usually the thrombolytic agent of choice, but t-PA may be indicated if the patient has previously reacted to SK or has received SK in the last 5 days to 1 year.

Give streptokinase 1.5 million units in 100mL 0.9% saline IVI over 1h. This regimen decreases mortality by ~43% (from 13% to 8%).[2] Standard t-PA (alteplase) regimen: t-PA 1.5mg/kg over 3h with heparin (eg 5000u IV bolus, then 1000u/h IVI for 24h; monitor APTT daily).[3] SK side-effects: BP↓ (use IV fluids and raise legs); anaphylaxis is rare; overall incidence of stroke is not increased.

Is thrombolysis working? If pain is uncontrolled, especially with continuing ST elevation, consider re-thrombolysis (no bolus), give diamorphine 5–10mg IV as needed. Consider immediate angiography ± angioplasty.*

- ACE-i ↓mortality, eg ramipril 2.5mg/12h PO on day 3; ↑after 48h to 5mg/12h.[4]
- Continuous ECG monitoring with 4-hourly TPR and BP.
- 24h bed rest.
- Daily 12-lead ECG, 'cardiac' enzymes, and U&E for 2–3 days.
- Examine heart, lungs, and legs for complications daily.
- No smoking!

---

*Meta-analyses (*JAMA* 1997 **278** 2093) indicate that, in the future, angioplasty may become first-line management for acute MI, but at present this remains thrombolysis—until more *longterm* trials have been conducted comparing the two. There are also major resource implications associated with angioplasty.
1 GREAT 1992 *BMJ* ii 548 **2** LIMIT-2 1992 *Lancet* **339** 1553 **3** GUSTO 1993 *NEJM* **329** 673 (there may be very marginal benefit in t-PA, rather than SK, but the cost is ~$220,000/extra life saved, H Freidman 1993 *NEJM* **330** 504) ◄4► E-BM 1997 **2** 174 & ISIS-4 1995 *Lancet* **345** 669 & *BNF* 1998 i 90

Contraindications to thrombolysis in acute MI

- Risk of bleeding
  - General bleeding tendency
    - warfarin anticoagulation when INR may be >3.0
    - haemophilia
    - severe liver disease (including varices)
    - thrombocytopenia
  - Local bleeding tendency
    - stroke (<2 weeks or with residual disability); recent surgery
    - trauma
    - resuscitation (prolonged cardiopulmonary resuscitation)
    - eye bleeding (vitreous; not proliferative retinopathy)
    - peptic ulcer; GI bleeding; pregnancy; serious vaginal bleeding
    - tooth extraction (recently); TB with cavitation
- Hypertension
  - Systolic BP > 200mmHg
  - Diastolic BP >120mmHg
- Pre-existing thrombus which might embolize
  - Endocarditis
  - Aortic aneurysm

Note: if previous allergic reaction to streptokinase (SK) or SK previously given 5 days to 1 year ago, use another thrombolytic agent.

If thrombolysis is contraindicated, consider referral for immediate angiography ± angioplasty.

Generally now only give Strep once, and if been on it before — use t-PA.

Acute postero-lateral myocardial infarction

Complications of myocardial infarction

- Arrhythmias (p286–p293).
- Shock.
- Heart failure.

- Hypertension: if BP >200/100mmHg, ensure adequate relief of pain and anxiety. If BP is still raised, try nitrateás by IVI (p278) or oral β-blockers (p302). Do not treat lower BPs. There is also a rôle for IV β-blockers.
- Pericarditis, eg Dressler's syndrome (p696).
- DVT and PE; and systemic embolization.
- VSD: presentation is acute cardiac failure; treatment, surgical.
- Papillary muscle rupture: presents with acute pulmonary oedema due to mitral regurgitation; the treatment is urgent surgery.
- Cardiac rupture and subsequent tamponade is similarly devastating and usually irremediable without very rapid surgery.
- Left ventricular aneurysm occurs late, presenting as intractable LVF, arrhythmias, or embolization. ECG: persistently raised ST segments. CXR: bulge on the left heart border. Anticoagulate. Consider excision.

Subsequent management of MI

If uncomplicated, the patient may sit out of bed on day 2, walk freely on day 5 (discontinue heparin now), go home on day 5–7, and return to work after 4–12 weeks, depending on degree of heavy manual labour. He should not drive for 1 month and is responsible for informing his insurance company. If the infarct has been complicated (eg arrhythmia, post-infarct angina, or heart failure) or he is a professional driver, he should inform the driving licence authorities. Advise to increase exercise slowly; consider a planned fitness training programme. Specifically mention to him and his partner that sexual activity may be safely resumed. Avoid air travel for 6 weeks (longer if severe angina or heart failure).[1] Ask about any fears of returning to a normal life. Address modification of risk factors. Arrange for a lipid test (≥3 months post-MI, unless done within the first 24h).

The 5 good prognostic signs
- Normal heart size on CXR
- No post-MI pulmonary oedema
- No pre-existing hypertension
- No significant arrhythmias after day 1
- No post-MI angina

These patients are at very little risk; plan to discharge them on aspirin and a β-blocker (eg atenolol 50mg/24h PO).[2] Start an ACE inhibitor (p299) if there is clinical evidence of LVF or echo shows reduced ejection fraction.[4] Consider starting a statin if total cholesterol >4.8mmol/L or LDL >3.2mmol/L (p654). Review at 4–6 weeks to:
- Review symptoms, eg angina, shortness of breath, and palpitations. If angina recurs, treat it conventionally, perform an exercise test, and consider coronary angiography.
- Start an exercise-based cardiac rehabilitation programme.
- Consider ACE inhibitor (p299) if any LVF (known to ↓ mortality).[3]

Check fasting lipid profile at 3 months and review the need for a statin (p276 & p654). Statins may reduce subsequent cardiovascular morbidity as much as aspirin and β-blockers.

1 H Bethneli 1996 BMJ 312 3172 2 G O'Connor 1989 Circulation 80 234-44 4 AIRE (ramipril) group 1993 Lancet ii 821 & ISIS-4 1995 Lancet 345 969

Left bundle branch block

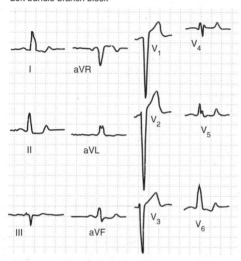

Right bundle branch block

✛ Arrhythmias

Rhythm disorders or arrhythmias are:

    common
    often benign (but may reflect underlying heart disease)
    often intermittent, causing diagnostic difficulty
    occasionally severe, causing cardiac compromise.

Causes: MI, cardiac ischaemia, dilated and hypertrophic cardiomyopathy, myocarditis, and aberrant conduction pathways. Other precipitants are drugs, electrolyte disturbance (K^+, Ca^{2+}, Mg^{2+}), and thyroid disease.

Presentation: Collapse, palpitations, 'funny turns', chest pain, ↓BP, LVF. Non-compromising arrhythmias, eg AF, are often an incidental finding.

Assessing suspected paroxysmal arrhythmia in an out-patient setting: Take a detailed history of palpitations (p52). Any precipitating factors or haemodynamic instability: chest pain, dyspnoea or collapse? Review drugs.

Tests: Blood for U&E, Ca^{2+}, Mg^{2+}, FBC, glucose, TSH. ECG: any signs of ischaemic heart disease, AF, or Wolff–Parkinson–White syndrome (p288)? Ambulatory ECG, eg 'cardiac memo' (p270). Do echocardiograms in those with unexplained arrhythmias if <50yrs old to exclude HOCM (p316; it causes broad-complex arrhythmias, p292) and mitral stenosis (causes AF). If a ventricular arrhythmia is documented, refer to a cardiologist for cardiac catheterization and electrophysiological studies. The arrhythmia may be stimulated and its therapeutic response to various drugs assessed.

Treatment: If normal rhythm on ECG during palpitations, reassure patient. If an arrhythmia is shown, treatment depends on type. The patient may be taught autonomic procedures, eg Valsalva manoeuvre for SVT. He may be started on oral drugs, eg verapamil (40–120mg/8h PO) or a β-blocker for SVT. Amiodarone is used for VT. Finally, permanent pacing may be used to overdrive tachyarrhythmias, to override bradyarrhythmias, or prophylactically in conduction disturbances (p294). Implanted automatic defibrillators are being evaluated. *Amiodarone:* Dose: 400mg/8h PO for 7 days, then 200mg/24h for 7 days. Maintain on 200mg/24h. SE: Corneal deposits, photosensitivity ('don't go out in the sun'), hepatitis, nightmares, INR↑, T4↑, T3↓ (amiodarone is 37.5% iodine). Monitor LFTs, T4, T3. If hyperthyroidism occurs, *concurrent* antithyroid drugs may be used.▨ Exogenous thyroxine (=levothyroxine) may be needed.

Periarrest arrhythmias

These are potentially dangerous arrhythmias which may quickly lead on to cardiac arrest. They can be classified by rate and QRS complex morphology:

    Bradycardia (rate <60bpm), see below
    Narrow complex tachycardia (rate >100bpm, QRS <120ms), p288
    Broad complex tachycardia (rate >100bpm, QRS >120ms), p292

Management is described in the ERC guidelines (p289 & 293). *In all cases:*
- Connect patient to a cardiac monitor and have a defibrillator at hand.
- Give oxygen and obtain IV access.
- Send blood to check for electrolyte abnormalities.
- If pulse disappears, move to cardiac arrest protocols (p771).

Bradycardia ECG shows a pulse rate <60 beats per minute.
Diagnostic table and management algorithm are given opposite.

Sick sinus syndrome Common in elderly. Sinus node dysfunction causes bradycardia ± arrest, sinoatrial block or SVT alternating with bradycardia/asystole (tachy–brady syndrome). AF and thrombo-embolism may occur. *Tests:* 24h ECG ± exercise ECG. *Management:* Pace if symptomatic.▨

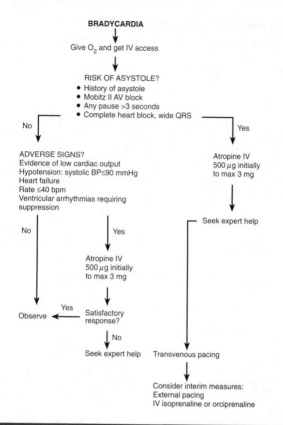

BRADYCARDIA

Give O$_2$ and get IV access

RISK OF ASYSTOLE?
- History of asystole
- Mobitz II AV block
- Any pause >3 seconds
- Complete heart block, wide QRS

No

ADVERSE SIGNS?
Evidence of low cardiac output
Hypotension: systolic BP≤90 mmHg
Heart failure
Rate ≤40 bpm
Ventricular arrhythmias requiring
suppression

No

Yes

Yes

Atropine IV
500 µg initially
to max 3 mg

Atropine IV
500 µg initially
to max 3 mg

Satisfactory
response?

Observe

No

Seek expert help

Seek expert help

Transvenous pacing

Consider interim measures:
External pacing
IV isoprenaline or orciprenaline

Diagnosis of bradycardias

Sinus bradycardia: Constant P-R interval <200ms (1 big ECG square).
Sinus node disease: eg sick sinus syndrome (see opposite).
AV node block
- First degree block: constant P-R>200ms. No treatment needed.
- Second degree block:
  - Mobitz type I (Wenckebach): progressively lengthening P-R followed by a dropped QRS
  - Mobitz type II: constant P-R with dropped beats
  - 2:1 or 3:1 block: only every 2nd or 3rd P wave is followed by a QRS complex.

  Exclude digoxin toxicity and β–blockade. The decision to pace is based on the symptoms.
- Third degree block: P-P and R-R intervals constant but unrelated. Pacing is essential, even if asymptomatic.

Narrow complex tachycardia

ECG shows a QRS complex of <120ms at a rate of >100bpm.

Principles of management:

- Identify the underlying rhythm and treat accordingly.
- If the patient is compromised ('adverse signs' opposite), DC cardiovert.

Diagnosis and management: See algorithm opposite.

Like carotid sinus massage, adenosine causes transient block of conduction via the atrio-ventricular (AV) node (t½ =10–15sec). It works in 2 ways:

by cardioverting a junctional tachycardia to sinus rhythm,

by transiently slowing ventricles to show the underlying atrial rhythm.

Give adenosine as a fast bolus into a large (eg antecubital) vein followed by a 10mL saline flush. Give 3mg, then 6mg, then 12mg, then 12mg at 2 min intervals while recording a hard copy of the rhythm. Warn patient they may feel temporarily unwell (eg chest tightness). Adenosine may exacerbate bronchospasm in asthmatics, is antagonized by theophylline, and augmented by dipyridamole—give half the dose.

Identification of the underlying rhythm can be difficult so enlist the help of an expert where possible.

Sinus tachycardia: Reviewing the patient may reveal the cause eg infection, shock, MI, pain (see p268). Adenosine may slow the ventricular rate transiently. Treatment is directed at the underlying cause.

Atrial fibrillation: Look for irregular timing of the QRS complexes and lack of P waves. Treat as on p290.

Atrial flutter: This can be particularly difficult to differentiate from an SVT. When the ventricular rate is 150bpm, always suspect atrial flutter with 2:1 block. Adenosine usually reveals the characteristic sawtooth baseline. Treat as on p290.

Junctional tachycardia: The normal AV node has a long refractory period, preventing a fast atrial rate being conducted to the ventricles, thus allowing adequate diastolic filling time. Some people have a second conduction pathway between the atria and ventricles allowing a circuit to be set up. There are two types of junctional tachycardia (1) intra-AV nodal re-entry tachycardia (AVNRT), where the entire tachycardia circuit is confined to the AV node and its surrounding myocardium, and (2) AV re-entry tachycardia (AVRT), where there is an additional abnormal pathway between the atrium and the ventricle completing the circuit. Because of the refractory period of the normal AV node, a ventricular rate of 150 with narrow QRS complexes is rarely exceeded except in a junctional tachycardia (150–250/min).

With adenosine, a junctional tachycardia will cardiovert, at least momentarily, to sinus rhythm. If it recurs, longer-acting treatment may be required, eg verapamil (if not β-blocked, WPW or in VT). Also consider amiodarone and overdrive pacing.

Wolff–Parkinson–White (WPW) syndrome (ECG on p295.) This involves a congenital accessory conduction pathway (bundle of Kent) between atrium and ventricle. ECG shows rapid conduction down the accessory pathway (short P–R interval) followed by initially slow depolarization through the ventricle (slurred upstroke or 'delta wave' into the QRS complex: seen only at rest, not during the SVT). WPW predisposes to an AV re-entry tachycardia (treat with verapamil), and to AF which is worsened by digoxin and verapamil, but improved by amiodarone, flecainide, or DC shock. Refer for electrophysiological studies and ablation of the accessory pathway.

Rare causes of narrow complex tachycardia: digoxin-induced atrial tachycardia, COPD–related multifocal atrial tachycardia.

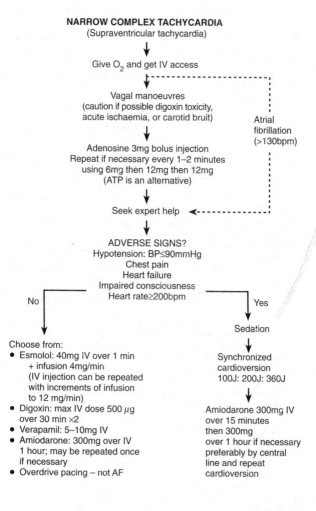

NARROW COMPLEX TACHYCARDIA
(Supraventricular tachycardia)

↓

Give O₂ and get IV access

↓

Vagal manoeuvres
(caution if possible digoxin toxicity,
acute ischaemia, or carotid bruit)

↓

Adenosine 3mg bolus injection
Repeat if necessary every 1–2 minutes
using 6mg then 12mg then 12mg
(ATP is an alternative)

↓

Seek expert help ◄ - - - - - - - - - -

Atrial
fibrillation
(>130bpm)

↓

ADVERSE SIGNS?
Hypotension: BP≤90mmHg
Chest pain
Heart failure
Impaired consciousness
Heart rate≥200bpm

No ──────┐   ┌────── Yes

↓   ↓

Choose from: Sedation
• Esmolol: 40mg IV over 1 min   ↓
  + infusion 4mg/min   Synchronized
  (IV injection can be repeated   cardioversion
  with increments of infusion   100J: 200J: 360J
  to 12 mg/min)   ↓
• Digoxin: max IV dose 500 μg   Amiodarone 300mg IV
  over 30 min ×2   over 15 minutes
• Verapamil: 5–10mg IV   then 300mg
• Amiodarone: 300mg over IV   over 1 hour if necessary
  1 hour; may be repeated once preferably by central
  if necessary   line and repeat
• Overdrive pacing – not AF   cardioversion

✛ Atrial fibrillation and flutter

Atrial fibrillation is an ineffective, chaotic, irregular and rapid (300–600/min) atrial rhythm. Its discharges approach the AV node from varying angles at varying intervals, thus resulting in a totally irregular ventricular rate. It is common in the elderly (up to 9%) and is often asymptomatic. The chief risk is embolic stroke (~4%/year); this is much reduced (eg to ~1%/yr[1]) by warfarin anticoagulation.

Common causes: Myocardial infarction and ischaemia, mitral valve disease (commoner in stenosis), hyperthyroidism (may be only sign), BP↑.

Rare causes: Cardiomyopathy, constrictive pericarditis, sick sinus syndrome, bronchial carcinoma, atrial myxoma, endocarditis, haemochromatosis, sarcoid. 'Lone' AF means none of the above causes.

The Patient There may be palpitations or an *irregularly irregular pulse*, ie the irregularity doesn't follow a pattern. The first heart sound is of variable intensity. The rate at the apex (p40) is greater than at radial artery.

Differential diagnosis: Variable AV block; runs of ventricular or atrial ectopics.

Diagnosis is on ECG: Chaotic baseline with no P-waves, and irregularly irregular but normally shaped QRS complexes.

Management: If managing any associated acute illness (eg MI, pneumonia) does not produce sinus rhythm within 48h, consider at least one go at DC cardioversion (this requires GA or heavy sedation): warfarinize for 3 weeks before DC shock (100J → 200J) and for 4 weeks after. If this fails, treat as chronic AF. Some attempt chemical cardioversion with amiodarone (but warfarin interacts) while awaiting DC shock, which may then be unnecessary.

Chronic AF: The aim is control of ventricular rate, not sinus rhythm.
- Use digoxin: oral loading dose 0.5mg × 3 doses in 2 days; maintenance 0.25mg/24h PO. In the elderly, load with 0.75mg in total and use a maintenance dose of ~0.125mg/24h. (Amiodarone also has a place here.)
- If still too fast, check concordance (p3) and serum level; cautiously ↑ dose — ± low-dose β-blocker (eg propranolol 10–20mg/8h PO or sotalol).▢
- Discuss risks and benefits of anticoagulation with the patient. In general, expect to use warfarin, aiming for INR of 2.5–3.5[1]◆ (p597). But if the patient is reluctant, or the risk of emboli is small (eg lone AF with normal echo and no past emboli or TIA[2]), or the risk of bleeding is high ± warfarin contraindicated (eg on NSAIDs, or past peptic ulcer) aspirin ~300mg PO with food may be acceptable and avoids doctor-dependency (stroke rate in the elderly is 4.6%/year on aspirin vs 4.3% for warfarin).[3]

Paroxysmal AF: Sotolol 80mg/24h PO (after ≥48h ↑dose to 80mg/12h ± further slow increases, up to 160mg/12h; monitor Q–T interval) or amiodarone (load with 200mg/8h PO for 1 week, 200mg/12h for 1 week, then maintenance 100–200mg/24h) may maintain patient in sinus rhythm.

Atrial flutter is a regular circus movement of continuous atrial depolarization with a period of 300/min. The AV node cannot conduct that fast, so there is usually 2:1 or 3:1 block. ►Always consider flutter first if a patient has a regular tachycardia of 150/min.
Flutter ECG: regular sawtooth baseline at a rate of 300/min. This may be difficult to see in 2:1 block, but may be revealed by carotid sinus massage (or adenosine IV, p288) which can increase the block.
Treatment: treat in the same way as atrial fibrillation.
Some patients seem to vary between flutter and fibrillation.

1 Stroke in AF group 1997 E-BM 2 19 2 M Ezekowitz 1992 NEJM 327 1406 3 Throm Haemost 1997 78 377

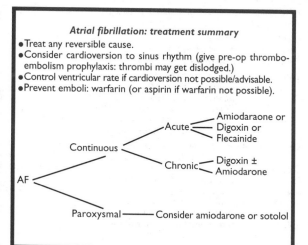

Atrial fibrillation: treatment summary
- Treat any reversible cause.
- Consider cardioversion to sinus rhythm (give pre-op thrombo-embolism prophylaxis: thrombi may get dislodged.)
- Control ventricular rate if cardioversion not possible/advisable.
- Prevent emboli: warfarin (or aspirin if warfarin not possible).

Atrial fibrillation

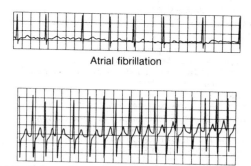

Atrial fibrillation with a rapid ventricular response. Diagnosis is based on the totally irregular ventricular rhythm.

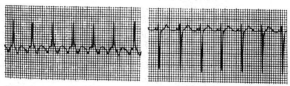

Atrial flutter with 2:1 AV block. Lead aVF (on left) shows the characteristic saw-tooth baseline whereas lead V_1 (on right) shows discrete atrial activity, alternate 'F' waves being superimposed on ventricular T waves.

ECG shows QRS complexes of >120ms (>3 small squares)+ rate of >100bpm.

▶The commonest cause of a wide complex tachycardia is ventricular tachycardia (VT).

Principles of management:
- If in doubt, treat as for VT and DC shock.
- Identify the underlying rhythm and treat accordingly.

Classification: ventricular tachycardia
ventricular fibrillation
ventricular extrasystoles (ectopics)
Torsade de pointes (ECG on p295)
supraventricular tachycardia with conduction block
eg AF, atrial flutter, junctional tachycardia

Identification of the underlying rhythm can be difficult so enlist the help of an expert where possible. A conscious patient does not exclude VT. Diagnosis is based on the history (ischaemic heart disease increases the likelihood of a ventricular arrhythmia over an SVT with aberrant conduction), a 12–lead ECG and the response to adenosine (p290). ECG findings in favour of an SVT with aberrant conduction include:
- The presence of P-waves *associated with* the QRS complex.
- No fusion or capture beats (diagnostic of ventricular origin).
- QRS <0.14sec.
- Same QRS morphology as in sinus rhythm.
- Normal axis.
- Classical LBBB or RBBB QRS morphology.

If all complexes have similar polarities in the chest leads ('concordance'), suspect VT.

Management: This depends primarily on the state of the patient (see 'adverse signs' opposite). Remember to:
- Connect patient to a cardiac monitor and have a defibrillator at hand.
- Give oxygen and obtain IV access.
- Send blood to check for electrolyte abnormalities.
- If pulse disappears, move to cardiac arrest protocol (p771).

See *Resuscitation Council Guidelines* (opposite). If the tachycardia does not respond to this, seek expert advice and consider:
- Procainamide 25–100mg IV over 2min up to 1g (ECG monitoring). Stop if BP falls below 100mmHg. Oral maintenance is 250mg/6h.
- Overdrive pacing.

Ventricular fibrillation (VF) (ECG on p295.) See guidelines on p771.

Ventricular tachycardia (VT) (ECG on p295.) Defined as ≥3 successive ventricular extrasystoles at a rate >100/min (2 is a called 'salvo').
Prevention of recurrent VT: Surgical isolation of the arrhythmogenic area or implantation of tiny automatic defibrillators may help.

Ventricular extrasystoles (ectopics) are the most common post-MI arrhythmia but they are also seen in healthy people (≤10/h). Post-MI they suggest electrical instability, and there is a risk of VF if the 'R on T' pattern (ie no gap before the T-wave) is seen. If frequent (>10/min), treat with lignocaine (=lidocaine). Otherwise, just observe patient (check U&E). ▣

Torsade de pointes (ECG on p295) Looks like VF but is VT with a varying axis. It is usually due to anti-arrhythmics which prolong the Q–T interval. Consider stopping anti-arrhythmics, giving IV Mg^{2+} and overdrive pacing.

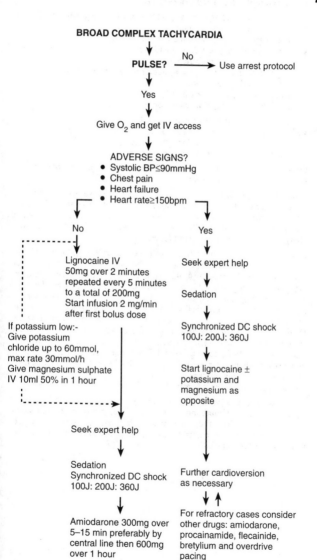

BROAD COMPLEX TACHYCARDIA

PULSE? → No → Use arrest protocol

Yes

Give O₂ and get IV access

ADVERSE SIGNS?
- Systolic BP≤90mmHg
- Chest pain
- Heart failure
- Heart rate≥150bpm

No

Lignocaine IV
50mg over 2 minutes
repeated every 5 minutes
to a total of 200mg
Start infusion 2 mg/min
after first bolus dose

If potassium low:-
Give potassium
chloride up to 60mmol,
max rate 30mmol/h
Give magnesium sulphate
IV 10ml 50% in 1 hour

Seek expert help

Sedation
Synchronized DC shock
100J: 200J: 360J

Amiodarone 300mg over
5–15 min preferably by
central line then 600mg
over 1 hour

Yes

Seek expert help

Sedation

Synchronized DC shock
100J: 200J: 360J

Start lignocaine ±
potassium and
magnesium as
opposite

Further cardioversion
as necessary

For refractory cases consider
other drugs: amiodarone,
procainamide, flecainide,
bretylium and overdrive
pacing

Pacemakers

Pacemakers supply electrical initiation to contraction. They may dramatically benefit even a very old patient. The pacemaker lies subcutaneously where it may be programmed through the skin as needs change, eg for different rates. They last 7–15 years.

Indications for temporary pacemakers—See p802 for further details and insertion technique.
- Symptomatic bradycardia, uncontrolled by drugs.
- Suppression of drug-resistant VT and SVT□ (overdrive pacing; do on ITU).
- Acute conduction disturbances:
    After acute *anterior* MI, prophylactic pacing is required in:
    2nd or 3rd degree AV block;
    Bi- or tri-fascicular block (p266).
After *inferior* MI, only act on these for symptoms.

Indications for permanent pacemakers
- 2° (Mobitz type II) and 3° heart block (atrioventricular block).
- Symptomatic bradycardias (eg sick sinus syndrome, p286).
- Occasionally useful in suppressing resistant tachyarrhythmias.

Some say persistent bifascicular block after MI requires a permanent system: this remains controversial.

Insertion is under local anaesthetic. *Pre-operative assessment:* FBC, platelets, clotting screen, HBsAg. Insert IV cannula. Consent. Consider premedication. Give antibiotic cover (eg flucloxacillin 500mg IM and benzylpenicillin 600mg IM) 20mins before, and 1 and 6h after. Before discharge, check position (CXR) and function.

ECG of paced rhythm Check each vertical pacing spike is followed immediately by a wide QRS complex. If the system is on 'demand' of 60 beats/min, a pacing spike will only be seen if the natural beats are coming less frequently than 60/min. If it is cutting in on a more rapid natural rate, its sensing mode is malfunctioning. If it is failing to cut in at slower rates, its pacing mode is malfunctioning, ie the lead is dislodged (either end), or the pacing threshold is high, or the lead (or insulation) is faulty. *Dual chamber pacemakers* pace atria and *then* ventricles, helping stroke volume and, via their sensory system, allowing rates to rise with exercise, if sinus node function is normal. They cost much more, but may be needed for patients to exercise and enjoy life. Because of the extra cost, in the UK NHS, many purchasers will only buy very few of these, for their youngest patients. This is a good (or bad) example of ageism at work.

Post-op Inspect for wound haematoma, dehiscence, or twitchings during the first week. Count apex rate (p40). If this is 6 or more beats-per-minute slower than the rate quoted for the pacemaker, suspect malfunction. Other problems: lead fracture; pacemaker interference (eg from patient's muscles). Driving rules: *OHCS* p468.

3-letter pacemaker codes—eg 'VVI' or 'DDD'

The 1st letter = the chamber paced (Atrium, Ventricle, or both, ie Dual).
The 2nd letter = the chamber sensed (Atrium, Ventricle, or both, ie Dual).
The 3rd letter = mode of response to sensing (I=inhibited output, T=Triggered, D=Inhibited and triggered)—so DDD, for example, means paced and sensed in atrium and ventricle, with atrial rate-sensing triggering the ventricular rate, to a preset upper limit (enabling paced hearts to beat faster when an intruder enters the room, but also, unfortunately, when there is an atrial tachyarrhythmia; this is *not* a feature of DDI).

(An 'R' after a code refers to various sensor input rate adjustments.)

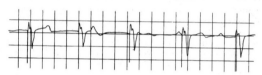

ECG of paced rhythm.

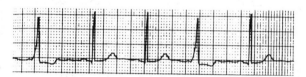

ECG of Wolff–Parkinson–White syndrome (p288) in 1st & 4th beats; compared with the other beats, it can be seen how the delta wave both broadens the ventricular complex, and shortens the PR interval.

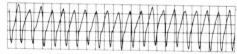

ECG of ventricular tachycardia with a rate of 235 per minute (p292).

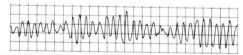

ECG of ventricular fibrillation (p771).

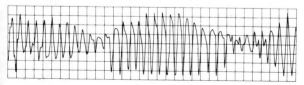

ECG of tosade de pointes tachycardia (p292).

⚕ Heart failure—basic concepts

This is a syndrome of fluid retention causing dyspnoea on exertion (or lying flat) and oedema due to insufficient cardiac output. It may complicate many different heart diseases. *A common mistake is to fail to look for the cause.* As venous (ie filling) pressure rises, there is pulmonary and peripheral congestion—hence the term congestive cardiac failure (CCF).

Classification Either (i) high-output, low-output, and fluid overload; or (ii) left or right ventricular failure (RVF or LVF).

High-output failure The heart's output is normal or increased in the face of much increased needs. Failure occurs when cardiac output fails to meet needs. It will occur with a normal heart, but even earlier if there is heart disease. Causes: heart disease with anaemia or pregnancy, hyperthyroidism, Paget's disease, arteriovenous malformation, beriberi. Consequences: initially features of RVF; later LVF becomes evident.

Low-output failure The heart's output is inadequate (eg ejection fraction <0.35), or can only be adequate with high filling pressures. Causes:
● *Excessive preload:* Eg mitral regurgitation or fluid overload. Fluid overload may cause LVF in a normal heart if renal excretion is impaired or big volumes are involved (eg IVI running too fast). It is easily caused if there is simultaneous compromise of cardiac function and in the elderly.
● *Pump failure due to:*
  —*Heart muscle disease:* Ischaemic heart disease; cardiomyopathy (p316).
  —*Restricted filling:* Constrictive pericarditis, tamponade, restrictive cardiomyopathy. This may be the mechanism of action of fluid overload: an expanding right heart impinges on the LV, so filling is restricted by the ungiving pericardium (the mechanism invoking a 'hump in the Starling curve' is now said to be an error based on an artefact).
  —*Inadequate heart rate:* β-blockers, heart block, post MI.
  —*Negatively inotropic drugs:* Eg most anti-arrhythmic agents.
● *Chronic excessive afterload:* Eg aortic stenosis, hypertension.

Left ventricular failure is dominated by *pulmonary oedema*. The *symptoms* are exertional dyspnoea, orthopnoea, paroxysmal nocturnal dyspnoea, wheeze (cardiac 'asthma'), cough (± pink froth), haemoptysis, fatigue. The *signs* are tachypnoea, tachycardia, end inspiratory basal crackles, S_3 (p260), pulsus alternans (alternating large and small pulse pressures), cardiomegaly, cyanosis, and pleural effusion. Peak expiratory flow rate may be low, but if it is <150L/min, suspect COPD or asthma.

Tests CXR shows prominent upper lobe veins (upper lobe diversion), diffuse patchy lung shadows often basal but sometimes perihilar 'bat's wings' or occasionally unilateral (if nursed on one side), or nodular (especially if pre-existing COPD), fluid in the fissures, pleural effusion, cardiomegaly, Kerley B lines (variously attributed to interstitial oedema[1] and engorged peripheral lymphatics[2]), peribronchial cuffing. ECG may elucidate cause (look for evidence of infarction, ischaemia or ventricular hypertrophy). *Echocardiography* is the key diagnostic test[3] and, ideally, it should be advised whenever the diagnosis or cause of heart failure is uncertain—which is often. ▣ *Endomyocardial biopsy* is rarely needed.

Right ventricular failure This causes peripheral oedema (p50), abdominal discomfort, nausea, fatigue, and wasting (often with weight gain). *Signs:* Raised JVP, hepatomegaly, pitting oedema, and ascites.

Communication As the term heart *failure* brings ideas of inescapable catastrophe to patients, we avoided this term, preferring 'congestion', until it was clear that our more intelligent patients, discovering the true name of their condition by other means, felt patronized. As ever, *know your patient* and communicate accordingly.

1 *Oxford Textbook of Medicine* (OTM) p2833 2 *OTM* (1996) p2502 3 HJ Dargie 1994 *BMJ* i 321

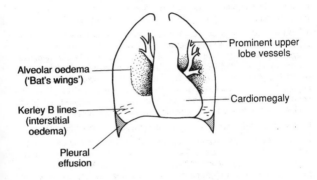

The CXR in left ventricular failure

✚ Heart failure: long-term management

- Treat causes if possible, eg valve lesions, or hypoxia in cor pulmonale.
- Treat exacerbating factors (anaemia, thyroid disease, infection, ↑BP).

- Restrict salt and alcohol intake (if the latter is excessive).
- Maintain optimal weight and good nutrition (p104). • Stop smoking.
- Try to avoid NSAIDs: they cause fluid retention and may interact with diuretics and ACE inhibitors to cause chronic renal failure.

Drugs: 4 types of drugs are used: 1 Diuretics 2 ACE inhibitors 3 Vasodilators such as nitrates 4 Inotropes (digoxin). A 5th option gaining favour is $\alpha + \beta$ blockade with carvedilol—which can save lives not by an immediate pharmacological effect, but 'by improving the biology of the heart long-term'.[1] If symptoms are mild, start with a thiazide diuretic, eg bendrofluazide (=bendroflumethiazide) 2.5mg/24h PO. Once stabilized, start an ACE-i (p299; this improves symptoms *and* prognosis; risk of MI↓); increase its dose as needed (eg captopril 25mg/8h PO).[2] If inadequate, swap thiazide for a loop diuretic, eg frusemide (=furosemide) 40mg/24h PO, up to 160mg, and, if needed, add digoxin[3] (p276) ± vasodilator, eg modified-release isosorbide mononitrate eg 60mg/24h PO.

Follow-up and avoiding diuretic-induced hypokalaemia: Check body weight, BP, clinical condition, and U&E before and 1 week or so after starting any drugs, and, ideally every 6 months once K⁺ is stable. K⁺-sparing diuretics are rarely needed (mild hypokalaemia is usually harmless[4]) unless:
- K⁺ <3.2mmol/L • Known predisposition to arrhythmias. • Concurrent digoxin (its cardio-toxicity is augmented by K⁺↓) • Pre-existing K⁺-losing conditions, eg cirrhosis. Dose example: amiloride 5mg/24h PO (= co-amilofruse if combined with 40mg frusemide [=furosemide]).

If HCO₃⁻↑, ± malaise, thirst or hypotension, suspect over-diuresis.

Heart failure and sexual intercourse Reassure that if he can mount 2 flights of stairs reasonably quickly, sex should be fine. If dyspnoea and angina are a problem, keep a nitrate spray by the bed. Activity is least likely to cause symptoms if engaged in after a good night's sleep with the least affected partner doing most of the work.[4] The most provocative occasion will be sex with a brand new partner, after a hot bath, on a full stomach.

Intractable heart failure Reassess cause and patient's concordance (p3) with your regimen. Aim to regain lost ground and improve the patient to his former out-patient-manageable state: so admit to hospital for:
- Strict bed rest. • Bedside commode. • Avoid straining at stool.
- DVT prevention: heparin 5000u/8h SC. Use antithrombo-embolic stockings.
- IV frusemide (<4mg/min—by this route it is a venodilator too).
- Consider the diuretic metolazone, eg 5–20mg/24h PO.
- Daily weight, and frequent U&E (K⁺↓).
- Alter ACE-inhibitor/vasodilator dosage to maximum tolerated. Sometimes a compromise is struck—accepting some oedema or exercise limitation in order to avoid unacceptable symptoms of low output.
- *In extremis,* a period on IV inotropes (see p768) to tide him over an acute exacerbation. But it may be very difficult to wean him off it. Similarly, opiates *may* have a rôle here (symptoms↓ + venodilatation).
- Finally, consider the patient for heart transplantation.

Acute heart failure (pulmonary oedema) See p772.

---

1 M Packer 1996 NEJM 334 1349—N=1094; here carvedilol ↓death rate by 65%—but there is a query over the results due to excess deaths with carvedilol during the pre-trial run-in period (E&M 1996 i 212) ...nsensus 1987 NEJM 316 1429 3 R Jaeschke 1990 *Am J Med* 88 279–86; meta-analyses say 12% of ...in heart failure in sinus rhythm benefit from digoxin (see p276). 4 *Drug Ther Bul* 1991 29 87

How to start ACE-inhibitors

►Most patients tolerate angiotensin-converting enzyme inhibitors very well, and with all the evidence suggesting that they will live longer and feel better, it is our job to use them when appropriate. Nevertheless, be sure to address the following, so that contraindications are not missed, and risks of first-dose hypotension are reduced.

Is there a contraindication or problem[P] with ACE inhibition?

Ask about: –symptomatic hypotension (faints, dizziness)

–interacting drugs:[P] NSAIDs (↑risk of renal damage); potassium salts/cyclosporin/K^+-sparing diuretics (all risk hyperklaemia); Li^+ (levels↑)

–pregnancy or breast feeding

–angio-oedema, collagen disease, porphyria

Look for: –renal artery* or aortic stenosis; BP↓

Is there a high-risk condition? *Specialist help ± admission may be needed*

Ask about: –symptoms of severe heart failure (shortness of breath on minimal exertion); frusemide of over 80mg per day (or equivalent)

–symptoms of intermittent claudication (risk of renal artery stenosis*)

–history of severe COPD or cor pulmonale

Look for: –systolic BP <90mmHg

–signs of severe heart failure, atherosclerosis (bruits), or COPD

Test for: –U&E imbalance: Na^+<130mmol/L; K^+>5.5mmol/L; creatinine >200μmol/L; FBC: rare neutropenia

Then. . . Stop diuretics and K^+ supplements.

Explain about risk of dizziness (first-dose hypotension): advise to lie down for 1h after first few doses.

Start with small dose, eg perindopril 2mg nocte PO Increase until symptoms resolve or side-effects supervene (BP↓) or creatinine rises, eg up to 2mg/12h.

Review in ~1 week for assessment; repeat U&E.

*If renovascular renal failure precludes use of ACEi (ACEi may worsen GFR here) and frusemide is providing no answer, consider maximal vasodilatation with nitrates and hydralazine: seek expert advice.

⚕ Hypertension

▶This is a major risk factor for stroke and myocardial infarction. It is often symptomless, so screening is vital—*before* damage is done. When taking BPs, be sure the cuff is wide enough (>½ the arm's circumference).

Value judgments There is no BP value above which you must always treat, and below which you can safely leave alone—you must take into account family history, age, smoking, and lipid (see *risk equation*, p740)—and more complex matters such as the value a patient sets on life. If he is agreeable, bring the spouse/partner in on the decision. No one remembers to take antihypertensives all the time, and the spouse may be more motivated to get treatment right. If the patient does not set the value of his life at a pin's worth, you may need to treat his depression, anger, or pain before talking about antihypertensives. So the first rule is: *know your patient*. Don't think of this as another chore to tick off; dialogue is our reward for all those boring things we do in a day, and helps keep us sane.

Patients' views of the balance of risk to benefit of treatment are critical. Be sure he is well-informed. It is unacceptable to cause significant side-effects in people who thought they were healthy before they met you: most of us live in the here-and-now, and relate with difficulty to the stranger who is us in 20 years. The British Hypertension Society suggests drugs are needed if *sustained* diastolic >100mmHg on ≥3 readings each a week apart. Drugs may also be indicated if diastolic *sustained* at >90mmHg over 6 months, if systolic >160mmHg, OR end-organ damage:
●Left ventricular hypertrophy ●PMH myocardial infarct ●PMH stroke/TIA
●Peripheral vascular disease ●PMH angina ●Renal failure
If *no* end-organ damage and diastolic 90–99mmHg for >½yr, treat if risk factors present, ie ♂, +ve family history; smoker; diabetes; lipids↑. (Systolic BP ≥200mmHg also prompts drugs even if no risk factors or end-organ damage or raised diastolic BP.) *BP in the elderly (65–80yrs)*: 3 trials support treatment if systolic ≥180mmHg. Note: if BPs are labile or equivocal, patient-worn 24h ambulatory BP measurement *may* be useful.▣

Causes In 95% the cause is unknown ('essential')—but alcohol and obesity may play an important part. Causes in the remaining 5%:
Renal disease: Renal artery stenosis (atheroma or fibromuscular hyperplasia, p397), polycystic kidneys, chronic pyelonephritis, glomerulonephritis, polyarteritis nodosa, systemic sclerosis (p670).
Endocrine disease: Cushing's (p548) and Conn's syndromes (p554), phaeochromocytoma (p554), acromegaly, hyperparathyroidism, DM.
Others: Coarctation, pre-eclampsia (OHCS p96), steroids.

Presentations Headache, stroke, heart failure, MI, renal failure (lethargy, proteinuria), patchy or distorted vision. Always check for retinopathy—either *arteriopathic* (arteriovenous *nipping*: arteries nip veins where they cross) or *hypertensive* (arteriolar vasoconstriction and leakage producing *retinal ischaemia with microinfarcts* (eg cotton-wool spots, macular oedema, haemorrhages and, rarely, *papilloedema*—see p676).

Look hard for a cause in the young, severe hypertensive; be more restrained in the older patient (diagnostic yield and treatment benefits will be less). Start by talking to the patient. Is he or she aware of the hypertension? Episodic feelings 'as if about to die' or headaches, or sweats or palpitations, suggests phaeochromocytoma (p554). Next do a full cardiovascular examination. Assess degree of end-organ damage with ophthalmoscopy (dilate with 1% tropicamide if poor view), ECG, CXR, U&E.
Also do U&E, Ca^{2+}, creatinine, fasting glucose and cholesterol, MSU (protein, blood). Sometimes consider renal ultrasound, IVU, renal arteriography, 24 hour urinary VMA × 3, urinary free cortisol (p550).

Management of hypertension ®

Look for and treat underlying causes (eg pain, obesity, alcohol↑, see p300).

Treatment goal BP <160/90*—and a happy, well-informed patient.

Non-drug treatment ●Stop smoking (to ↓arteriopathy, not BP). If obese, explain about optimum weight; find a good diet (p482); review current diet. 'Weight-Watchers' self-help helps more than doctors here. ●Cut alcohol intake to ~1u/day. ●Encourage regular exercise. ●Avoid heavy salting of food. ●↑Dietary K+ (eg 5 pieces of fruit/day). ●Reduce stress. Consider relaxation therapy (eg slow breathing, muscle relaxation and mental relaxation by imagining pleasant experiences ± cognitive strategies to cope with stress, and knowledge of how to deal with hostile feelings). This may be done in groups with the leader setting regular homework. Typical falls in BP are 6–26mmHg (systolic) and 5–15mmHg (diastolic) in those 50% of trials showing a benefit.

Drugs Explain the need for long-term care, aiming to make him live longer. "See your doctor about side-effects: don't just stop the tablets". Older drugs have more side-effects, but trials used these drugs, and they saved lives. Ca²⁺-channel blockers have been validated in one big trial in the elderly,¹ but we do not know if newer ACE-i and angiotensin II receptor blockers (eg losartan▧) can save as many lives. *Here is one approach:*
●Bendrofluazide (=bendroflumethiazide) 2.5–5mg PO mané, or β-blocker, eg atenolol 50–100mg/24h PO (if no asthma, heart failure, or claudication).
●If inadequate, add or replace with an angiotensin converting enzyme inhibitor (ACE-i), eg lisinopril 2.5–20mg/24h PO (max 40mg/day) or enalapril (same dose). See p299 for starting regimen. ACE-i may be first choice if co-existing LVF. ACE-i are first choice in diabetics (helps prevent renal failure); also in some older patients, as β-blockers frequently cause side-effects.
●If uncontrolled, add a calcium antagonist (eg amlodipine 5mg/24h PO). SE: flushing, fatigue, gum hyperplasia, oedema—see warning on p276.
●If the hypertension is still not controlled, seek expert help. Agents such as methyldopa, prazosin, minoxidil, or hydralazine may be needed.
Note: *thiazides* (eg bendrofluazide/bendroflumethiazide) are somewhat out of favour due to impotence, the ultimate negative QALY (p12); other SE: gout, K+↓, cholesterol↑, glucose↑—but may suit the elderly. *Methyldopa* often fails due to drowsiness (or haemolysis), and *hydralazine* will cause tachycardia (unless given with a β-blocker), and can cause SLE.

Side-effects often dictate choice. With β-blockers and diuretics, 80% of SE occur in first year. If one first-line drug does not suit, try another.

Malignant hypertension Its hallmark is fibrinoid necrosis. Untreated, 90% die in 1 year; treated, 60% survive 5yrs. *Detection:* Universal screening from aged 20yrs. *Presentation:* LVF, encephalopathy (fits, coma), renal failure, headache, BP↑↑ ± severe retinopathy (p300). Do CT if acute CNS signs make it hard to rule out stroke. *Treatment:* Bed rest; nifedipine 10–20mg/8h; start by biting a 10mg capsule and swallowing it. BP starts to fall gently after ½h. *Frusemide* if LVF (p772). Avoid sudden drops in BP as cerebral autoregulation↓ (so stroke risk↑). If minute-by-minute BP control is essential (eg during fits), take to ITU, and use nitroprusside: 0.3µg/kg/min IVI titrated up to 6µg/kg/min (eg 50mg in 1L dextrose 5%; expect to give 100–200mL/h for a few hours only, to avoid cyanide risk). Do BP every minute (intra-arterial monitoring if available) until stable, then every 30min. Aim for diastolic BP of 100–110mmHg. Cover burette with reflective foil to stop photodeactivation. *Labetalol* is an alternative IV drug (eg 50mg IV over 1min, repeated every 5min, max 200mg), as is *hydralazine* (5–10mg over 20min; repeat after 30min if needed).

*The lower the better; William Blake knew the problem here: *you cannot tell what is far enough without going too far*. ▶beware falls and faints; ∴ you've got to *guess* when to stop 1 J Staessen 1997 *Lancet* 1997 **350** 757

160-95

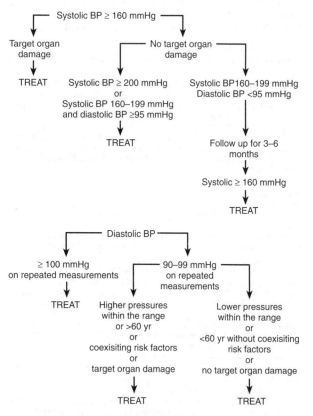

Guidelines for the management of essential hypertension – adapted from the British Hypertension Society Guidelines *BMJ* 1993 306, 983–987.

Examples of coexisting risk factors: diabetes mellitus, angina, hyperlipidaemia

To calculate how risk factors interact, see the risk equation on p740.
See also USA Joint National Committee regimen (JNV vi) 1997 *Arch Int Med* 157 2413 & *Lancet* 1998 251 288

Rheumatic fever

This systemic illness is due to cross-reactivity with Group A β-haemolytic streptococci (eg after throat infection). In the susceptible 2% of the population, there may be permanent damage to heart valves—and ↑risk of subsequent endocarditis. It is common in the Third World, and rare in the West. Pockets of resurgence are appearing in the USA. It usually follows a latent period of 2–4 weeks. Peak incidence: 5–15yrs.

Diagnosis This is based on the *revised Jones criteria* and can be made in the presence of evidence of previous streptococcal infection plus 2 major criteria or 1 major and 2 minor criteria.

Evidence suggesting recent streptococcal infection (1 is enough):
- Recent scarlet fever.
- Positive growth from throat swab.
- Increase in antistreptolysin O titre (ASOT) >200u/mL.

Major criteria:
- Carditis (endo-, myo-, or pericarditis), eg sleeping tachycardia, changing murmurs (eg mitral or aortic regurgitation, or Carey Coombs' murmur—p262), pericardial rub, heart failure, cardiomegaly, conduction defects (45–70%). An apical systolic murmur may be the only sign.[1]
- Migratory ('flitting') polyarthritis—red and very tender joints (75%).
- Sydenham's chorea—10% (St Vitus' dance, OHCS p758); commoner if ♀. These odd darting movements are usually a late sign, which may be preceded by emotional lability and uncharacteristic behaviour.[2]
- Subcutaneous nodules (2–20%).
- Erythema marginatum (2–10%)—trunk, thighs, arms (p678).

Minor criteria:
- Raised ESR or C-reactive protein (CRP).
- Arthralgia (but not if arthritis is one of the major criteria).
- Fever.
- History of previous rheumatic fever or rheumatic heart disease.
- Prolonged P-R interval (but not if carditis is major criterion).

Management
- Bed rest until CRP normal for 2 weeks—may be 3 months.
- Benzylpenicillin 600mg IM stat then penicillin V 250mg/6h PO.
- Analgesia for carditis/arthritis: NSAIDs (p664) or aspirin 90mg/kg/day PO (in 4-hourly divided doses; up to 8g) for 2 days then 70mg/kg/day for 6 weeks. Monitor blood levels. Watch for toxicity: ototoxicity, hyperventilation and metabolic acidosis, GI upset. Steroids are thought not to have a major impact on sequelae, but they may improve symptoms.[1,2]
- Immobilize joints in severe arthritis.
- Haloperidol (0.5mg/8h PO) for the chorea.

Prognosis 60% who have carditis develop chronic rheumatic heart disease. This correlates with the severity of the carditis—eg mild carditis and no cardiomegaly will heal completely in ~80% of patients, if recurrent rheumatic attacks are prevented.[3] Average acute attacks last 3 months. Recurrence may be precipitated by future streptococcal infection, pregnancy, or the contraceptive pill. Of the 60% with cardiac complications, sequelae affect mitral, aortic, tricuspid, and pulmonary valves in 70%, 40%, 10%, and 2% respectively. Incompetent lesions may develop with the attack and may regress; stenoses may develop years later.

Secondary prophylaxis After rheumatic fever, give twice-daily penicillin V PO until 25 years old. Thereafter, give antibiotics for dental and other surgery for life (p314). In penicillin allergy, use erythromycin.

1 G Stollerman 1995 *Lancet* 346 391 2 D Kanabar 1996 *Lancet* ii 1000 3 D Albert 1995 *Medicine* 74 1–12

Mitral valve disease

►Defer replacing a mitral valve until symptoms demand.

Mitral stenosis *Cause:* Rheumatic heart disease.

Symptoms: Dyspnoea, palpitations, fatigue; with pulmonary hypertension: haemoptysis, recurrent bronchitis, right heart failure and sometimes chest pain (but suspect other causes of pain).

Signs On inspection: Peripheral cyanosis (if on cheeks = 'malar flush').

Palpation: Pulses are of normal character; irregular if AF from an enlarged left atrium; left parasternal heave (from pulmonary hypertension causing RVH); undisplaced, tapping apex beat (ie palpable S₁, see p260 & p40).

Auscultation: Loud S₁; opening snap (after S₂, from abrupt checking of the valve opening—like the crack of a sail struck by a strong wind) preceding a rumbling mid-diastolic murmur (best heard at the apex, p40), presystolic accentuation murmur. Pulmonary hypertension (p366) and Graham Steell murmur (p262) may occur.

Severity: The more severe the stenosis, the worse the dyspnoea; the larger the left atrium, the longer the murmur, and the closer the opening snap is to S₂. Typically, symptoms start if the valve area is < 1.25cm².

Tests: ECG: P mitrale if in sinus rhythm, but usually in AF; right ventricular hypertrophy. CXR: large left atrium, appearing as a 'second' cardiac shadow as if behind the heart and splaying the carina, pulmonary oedema and, later, mitral valve calcification. Echocardiography is diagnostic (is the mid-diastolic closure rate of the anterior cusp <50mm/sec?). Significant stenosis exists if the valve orifice is < 1cm²/m² body surface area.

Management: If AF, anticoagulate (p596); diuretics and digoxin (p298 & p276) for symptoms. If this is inadequate, mitral valvotomy or balloon valvuloplasty (if valve is still pliant and not calcified), or replacement. Endocarditis prophylaxis (p314). Regular penicillin to ward off recurrent rheumatic fever if <25yrs old (p304). Ensure well-nourished (p104).

Complications: Pulmonary hypertension; emboli, from mural thrombus, eg on McCallum's patch, just above the posterior mitral valve cusp.

Mitral regurgitation *(incompetence) Causes:* Congenital, rheumatic fever, mitral valve prolapse, ruptured chordae tendinae/papillary muscle after MI, or dysfunction (in ventricular dilatation), endocarditis, cardiomyopathy (any), rheumatoid arthritis, possibly fenfluramine and phentermine.

Symptoms: Dyspnoea, fatigue. *Signs:* Displaced, forceful apex (p40), soft S₁, loud S₃, pansystolic murmur at apex radiating to axilla. Sometimes AF.

Severity: The more severe, the larger the left ventricle. Eventually, left ventricular failure occurs.

Tests: CXR: large heart. Echocardiography may reveal cause and extent of ventricular dilatation. *Doppler echocardiography* is semi-quantitative in assessing regurgitation.

Management of mitral incompetence: Anticoagulation in AF. Digoxin, diuretics, and surgery if severe. Antibiotics to prevent endocarditis.

Mitral valve prolapse *Prevalence:* ~5%. It may be asymptomatic or be associated with atypical chest pain, palpitations, syncope, postural hypotension, and emboli. There may be a mid-systolic click and/or a late systolic murmur. There is catecholamine excess and hyperresponsiveness and the syndrome may be, in part, a neuroendocrinopathy. *Tests:* Echocardiography is diagnostic. ECG may show inferior T-wave inversion. Very rarely VF may cause sudden death, and it is recommended that those with syncope or ventricular arrhythmias should be referred for invasive electrophysiology. *Treatment:* β-blockers may help palpitations and chest pain. There is risk of endocarditis, so give antibiotic prophylaxis, eg if there is regurgitation or thickened (myxomatous) valve leaflets.

Aortic valve disease

Aortic stenosis (AS) *Causes:* Congenital or rheumatic heart disease, bicuspid valve, degenerative calcification, hypertrophic cardiomyopathy.

Symptoms: Angina, dyspnoea, syncope, dizziness, sudden death.

Signs: Slow rising, small volume pulse; narrow pulse pressure (difference between systolic and diastolic pressures); heaving undisplaced apex beat (p40). In mild stenosis, S_2 is normally split, with A_2 preceding P_2. As stenosis worsens, A_2 is increasingly delayed, giving first a single S_2 and then reversed splitting. If there is aortic valve calcification, A_2 becomes ever softer and may disappear totally. There may be an S_4, ejection click (in pliable valves), and an ejection systolic murmur, loudest in the aortic area (but sometimes elsewhere) which radiates to the carotids and apex.

Tests: ECG: Left ventricular hypertrophy with strain. CXR: Post-stenotic dilatation of ascending aorta; calcification on valve (best seen at fluoroscopy). 2D-echo/Doppler is diagnostic, and may estimate the gradient across the valve quite well. If angina is prominent, coronary angiography should be done to show coronary artery disease. Angiography may not be needed if there is no angina.

Management: These patients are at great risk of Stokes–Adams attacks and sudden death. Prompt valve replacement is normally required if attacks or other symptoms occur. The management of asymptomatic significant AS is an unresolved problem: most cardiologists would advise replacement if the systolic gradient across the valve was >50mmHg. If the patient is not fit for surgery, percutaneous transluminal valvuloplasty may be attempted. Antibiotic prophylaxis against endocarditis is essential (p314) as is good nourishment pre-operatively (p104).

Aortic sclerosis is senile degeneration not associated with left ventricular outflow tract obstruction. There is an ejection systolic murmur, but the character of the pulse remains normal. These patients do not have ejection clicks or abnormal S_2.

Aortic regurgitation 'Common' and	*Rarer causes:*	Spondylitis
Rheumatic heart disease	Takayasu's dis (p708)	Reiter's
Aortic dissection	Ehlers–Danlos (OHCS p746)	Marfan's
Endocarditis; syphilis	Aortic cusp fenestration	SLE (p672)
Congenital, eg with: –VSD	Relapsing polychondritis	BP↑
–bicuspid aortic valve	Osteogenesis imperfecta	Aortitis
–subvalvular aortic stenosis	Calcific valve disease	Trauma

Some slimming drugs *may* also be causative (fenfluramine, phentermine).

Symptoms: Dyspnoea, palpitations (due to extrasystoles).

Signs of a wide pulse pressure: Collapsing (water-hammer) pulse. Corrigan's sign—visible neck pulsation. De Musset's sign—head nodding. Visible capillary pulsations (eg seen in nail beds—Quincke's sign).

Other signs: Duroziez's sign is a femoral diastolic murmur reflecting flow of blood *backwards* up the aorta in severe aortic regurgitation. To elicit this, make this backflow turbulent by pressing on the femoral artery distal to the point of listening. Hyperdynamic displaced apex beat (p40); high-pitched early diastolic murmur; Austin Flint mid-diastolic murmur (due to regurgitant stream vibrating the anterior mitral cusp).

Investigations: CXR: cardiomegaly. Doppler echo is diagnostic. M-mode and 2D show the degree of ventricular dilatation.

Management: Try to replace valve before significant impairment of left ventricular function. Endocarditis prophylaxis (p314).

Right heart valve disease

Tricuspid stenosis *Cause:* Rheumatic fever; mitral disease always co-exists. *Features:* Oedema; giant *a* wave, small *v* wave, and slow *y* descent in JVP (p258); opening snap, early diastolic murmur (left sternal edge in inspiration). Echocardiography with Doppler may be diagnostic.
Treatment: Diuretics—and sometimes surgical repair.

Tricuspid regurgitation usually occurs with RV enlargement (p366). *Causes:* Endocarditis (IV drug abusers), carcinoid, rheumatic, congenital (eg Ebstein's anomaly, *OHCS* p746); slimming drugs, p308.

The Patient: Look for: oedema, systolic waves in JVP, pulsatile hepatomegaly (leads to jaundice ± fibrosis), systolic propulsion of the eyeballs; ascites, parasternal RV heave, pansystolic murmur heard best at lower sternal edge in inspiration. Also features of underlying condition (eg dyspnoea). *Management:* Diuretics, vasodilators. *Surgery:* Annuloplasty, replacement (but 20% operative mortality). Treat the underlying cause.

Pulmonary stenosis Usually congenital, eg Fallot's tetralogy (*OHCS* p748). Other: rheumatic, carcinoid. *Signs:* Prominent *a* waves in JVP (↑ in inspiration); RV heave at left sternal edge; S₂ may at first be widely split, but, in severe stenosis, the pulmonary component may be inaudible, so no split is heard; ejection systolic murmur (loudest to left of upper sternum), radiating to left shoulder; pulmonary ejection click augmented by expiration (in mild stenosis); ECG: RVH. CXR: dilated pulmonary artery.

Pulmonary regurgitation is caused by any cause of pulmonary hypertension (p366). It causes a decrescendo murmur in early diastole at the left sternal edge (the Graham Steell murmur).

Cardiac surgery

Closed mitral valvotomy is used in stenosis of uncalcified valves (ie loud S₁, prominent opening snap). A finger inserted in the left atrium dilates the valve orifice. Overenthusiasm leads to regurgitation. This procedure may be repeated. **Open mitral valvotomy** is under direct vision at bypass. Balloon valvuloplasty is gaining popularity.

Valve replacements may be pig aortic valves (Carpentier–Edwards xenografts—can replace any heart valve). Unlike metal valves, no permanent anticoagulation is needed (useful if elderly or pregnant). Metal valves last longer, eg ball-and-cage Starr–Edwards or single tilting discs (Björk–Shiley, Medtonic–Hall). St Jude valves have 2 tilting discs; all risk thromboembolism, haemolysis, leaks, and endocarditis (prophylaxis, p314).

▶If a patient with a valve prosthesis deteriorates suddenly, assume the valve has clotted (or broken)—particularly if the heart sounds are odd, quiet, or absent: get expert help urgently. Also, think of endocarditis. Note: there is little to choose between tissue or mechanical valves in terms of survival. Some people find the mechanical device rather noisy.[1]

Cardiac transplantation Consider this when cardiac disease is *severely* curtailing quality of life, and survival is not expected beyond 6–12 months. 5-year survival can be ~70%. CI: recent lung infarction; significant peripheral vascular or cerebrovascular disease; severe systemic disease; active infection (contraindication to immunosuppression); HIV+ve.

Pre-op assessment FBC, platelets, ESR, clotting, U&E, LFTs, HBsAg, CMV serology, CXR, ECG, crossmatch 10 units, MSU, swab nose and groin.

1 British Heart Foundation *Factfile* 1994 **9** 1

Coronary artery bypass grafts

This is an option for angina if drugs fail, or there is left mainstem disease (here it saves lives), and angioplasty (p278) is unsuitable or has failed.

Surgery is planned in the light of angiograms. The heart is stopped and blood pumped artificially by a machine outside the body (cardiac bypass). (Minimally invasive thoracotomies not requiring this are well-described,[1,2] but have not yet been validated in randomized trials.)

The patient's own saphenous vein is used as the graft. One end is attached to the aorta, the other to a coronary artery distal to the stenosis. Several grafts may be placed.

>50% of vein grafts close in 10 years (low-dose aspirin helps prevent this). Internal mammary artery grafts last longer (but may cause chest-wall numbness).

After CABG: If angina persists (from poor run-off from the graft, distal disease, new atheroma, or graft occlusion) add in drugs, and consider angioplasty (repeat surgery is dangerous). Mood, sex, and intellectual problems are common early—rehabilitation helps:
- Exercise: walk→cycle→swim→jog
- Drive at 1 month: no need to tell DVLA if non-HGV licences, *OHCS* p468
- Get back to work eg at 3 months
- Attend to: smoking; BP; lipids
- Aspirin 75mg/24h PO for ever

1 M Massimo 1998 *BMJ* i 88 2 GD Angelini 1996 *NEJM* 347 757

Infective endocarditis

▶*Fever + new regurgitant murmur = endocarditis until proven otherwise.*

Classification

1 50% of all endocarditis is on normal valves. It follows a more acute course presenting with acute heart failure.

2 Endocarditis on rheumatic, degenerative or congenitally abnormal valves tends to run a subacute course.

3 Endocarditis on prosthetic valves may be 'early' (acquired at implantation, very bad prognosis) or 'late' (acquired haematogenously). Lifetime risk: 1–4%. Infected prosthetic valves must usually be replaced.

Pathogenesis Any bacteraemia, eg any dentistry/poor dental hygiene, GU manipulation, or surgery exposes valves to colonization. In 60% no cause is found. The commonest organism, *Strep viridans* (35–50%), typically runs a subacute course. Others include other streptococci (mainly *Enterococcus faecalis*) and *Staph aureus* (20% of all cases, but 50% acute endocarditis). Rarely other bacteria, fungi, *Coxiella*, or *Chlamydia*. Non-bacterial causes are SLE (Libman–Sacks endocarditis); malignancy. Vegetations may embolize. Right heart endocarditis is commonest in IV drug abusers. It may cause pulmonary abscesses. Endocarditis is associated with vasculitis.

The Patient with chronic endocarditis may suffer 4 phenomena: a) *Infective:* Fever, weight↓, malaise, night sweats, clubbing (PLATE 7), splenomegaly, anaemia, mycotic aneurysms; b) *Heart murmurs ± heart failure;* c) *Embolic:* eg stroke; d) *Vasculitic:* Microscopic haematuria, splinter haemorrhages, Osler's nodes (painful lesions on finger pulps), Janeway lesions (palmar macules), Roth's spots (retinal vasculitis), even renal failure.

The 4 cardinal signs are: fever, haematuria, splenomegaly, and murmurs.

Diagnosis can be difficult. Take 3 *blood cultures* at different times and from different veins, preferably when the fever is rising. The first 2 sets of blood cultures are positive in >95% of culture-positive endocarditis. ESR high. Normochromic, normocytic anaemia. CXR: cardiomegaly. *Transthoracic echocardiography* may show vegetations, but only if >3mm (transoesophageal echo is more sensitive and has a high negative predictive value). Do *urinalysis* for haematuria. *Strep bovis* endocarditis is associated with colonic carcinoma, and should prompt colonoscopy. The *Duke criteria*[1] for definite diagnosis of endocarditis are given opposite.

Management Liaise with a microbiologist and a cardiologist.
● Antibiotics—for streps: benzylpenicillin 1.2g/4h IV + gentamicin (eg 1mg/kg/8h IV for ≥2wks, see p750), then amoxicillin 1g/8h PO for 2 wks. *Staph aureus:* flucloxacillin 2g/6h IV + gentamicin (p750), then flucloxacillin alone for ≥2wks. For either in penicillin allergy: vancomycin 1g/12h IV slowly + gentamicin. *Staph epidermidis:* vancomycin + rifampicin. Do MBCs (minimum bactericidal concentrations) & gentamicin levels (p750).
● If blind therapy required: benzylpenicillin eg 1g/4h IV + gentamicin (p750); if acute, add flucloxacillin 2g/6h IV.
● Consider surgery (eg valve replacement under vancomycin cover) if:[2]
 —Worsening LVF —Valvular obstruction —Repeated emboli
 —Fungal endocarditis —Persistent bacteraemia —Myocardial abscess
 —Unstable infected prosthetic valve

Prognosis 30% mortality with staphylococci; 14% with bowel organisms; 6% with sensitive streptococci.

1 DT Durack *Am J Med* 1994 96 200 2 NJ Beeching 1994 *Infectious Diseases* 1994 Wolfe

---

The Duke clinical criteria for diagnosing infective endocarditis

Major criteria:
- Positive blood culture —typical organism in 2 separate cultures **or**
  —persistently positive blood cultures (>12hr apart, 3 or majority of 4 or more)
- Endocardium involved —positive echocardiogram (<u>vegetation, abscess, dehiscence of prosthetic valve</u>) **or**
  —<u>new valvular regurgitation</u> (change in murmur not sufficient)

Minor criteria:
- Predisposition (cardiac lesion or IV drug abuse)
- Fever >38°C
- Vascular/immunological phenomena
- Positive blood cultures that do not meet major criteria
- Positive echocardiogram that does not meet major criteria

How to diagnose: Definite infective endocarditis: 2 major **or**
1 major and 3 minor **or**
All 5 minor criteria (if no major criterion is met)

Prevention of endocarditis[1]

Anyone with congenital, or rheumatic heart valve disease, or prosthetic valves is at risk of endocarditis and should take antibiotics before elective procedures which may result in bacteraemia. The recommendations of the *British Cardiac Society/Royal College of Physicians* are given below.[1]

Which valvular and other conditions?

Prophylaxis recommended	*Prophylaxis not recommended*
Prosthetic valve(s)	Mitral valve prolapse (no regurgitation)
Previous endocarditis, even if no other heart disease	Functional/innocent murmur
Any acquired valve disease	
Mitral valve prolapse with regurgitation	
Those with septal defects	

Which procedures?

Prophylaxis recommended	*Prophylaxis not recommended**
Dental procedures causing gingival bleeding, eg scaling	Flexible bronchoscopy
Upper respiratory tract surgery	Diagnostic upper GI endoscopy
Sclerotherapy of oesophageal varices	Trans-oesophageal echocardiography
Oesophageal dilatation	Cardiac catheterisation
Surgery/instrumentation of lower bowel, gall bladder, or GU tract	Caesarean section or normal delivery
Obstetric/gynaecological procedures in high-risk patients	

Which regimen?

●Dental and upper respiratory tract procedures:

	No penicillin allergy	*Penicillin allergy or >1 exposure in past month*
Low/moderate-risk patients	Amoxicillin 3g PO 1h pre-op	Clindamycin 0.6g PO 1h pre-op
Special risk patients (prosthetic valve and GA, previous endocarditis)	Amoxicillin 1g IV *plus* Gentamicin 120mg IV pre-op *and* Amoxicillin 0.5g PO 6h post-op	Vancomycin 1g IV over 100 minutes Gentamicin 120mg slowly IV pre-op**

●Genitourinary procedures: antibiotics as for special risk dental patients above. If urine is infected, cover this organism too.

●Gastrointestinal, obstetric and gynaecological procedures: prophylaxis is only needed if a prosthetic valve is present or he/she has had endocarditis in the past (then as for special risk dental patients above).

1 *Valvular Heart Disease Investigation and Management,* Royal College of Physicians, 1996
*Prophylaxis may be advisable for these procedures in high-risk patients.**
The BNF suggests teicoplanin as a possible substitute for vancomycin.

Diseases of heart muscle

Cardiomyopathies are disorders of heart muscle. There are 3 kinds:

• *Idiopathic congestive (dilated) cardiomyopathy:* (Ventricle size↑; contractility↓) *Prevalence:* 0.2%. *Mortality:* 40% in 2yr (sudden death, cardiogenic shock). *Typical patient:* A young man with RVF, LVF, cardiomegaly, AF, ± emboli. Diagnose by excluding ischaemia, valvular, BP↑, pericardial, and specific heart muscle diseases (below). *Echocardiography* shows a *globally* hypokinetic, dilated heart. Other tests show no or nonspecific abnormalities.

Management: As for heart failure. Consider transplantation.☐

• *Hypertrophic (obstructive) cardiomyopathy (HOCM)* implies hypertrophy of ventricular muscle (usually septum and LV, >2 standard deviations from the mean) of no known cause, usually leading to gradually falling LV function or, rarely (<2.5% per year), sudden death (risk ↑ by hard exercise and anaesthesia, also family history of sudden death; paroxysmal AF or ventricular tachycardia). *Prevalence:* 0.2%. 25% are associated with subaortic obstruction and/or systolic anterior motion of the mitral valve. 70% are associated with mutations in genes proteins encoding eg β-myosin (chromosome 14), α-tropomyosin (chromosome 15) and troponin-T (chromosome 1).

Inheritance is typically autosomal dominant, but ½ are sporadic.

Screening relatives: This may yield mixed blessings: helpful preventive measures, but possible life insurance refusal.

Symptoms: Often none, or dyspnoea (eg paroxysmal nocturnal dyspnoea), exertional or atypical chest pain, faints (15–25%, eg from arrhythmias), palpitations, and features of right heart failure.

Signs: Often none, or jerky pulse (rapid upstroke), double impulse at apex (p40), S3, S4, late systolic murmur (outflow tract obstruction ± mitral regurgitation). Atrial fibrillation is seen in ~5%. ECG: LVH, LBBB.

Echocardiography is usually diagnostic: Asymmetrical septal hypertrophy, systolic anterior movement of mitral valve, midsystolic closure of aortic valve. Cardiac catheterization shows a small banana-like LV cavity + thickened papillary muscles and trabeculae; cavity obliteration in systole.

Management: β-blockers or verapamil for chest pain. Amiodarone 100–200mg/day for arrhythmias (improves prognosis). Try to maintain sinus rhythm, as the loss of atrial kick is serious. Dual chamber pacing may be tried in outflow obstruction. Finally consider septal myectomy. In paroxysmal AF, anticoagulate.

• *Restrictive cardiomyopathy* is due to endomyocardial stiffening, with signs as in constrictive pericarditis (p318). It is commonest in the Tropics where it is due to idiopathic fibrosis. Commonest UK cause is amyloid.

Specific heart muscle diseases behave like dilated cardiomyopathy. But amyloid and carcinoid may be restrictive; amyloid and cardiac involvement in Friedreich's ataxia may resemble HOCM. *Chief causes:* Ischaemia, BP↑ (may present in failure with normal BP: examine fundi to reveal signs of earlier hypertension). *Others:* Infection (rheumatic fever, IE, TB, Lyme disease); alcohol; cocaine; 'ecstasy'; post-partum; smoking; connective tissue diseases; diabetes; hyper- or hypothyroidism; acromegaly; Addison's; phaeochromocytoma; haemochromatosis; sarcoid; Duchenne muscular dystrophy; myotonic dystrophy; irradiation; cytotoxics; storage diseases.

Acute myocarditis is inflammation of the myocardium and may present similarly to myocardial infarction. Typical cause: viral eg *Coxsackie*; also Lyme disease, diphtheria, other infections, rheumatic fever, drugs.

The Patient: Faints, pulse↑, angina, dyspnoea, arrhythmia, heart failure.

Tests: Exclude MI + pericardial effusion. Consider viral or Chagas' serology.

Management: Supportive. These patients may recover spontaneously or develop intractable heart failure.☐

Cardiac myxoma

We all need to know when to suspect left atrial myxoma even though it is rare (prevalence ≤5/10,000) because it is dangerous but very treatable—and patients may present confusingly (eg on general surgical 'take'). Presentation may be as left atrial obstruction (like mitral stenosis), systemic emboli, AF, or fever, weight loss, ↑ESR, and clubbing (it's a very rare cause of this). ♀:♂ ≈ 2:1.

Signs distinguishing it from mitral stenosis are the occurrence of emboli (eg large enough to obstruct the aortic bifurcation) while the patient is in sinus rhythm. Auscultation may reveal a 'tumour plop', as the pedunculated tumour reaches the end of its tether. Auscultatory signs may vary according to posture. Whenever emboli are excised, put them under the microscope to see if myxoma cells are present.

Tests: Echocardiography is diagnostic. If a *right* atrial myxoma is diagnosed, it may be part of the Carney syndrome (multiple myxomas, centrofacial freckling ± Cushing's, acromegaly or Sertoli cell tumour).

Treatment: Excision.

Types of intracardiac mass *Benign tumours* *Malignant* Sarcoma
Thrombus; Vegetation Myxoma; teratoma Mesothelioma
Pericardial cyst; Hydatid Lipoma; neurofibroma Lymphoma

See *OTM* 3e 2472 **1** Cardiomyopathy Assoc^n: 40 The Metro Centre, Tolpits Lane, Watford, Herts WB1 8SB. UK tel. 01923 24997; also 1997 British Heart Foundation Factfile 5/97

Diseases of the pericardium

Pericarditis

Causes: •Infections—viruses (commonest cause, especially *Coxsackie*); TB (often rapid effusion, look for calcification); other bacteria; parasites. •Malignant pericarditis. •Uraemia. •Myocardial infarction (MI). •Dressler's syndrome (occurs about 10 days post-MI, p696). •Trauma. •Radiotherapy. •Connective tissue disease. •Hypothyroidism.

Symptoms: A sharp, constant sternal pain, relieved by sitting forward. It may radiate to the left shoulder, and sometimes down the arm or into the abdomen. It may be worsened by lying on the left, inspiration, coughing, and swallowing.

Signs: Pericardial friction rub may be heard—this is a scratchy, superficial sound heard best at the left sternal edge. Check for signs of tamponade: ↑JVP and pulsus paradoxus.

Tests: ECG: Concave-upwards (saddle-shaped) ST segments in all leads except AVR. Unlike an infarct, there are no reciprocal changes. (This classical pattern is quite rare.)
CXR: Normal unless there is an effusion.

Treatment: Treat the cause. Ibuprofen eg 400mg/8h after food, for pain. Consider steroids in resistant disease.

Pericardial effusion is accumulation of fluid in the pericardial sac, caused by anything that causes pericarditis.

The Patient may present with symptoms of left and right heart failure. If the effusion is so large as to cause the blood pressure to fall, *cardiac tamponade* has occurred (p768). It is characterized by tachycardia, hypotension, peripheral shutdown, pulsus paradoxus (fall of systolic blood pressure of >10mmHg on inspiration), and a high JVP which paradoxically rises with inspiration (Kussmaul's sign). Beck's triad: rising JVP; falling BP; small, quiet heart.

Differential diagnosis: MI and pulmonary embolism. Although tamponade is much less common, it must be remembered in high-risk situations, eg in the days following cardiac surgery.

CXR shows a large globular heart. ECG shows loss of voltages and alternating QRS morphologies (electrical alternans).

Echocardiography is diagnostic, showing an echo-free zone surrounding the heart. The fluid may not be evenly distributed.

Management: Treat causes. If there is tamponade the effusion should be drained urgently. See p769 for method (get help). Send fluid for culture, cytology, and haematocrit. It may be wise to leave a pericardial drain *in situ*.

Constrictive pericarditis is the encasement of the heart within a non-expansile pericardium. Usual cause: TB, but may follow any pericarditis.

The Patient: Signs are mainly of right heart failure with severe ascites, hepatosplenomegaly, JVP↑, rising paradoxically with inspiration, hypotension, pulsus paradoxus and a loud, high-pitched S_3 (pericardial knock). CXR shows a small heart (in 50%) and may show calcification.

Management: This is by surgical excision of the pericardium.

Saddle-shape ST elevation.

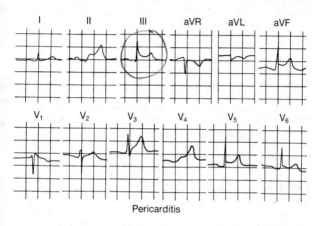

Pericarditis

Atrial septal defects (ASD)

Essence There is a hole connecting the atria. Often they are not detected until they cause symptoms in adult life. Ostium secundum holes (high in the septum) are commonest; ostium primum holes (opposing the endocardial cushions) are associated with AV valve anomalies.

Presentation The majority over 40 years old will have symptoms, namely arrhythmias (especially AF) and cardiac failure. Paradoxical emboli (embolus passing from right to left through the defect) are rare.

Signs There is wide and fixed splitting of S_2. There is a pulmonary ejection systolic murmur (increased flow across the valve). Pulmonary hypertension may cause pulmonary regurgitant murmurs (from pulmonary artery dilatation) or tricuspid regurgitant murmurs (both diastolic). ASDs should be suspected whenever murmurs are best heard in the 2nd intercostal space at the left sternal edge.

Complications Shunt reversal, as above. There is *no* significant increase risk of endocarditis (little turbulence in the low-pressure system).

Tests CXR: pulmonary plethora (peripheral 'pruning' with onset of pulmonary hypertension); globular heart. ECG: right bundle branch block with right (secundum) or left (primum) axis deviation. 2D-echocardiogram with Doppler colour flow. Cardiac catheter: RA O_2 >IVC O_2.

Treatment Best prognosis with operative correction in first 2 decades. Close ASD if physical signs (unless >65 years old, with a small shunt)—or Eisenmenger's syndrome is developing (p366).

Ventricular septal defects

Essence There is a hole connecting the two ventricles. When congenital (the commonest congenital heart defect) this is usually in the membranous part of the septum, rather than the muscular part. Acquired septal rupture occurs after myocardial infarction.

Presentation In adults, this ranges from an incidental finding to advanced pulmonary vascular disease (Eisenmenger's syndrome, p366). AF may occur—and, in some sites, aortic incompetence may be caused.

Signs The characteristic murmur is pansystolic, best heard at the 3rd/4th intercostal space. Small holes give loud murmurs, but are haemodynamically insignificant (*maladie de Roger*). There may be a systolic thrill, ± left parasternal heave. There may be pulmonary hypertension signs (loud P_2; pulmonary diastolic incompetent murmur).

Complications Reversal of shunt if a significant defect is left untreated (Eisenmenger's syndrome, p366); infective endocarditis (at point of maximal turbulence where the jet impinges on the right ventricular wall); ventricular ectopics; ventricular tachycardia.

Associations Down's syndrome; Turner's syndrome; Fallot's tetralogy (VSD, pulmonary stenosis, overriding aorta, and right ventricular hypertrophy—*OHCS* p746).

Investigations CXR: pulmonary plethora. ECG: normal or left axis deviation. 2D-echocardiogram with Doppler colour flow. Cardiac catheter: RV O_2 > vena caval O_2 and right atrial O_2.

Treatment Small defects can close spontaneously, even in adulthood. Otherwise, close if symptomatic, shunt >3:1, or a single attack of endocarditis. Endocarditis prophylaxis is vital for untreated defects (p314).

8. Chest medicine

Relevant pages in other sections:

Symptoms and signs: The respiratory examination (p28); chest deformities (p40); chest pain (p256); clubbing (p42; PLATE 7); cough (p42); cyanosis (p42); dyspnoea (p44); haemoptysis (p48); sputum (p58); stridor (p58).

Others: The chest film (p718); acute severe asthma (p776); pulmonary embolism (p774); pulmonary oedema (p772); acid–base balance (p630); tuberculosis (p198–200); pulse oximetry (p658); sinusitis (*OHCS* p554).

Points on examining the chest

Expansion (on inspiration) of one hemithorax reflects the tidal volume of that lung. *Tracheal position* indicates the position of the upper mediastinum. Increased *tactile vocal fremitus* (TVF, p28), increased *vocal resonance* (VR, p28), *bronchial breathing*, and *whispering pectoriloquy* all imply the presence of consolidation or fibrosis stretching from the chest wall to a large conducting airway. The combination of decreased TVF, decreased VR, and reduced breath sounds indicates that transmission of sound from a large airway to the chest wall is impaired, eg pleural effusion or bronchial occlusion.

Added sounds

Wheezes (= rhonchi) may be monophonic (a single note typically heard in only one part of the chest, signifying a partial obstruction in one airway) or polyphonic, multiple notes generalized throughout the chest (signifying widespread narrowing of airways of differing calibre eg asthma or COPD). In general, the higher the pitch of the wheeze, the narrower the airway it is coming from.

Crackles (= crepitations) Fine and high pitched if coming from distal air spaces (eg pulmonary oedema, fibrosing alveolitis); coarse and low pitched if they originate more proximally (eg bronchiectasis, in which condition the crepitations may be audible at the mouth and in both inspiration and expiration). Crepitations disappearing on coughing are of no significance (and are sometimes called 'rattles'—a non-standard term).

Pleural rubs occur with inflammatory conditions of the pleura eg adjacent pneumonia, pulmonary infarction.

The silent chest may represent severe bronchospasm in the pre-terminal asthmatic (or patients with COPD), with almost no air entering to cause wheezing. By now his P_aCO_2 will be rising. Delay at his peril.

CO_2 retention causes peripheral vasodilation, bounding pulses, flap, confusion, and finally narcosis.

Respiratory distress occurs when high negative intrapleural pressures are needed to generate air entry. It is indicated by nasal flaring, tracheal tug (pulling of thyroid cartilage towards sternal notch in inspiration), the use of accessory muscles of respiration, intercostal, subcostal and sternal recession, and pulsus paradoxus (systolic BP falls in inspiration by >10mmHg).

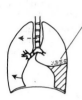

(There may be bronchial breathing at the top of an effusion.)

PLEURAL EFFUSION

Expansion: ↓
Percussion: Stony dull ↓
Air entry: ↓
Vocal resonance: ↓

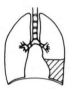

Trachea + mediastium central
Expansion ↓
Percussion note ↓
Vocal resonance ↑
Bronchial breathing ± coarse crackles
(with whispering pectoriloquy)

CONSOLIDATION

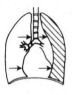

Expansion ↓
Percussion note ↓
Breath sounds ↓

EXTENSIVE COLLAPSE PNEUMONECTOMY /LOBECTOMY

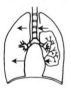

Expansion ↓
Percussion note ↑
Breath sounds ↓

PNEUMOTHORAX

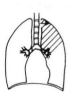

Expansion ↓
Percussion note ↓
Breath sounds bronchial ± crackles

FIBROSIS

Some physical signs

✠ The chest x-ray

Be systematic in your approach to the chest film. (See *Radiology*, p718.)

The heart Normally < ½ the width of the thorax, but may appear smaller in the hyperexpanded chest of COPD. Cardiomegaly and left ventricular failure results in characteristic x-ray appearances (p772, p296).

The mediastinum may be enlarged on a PA CXR in many disorders. A lateral chest film is essential to localize (and helps elucidate) any masses:
- *Superior mediastinum*—thymoma, retrosternal thyroid, paraoesophageal (Zenker's) diverticulum.
- *Anterior and middle mediastinum*—dermoid cyst, teratoma, bronchogenic cyst, pericardial cyst, Morgagni diaphragmatic hernia.
- *Posterior mediastinum*—neurogenic tumours, any paravertebral mass, Bochdalek diaphragmatic hernia, achalasia, hiatus hernia.
- *Any section*—aortic aneurysm, lymph nodes (lymphoma, metastases).

The hila The left should be slightly higher. They can be pulled up or down by fibrosis or collapse (p718), or enlarged by pulmonary arterial hypertension, or lymphadenopathy (eg from TB, sarcoid, lymphoma, or metastases). Hilar calcification suggests TB, silicosis, or histoplasmosis.

The diaphragm The right side is usually slightly higher. An apparently elevated hemidiaphragm may be due to loss of lung volume, phrenic nerve palsy, subpulmonic effusion, subphrenic abscess, hepatomegaly, or diaphragmatic rupture (eg post-traumatic).

Diffuse lung disease produces the most interesting CXRs and often the most difficult to interpret. Try to categorize the pattern into nodular (small or large, equal size, or varying), reticular (a network of thin lines) or alveolar ('fluffy') or often a combination of all three.

Nodular shadows
- Viral pneumonia (varicella)
- Septic emboli
- Granulomas (miliary TB, sarcoidosis, histoplasmosis, hydatid, Wegener's)
- Mitral stenosis (microlithiasis pulmonale due to pulmonary haemosiderosis)
- Malignancy (metastases, lymphangitis carcinomatosis, bronchoalveolar ca)
- Pneumoconioses (except asbestos—linear shadow), Caplan's syndrome

Reticular shadows
- Fibrosis of chronic infections (TB, histoplasmosis)
- Sarcoid, silicosis, asbestosis
- Early LVF
- Malignancy (lymphangitis carcinomatosa)
- Extrinsic allergic alveolitis
- Cryptogenic fibrosing alveolitis
- Autoimmune diseases, eg Wegener's, SLE, PAN, CREST (p670), rheumatoid

Alveolar shadows ('Alveolar filling pattern')
- Pulmonary oedema (p772), haemorrhage (p48) or infection
- Smoke inhalation (p805)
- Drugs (heroin, cytotoxics, p690)
- ARDS (acute respiratory distress syndrome, p350)
- O_2 toxicity
- Fat emboli (suspect this if, on day 3–10 after a fracture there is sudden dyspnoea, fever, confusion, coma, petechial rash, DIC or ARDS).
- DIC (disseminated intravascular coagulation, p598)
- Renal or liver failure (p388 and p504)
- Head injury (p778), or after neurosurgery
- Alveolar proteinosis (p330)
- Near drowning (OHCS p682)
- Heat stroke (p766)

Left upper-lobe collapse

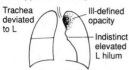

Trachea deviated to L

Ill-defined opacity

Indistinct elevated L hilum

Sharply-defined posterior border due to anterior displacement of oblique fissure

Left lower-lobe collapse

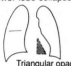

Triangular opacity visible through the heart with loss of medial end of diaphragm

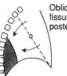

Oblique fissure displaced posteriorly

Lingular consolidation

Indistinct L heart border

Right upper lobe collapse

Trachea deviated to R

Horizontal fissure and R hilum displaced upwards

Triangular opacity with well-defined margins

Right middle lobe collapse

Horizontal fissure displaced down
Ill-defined opacity adjacent to R heart border
Loss of R heart border

Well-defined triangular opacity running from hilum

Right lower-lobe collapse

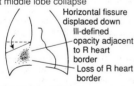

Horizontal fissure displaced downwards

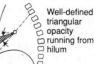

Oblique fissure and hilum displace posteriorly

Well-defined posterior opacity

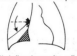

Well-defined opacity adjacent to R heart border (R heart border still visible)

Bedside tests in chest medicine

Arterial blood gas analysis gives information about:

- *Ventilatory efficiency:* P_aCO_2 >6.5kPa diagnoses *hypoventilation*; P_aCO_2 <4.5kPa diagnoses *hyperventilation*. Example: in severe asthma, at first the patient hyperventilates to maintain his P_aO_2—he has a low P_aCO_2. As he tires, he hypoventilates—his P_aCO_2 becomes normal then rises. A normal P_aCO_2 is thus a danger sign in asthma.

- *Oxygenation:* P_aO_2 is principally dependent on the ventilation:perfusion ($\dot{V}/\dot{Q}$) balance which is upset in almost all lung diseases. P_aO_2 is also affected by inspired O_2 concentration (F_iO_2), ventilatory efficiency, and the affinity of blood for O_2. A P_aO_2 <8kPa defines *respiratory failure* (see p352). As a rough estimate, the *alveolar:arterial O_2 concentration gradient* (A–a gradient) = $F_iO_2 - (P_aO_2 + P_aCO_2)$. At 25 years old, the normal range is 0.2–1.5kPa; at 75 years, 1.5–3.0. Larger gradients suggest *impaired gas exchange*. For practical purposes, if the units are kPa, F_iO_2 (partial pressure of inspired oxygen) equals its %: ie 20kPa if breathing air.

- *Acid–base status:* See p630.

See p353 for the clinical scenarios necessitating blood gas measurement.

Sputum examination This involves inspection, microscopy to look for bacteria, particulate matter, and malignant cells, and culture. *Gram stain:* See p183. Bacteria are only likely to be pathogenic if intracellular or present in large numbers. Make sure the sample you send for analysis is sputum, not saliva. Physiotherapists may help with sputum production, sometimes loosening secretions with a hypertonic saline nebulizer.

Spirometry measures functional lung volumes. *Obstructive* spirometry implies that FEV$_1$ (forced expiratory volume in first second) is reduced more than the forced vital capacity. *Causes:* ●Asthma ●COPD ●Tumours. *Restrictive* implies a small FVC—often associated with a normal (~70%) or increased ratio of FEV$_1$:FVC. *Causes of restrictive spirometry:* ●Chest wall problems ●After lung surgery ●Pulmonary oedema/effusion ●Lung fibrosis.

In asthma, *peak flow rate* is closely related to FEV$_1$, and the pattern is obstructive. Peak flow meters are prescribable in the UK, and their use in the home monitoring of asthma is very common—and not entirely straightforward: to persuade patients to monitor themselves when they are well, you can end up encouraging their obsessive traits; and when they are falling ill with asthma, they can abandon the peak flow meter, because it is depressing to do badly at anything. This does not mean that peak flow meters should be discarded, but these issues might usefully be addressed with patients. It is a moot point whether all this puffing saves lives and provides universal benefit.

The disposable end tidal carbon dioxide detector (Easy Cap™) This uses a chemical pH indicator (metacresol) to detect the presence of CO_2 in expired gases. The colour varies from mauve to yellow with inspiration and expiration (respectively). Mauve indicates a CO_2 of <0.5%; tan ≈0.5–2%; yellow ≈2–5%. The device's *cyclical* colour change may be used to distinguish oesophageal from tracheal intubation—except that gastric fluid contamination produces a *permanent* orange colour which may be falsely reassuring. Also, if the patient is being resuscitated with lignocaine (=lidocaine) or adrenaline (=epinephrine) given via an endotracheal tube (p770), a permanent yellow colour occurs. The device does not work if wet, or very cold. After ~2h replacement is needed. It is not reliable when used in cardiopulmonary resuscitation.

Pulse oximetry See p658.

Normal Peak Expiratory Flow Rates

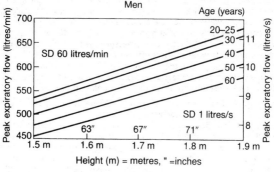

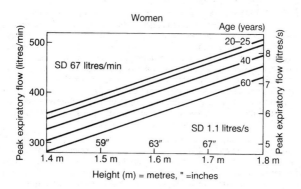

Examples of spirograms

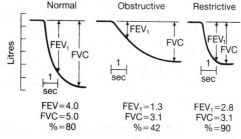

J West 1982; in *Harrison's Principles of Internal Medicine* 11 ed, ed E Brunnward *et al.*, p1055, McGraw-Hill, New York. Reproduced with permission.

Further investigation in chest medicine

Lung function tests FEV₁, FVC, PEFR (see p328). *Total lung capacity* (TLC) and, more so, *residual volume* (RV) are increased in obstruction because of air trapping. Obstruction may be so severe that the spirogram no longer shows the typical pattern. *Flow volume loop* measures peak flows at various lung volumes: flows are most affected at low volumes in distal obstruction (eg asthma) and at high volumes in proximal obstruction (eg trachea). *Transfer factor* (TCO, DLCO) measures gas transfer by assessing carbon monoxide uptake. Abnormalities are nonspecific, but it is a good test of gas exchange in interstitial disease. The effect of *bronchodilators* on obstruction may be assessed: 10% increase in any of FEV₁, FVC, or vital capacity (VC) is useful. Similarly >15–20% increase in FEV₁/FVC.

Fibre-optic (flexible) bronchoscopy is done using topical anaesthesia to the nasopharynx and larynx. The instrument may be introduced via the nostril. It allows examination as far as the subsegmental bronchi. *Uses:* Direct examination of airways; obtaining biopsies, cytological brushings, traps for bacteriology and cytology; bronchoalveolar lavage; removal of foreign bodies. *Preparation for bronchoscopy:* CXR, spirometry, HIV/HBsAg serology (for biopsy: clotting studies, platelets, urea). Blood gases may be needed (bronchoscopy is hazardous in hypoxia; use O₂).

Bronchoalveolar lavage is performed by wedging the tip of the bronchoscope into a subsegmental bronchus, then instilling and aspirating a known volume of buffered saline into the distal airway. It may be diagnostic in *pneumocystis carinii* infections (HIV associated); TB; viral or fungal infections, eg in the immunosuppressed or on ITU; pulmonary haemosiderosis; eosinophilic granuloma and alveolar proteinosis. It may also help differentiate certain interstitial diseases, eg extrinsic allergic alveolitis and sarcoidosis usually produce a highly lymphocytic lavage. It is used therapeutically to wash out secretions. This is the treatment for alveolar proteinosis because its characteristic phospholipid/proteinaceous secretions are too sticky to be expectorated.[1]

Lung biopsy may be obtained in several ways. *Percutaneous needle biopsy* under radiological imaging is useful for discrete peripheral lesions. *Bronchial biopsy* is helpful in diagnosing proximal lesions, usually tumours. *Transbronchial biopsy* at bronchoscopy may help diagnosis of diffuse lung disease such as sarcoidosis. Surgical *open lung biopsy* may be considered.

Surgical procedures *Rigid bronchoscopy* provides a wide lumen, better for controlling haemorrhage, large biopsies, and removal of viscid secretions (eg proteinosis) and foreign bodies. *Mediastinoscopy* allows examination and right hilum biopsy. *Mediastinotomy* allows similar access to the left hilum. *Thoracoscopy* allows examination and biopsy of pleural lesions. *Open lung biopsy* can diagnose and stage interstitial lung disease.

Radiology CXR p326. *Conventional tomography*, for long used to define hilar and other masses, has now been superseded by *computerized tomography* to visualize mediastinum, hilum, pleura and lung parenchyma. *Bronchography* entails instilling radio-opaque material in airways. Patients dislike it, but it may be useful for defining the extent of bronchiectasis if surgery is contemplated—a CT (p736) scan is usually a better option.

---

1 Suspect this rarity in those with an atypical pneumonia (the protein material may harbour nocardia, CMV, candida, mucor, mycobacteria, histoplasma or aspergillus species) whose CXR seems to show pulmonary oedema (alveolar filling pattern), yet in whom there is no sign of cardiac disease (eg no cardiomegaly, and a normal ECG).

Lung volumes: physiological and pathological[1]

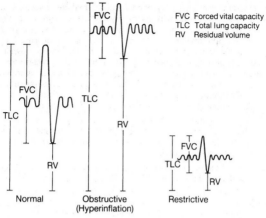

FVC Forced vital capacity
TLC Total lung capacity
RV Residual volume

Flow volume loops[2]

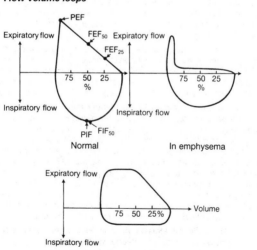

1 After D Flenley 1987 *Med Intl* 1 (20) 240 2 After B Harrison in *Thoracic Medicine* 1981, ed P Emerson, Butterworths, London; and B Harrison 1971 *thorax* 26 579

PEF = peak expiratory flow; FEF_{50} = forced expiratory flow at 50% total lung capacity; FEF_{25} = forced expiratory flow at 25% total lung capacity; PIF = peak inspiratory flow; FIF_{50} = forced inspiratory flow at 50% total lung capacity.

╫ Pheumonia

The Patient *Symptoms:* Dyspnoea, cough, malaise, anorexia, fever, sweats, rigors, pleuritic pain, haemoptysis (less common); confusion (may be the *only* sign in the elderly, in whom you must have a high index of suspicion). Sputum may be scant at first, then green, or 'rusty' (classically in pneumococcal pneumonia). *Signs:* Patient looks unwell and flushed; tachypnoea (a valuable early sign in the elderly); tachycardia; rigors and a high temperature in the young; Herpes labialis (pneumococcal pneumonia); reduced expansion on the affected side; pleural rub; signs of consolidation (dull percussion note, ↑vocal fremitus/resonance, bronchial breathing) or just localized inspiratory crepitations.

Classification guides blind therapy. First classify by source of infection:
1 Community acquired. 2 Nosocomial (>48h after hospital admission).
3 Aspiration (stroke; impaired consciousness; oesophageal disease).
4 Immunocompromised patient.

Now decide if the pneumonia is primary (patient previously well) or secondary (with a predisposing condition). Finally, assess severity (opposite).

Bacteriology *Community-acquired primary:* Streptococcus pneumoniae is the commonest. *Mycoplasma pneumoniae* and other 'atypical' bacteria affect children and young adults almost exclusively (p334). *Secondary:* Staphylococcus aureus, Haemophilus influenzae, Streptococcus pneumoniae, viral and other bacteria cause pneumonia on the back of influenza epidemics. All of these are seen in COPD along with Pseudomonas. *Nosocomial:* Most commonly gram-negative enterobacteria or Staph. aureus but also Pseudomonas; Klebsiella; Bacteroides; Clostridia. *Aspiration:* Anaerobes from the oropharynx. *Immunocompromised:* Pneumocystis carinii; Strep. pneumoniae; H. influenzae; Staph. aureus; Moxarella catarrhalis; Mycoplasma; Gram-negatives.

Differential Pneumonia presenting as above is a fairly clear-cut diagnosis, but pulmonary infarction, pulmonary oedema, bronchial carcinoma and alveolitis (very fine 'velcro' crepitations) may present similarly. Acute pancreatitis and subphrenic abscesses can mimic a lower lobe pneumonia. If fever and cough but no localizing signs consider acute bronchitis.

Tests Aim to confirm diagnosis and identify the organism. CXR; blood gases or pulse oximetry; U&E; FBC (differential WCC); LFTs; blood cultures; sputum culture and microscopy; pleural fluid culture and microscopy serology for atypicals: *Legionella, Mycoplasma, Chlamydia, Coxiella* (send 10mL clotted blood on admission and a convalescent sample 10 days later to demonstrate an antibody rise). If the patient is very ill and is not responding to treatment, microbiological specimens may be obtained by bronchoscopy (bronchial washings) or by percutaneous lung aspiration. In some centres *countercurrent immunoelectrophoresis* (CIE) is done on blood, urine, sputum, or CSF to identify pneumococcal antigen (not affected by antibiotics). Consider also: ECG, cardiac enzymes.

Complications Pleural effusion (if empyema, often loculated); lung abscess; septicaemia; metastatic infections; respiratory failure; jaundice.

Preventing pneumococcal infection Offer pneumococcal vaccine (23-valent Pneumovax II®, 0.5mL SC) to those with: ●Chronic heart or lung conditions ●Cirrhosis ●Nephrosis ●Diabetes mellitus ●Immunosuppression (eg splenectomy, AIDS, or on chemotherapy). CI: pregnancy, lactation, fever. If high risk of fatal pneumococcal infection (asplenia, sickle-cell disease, nephrosis, post-transplant), revaccinate after 6yrs (3–5yrs in children >2yrs old), unless they had a severe vaccine reaction.

Management See pages 336 and 337.

Features of community-acquired pneumonia associated with an increased risk of death[1]

Clinical
- Tachypnoea (respiratory rate $\geq$30/min)
- Hypotension (diastolic <60mmHg)
- Age $\geq$60 years
- Underlying disease
- Confusion
- Atrial fibrillation
- Multilobar involvement

Laboratory
- Serum urea $\geq$7mmol/L
- Serum albumin <35g/L
- Hypoxia P_aO_2 $\leq$8kPa
- Leucopenia <4000 $\times$ 10^9/L
- Leucocytosis >20,000 $\times$ 10^9/L

1 British Thoracic Society, London 1993 *Brit J Hosp Med* **49** 346

'Atypical' and *Pneumocystis* pneumonia

►Suspect this when chest symptoms are slow to resolve or if the CXR is much worse than symptoms. Ask yourself: *Is he immunocompromised?* Remember that identification of the infectious agent responsible for a pneumonia must *not* be allowed to delay blind treatment—therapy can always be changed once serology or culture results come back.

Chlamydia pneumoniae The commonest chlamydial infection.[1] Person-to-person spread occurs (no animal needed) causing a biphasic illness: pharyngitis, hoarseness, otitis, then pneumonia. *Tests:* Serology (nonspecific).[2] *Treatment:* Erythromycin 500mg/6h PO for ~10 days.

Chlamydia psittaci causes psittacosis *via* parrots, poultry, pigeons and sheep. *Incubation:* 4–14 days. *Presentation:* Flu-like illness ± anorexia, lethargy, arthralgia, D&V, headache, pneumonia (rigors, dry cough, crepitations). Extra-pulmonary features are legion but rare, eg SBE/IE, nephritis, meningoencephalitis, and hepatosplenomegaly. CXR: Patchy consolidation. *Diagnosis:* Serology. *Treatment:* Tetracycline 250–500mg/8h PO for 21 days, or erythromycin. Try to remove the source. Relapses occur. (Pigeon fancier's lung, an extrinsic allergic alveolitis, is unconnected.)

Mycoplasma pneumoniae Between epidemics (eg 4-yearly) it is rare. *Incubation:* 12–14 days. *The Patient:* Dry, persistent cough. *Tests:* WCC ↔, bilateral patchy consolidation on CXR; 80% have 4-fold↑ in antibody titre; cold agglutinins suggest recent infection. *Complications:* Haemolytic crises; D&V; skin signs (erythema multiforme, Stevens–Johnson syndrome); arthralgia; myalgia; meningoencephalitis or myelitis; Guillain–Barré. *Treatment:* Erythromycin, eg 500mg/6–12h PO for >1 week. An alternative is tetracycline 250–500mg/8h PO or IV. Relapse is common.

Legionella pneumophila Multiplies in warm, still water, eg the tanks of air-conditioning systems, then are released as an aerosol. *The Patient:* Often just returned from holiday in a hotel abroad. Incubation 2–10 days. ♂:♀ ≈ 3:1. *Symptoms:* Mild flu-like illness or pneumonia with abrupt onset of high fever, shivers, headache and myalgia. Confusion, delirium, nausea, vomiting, diarrhoea, abdominal pain, and bloody PR may precede chest problems. The patient may be very ill. CXR: 90% show consolidation. Neutrophilia and lymphopenia. U&E: Na$^+$↓ and Ca^{2+}↓ are common. Myoglobinuria may be present. *Diagnosis:* Serology or immunofluorescence. *Treatment:* Erythromycin 500mg–1g/6h IVI (1 week) then PO (3 weeks) + rifampicin if severe. *Mortality:* 5–15% in the previously well.

Other causes: TB, influenza (p206), CMV, measles, varicella, *Coxiella burnetii* (Q-fever, p236), aspergillosis (p340), actinomycosis.

Pneumocystis carinii pneumonia (PCP) This variously classed fungus/protozoa causes pneumonia if immunocompromised (eg AIDS, on steroids). *Presentation:* Tachypnoea, exertional dyspnoea, dry cough, respiratory failure (± cyanosis), fever. *Diagnose* from setting, induced sputum, bronchoalveolar lavage, or lung-tissue microscopy. CXR: normal, or diffuse bilateral alveolar shadows, sparing lower zones—or ground-glass appearance. *Treatment:* Trimethoprim (TMP)/sulfamethoxazole (SMX) 2 double-strength (DS) tablets (TMP 160mg/SMX 800mg)/8h PO × 21 days (serum TMP levels 5–8µg/mL, if available). IV dose: 5mg/kg/6h. SE: rash—do not always stop TMP/SMX. Alternative: dapsone 100mg PO/24h + TMP 5mg/kg/6h PO or pentamidine 4mg/kg/day IV over 2h × 21 days. Consider prednisolone if P$_a$O$_2$ <70mmHg: 40mg/12h PO × 5d (start just *before* first dose of TMP/SMX) then daily for 5d, then 20mg/24h for 11d. If history of PCP or CD4 <200 cells/mL, give prophylaxis (1 TMP/SMX DS tab PO daily or thrice-weekly).[3]

1 SJ Bourke 1993 *BMJ* i 1219   2 M Sillis 1993 *BMJ* ii 63   3 J Sanford 1997 *GAT* ISBN 099377530x

Management of pneumonia

- When two or more of 1) Respiratory rate ≥30/min 2) Diastolic <60mmHg 3) Serum urea >7mmol/l are present discuss the patient with your senior cover and consider early transfer to ITU. Other indications for transfer: P_aO_2 <8kPa breathing >60% O_2; P_aCO_2 >6.4kPa; exhausted or unconscious; respiratory or cardiac arrest; shock.
- Antimicrobials: see below and opposite.
- Treat septicaemic shock if present (p766).
- Monitor pulse, BP, temperature and respiratory rate 4-hourly until the patient improves. Monitor oxygen saturation with pulse oximetry.
- Analgesia for pleuritic pain (eg NSAID).
- Fluids (IV if necessary) to rectify dehydration and maintain an adequate urine output (>1.5 litres/24h). Losses are increased in febrile patients but free water clearance is impaired, so beware of overhydration.
- Oxygen to keep P_aO_2 >8kPa but take care in COPD (see p348).
- Physiotherapy is not helpful unless there are copious secretions.

Antimicrobials: general points
- If the patient is very ill, take blood cultures then start 'blind' therapy immediately. Do *not* wait for culture results or advice from seniors.
- Use IV therapy in very ill patients, in those who can't swallow, and those who may not properly absorb oral antibiotics.
- If mild and uncomplicated, treat for at least 5 days but longer if needed. Treat atypical pneumonias for longer (p334).
- If in doubt about the sensitivities of local pathogens, prescribing policies, or the significance of an equivocal culture growth, take advice from your local microbiologist.

Choice of blind therapy depends upon 1) The source of the infection (community-acquired; nosocomial; aspiration; immunocompromised patient); 2) The severity of the infection; 3) The likely pathogen; 4) Antibiotic sensitivities of local pathogens.

Lung abscess

Lung abscesses are cavitating areas of localized, suppurative infection within the lung associated with necrosis of parenchyma.

Causes 1) Inadequately treated pneumonia (especially *Staph*, *Klebsiella*). 2) Aspiration eg alcoholism, bulbar palsy, achalasia, oesophageal obstruction. Affects the right lung most often. 3) Bronchial obstruction (tumour, foreign body) causing pooling of lung secretions behind the obstruction which becomes infected. 4) Pulmonary infarction. 5) Septic emboli (subacute bacterial endocarditis, septicaemia, IV drug abuse). Usually multiple. 6) Spread of a subphrenic or hepatic abscess.

The Patient *Symptoms:* Swinging fever; cough, often with plentiful bloodstained, foul-smelling, purulent sputum; pleuritic chest pain; haemoptysis; malaise; ↓weight. *Signs:* Clubbing (PLATE 7); anaemia; localized crepitations; empyema develops in 20–30%.

Tests CXR: Walled cavity often with a fluid level (different place on decubitus film). *Blood tests:* Cultures; Hb↓; ESR ↑. Sputum culture (include mycobacteria, fungi, and anaerobes). If lesion on CXR is not in the apical segment of the lower lobe or the posterior segment of the upper R lobe (suggestive of aspiration) then do bronchoscopy to exclude obstruction.

Treatment Antibiotics as indicated by sensitivities. In aspiration, anaerobes dominate, so start benzylpenicillin 2–3mu/6h until there is clinical improvement when oral therapy can be started. Continue for 4–6 weeks. Postural drainage helps clear the pus. Surgery is rarely necessary.

Empirical treatment for pneumonia

Setting	Organisms	Empiric antibiotics
Normal immunity *Community-acquired*		
• Out-patient	Strep pneumoniae Mycoplasma pneumoniae Chlamydiae pneumoniae Haemophilus influenzae Legionella pneumophila	Erythromycin 500mg/6h PO *or* Azithromycin or clarithromycin; consider adding co-amoxiclav or 2nd/3rd generation cefalosporin (p178) if severe or co-morbid illness.
• In-patient, if very ill	Same as above	Erythromycin ½–1g/6h IV *plus* 2nd/3rd generation IV cefalosporin, eg cefuroxime 1.5g/8h; ceftriaxone 2g/day
Impaired host defences		
•COPD	Strep pneumoniae, H influenza, Moraxella catarrhalis	Amoxicillin 250–500mg/8h PO *or* Doxycycline 100mg/12h PO
•Post-influenza	Strep pneumoniae, H influenzae, Staph aureus	Amoxcillin/clavulanic acid PO or cefuroxime
•Aspiration	Strep pneumoniae, Anaerobes (Bacteroides sp. peptostreptococci, fusobacterium)	Clindamycin 450–900mg/8h IV *or* Cefoxitin 2g/8h IV
•Nosocomial	Gram negative bacilli, Enterococci, Legionella, Staph aureus	*2nd/3rd gen. cefalosporin IV *or* Antipseudomonal penicillin IV + antipseudomonal aminoglycoside (eg mezlocillin 4g/6h)+gentamicin (p750)
•Neutropenic	Gram positive cocci, Gram negative bacilli, Aspergillus species	Antipseudomonal penicillin or 3rd generation cefalosporin *plus* Antipseudomonal aminoglycoside For fungal infection, see p244
•Severe/sepsis	Strep pneumoniae, Staph aureus, Gram negative bacilli,*	*Vancomycin 1g/12h IV or ticarcillin + co-amoxiclav + 3rd generation cefalosporin

*If Legionella is possible add erythromycin 500–1000mg/6h IV.

1 J Bartlett 1995 NEJM 333 1618

Bronchiectasis

►Consider this in any recurrent or persistent chest infection.

Pathology Irreversibly dilated bronchi act as sumps for persistently infected mucus which is expectorated daily. *H influenzae* and *Strep pneumoniae* are commonest agents but *Pseudomonas aeruginosa* is also seen.

Causes *Congenital:* Cystic fibrosis, Kartagener's syndrome (bronchiectasis, sinusitis, dextrocardia). *Post-infection:* TB, measles, pertussis, pneumonia. *Other:* Bronchial obstruction, allergic bronchopulmonary aspergillosis, (ABPA, p340), hypogammaglobulinaemia, gastric aspiration.

The Patient Asymptomatic with winter exacerbations (fever, cough, purulent sputum, pleuritic chest pain, dyspnoea) or if more severe, persistent cough and sputum; haemoptysis, clubbing, low-pitched 'leathery' inspiratory *and* expiratory crackles (eg audible at mouth), and wheeze.

Tests CXR: cystic shadows, fluid levels, thickened bronchial walls (tramline and ring shadows), collapse; CT to assess extent of disease (bronchography used to be done); sputum culture; spirometry (lung damage, reversible airway obstruction); serum immunoglobulins; CF sweat test; skin-prick test for aspergillus; bronchoscopy if suspected obstruction.

Management 1 Physiotherapy—twice-daily postural drainage.
2 Antibiotics—short courses for intermittent exacerbations (eg doxycycline 200mg PO on day 1, then 100mg/24h for 7–14 days; or 5 days of high-dose amoxicillin 3g/12h); prophylaxis if frequent recurrence; continuous therapy if persistently infected (given PO, IV or by nebulizer).
3 Bronchodilators, for reversible airway obstruction.
4 Surgical excision (for localized disease) is rarely needed.

Complications Haemoptysis (can be life-threatening); respiratory failure; cor pulmonale; pneumothorax; brain abscess; amyloidosis.

Cystic fibrosis (CF)   See OHCS (Paediatrics, p192)

One of the commonest autosomal recessive diseases (~1 in 2500). Caused by mutation of the cystic fibrosis transmembrane conductance regulator gene (CFTR) on chromosome 7 rendering cells relatively impermeable to chloride. Secretions are high in salt and low in water making them viscid and likely to clog mucosal surfaces and block glands.

The Patient *As a neonate:* Meconium ileus can occur. *As a child or young adult:* Recurrent chest infections, bronchiectasis, pancreatic insufficiency (steatorrhoea, failure to thrive, good appetite), DM, distal intestinal obstruction syndrome (meconium ileus equivalent). Fertility problems.

Tests CXR: shadowing suggesting bronchiectasis, especially in upper lobes. Malabsorption screen. Glucose tolerance test. Spirometry. Sputum culture. Skin test for *Aspergillus* (20% develop allergic bronchopulmonary aspergillosis—p340). ►Sweat Na^+ or chloride >70mmol/l on 2 occasions.

Management 1 *Immunize* (measles, influenza, pneumococcus, p332).
2 *High calorie diet with pancreatic enzyme and vitamin supplements* (A, D, E, K).
3 *Chest management:* as for bronchiectasis, with appropriate antibiotics (*Staph* is commonest in children, *Pseudomonas* species in adults, OHCS p192).
4 *?Heart–lung transplantation* (5yr survival ~50%). *The future:* Trials of recombinant human DNase-I have shown it ↓sputum viscosity, improving lung function in the short-term. Gene transfer using adenovirus or liposome vectors to introduce the normal gene into respiratory mucosa (nasal) has been demonstrated but thus far no benefit has been shown.

Prognosis Improving. Median survival 30 years, 75% adult sufferers are active and employed. Permanent colonization by Pseudomonas is a poor prognostic indicator. Genetics and prenatal tests: OHCS p192.

Fungi and the lung

Aspergillus fungi These affect the lung in 4 ways: *mycetomas; pneumonia* in the immunocompromised; as an atopic (type I) phenomenon in *asthma*; or as *allergic bronchopulmonary aspergillosis* (a type III reaction).

Mycetoma (Aspergilloma): A tangled mass of hyphae, fibrin, and inflammatory cells, which accumulates in a lung cavity, often after TB. Usually asymptomatic, it may cause cough and haemoptysis (which may be torrential)—but lung invasion is rare. CXR: round opacity, usually in the upper zone, surmounted by a thin dome of air. Organisms may be cultured from sputum, and *Aspergillus* precipitins are present in high titre. Treatment is only required for symptoms (usually severe haemoptysis) and surgical excision is the most effective, although mortality is high because most patients have poor lung function. Local instillation of antifungal drugs (via a CT-guided catheter) often yields at least partial success in carefully selected patients—eg in partly controlling massive haemoptysis.[1] The systemic route is also problematic.

Allergic bronchopulmonary aspergillosis (ABPA): This results from an allergic reaction to *Aspergillus fumigatus.* Early on, the allergic response causes bronchoconstriction, but as the inflammation persists, permanent damage occurs, causing bronchiectasis (classically proximal). The clinical picture is of wheeze, cough (productive of plugs of mucus), dyspnoea, and 'recurrent pneumonia'. ABPA should be suspected in asthmatics who have transient shadows on CXR and eosinophilia. The shadowing may be permanent and proximal bronchiectasis is seen. A positive skin-prick test confirms hypersensitivity. Serum precipitins are present but rarely in high titre. Serum IgE is raised, as is the peripheral eosinophil count. It is almost impossible to eradicate the fungus, so prednisolone 30–45mg per 24h PO is given to reduce inflammation until clinically and radiographically clear. Some maintain patients on prednisolone 20mg on alternate days. Sometimes bronchoscopic aspiration of mucus plugs is needed.

Invasive aspergillosis: This only occurs in the immunocompromised, and should be considered in the differential diagnosis of any focal infection or septicaemia in such a patient. Diagnosis may only be made at biopsy—or autopsy. Treat with amphotericin B.

Using amphotericin B: First give a test dose, 1mg in 20mL 5% dextrose IV. If there is no reaction, give 0.3mg/kg IV over 6h on day 1 in ~50mL of 5% dextrose (at pH >4.2—check the pH of the dextrose). Then increase by 0.1–0.2mg/kg increments per day until 1mg/kg/24h (given over 6h at a concentration of 10mg/100mL; max dose: 1.5mg/kg/24h).

Do not give any other drug in the same IVI. SE: anaphylaxis, arrhythmias, seizures (all after rapid infusion). Nephrotoxicity (common), vomiting, phlebitis, hypokalaemia, anaemia, fevers, and weight loss. Monitor K^+ and renal function daily. Ambisome® is liposomal amphotericin (less nephrotoxic, fewer side-effects, much more expensive; dose example:[2] start with 1mg/kg/day IVI over 1h, increase by 1mg/kg/day up to 3mg/kg/day or more. Ambisome® may be reserved for those intolerant of conventional amphotericin).

1 CA Kauffman 1996 *Lancet* 347 1640   2 *Drug Ther Bul* 1993 31 93

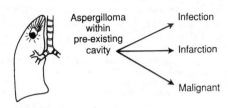

Aspergilloma within pre-existing cavity

→ Infection

→ Infarction

→ Malignant

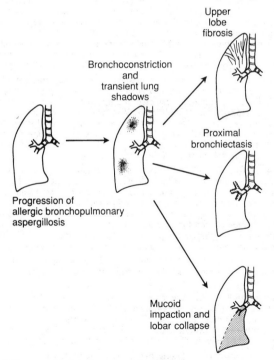

Progression of allergic bronchopulmonary aspergillosis

Bronchoconstriction and transient lung shadows

Upper lobe fibrosis

Proximal bronchiectasis

Mucoid impaction and lobar collapse

After PJ Kumar and ML Clark 1990 *Clinical Medicine* 2 ed, p688, Baillière Tindall

Lung malignancy

Bronchial carcinoma ≈19% of all cancers and 27% of cancer deaths. Incidence is increasing. The major risk factor is cigarette smoking:[1]

Cigarettes/day	0	1–14	5–24	≥25
Male deaths/yr/1000	0.07	0.78	1.27	2.51

Other risk factors: Age, ♂ sex, asbestos, radiation, chromium, iron, iron oxides. Chronic inflammation predisposes to alveolar cell carcinoma.

Histology 4 types: squamous (35% of cases); adenocarcinoma (20%); large cell (19%); small (oat) cell (25%). Figures depend on the smoking history of the population. Adenocarcinomas are *not* smoking related.

The Patient *Symptoms:* Cough 80%; haemoptysis 70%; dyspnoea 60%; chest pain (often mild) 40%; wheeze 15%; recurrent or slow to resolve pneumoni; weight↓. *Signs:* Clubbing (PLATE 7); supraclavicular nodes; monophonic wheeze; stridor; rib or back tenderness; signs of complications.

Complications *Intrathoracic:* Pleural effusion; recurrent laryngeal or phrenic nerve palsies; SVC obstruction; brachial neuritis and Horner's syndrome (Pancoast's tumour); rib erosion; pericarditis; AF. *Metastases:* Brain, bone, liver, adrenals. *Non-metastatic: Ectopic secretion:* SIADH (↓Na⁺); ACTH; PTH (↑Ca²⁺). Less commonly: β-HCG (*OHCS* p78); erythropoietin; β-endorphin; glucagon. *Neurological:* Neuropathy; myelopathy; (dermato-)myositis; encephalopathies including cerebellar degeneration; Eaton–Lambert myasthenic syn (p472). *Other:* ↓Weight; anaemia; thrombophlebitis migrans; bleeding disorders; hypertrophic pulmonary osteoarthropathy (painful, swollen wrists and ankles; x-ray shows onion-skin appearance at ends of long bones. Always with clubbing).

Tests CXR   : Masses; mediastinal lymphadenopathy; consolidation; pleural effusion. *Histology:* Bronchoscopy allows biopsy/brushings of 80%. Peripheral lesions are sampled by percutaneous fine needle aspiration or biopsy, as are lymph nodes. Aspirate pleural effusions and do cytology. *Are there metastases?* CT thorax. If there is mediastinal lymphadenopathy and surgery is indicated, do mediastinoscopy or mediastinotomy to confirm nodes are malignant. Do an isotope bone scan if bone pain or ↑alk phos. Abdominal CT may be helpful.

Treatment *Non-small-cell tumours:* If no metastatic or pleural spread (~25%) consider excision. Radical radiotherapy is an option in the inoperable. *Small-cell tumours* are almost always disseminated and rarely operable. Chemotherapy (eg doxorubicin + cyclophosphamide + etoposide) may extend life by ~4 months. *Palliation:* Most patients. Radiotherapy is used for bronchial obstruction, SVC obstruction, bony pain, or distressing haemoptysis. Methadone linctus 2mg/4h helps cough. Drain symptomatic effusions and consider pleurodesis.

Prognosis *Non-small cell:* 50% 2-yr survival without spread, 10% with spread. *Small cell:* Median survival: 3 months untreated; 1–1½yrs if treated.

Other tumours *Bronchial adenoma:* Mostly carcinoid; slow-growing, metastasize late; often operable. *Mesothelioma:* Arises in the pleura. If malignant there is usually a remote history of asbestos exposure but the relationship is complex.[2,3] *Signs:* Chest pain, dyspnoea, bloody effusion. Diagnosis needs pleural biopsy (eg thoracoscopic). Prognosis is very poor (~2yrs; >650 deaths/year in the UK). Treatment is symptomatic.

Stopping smoking ►You *can* help people quit; most smokers want to, and it *does* pay: former smokers of <20 cigarettes/day take 13y to reach risk of non-smokers. *Practical help: OHCS* p452. Smokers dying aged 35–69yrs don't just miss a few years' life: *a quarter of a century is more likely.*[1]

1 R Doll 1994 BMJ ii 901,1976 BMJ ii 1525 2 T Eisen 1995 *Lancet* 345 1285 3 R Damhuis 1995 *Lancet* 345 1233

Coin lesions of the lung

Malignancy (1° or 2°)	Arteriovenous malformation
Abscesses (p334)	Encysted effusion (fluid, blood, pus)
Granuloma	Cyst
Carcinoid tumour	Foreign body
Pulmonary hamartoma	Skin tumour (eg seborrhoeic wart)

TNM staging for lung cancer

Primary tumour (**T**)	TX	Malignant cells in bronchial secretions, no other evidence of tumour
	Tis	Carcinoma *in situ*
	T0	None evident
	T1	≤3cm, in lobar or more distal airway
	T2	>3cm, and >2cm distal to carina *or* any size if pleural involvement *or* obstructive pneumonitis extending to hilum, but not all the lung.
	T3	Involves the chest wall, diaphragm, mediastinal pleura, pericardium or <2cm from, but not at, carina
	T4	Involves the mediastinum, heart, great vessels, trachea, oesophagus, vertebral body, carina, *or* a malignant effusion is present
Regional nodes (**N**)	N0	None involved (after mediastinoscopy)
	N1	Peribronchial and/or ipsilateral hilum
	N2	Ipsilateral mediastinum or subcarinal
	N3	Contralateral mediastinum or hilum, scalene, or supraclavicular
Distant metastasis (**M**)	M0	None
	M1	Distant metastases present

Stage	Tumour	Lymph nodes	Metastasis
Occult	TX	N0	M0
I	Tis, T1 or T2	N0	M0
II	T1 or T2	N1	M0
IIIa	T3	N0 or N1	M0
	T1–T3	N2	M0
IIIb	T1–T3	N3	M0
	T4	N0–N3	M0
IV	T1–T4	N0–N3	M1

┼┼┼ Bronchial asthma

►Respect asthma: *people still die from it.* See p776 for emergency treatment.
In asthma, there is widespread airways obstruction, which, in the early stages
at least, is episodic and reversible. The 3 factors which narrow airways:

• *Mucosal swelling/inflammation* caused, in part, by mast cell and basophil
degranulation, releasing prostaglandins, cysteinyl leukotrienes,[1] histamine, ±
other inflammatory mediators (responds to steroids and antileukotrienes)
• ↑*Mucus formation* •*Bronchial muscle contraction* (responds to β_2-agonists).

Prevalence Up to 8% of people are episodic wheezers in some populations and the condition was probably under-recognized in the past.

Symptoms Intermittent wheeze, dyspnoea or cough (eg at night; this
may be the *only* symptom). In your history ask specifically about:
• *Disturbed sleep:* Quantify as nights/week—a sign of serious asthma.
• *Exercise:* Quantify the distance to breathlessness.
• *Days per week off work or school.*
• *Diurnal variation* in symptoms or peak flow (if measured). Marked
morning dipping of peak flow is common and can tip the patient over
into a serious attack, despite having normal peak flow at other times.
• *Precipitants:* Emotion, exercise, infection (often rhinovirus or coron-
avirus URTI), allergens, drugs eg NSAIDs/aspirin, β-blockers, cold air.
• *Other atopic disease:* Eczema, hay fever, allergy himself or in the family?
• *Acid reflux:* This has a known association with asthma.[2]
• *Occupation:* If symptoms remit at weekends or holidays something at
work may be a trigger. Ask the patient to measure his peak flow at
work and at home (at the same time of day) to confirm this.
• *The home (especially the bedroom):* Pets? (are they allowed in the bedroom?) carpet? (if you dare, ask how often it is vacuumed) feather
duvets? floor cushions and other 'soft furnishings'?

Signs: Widespread polyphonic, high-pitched wheezes (airways of varying
size—chiefly small calibre). Chronic asthma may give a 'barrel chest' with
indrawn costal margins (Harrison's sulci). ►Life-threatening signs: p776.

Tests *Chronic asthma:* Teach self-monitoring with a peak flow meter
(p348). CXR: hyperinflation (>6 ribs visible above each hemidiaphragm);
spirometry (↓FEV$_1$/FVC); residual volume (↑suggests air trapping). Test for
aspergillus (serology). Skin prick tests can help identify allergies but rarely
alter management. *Acute:* Investigations aim to assess severity, identify precipitants, eg infection; rule out complications, eg pneumothorax.

Differential diagnosis Pulmonary oedema ('cardiac asthma': crepitations need not be audible); COPD (often co-exists or has a reversible
component); large airway obstruction (may cause stridor) eg foreign
body; tumour; SVC obstruction; pneumothorax; pulmonary embolism;
bronchiectasis; obliterative bronchiolitis. Clearly this differential must
be considered carefully in the elderly presenting with possible asthma.

Natural history Most childhood asthmatics (described in OHCS p270)
either grow out of asthma in adolescence, or suffer much less as adults.
A significant number of people develop chronic asthma late in life.
Mortality: Death certificates give a figure of 2000/year (UK): more careful surveys more than halve this figure.◨ 50% are >65 years old.

Treatment See p346. Emergency treatment of severe asthma: p776.

---

1 This is the reason behind giving antileukotrienes (only recently available, eg montelukast 10mg PO
at night—a selective CysLT$_1$ receptor antagonist) but they seem less effective than steroids; although
they are of use in some patients, and seem to have fewer SEs: their exact rôle has yet to be defined.
2 Other associations: PAN; Churg-Strauss syndrome (p674); bronchopulmonary aspergillosis (ABPA, p340).

Examples of serial peak flow charts

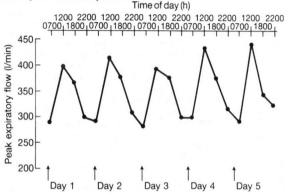

Classical diurnal variation of asthma
Arrows point to morning 'dips'

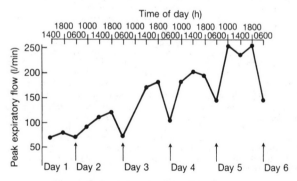

Recovery from severe attack of asthma
Predicted PEFR was 320 l/min
Arrows point to early morning 'dips'

After B Harrison 1981 *Thoracic Medicine*, ed P Emerson, Butterworths, London

✛✛✛ Management of bronchial asthma[1]

▶*Full symptom control* is the aim. Rarely be satisfied with less.

Behaviour Stop smoking and avoid *relevant* allergens. Educate patients to manage their disease using written self-management plans enabling the patient to alter medication in response to changes in symptoms or peak flows. Include specific advice about what to do in an emergency. ▶Avoid all β-blockers and NSAIDs: they can worsen asthma.

British Thoracic Society guidelines[1] Check inhaler technique; address the patient's fears; prescribe a peak flow meter and monitor the response to treatment. Start at the step most appropriate to severity; moving up if needed, or down if control is good for >3 months. Rescue courses of oral prednisolone may be needed (and given) at any time.

Step 1: Occasional short-acting inhaled β-agonist as needed for symptom relief. If used > once daily and inhaler technique is good, go to step 2.

Step 2: Add inhaled beclomethasone* or budesonide 100–400µg/12h or fluticasone 50–200µg/12h. Nedocromil sodium or cromoglicate can be tried first but if they don't control symptoms change to inhaled steroids.

Step 3: ↑Inhaled beclomethasone*/budesonide to 800–2000µg/24h or ↑fluticasone to 400–1000µg/24h by large volume spacer. Alternatively, try salmeterol 50µg/12h plus 100–400µg/12h beclomethasone*/budesonide or 50–200µg/12h fluticasone. Add slow-release theophylline, eg 250mg/12h PO to step 2 if problems with steroid doses (rare).

Step 4: Add one of: inhaled long-acting β-agonists, slow-release theophylline, inhaled ipratropium, long-acting β-agonist tablets, high-dose inhaled bronchodilators, cromoglicate, nedocromil (in order) to step 3.

Step 5: Check compliance; add regular oral prednisolone (1 daily dose).

Drugs *β₂ adrenoreceptor agonists* relax bronchial smooth muscle, acting within minutes. Salbutamol is best given by inhalation (aerosol, powder, nebulizer), but may also be given PO or IV. SE: tachyarrhythmias, ↓K⁺, tremor, anxiety. Salmeterol is a long-acting inhaled β₂ agonist that can help nocturnal symptoms and and reduce morning dips.[2] It is an alternative to ↑steroid dose when symptoms are uncontrolled.[2] SE: *paradoxical bronchospasm, tolerance, arrhythmias.*

Corticosteroids are best inhaled, eg beclomethasone* spacer (or powder), but may be given PO or IV. They act over days to ↓bronchial mucosal inflammation. The patient should gargle after inhaled steroids to prevent oral candidiasis. Oral steroids are used acutely (high-dose, short courses, eg prednisolone 30–40mg/24h PO for 7 days) and longer-term in lower dose (eg 7.5mg/24h) if control is not optimal on inhalers.

Aminophylline (metabolized to theophylline) may act by inhibiting phosphodiesterase, thus ↓bronchoconstriction. It is given PO as a prophylactic agent at night to prevent morning dipping. It is also useful as an adjunct if inhaled therapy is inadequate. In acute severe asthma, it may be given IVI. It has a narrow therapeutic ratio, causing arrhythmias, GI upset and fits in the toxic range. Check theophylline levels (p751), and do ECG monitoring if IV therapy is used. *Antileukotrienes:* See p344.

Anticholinergics (eg ipratropium) may ↓muscle spasm synergistically with β₂ agonists. They may be of more benefit in COPD than in asthma. Try each alone, and then together; assess with spirometry.

Cromoglicate May be used as prophylaxis in mild and exercise-induced asthma (always inhaled), especially in children. It may precipitate asthma.

Pitfalls ●Failure to prescribe steroids soon enough.
●Failure to notice severe morning dips in peak flow. Always ask about nocturnal waking: it is a sign of dangerous asthma.
●Failure to admit those with moderately severe attacks to hospital.

1 BTS Guidelines *Thorax* 1997 **52** S1 11 2 *Drug Ther Bul* 1997 **35** 1 *New name: beclometasone

Doses of some inhaled drugs used in bronchoconstriction

	Inhaled aerosol	Inhaled powder	Nebulized *(under close supervision)*
Salbutamol			
single dose	100µg or 200µg	100µg or	1mg/mL or 5mg/mL
recommended regimen	200µg/6h	400µg/6h	2.5–5mg/6h
Terbutaline			
single dose	250µg	500µg*	2.5mg/mL
recommended regimen	≤500µg/4h	500µg/6h	5–10mg/6–12h
Salmeterol			
single dose	25µg	50µg	–
recommended regimen	50–100µg/12h	50–100µg/12h	–
Ipratropium bromide			
single dose	18µg or 36µg	–	250µg/mL
recommended regimen	18–72µg/6h	–	100–500µg/6h
Beclomethasone (=beclometasone)			
Becotide®			
single dose	–	100µg or 200µg	50µg/mL
recommended regimen	–	200µg/6–8h up to 800µg/12h	100µg/12h
Becotide 50®			
single dose	50µg	–	–
recommended regimen	100µg/6–8h or 200µg/12h		
Becotide 100®			
single dose	100µg	–	–
recommended regimen	100µg/6–8h or 200µg/12h		
Becloforte®			
single dose	250µg		
recommended regimen	250µg/6h or 250–1000µg/12h 500µg/12h**		

*as Turbohaler®—which is easier to use than the comparable form of salbutamol (Diskhaler®).

**Max dose: 1500–2000µg/day—when significant systemic absorption occurs, and the patient should carry a steroid card.[1] Note: systemic absorption (via the throat) is minimized if inhalation is through a large-volume device, eg Volumatic® or Integra® (for Becloforte®) devices. The latter is more compact. Static charge on some devices reduces dose delivery, so wash in water before doses. It is pointless to squirt many puffs into the device: it is best to repeat single doses—and be sure to inhale *as soon as the drug is in the spacer* (BMJ 1997 i 1061). SE: local (oral) candidiasis (p500); ↑rate of cataract if lifetime dose ≥2g beclomethasone (EBM 1998 3 24).

1 *Drug Ther Bul* 1990 **28** 45 Inhalers used to use fluorocarbons as propellants, but manufacturers are switching to other agents to protect the ozone layer. Patients need to know that their inhalers may taste different, and that they will not have been harmed by the fluorocarbons.

348

Essence COPD includes the spectrum of chronic bronchitis and emphysema. *Chronic bronchitis* is defined *clinically* as sputum production on most days for 3 months of 2 successive years. It may cause obstruction by narrowing the airway lumen with mucosal thickening and excess mucus. *Emphysema* (defined *histologically*) is the dilation of the air spaces by destruction of their walls. It causes obstruction by decreasing the lungs' elastic recoil, which normally holds the airways open in expiration. The two co-exist in varying proportions in COPD.
Causes: smoking, α_1-antitrypsin deficiency (p650).

Symptoms Cough, sputum, dyspnoea, and wheeze. **Signs** Hyperinflation, descended trachea (decreased distance between thyroid cartilage and sternal notch), prolonged expiratory phase, respiratory distress (p324), quiet breath sounds (quietest over bullae), wheezes, cyanosis, and cor pulmonale (p366). (If haemoptysis or clubbing, consider malignancy.)

Pink puffers and **blue bloaters** Some patients with COPD have ↑alveolar ventilation, and normal or low P_aCO_2 and a near normal P_aO_2. They are breathless but not cyanosed, ie 'pink puffers'. They may progress to type I respiratory failure (p352). Other COPD patients have ↓alveolar ventilation, with a high P_aCO_2 and low P_aO_2. They are cyanotic, and if cor pulmonale develops (p366), become 'blue and bloated', ie cyanosed but not breathless. Their respiratory centres are relatively insensitive to CO_2 and they rely on their hypoxic drive to maintain respiratory effort. It is dangerous to give these patients supplemental oxygen without careful observation, as hypoventilation or apnoea may result. These extremes are ends of a spectrum; most patients fall in between.

Tests—*CXR*: Hyperinflation (>6 anterior ribs seen above diaphragm in mid-clavicular line), flat hemidiaphragms, large central pulmonary arteries but reduced peripheral vascular markings, bullae.
Lung function tests: Obstruction with air trapping (FEV_1/ FVC ≪70%); RV (residual volume) and TLC (total lung capacity)↑; DLCO (p330) ↓in emphysema (unlike asthma). FBC: Secondary polycythaemia.

Acute exacerbations Look for dyspnoea + features dependent on cause:
●Infection   ●Left ventricular failure   ●Inspissated secretions & collapse
●Sedatives   ●Pulmonary embolism   ●Pneumothorax
Management: Take blood for: FBC, U&E, arterial blood gas (ABG) + culture if pyrexial. Give O_2 (according to ABG, p352; start at 28%) and nebulized salbutamol 2.5mg and ipratropium 500μg. Consider a cardiac monitor. Give ~20mg prednisolone (40mg if already on steroids), and hydrocortisone 100mg IV if very unwell, unless known not to be steroid-responsive. Start physiotherapy and antibiotics (p332). If the patient is *beginning* to tire and pH <7.35, consider *non-invasive* intermittent positive pressure ventilation (NIPPV, via nasal or full face mask, + flow generator). This reduces deaths and hospital stay.[1] Finally, consider ventilation on ITU. Liaise with GP prior to discharge regarding smoking, pneumococcal and annual flu vaccinations (p332), and reducing steroids. Consider a spare supply of antibiotics to pre-empt emergencies. *Long-term plan* to include:
●Spirometry (p328). ●?Domiciliary O_2, eg for non-smokers if resting P_aO_2 <7.3kPa, FEV_1 <1.5L, and FVC <2L. O_2 concentrators are prescribable by UK GPs. If P_aO_2 maintained ≥8.0kPa for ≥15h a day, mortality falls by 50%.
●Aim for maximal bronchodilation with drugs (p347).
Complications: Pulmonary hypertension and polycythaemia (p366).

Dying horribly with respiratory failure: This is all too common an occurrence—and because COPD is not a cancer, the well-known principles of palliation do not come to mind, but are *just* as relevant.

1 DR Baldwin 1997 *BMJ* i 163

Self-administration of inhaled drugs

This is the cornerstone of therapy for asthma and COPD. Many find it difficult, eg because they are badly taught.

Shake the inhaler (to mix drug with propellant). The patient should exhale fully. Then, putting the mouthpiece between his teeth, press the canister once just *after* beginning to inhale through the mouth. He should hold his breath in inspiration for 10 seconds if possible. If the patient cannot master the technique, alternatives include: a 'spacer' (which is first filled from the canister with the aerosolized bronchodilator and the breath is then taken from it); several breath-activated devices for inhaled powders eg Rotahaler®; the breath-activated aerosol inhaler (avoiding the need to coordinate breathing and hand movements); and the nebulizer in which an aqueous solution of the drug is mixed with saline and aerosolized by passing air through it from an air compressor.

►*Always assess your patient's inhaler technique.* Omitting to do so may be as effective as forgetting to write the prescription.

Advise taking a bronchodilator several minutes before an inhaled steroid so that the steroid may have greater access to the airways.

British Thoracic Society 1997 Guidelines for severe but stable COPD

- Severe COPD means FEV_1 <40% of predicted and breathless at rest.
- Give regular short-acting inhaled β_2-agonists (eg salbutamol, p347) *and* anticholinergics (eg ipratropium bromide, p347).
- Trial of steroids: prednisolone 30mg/24h PO for 2 weeks, assessing change in FEV_1 (+ve test if it rises by >200mL *and* is >15% above baseline). If +ve, give steroids (via an inhaler or as tablets), monitoring response.
- Nebulizers should only be advised after specialist assessment.
- If symptoms fail to respond, oral theophyllines may have a rôle.
- Give antibiotics (p337) if ↑sputum volume, or it becomes purulent.
- Long-term O_2 therapy if P_aO_2 <7.3kPa and FEV_1 <1.5L.
- Only give long-acting bronchodilators (eg salmeterol p346–7) if there is objective evidence of improvement.
- Life-style advice: *no smoking; do regular exercise;* ↓*obesity; treat depression.*
- Prevention: *pneumococcal vaccination* and *annual 'flu vaccinations.*
- When to refer: severe COPD; at onset of cor pulmonale; <40yrs old (α_1-antitrypsin↓, p650); lung bullae; rapid ↓in FEV_1; diagnostic doubt.

1 *Thorax* 1997 52 (suppl 5 1–32) NB: *mild COPD* = FEV_1 60–80%; *moderate* =40–60% (no long-term O_2 is needed here, and *either* anticholinergics *or* short-acting β_2-agonists are recommended, not both).

Acute respiratory distress syndrome

Acute respiratory distress syndrome (ARDS) is acute respiratory failure with non-cardiogenic pulmonary oedema that occurs secondary to severe insults to the lungs or other organs. *Synonyms* adult respiratory distress syndrome (ARDS); acute lung injury (ALI).

Pathophysiology Increased permeability of pulmonary microvasculature causes leakage of proteinaceous fluid across the alveolar–capillary membrane. This may be one manifestation of a more generalized disruption of endothelium, resulting in hypoxia and multiple organ failure.

Risk factors These are legion but the commonest are sepsis, major trauma, hypovolaemic shock, and severe chest infection (see opposite for others). The more risk factors, the greater the chance of ARDS.

Ask about Recent injury and ↑dyspnoea (eg some time after the precipitating event). **Signs** Cyanosis (hypoxia refractory to O_2), tachypnoea, pulse↑, peripheral vasodilatation. Bilateral fine inspiratory crackles.

CXR Bilateral alveolar shadowing, often with air bronchograms.

Diagnostic criteria One recent consensus requires these 4 to exist: 1 Acute onset. 2 CXR: bilateral infiltrates. 3 Pulmonary capillary wedge pressure <19mmHg or a lack of clinical congestive heart failure. 4 Refractory hypoxaemia with P_aO_2: F_iO_2 <200 for ARDS. Others include total thoracic compliance <30mL/cm H_2O.

Management—on ITU Treat the underlying cause and give supportive therapy to maintain O_2 delivery while lung function improves.
- *Sepsis:* Identify organism/antibiotic sensitivity then treat. If clinically septic but no organisms cultured, use broad spectrum antibiotics (p337).
- *Circulatory support:* Pulmonary artery catheterization aids haemodynamic monitoring. Maintain cardiac output and O_2 delivery with dobutamine 2.5–10µg/kg/min. Correct anaemia. Consider treating pulmonary hypertension with low-dose (20–120ppm) nitrous oxide, a selective pulmonary vasodilator. Vigorous lung drying out is no help but avoid fluid overload. Haemofiltration may be needed in renal failure but is sometimes also used to achieve a negative fluid balance.
- *Respiratory support:* Those with mild lung injury may only need continuous positive airway pressure (CPAP) to maintain adequate oxygenation but most patients require positive-pressure ventilation. The large tidal volumes (10–15mL/kg) produced by conventional ventilation plus reduced lung compliance in ARDS may, however, lead to high peak airway pressures and pneumothorax. Positive end-expiratory pressure (PEEP) increases oxygenation but at the expense of venous return, cardiac output, and perfusion of the kidneys and liver. Newer approaches include inverse ratio ventilation (more time spent in inspiration than expiration), high-frequency jet ventilation, and permissive hypercapnia, (well tolerated). These techniques all keep mean airway pressures high enough to recruit alveoli but avoid high peak airway pressures.
- *Other:* Start enteral feeding early and give stress ulcer prophylaxis. Steroids given in the acute phase do not improve mortality.

Prognosis Early diagnosis and institution of therapy improves prognosis. Overall mortality is 50–75% but varies with the precipitating condition—opportunistic pneumonia 86%, trauma 38%. Mortality increases with the number of organ systems in failure—any 3 organs in failure for over a week is almost always fatal. The older the patient, the worse their prognosis. Survivors may be left with a reduced vital capacity and some obstructive lung disease but others regain good lung function.

Risk factors for acute respiratory distress syndrome

Sepsis	Massive transfusion
Hypovolaemic shock	Burns (p804)
Trauma	Smoke inhalation (p805)
Pneumonia	Near drowning
Diabetic ketoacidosis	Acute pancreatitis
Gastric aspiration	DIC
Pregnancy	Head injury
Eclampsia	ICP↑
Amniotic fluid embolus	Fat embolus
Drugs/toxins	Heart/lung bypass
Paraquat, heroin, aspirin	Tumour lysis syndrome (p686)
Pulmonary contusion	

1 GR Bernard 1994 *J Critical Care* 9 72   2 M Sair, T Evans 1995 *Medicine* 23:9 388

Respiratory failure

Respiratory failure occurs when gas exchange is inadequate, causing hypoxia. It is defined by a P_aO_2 <8kPa (normal 10.7–13.3kPa). Levels of CO_2 are used to divide respiratory failure into two types. In type I, P_aCO_2 is <6.5kPa, while in type II P_aCO_2 is >6.5kPa (normal 4.7–6.0kPa). Respiratory failure may be transient, eg only when asleep, and a patient may fluctuate between types I and II.

Type I Hypoxia with normal or low P_aCO_2. It is caused by ventilation–perfusion mismatch. Despite compensatory vasoconstriction in hypoxic areas of lung, some mixed venous blood still flows to underventilated alveoli (physiological shunting), eg pneumonia, acute asthma, pulmonary fibrosis or oedema; also anatomical shunts where venous blood bypasses ventilated alveoli (R–L intracardiac shunts, lung AVM). Hyperventilation cannot compensate as blood leaving unaffected alveoli is already almost 100% saturated (sigmoid oxyhaemoglobin dissociation curve). Removal of CO_2 is increased (linear curve), hence the normal or low P_aCO_2.

The Patient may be *restless, agitated, sweating,* and *confused* (if severe). *Signs:* *Pulse↑; central cyanosis* (reliably evident when saturation <80% or P_aO_2 <7kPa so it indicates *severe* hypoxia). If long-standing hypoxia: *pulmonary hypertension* (leads to *cor pulmonale,* p366) and *polycythaemia.*

Management 1 Treat the cause 2 Supplemental oxygen sufficient to correct hypoxia. ►There is no need to give low concentrations (see below).

Type II Hypoxia with hypercapnia indicating overall alveolar ventilation inadequate for metabolic needs. Any V̇/Q̇ mismatch will influence P_aO_2.

Causes: 1 *Reduced respiratory drive:* Sedative drugs, CNS tumour, or trauma. 2 *Neuromuscular:* Myasthenia gravis, cervical cord lesion, diaphragmatic paralysis, Guillain–Barré syndrome. 3 *Thoracic wall:* Flail chest, kyphoscoliosis. 4 *Airway/lung:* COPD, asthma, pneumonia, pulmonary fibrosis, epiglottitis, obstructive sleep apnoea (p362).

The Patient may show signs of the underlying cause. Acute hypercapnia causes *restlessness, flapping tremor, warm limbs, bounding pulse.* As CO_2 rises further, *CO_2 narcosis* supervenes, characterized by *drowsiness, papilloedema* (cerebral vasodilatation), *↓tendon reflexes, miosis, confusion* and eventual *coma.* Chronic hypercapnia is better tolerated but produces *early-morning headaches.* Sleep quality is poor causing *tiredness, decreased intellectual performance,* and even *personality change.*

Management: Depends on cause and timescale. *Acute CO_2 retention* causes uncompensated respiratory acidosis (p630). *Causes:* sedative drugs, acute asthma, pneumonia, pulmonary oedema. 1 Ensure a patent airway. 2 Treat underlying cause. 3 Assess respiratory drive. Is the patient trying to breathe? If not, is it due to sedatives eg opiates? Consider naloxone. 4 Correct hypoxia with high concentration O_2. 5 Assisted ventilation. ►CO_2 retention in acute respiratory disease eg asthma or pneumonia indicates exhaustion and impending death. *It is a medical emergency.*

Chronic CO_2 retention causes a compensated respiratory acidosis with renal retention of HCO_3^- and a relatively normal pH. Causes: see above; typically COPD. 1 Treat underlying cause. 2 Controlled oxygen (24–28%). High-dose O_2 with complete correction of hypoxia may decrease respiratory drive and increase CO_2 retention, therefore titrate O_2 against blood gases. 3 Consider a respiratory stimulant (doxapram 1–4mg/min IV) provided the patient isn't tachypnoeic or exhausted. *Use of doxapram in an exhausted patient simply worsens exhaustion.* 4 Consider assisted ventilation (eg NIPPV, p354). This can buy time to treat an underlying condition but may be inappropriate in end-stage lung disease.

When to consider arterial blood gas measurement

In this clinical scenario:
  Any unexpected deterioration in an ill patient.
  Anyone with an acute exacerbation of a chronic chest condition.
  Anyone with impaired consciousness.
  Anyone with impaired respiratory effort.

Or if any of these signs or symptoms are present:
  Bounding pulse, drowsy, tremor (flapping), headache, pink palms,
    papilloedema (signs of CO_2 retention).
  Cyanosis, confusion, visual hallucinations (signs of hypoxia).

Or to monitor the progress of a critically ill patient:
  Monitoring the treatment of known respiratory failure.
  Anyone ventilated on ITU.
  After major surgery.
  After major trauma.

To validate measurements from transcutaneous pulse oximetry
  Pulse oximetry (p658) *sometimes* suffices when it is not critical to
  know P_aCO_2. Even so, it is wise to do periodic blood gas checks.

Learn arterial puncture from an expert (local anaesthesia *does* ↓pain).

Mechanical ventilation[1] See also *Pulse oximetry*, p658

Indications Deteriorating gas exchange due to a reversible cause of respiratory failure, eg pneumonia, pulmonary oedema, exacerbation of COPD, massive atelectasis, exhaustion, neuromuscular weakness (eg Guillain–Barré, myasthenia gravis), head injury, cerebral hypoxia (asphyxiation, cardiac arrest), chest trauma or burns, and the need for airway protection.

Intubation (An *aide-mémoire*, only: learn from an expert; intubation is not needed eg for CPAP and BIPAP.) Choose an endotracheal tube with the largest feasible internal diameter, to decrease airflow resistance, facilitate pulmonary toilet, and/or permit bronchoscopy (ideally ≥7.5mm).
- Sedate (± paralyse) patient. Bag-and-mask ventilate with high-flow O_2.
- Intubate patient. If unsuccessful after 30secs, stop, and reoxygenate.
- Once intubated, inflate cuff. Check for placement by auscultation over chest (both sides!) and stomach during bag ventilation. Verify with CXR.
- Secure tube with tape and note distance inserted. Suction the airway.
- Begin mechanical ventilation.

Modes Positive pressure ventilation actively blows air into the lungs. *Continuous positive airways pressure (CPAP)* provides a *constant positive pressure* throughout the respiratory cycle. This re-expands collapsed alveoli, increasing functional residual capacity (FRC) and compliance. The work of breathing is reduced and gas exchange improves. A high-flow O_2-air mixture is breathed through a tightly fitting mask or via the nose.

BIPAP is a similar device that allows one to set a higher pressure for inspiration and a lower pressure for expiration. The ventilator triggers on the patient's initiation of inspiration. The patient must be able to protect their airway and generate enough effort to trigger the machine.

Assist-control (A/C) is a *volume*-targeted mode of ventilation which delivers a selected tidal volume (TV) at a pre-determined rate. By controlling both of these variables there is greater control in the amount of ventilation that a patient receives. If the patient is initiating breaths at a spontaneous rate above the machine-set rate, the ventilator 'assists' the patient by assuring a full TV with every breath. Because a full TV is delivered by the ventilator with each patient-initiated breath, tachypnoea may lead to severe respiratory alkalosis (p630) and dynamic hyperinflation.

Simultaneous intermittent mandatory ventilation (SIMV), also a *volume*-targeted mode, delivers a fixed rate of machine-set TV breaths and allows the patient to take additional spontaneous breaths, *with patient-determined TVs*. This mode gives the patient the flexibility to adjust his minute ventilation to meet his metabolic demands.

Pressure support ventilation (PSV) is a *pressure*-targeted mode in which the patient breathes at a spontaneous rate while the TV is determined by a machine-set inflation pressure *and* thoracic compliance. Note: adequate minute ventilation is *not* ensured with PSV. Monitor exhaled tidal volumes.

Intermittent negative pressure ventilation (INPV) works by 'sucking' out the chest wall and is used in patients with chronic hypoventilation (eg polio, kyphoscoliosis or muscle disease). Some manage for months on their own after a few weeks of INPV. 'Iron lung' alternatives include thoracic cuirass ventilators and other devices which may be custom built.

Nasal intermittent positive pressure ventilation (NIPPV): This is a non-invasive technique useful in COPD if the patient is *beginning* to tire, and pH <7.35, and full mechanical ventilation is not required. Intermittent positive pressure is delivered via nasal or full face mask and flow generator. This is generally an acceptable way to reduce deaths and hospital stay.

Managing ventilators is an art best learned by expert guidance at the bedside.

1 M Tobin 1994 *NEJM* **330** 1056

✛ Pulmonary embolism (PE) ►Emergency care: p774

These may be small (<u>intermittent dyspnoea</u>), medium, or large (<u>sudden collapse with pleuritic pain</u>—p774). Medium-sized emboli typically present with <u>chest pain (not always pleuritic)</u> and dyspnoea: there may be no sign of any causative DVT. <u>Think of PE whenever you are diagnosing myocardial infarction: they are hard to distinguish.</u> Tests: ECG: rate↑; often the only sign; $S_I Q_{III} T_{III}$ pattern (p268) is rare; $P_aO_2\downarrow$, V/Q scan (p732) ± spiral CT (p736) ± angiography; CXR: normal—or wedge-shaped pulmonary infarct.

The typical at-risk time is in the days <u>following surgery</u> (particularly orthopaedic or gynaecological). Other at-risk contexts: <u>immobility</u>; <u>smokers on the Pill</u>; <u>malignancy</u> (especially pelvic); <u>thrombophilia (p620)</u>.

Treatment Give O_2 (100%, unless COPD) and pain relief (morphine, eg 10mg IV). <u>Anticoagulate (p596)</u>; <u>thrombolysis may be needed</u> (p356). Get help if thrombophilia is possible (p622), eg if no post-op 'excuse'.

Pneumothorax

This is accumulation of air in the pleural space.

Causes Often spontaneous (especially in young thin men) due to rupture of a pleural bleb. Other causes include trauma (especially iatrogenic, eg CVP lines), asthma, COPD, positive pressure assisted ventilation, TB, pneumonia and abscess, lung carcinoma, cystic fibrosis, sarcoidosis, fibrosing alveolitis and any diffuse lung disease, and ascent in aeroplanes. In USA cities, AIDS-associated pneumocystosis is the leading cause.

The Patient There may be no symptoms (especially in fit people with small pneumothoraces) or there may be dyspnoea or pleuritic pain (may be transient). Signs: look for ipsilateral decreased breath sounds in a resonant chest. There may be hyper-resonance, but this is hard to detect. Also: diminished expansion and breath sounds. The mediastinum may be shifted away from the side of a tension pneumothorax.

CXR pneumothorax shows as an area devoid of lung markings peripheral to the edge of the collapsed lung (do not confuse this with the medial edge of the scapula). It may be better demonstrated in an expiratory film when the lung is deflated. It may be missed in a supine film.

Management[1] Small pneumothoraces (ie a small rim of air around a lung) usually need no treatment. If no chronic lung disease, send home with an appointment for the chest clinic in 7–10 days. Advise the patient that flying is dangerous. Admit all others. Moderate (lung collapsed ½-way towards heart border) and complete pneumothoraces (airless lung, separate from diaphragm) need simple aspiration:
- Under 1% lignocaine (=lidocaine) anaesthesia insert a 16G cannula in 2nd intercostal space in the midclavicular line (or 4–6th space, midaxillary line).
- Enter pleural space; withdraw needle's point. Connect to 50mL syringe with Luer lock and 3-way tap. Aspirate up to 2.5 litres of air (50mL×50).
- Stop if resistance is felt, or if the patient coughs excessively.
- Request CXR in inspiration. If the pneumothorax is gone or is small, you have succeeded. If you fail after a 2nd attempt, use an underwater drain, p800. (Never clamp these drains: this impairs successful inflation.)
- If a drain is used, remove 24h after bubbling has stopped. Then do CXR.
- If a drain continues to bubble, it may be dislocated, or air may be leaking around it, or a bronchopleural fistula may exist. Pleurodesis, pleurectomy or surgical closure may be the answer to persistent leaks.

1 British Thoracic Society Guidelines 1993 *BMJ* ii 114

Right axis deviation
RBBB . AF.

Tension pneumothorax

This is an emergency. Air drawn into the pleural space with each inspiration has no route of escape during expiration. The mediastinum is pushed over into the contralateral hemithorax. Unless the air is rapidly removed, cardiorespiratory arrest will occur.

Signs: Respiratory distress, tachycardia, hypotension, distended neck veins, trachea deviated away from side of pneumothorax.

Treatment: ►►To remove the air, insert a large-bore (14–16G) needle with a syringe, partially filled with 0.9% saline, into the second intercostal interspace in the midclavicular line on the side of the suspected pneumothorax. Do this *before* requesting a CXR. Remove plunger to allow the trapped air to bubble through the syringe (with saline as a water seal) until a chest tube can be placed. See p800.

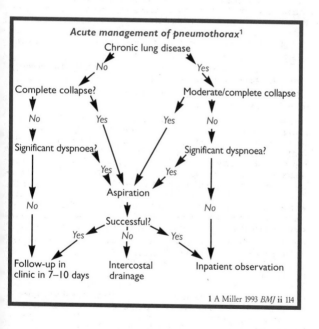

Acute management of pneumothorax[1]

1 A Miller 1993 *BMJ* ii 114

Pleural effusion

A pleural effusion is fluid in the pleural space. Simple effusions can be divided by their protein concentration into *transudates* (<30g/L) and *exudates* (>30g/L). Blood in the pleural space is a *haemothorax*; pus in the pleural space is an *empyema*, and chyle (lymph with fat) is a *chylothorax*. Both blood and air in the pleural space is called a *haemopneumothorax*.

Causes Classifying an effusion as a transudate or an exudate can narrow down the list of causes, but if protein content is borderline the distinction is less useful. *Transudates:* May be due to ↑venous pressure (heart failure, constrictive pericarditis, fluid overload), or hypoproteinaemia causing reduced capillary oncotic pressure (liver disease, nephrotic syndrome, malabsorption). They also occur in hypothyroidism. Transudates are usually bilateral, but if unilateral typically affect the right.
Exudates: Mostly due to increased leakiness of pleural capillaries secondary to inflammation (infection including TB, rheumatoid arthritis, SLE, pancreatitis, pulmonary infarction, drug-induced, asbestos) or neoplasia (metastatic carcinoma, bronchogenic carcinoma, mesothelioma, Meigs' syndrome, lymphoma) but pulmonary vessel obstruction (lymphangitis carcinomatosis) can also be responsible. They are usually unilateral in focal disease but bilateral in diffuse lung disease and systemic disease.

Symptoms Dyspnoea with large effusions; pleuritic chest pain with small effusions; symptoms of underlying cause. May be asymptomatic.

Signs Stony dull percussion note; absent breath sounds; tactile vocal fremitus↓, and vocal resonance↓. Above the effusion where lung is compressed, there may be bronchial breathing and bleating vocal resonance (aegophony). There is mediastinal shift *away* from large effusions and reduced chest wall expansion on the affected side. Early on, there may be a pleural rub. Look for signs of associated disease, eg cardiac failure.

CXR Small effusions blunt the costophrenic angles, larger ones are seen as water-dense shadows with concave upper borders. A completely horizontal upper border implies that there is also a pneumothorax.

Ultrasound Useful for identifying the presence of pleural fluid but also for guiding diagnostic or therapeutic aspiration.

Diagnostic aspiration Draw off 30mL using a 21G needle inserted just above the upper border of an appropriate rib (avoids neurovascular bundle). Use the CXR and percussion for guidance or ultrasound if the tap is difficult. Send fluid for cytology (mesothelial cells, lymphocytes, neutrophils); biochemistry (protein, glucose, pH, LDH, amylase); bacteriology (microscopy and culture, including for TB); immunology (rheumatoid factor, ANA, complement). See opposite for pleural fluid analysis. *Other tests:* If pleural fluid analysis is inconclusive, consider parietal pleural biopsy with an Abrams' needle. It improves diagnosis of TB but thoracoscopy is better still, allowing direct inspection of the pleural cavity and biopsy of suspicious areas. Diagnostic yield in both malignancy and TB is 80–100%.

Management is of the underlying cause. If the effusion is symptomatic, it should be drained, repeatedly if necessary. The fluid is best removed slowly (≤2 litres/24h). It may be aspirated in the same way as a diagnostic tap, or an indwelling chest drain may be inserted (see p800). *Empyemas* are drained (ultrasound or CT guided). Streptokinase 250,000u in 20–100mL of 0.9% saline is used to break down pleural adhesions.[1,2] Persistent collections and increasing pleural thickness (on ultrasound) requires surgery.[1] Thoracoscopic pleurodesis with talc is the most effective form of chemical pleurodesis for troublesome malignant effusions.

1 MF Muers 1997 *Lancet* 349 1491   2 RJO Davies 1997 *Thorax* 52 416–21

Pleural fluid analysis

Gross appearance

Turbid yellow	Empyema
Haemorrhagic	Pulmonary infarction, trauma, malignancy
Straw-coloured	Transudate

Cytology

Neutrophils ++	Bacterial infection
Lymphocytes ++	2° Malignancy, lymphoma, TB
Mesothelial cells ++	Pulmonary infarction
Abnormal mesothelial cells	Mesothelioma
Multinucleated giant cells	Rheumatoid
Lupus erythematosus cells	SLE

Biochemistry

Protein <30g/L	Transudate
>30g/L	Exudate
Glucose <3.3mmol/L	Infection, rheumatoid, malignancy
pH >7.3	Infection, rheumatoid, malignancy
LDH↑	Infection
Amylase↑	Pancreatitis

Immunology

Rheumatoid factor	Rheumatoid, others
ANA	Connective tissue disease
Complement levels↓	Rheumatoid, SLE, malignancy, infection

Sarcoidosis

A disease of unknown cause characterized by non-caseating granulomata. It may affect any organ and occur at any age, but most commonly affects the chests of young adults. Incidence: 1–64/100,000/yr. Blacks are

more often and more severely affected, often by extrathoracic disease.

Presentation Acute sarcoidosis (Löfgren's syndrome): erythema nodosum, bilateral hilar lymphadenopathy (BHL) on CXR, swinging fever, polyarthralgia. Insidious onset: BHL may be an incidental finding in asymptomatic patients or be accompanied by mild respiratory or systemic symptoms such as the gradual onset of exertional dyspnoea, non-productive cough, malaise, tiredness, and weight loss. Parenchymal lung disease may be present ± BHL, the pulmonary infiltrates appearing as diffuse, bilateral mottled shadows on CXR. This may be asymptomatic (crepitations are also rare) but if progressive fibrosis develops, increasingly severe exertional dyspnoea and a persistent, dry cough result. Significant fibrosis appears as upper lobe reticular shadowing and causes dyspnoea and hypoxia at rest, cor pulmonale, and eventually congestive heart failure.

Diagnosis Relies on compatible clinical, radiological, and histological findings. CT is useful for demonstrating perivascular nodularity of lungs. Check for TB by examination of sputum/lavage for acid-fast bacilli and tuberculin test (but sarcoid can make the test −ve in those previously +ve). Non-caseating granulomata in biopsy material confirm diagnosis. Multiple transbronchial biopsies offer a high yield in thoracic sarcoid but when biopsy is inappropriate, a Kveim–Siltzbach test can be done. A suspension of human sarcoid spleen tissue is injected intradermally.* If the test is +ve, non-caseating granulomata are seen at the injection site at 4–6 weeks. Positive tests are not exclusive to sarcoidosis and unfortunately occur most in clinically overt disease. Abnormal vitamin D synthesis can cause hypercalciuria and hypercalcaemia (only rarely symptomatic) while lung function tests may show reduced lung volume and compliance, impaired gas transfer and a restrictive ventilatory defect. *Monitoring disease activity:* Clinical, serial radiographs, lung function tests, serum ACE levels (↑in active sarcoid), Ca^{2+}.

Other causes BHL: TB; lymphoma; cancer; fungi. *Other granulomatous diseases:* TB; brucella; berylliosis; primary biliary cirrhosis; allergic alveolitis; drugs; leprosy; mycoses; *toxoplasma; leishmania;* Hodgkin's; Wegener's; Crohn's.

Treatment ►No therapy cures sarcoidosis and there is no proof that palliative therapy alters final outcome. *Indications:* Symptomatic pulmonary fibrosis; worsening pulmonary infiltration or infiltration with breathlessness/impaired lung function; persistent Ca^{2+}↑ or hypercalciuria (avoids renal failure/nephrocalcinosis); some extrathoracic disease. *Always* treat uveitis to prevent blindness (cyclopentolate and steroid eye-drops—fluorometholone is least likely to cause glaucoma).
Systemic therapy: Prednisolone (20–40mg/24h) PO for 4–6 weeks. If no response, discontinue. Wean down responders to a low maintenance dose (eg 15mg/24h) over 6 months. After 6 months maintenance, attempt withdrawal. Relapse is common (especially in blacks) and requires reinstitution of therapy. Where steroids are contraindicated, hydroxychloroquine is an option. Low-dose methotrexate or azathioprine can be used to reduce steroid exposure but are of questionable long-term benefit.
Acute sarcoidosis: Bed rest, NSAIDs, corticosteroids only if needed.

Prognosis Remits without treatment in 2/3 whites, 1/3 blacks. Pulmonary sarcoid will eventually resolve to leave a clear CXR in 2/3 but this is less likely with extrathoracic disease. Löfgren's syndrome has the best prognosis as 90% can expect complete remission within 2 years. A minority of patients are left disabled. Mortality is <3% of diagnosed patients.

*Available in UK from PHLS (OTM 1996): special precautions are in place to prevent pathogen transmission

Extrathoracic sarcoidosis

Skin   Erythema nodosum; nodules; lupus pernio (blue-red rash on nose, cheeks, digits); scar infiltration.

Eyes   Enlarged lacrimal glands; hypopyon (WBC in the anterior chamber); uveitis, anterior or posterior. The latter causes most of the visual loss, and consists of perivascular cuffing of retinal equatorial veins which appear like candle wax dripping (*tache de bougie*).

Bones   Arthralgia; dactylitis; osteopenic 'punched out' lesions.

Heart[1]   Always think of sarcoid when you know there's something wrong with the heart, but you don't know what—and you've excluded coronary artery disease. There may be no symptoms, or: sudden death; ventricular tachycardia; complete heart block; congestive cardiomyopathy; heart failure; pericardial effusion; perfusion defects—on ^{210}thallium myocardial scintigraphy they may diminish on exercise—unlike other perfusion defects. *Have low thresholds for doing echoes, 24h ECGs, and inserting pacemakers.*

CNS   Cranial and peripheral nerve palsies (especially VII); space occupying lesions (± seizures) or diffuse CNS disease; granulomatous meningitis; pituitary (eg diabetes insipidus).

Kidney   Hypercalcaemic nephropathy; renal calculi.

General   Lymphadenopathy; hepatosplenomegaly; fever; malaise.

1 DN Mitchell 1997 BMJ i 320

Obstructive sleep apnoea syndrome (OSAS)

In this disorder, also called Pickwickian syndrome, there is intermittent and recurrent closure of the pharyngeal airway, with partial or complete cessation of breathing during sleep. This apnoea is terminated only by partial arousal. The typical patient is a middle-aged fat man who presents because of snoring or daytime somnolence. The spouse or partner usually describes the patient stopping breathing frequently during sleep; also:
- Snorts loudly in sleep
- Daytime somnolence
- Poor sleep quality
- Morning headache
- Decreased libido
- Cognitive performance↓

Type II respiratory failure (p352) may be evident, if there is associated COPD. There is also ↑risk of road accidents and (possibly[1]) heart disease.

Tests Polysomnography (monitoring oxygen saturation, airflow at the nose and mouth, ECG, EMG chest and abdominal wall movement during sleep). Simpler studies (oximetry and video recordings) will often be all that is required for diagnosis. The occurrence of 15 or more episodes of apnoea or hypopnoea during 1h of sleep is the conventional indicator of significant sleep apnoea, but then symptoms occur with lower or normal apnoea rates when snoring alone is provoking sleep disruption.

Management ●Continuous positive airway pressure (CPAP) via a nasal mask during sleep is the best device when symptoms justify this cumbersome impertinence. ●Weight reduction *may* help. ●Tonsillectomy, uvulopalatopharyngoplasty, and tracheostomy are very rarely needed.

Extrinsic allergic alveolitis

Essence Inhaled antigens provoke a hypersensitivity reaction in the lungs of sensitized individuals. Allergens are usually spores of microorganisms (eg *Micropolyspora faeni* in farmer's lung) or avian proteins (eg droppings or feathers in bird fancier's lung or pigeon breeders' disease).

Symptoms *4–8h post-exposure* Fever, malaise, dry cough, and dyspnoea. *Chronic:* Gradually increasing malaise, weight↓, exertional dyspnoea, and fine crepitations. Chronic disease may follow or be independent of acute episodes, which themselves may have no complications.

Pathology *Acute:* Mostly type III immune-complex mediated alveolitis. *Chronic:* Predominantly type IV (cell mediated) with lymphocyte infiltration, granulomata, giant cells, exudates, and bronchiolitis obliterans.

Tests *Acute:* Neutrophilia (eosinophils usually ↔); ESR↑; serum precipitins detectable, eg ELISA IgG antibody to pigeon gammaglobulin; CXR: normal *or* widespread small nodules *or* ground-glass appearance; spirometry: slight and transient reduction in lung volumes and transfer factor. *Chronic:* Serum precipitins detectable; CXR: mainly upper zone shadowing due to fibrosis; RFTs: more marked restrictive changes and reduced gas transfer. Bronchoalveolar lavage fluid in acute or chronic disease shows a predominance of lymphocytes and mast cells.

Management Avoid exposure to allergens, failing which, wear a very fine mesh face mask or positive pressure helmet. Acute symptoms may be controlled by prednisolone 40mg/24h PO; when asymptomatic, reduce dose rapidly. In chronic disease, long-term steroids often achieve radiological and physiological improvement. In practice, in the face of overzealous advice about eliminating allergens, many patients with bird fancier's lung end up avoiding their doctors, not their birds—and frequently symptoms wane in spite of repeated exposure.

Note: Psittacosis and ornithosis are infections (zoonoses). They are not a cause of allergic alveolitis. See p334.

---

1 The link is weak making some commentators unsure as to whether to treat—but this misses the point that it is the hypersomnolence which is what most needs treating: J Stradling 1997 *BMJ* i 368

Fibrosing alveolitis

Essence A disease of unknown cause, characterized by increased numbers of inflammatory cells in alveoli and interstitium, with variable degrees of pulmonary fibrosis. A third are associated with connective tissue diseases (RA—10% of all fibrosing alveolitis, SLE, systemic sclerosis, mixed connective tissue disease, Sjögren's, poly/dermatomyositis)—or chronic active hepatitis, renal tubular acidosis, autoimmune thyroid disease, ulcerative colitis. The rest are 'cryptogenic' with putative agents being occupational exposure to metal and wood dust.[1]

The Patient Features include: progressive exertional dyspnoea; dry cough; general malaise; weight loss; arthralgia; finger clubbing (65%; PLATE 7); fine end-inspiratory crepitations ('Velcro® crepitations'); cyanosis.

Tests CXR: Bilateral diffuse nodular or reticulonodular shadowing favouring the lung bases. Honeycomb shadows develop as the disease progresses and lung volume is lost. *Hypergammaglobulinaemia.* ESR raised. ANA and *rheumatoid factor* are present in 35% of patients. *Respiratory function tests:* Reduced lung volumes (restrictive pattern) and reduced transfer factor. *Bronchoalveolar lavage:* Increased total cell count with increased proportion of neutrophils and/or eosinophils. Lymphocytes are occasionally raised and may indicate a favourable response to treatment. *Open lung biopsy* may be needed for diagnosis and staging.

Management 35% respond to immunosuppression, eg with prednisolone 60mg/24h PO or cyclophosphamide 100–120mg/24h PO + prednisolone 20mg PO on alternate days. Monitor response with CXR and lung function tests. Response to steroids may take 1–2 months, after which the dose may be cautiously reduced. Response to cyclophosphamide may take longer. The patient may be suitable for lung transplantation.[2]

Survival 50% die in 4–5yrs, but the range is wide (1–20yrs).

Other causes of lung fibrosis Respiratory distress syndrome (p350), chronic extrinsic allergic alveolitis (p362), eosinophilic granuloma, radiation, uraemia, bleomycin, busulfan, amiodarone, nitrofurantoin.

Mineral fibrosis

Simple coal worker's pneumoconiosis (CWP) results from pulmonary coal dust deposition. It is asymptomatic and causes no signs. CXR: multiple round opacities (1–5mm, mostly in upper zones). It may proceed to **progressive massive fibrosis (PMF)**, causing dyspnoea, black sputum, and a restrictive defect on spirometry (p328). CXR opacities are sausage-shaped (1–10cm).

Silicosis is similar radiographically, but is associated with egg-shell calcification of hilar nodes. Unlike CWP, silicosis is a risk factor for TB.

Asbestosis is also a progressive fibrotic lung parenchymal disease, clinically and radiographically like cryptogenic fibrosing alveolitis. This is distinct from the other asbestos-related chest conditions: pleural plaques (which may calcify), malignant mesothelioma, and bronchial carcinoma.

1 I Johnston 1996 *Lancet* 347 284   2 JH Dark 1998 *Lancet* 351 4

⚕ Cor pulmonale

Cor pulmonale is right heart failure caused by chronic pulmonary hypertension induced by chronic hypoxia secondary to diseases of the lung, its vessels, or the thoracic cage (or ventilatory problems, see opposite).

Typical presentation CCF ± infective bronchitis (dyspnoea, cyanosis). Blue-bloaters get cor pulmonale more often than (non-hypoxic) pink puffers, p348. Typical symptoms are exertional dyspnoea and fatigue—with other features depending on the interplay of these 3 phenomena:–

Pulmonary hypertension	Right heart hypertrophy	Right heart failure
Chest pain	Right ventricular heave	Peripheral oedema
Syncope	Dominant R wave in	Anorexia; nausea; JVP↑
Loud P₂	lead V₁ on ECG	from liver + GI eng-
4th heart sound		orgement; ascites
Pulmonary flow murmur		Tender smooth hep-
Diastolic murmur from		atomegaly
pulmonary regurgitation		Tricuspid regurgitation

Functional tricuspid regurgitation occurs because the right heart enlarges. It is recognized by a pansystolic murmur, v wave in the JVP, pulsatile liver; more rarely ascites and right-sided pleural effusion.

Tests Blood gases; blood/sputum cultures if infection suspected clinically. *CXR:* Enlarged right atrium and ventricle and prominent pulmonary artery.

ECG: P pulmonale (peaked P wave); right axis deviation; right ventricular hypertrophy/'strain': tall R in V₁; deep S in V₆; if severe, inverted T in V₁₋₄.

FBC: Haematocrit↑ from secondary polycythaemia in response to hypoxia.

Causes of pulmonary hypertension* *↑Pulmonary vascular resistance:* Any causes of chronic hypoxia (opposite), primary pulmonary hypertension, collagen vascular disease, drugs, toxins: crotolaria, denatured rape-seed oil.

High pulmonary blood flow: Left-to-right shunts (VSD, ASD, patent ductus) ↑pulmonary flow (∴ ↑pulmonary resistance, causing ↑right-sided pressure, which progressively decreases left-to right shunt). Eventually, right heart pressure becomes > left heart pressure, and the shunt reverses causing cyanosis. This is Eisenmenger's syndrome and is irreversible.

Chronic pulmonary venous hypertension: Chronic LVF or mitral stenosis.

Management In pulmonary hypertension that is irreversible or resistant to treatment, a steady decline towards cor pulmonale and death is likely. Try to reduce the work of the right heart by reducing pulmonary resistance and arterial pressure. Treat any underlying condition. *Treat infective exacerbations* vigorously (these may precipitate cardiorespiratory failure).

Continuous *oxygen therapy* for at least 15h/day reduces hypoxia, lowers pulmonary resistance, and increases survival. Home oxygen concentrators are prescribable by GPs in the UK (usually after assessment in a specialist respiratory unit) and oxygen may be piped into several rooms in the home (*of non-smokers only*). A transformation in the patient's quality of life is possible with careful selection of patients (find out if they would really use it—and don't wait until the patient is terminally ill).

Fluid overload is treated with *frusemide* (=furosemide), eg 40–160mg/ 24h PO) and appropriate potassium supplements (check U&E periodically). *Venesection* may be performed to ↓severe polycythaemia in the acute situation (↓ thrombosis and the work of the heart). Selected (usually young) patients should be considered for *heart–lung transplantation.*

*Not all causes of pulmonary hypertension are causes of cor pulmonale, which, by definition, presupposes a *primary* disease of the lungs, their vessels or the thoracic cage.

Causes of cor pulmonale

Lung disease
Asthma (severe, chronic)
Bronchiectasis
Pulmonary fibrosis

Pulmonary vascular disease
Multiple pulmonary emboli
Sickle-cell disease
Parasite infestation

Thoracic cage abnormality
Kyphosis
Scoliosis
Thoracoplasty

Neuromuscular disease
Myasthenia gravis
Poliomyelitis
Motor neurone disease

Hypoventilation
Sleep apnoea (p362)
Enlarged adenoids in children
Cerebrovascular disease

Relevant pages in other chapters:

Symptoms and signs: Frequency (p46); loin pain (p50); oedema (p52); oliguria (p52); polyuria (p52).

Also: Urinary retention (p134); catheters (p134); biochemistry of kidney function (p632); electrolyte physiology (p636); sodium (p636–8); potassium (p640); calcium (p642); urate and the kidney (p634); osteomalacia (p648); incontinence (p74); immunosuppressive drugs (p622).

In OHCS: Gynaecological urology (*OHCS* p70); bacteriuria and pyelonephritis in pregnancy (*OHCS* p160); obstetric causes of acute tubular necrosis (*OHCS* p160); chronic renal disease in pregnancy (*OHCS* p160); UTI in children (*OHCS* p188); urethral valves (*OHCS* p220); horseshoe kidney (*OHCS* p220); ectopic kidney (*OHCS* p220); hypospadias (*OHCS* p220); Wilms' nephroblastoma (p220); acute and chronic renal failure in children (*OHCS* p280); nephritis and nephrosis in children (*OHCS* p282); Potter's syndrome (*OHCS* p120).

Introduction to nephrology

One of the main problems in approaching nephrology is that there is no strict correlation between the clinical syndrome and pathology. This is because the kidney has a limited number of ways of responding to a multitude of pathogenic stimuli.

Presentation of renal disease There are 6 main presentations:

1 *Proteinuria and the nephrotic syndrome* A major cause of excessive protein in fresh midstream urine is glomerular disease—principally one of the glomerulonephritides. The nephrotic syndrome refers to the syndrome of proteinuria (≥3g/day), oedema and hypoalbuminaemia (via protein loss in the urine, and causing oedema).

2 *Nephritic syndrome* The central feature here is blood in the urine from glomerular bleeding. Other features include fluid retention, hypertension, a low urine output (because of low glomerular filtration rate), and a rising plasma urea and creatinine. The cause is typically glomerulonephritis or vasculitis.

3 *Acute renal failure* (ARF, p384, 386) ARF can result from acute damage to any part of the kidney or renal tract. The key point when faced with a patient in acute renal failure is to consider the range of possible causes before making the diagnosis of acute tubular necrosis (the most common cause). If renal tract obstruction, for example, is not treated quickly, perfect kidneys may be irreversibly damaged.

4 *Chronic renal failure* (p388) usually results from glomerular or interstitial disease, eg de novo or as a complication of diabetes mellitus.

5 *Pyelonephritis/urinary tract infection* (UTI, p374) UTI is common in women, and untreated, it may permanently damage the kidneys.

6 *Hypertension* A common effect of *chronic* renal failure of any cause.

Classification of renal disease by pathology The table shows the relationships between the 6 clinical syndromes and the 4 main types of pathology: *glomerulonephritis* (GN); *renal vascular disease* (small vessel disease—vasculitis, or large vessel disease, eg atherosclerosis and renal vein thrombosis—RVT); *obstruction to renal outflow*; and *interstitial disease*, ie *acute tubular necrosis* (ATN), and *acute interstitial nephritis* (AIN), chronic interstitial nephritis (cIN).

	GN	Interstitial disease			Vascular disease			Outflow tract
		AIN	ATN	cIN	Small	Large	RVT	obstruction
Nephrotic syndrome	++	0	0	0	(+)	0	+*	0
Nephritic syndrome	++	(+)	0	0	(+)	0	+	0
Acute renal failure	+	+	++**	0	+	+	(+)	++
Chronic renal failure	++	(+)	0	++	(+)	+	0	++
Pyelonephritis/UTI	0	0	0	0	0	0	+	+
Hypertension	(+)	(+)	0	(+)	(+)	(+)	0	+

*Renal vein thrombosis is a complication, not a cause of the nephrotic syndrome.
**ATN is the chief cause of acute renal failure, but you *must* look for other causes.

►If you suspect renal disease always obtain some fresh midstream urine for: 1 'dipstick' testing, 2 microscopy, and 3 culture.

Causes of abnormalities on ward test (eg Multistix®)

● **Haematuria** Causes of urinary red blood cells may be divided into:
Renal: Glomerulonephritis (p380); vasculitis (eg endocarditis, SLE, and other connective tissue diseases); interstitial nephritis; carcinoma (renal cell, transitional); cystic disease (polycystic disease, medullary sponge kidney); trauma; vascular malformations; emboli.
Extra-renal: Calculi; infection (eg cystitis, prostatitis, urethritis); trauma; neoplasm; bladder catheterization; post-cyclophosphamide.
Coagulation disorders: (or anticoagulants; if INR is in therapeutic range, it is wise to consider other causes). *Others:* Sickle trait/disease; vasculitis. *Work-up:* MSU, FBC, ESR, U&E, creatinine clearance, plain films+ultrasound, ?renal biopsy before cystoscopy in those <45yrs (p373). Note: free Hb and myoglobin make 'stix' +ve in the absence of red cells. Discoloured urine is also seen with porphyria, rifampicin, or beetroot ingestion.

● **Glycosuria** Causes: diabetes mellitus, pregnancy, sepsis, tubular damage (p398), or low renal threshold (check blood glucose).

● **Proteinuria** Rates vary through the day, so 24h samples may be needed, but collection is notoriously unreliable. One way round this (to monitor chronic proteinuria, and thus renal decline) is measuring the protein:creatinine ratio (P_u:C_u) in a spot morning urine.[1] *Causes of proteinuria:* UTI, vaginal mucus, DM, glomerulonephritis, nephrosis, pyrexia, CCF, pregnancy, postural proteinuria (2–5% of adolescents, rare if >30yrs)—protein excretion (generally <1g/24h) when upright, and normal in recumbency. *Rarer causes:* Hemolytic-uraemic syndrome, BP↑, SLE, myeloma, amyloid (p616). *Microalbuminuria:* See p396. Causes: DM; acute illness; arteriopathy.

● **Bile** See p484. ● **Nitrite** Suggests UTI (or a high-protein meal).

Microscopy Find a scrupulously clean slide. It need not be new.
1 Almost close the iris diaphragm of a light microscope.
2 Put a tiny drop of urine on a slide; cover urine with coverslip.
3 Open iris diaphragm a little and engage the × 40 objective.
4 Look for blood, pus, crystals, casts, cocci, and rods. A counting chamber helps to quantify bacteria: 1+ means a few bacteria in every square, 2+ means many bacteria in every square, 3+ means innumerable bacteria. UTI is very likely if 3+, and unlikely if <1+. If 1+ or 2+ bacteria, then UTI is very likely if there are >400 wcc/µl.[2]

RBCs: See *haematuria*, above; >2/mm³ is considered abnormal.
WBCs: Bacterial or chemical cystitis, urethritis, prostatitis, pyelitis, TB, analgesic nephropathy, stones. ≤15/mm³ may be normal.
Casts are best seen in counting chambers. The person who meticulously examines urines may do so for months and see no other variety than insignificant, transparent, jelly-baby-like *hyaline casts,* or *granular casts* (signifying a wide range of renal diseases, eg acute tubular necrosis or rapidly progressive glomerulonephritis, or no disease at all—simply the result of exercise). *Red cell casts* mean glomerulonephritis; they look greenish. *WBC casts* mean pyelonephritis.
Crystals: Combine to form stones (p376). To find a few crystals is common, eg in old or cold urine—when they may not signify any pathology.

24-h urine quantification Na⁺, K⁺, Ca²⁺, urea, creatinine, protein. Do simultaneous plasma creatinine for creatinine clearance (p632).

1 A Perna 1998 *BMJ* i 504—Kidney survival (over 1yr) was >95% in those with chronic non-diabetic renal failure if P_u:C_u <1.7 *vs* <80% if P_u:C_u >2.7   2 F Culclasure 1994 *Arch Int Med* 154 649

Urine microscopy

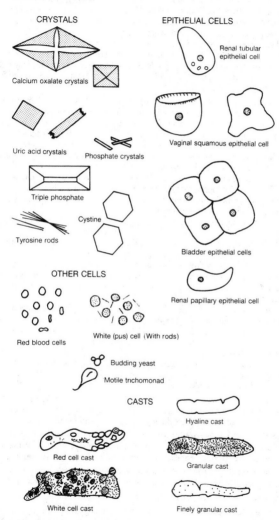

CRYSTALS

Calcium oxalate crystals

Uric acid crystals

Phosphate crystals

Triple phosphate

Tyrosine rods

Cystine

EPITHELIAL CELLS

Renal tubular epithelial cell

Vaginal squamous epithelial cell

Bladder epithelial cells

Renal papillary epithelial cell

OTHER CELLS

Red blood cells

White (pus) cell (With rods)

Budding yeast

Motile trichomonad

CASTS

Hyaline cast

Red cell cast

Granular cast

White cell cast

Finely granular cast

Principle source: M Longmore 1986 *An Atlas of Bedside Microscopy* Royal College of General Practitioners occasional paper No. 32

Radiology of the urinary tract

Plain abdominal films Look for: 1 Renal outlines—normal size 10–12cm and situated at T12–L2. 2 Abnormal calcification—90% of renal stones are radio-opaque; tumour; TB; nephrocalcinosis (p396).

Ultrasound is a key test in acute renal failure as it tests for dilatation of the ureters (the chief cause of reversible renal failure—requiring *prompt* surgical referral). Dilated ureters strongly suggest obstruction; but 5% of anuric patients with obstruction are not dilated (here diagnosis is usually malignancy); dilatation without obstruction occurs in relieved obstruction and pregnancy. *Other uses:* to show renal size—small kidneys are typical of chronic renal failure; to guide biopsy. Doppler ultrasound may help investigate haematuria. With plain x-ray, this is at least as good as IVU for investigation of haematuria.[1]

Intravenous urography (IVU = IVP) Preparation: laxatives; nil by mouth (unless uraemic or myeloma when dehydration is contraindicated) for 12h. Always look at the plain film for renal size and calcification anywhere in the urinary tract. *Nephrogram phase:* (Contrast reaches renal tubules: usually *immediate*—within the first min—and *brief*). Timing of the nephrogram may be capricious (and isotope renography may be preferred) but is said to be *intense* in obstruction and glomerulonephritis (GN); *prolonged* in obstruction, ATN (acute tubular necrosis), chronic GN and renal vein thrombosis; *absent* in a non-functioning kidney (infarction, severe GN); *delayed* in renal artery stenosis (specificity 80%; sensitivity 85% if unilateral).[2] Look for these abnormalities:

- Absent kidney: obscured by bowel gas or perinephric abscess, renal agenesis, nephrectomy (look for amputated 12th rib).
- Small kidney: (<10cm) chronic pyelonephritis, renal artery stenosis. Bilateral in chronic renal failure (chronic GN or pyelonephritis).
- Large kidney: (>14cm) hydronephrosis, tumour, renal vein thrombosis, post-contralateral nephrectomy. Bilateral in polycystic kidneys, and sometimes in: amyloidosis, myeloma, lymphoma, bilateral obstruction.
- Scarred outline: pyelonephritis, ischaemia, TB.
- Low kidney: (normal T12–L2) hepatomegaly, transplants, congenital.
- Pelvicalyceal filling defects: one calyx not seen in tumour, TB, partial nephrectomy. Irregular filling defect—clot or tumour. Smooth defect—papilloma, renal artery aneurysm, pressure from vessel.
- Some patterns:
  Obstruction: (p378) Prolonged and dense nephrogram, clubbed calyces, mega-ureter. *Chronic pyelonephritis:* Small scarred kidneys, thin cortex, clubbed calyces. *Papillary necrosis:* Linear breaks at papillary bases.

Micturating cystourethrogram The bladder is catheterized and filled with contrast. Usually carried out for the investigation of recurrent UTI. It shows ureteric reflux during micturition and bladder diverticula.

Retrograde ureteropyelography The ureters are catheterized and contrast injected. Used for non-functioning kidneys and to define the site of obstruction, eg papillary necrosis and non-opaque stones.

Renal arteriography via femoral arteries. Used for imaging: renal artery stenosis or occlusion, renal tumour circulation, and renal trauma.

Isotope renal scans (DMSA and DTPA scans) See p734.

Antegrade nephrostomy is used in diagnosing and relieving obstruction. The kidney is punctured, under ultrasound guidance, from the flank. A tube is placed in the renal pelvis. This relieves obstruction. After 2 days, 'contrast' passed down the tube reveals the site of obstruction.

1 J Spencer 1990 *BMJ* i 1074 2 A Raine & J Ledingham in *Oxford Textbook of Medicine* 3e 1996 15.28.1 (2547)

Renal biopsy

Renal biopsy should only be performed if knowing histology will influence management. The most common indication is in the nephrotic syndrome, and in acute nephritis.

Small kidneys are hard to biopsy and results usually unhelpful.
- Before biopsy: check FBC and clotting. Group and save serum.
- Check size and position of the kidneys by IVU or ultrasound—IVU will also ensure that there are 2 functioning kidneys.
- Biopsy is done with ultrasound guidance (prone position, breath held).
- Send samples for normal stains, immunofluorescence, and electron microscopy. Special stains (eg Congo Red for amyloid, if indicated).
- After biopsy the patient should rest in bed for 24h. Monitor pulse, BP, symptoms, and urine colour. The major complication is bleeding.

Normal kidney

Polycystic kidney

Spidery calyces

Chronic pyelonephritis

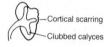
Cortical scarring
Clubbed calyces

Space occupying lesion

Stretched calyx

Chronic glomerulonephritis

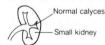
Normal calyces
Small kidney

Papillary necrosis

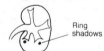
Ring shadows

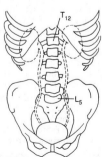

The course of the ureters

Urinary tract infection (UTI)

Most women will have ≥1 UTI in their lives. Men have longer urethras, and fewer UTIs. *Risk factors:* DM; pregnancy; impaired voiding (causes of obstruction, p378); GU malformation; GU instrumentation; urethral reverberations at sexual intercourse; diaphragm use; ↓oestrogen (menopause).

Definitions *Bacteriuria:* any bacteria in urine uncontaminated by urethral flora. It may be asymptomatic (*covert*). If there are >10⁸ organisms/litre (of a pure culture) bacteriuria *is significant.* UTI denotes bacteriuria, with features of GU inflammation at particular sites—eg kidney (*pyelonephritis*), bladder (*cystitis*), prostate (*prostatitis*), or urethra (*urethritis*—non-gonococcal urethritis is the commonest cause of male GU infection, p220). Acute and chronic pyelonephritis are separate entities: *acute pyelonephritis* is acute kidney infection with symptoms of fever, chills, rigors, and flank pain with tenderness. *Chronic pyelonephritis* presents as chronic renal failure or one of its complications, and probably arises from childhood UTIs associated with reflux and renal scarring (OHCS p188). It may be shown on IVU (p372). *Urethral syndrome:* (Women only.) Symptoms of urgency, frequency and dysuria (ie painful micturition) in the absence of readily identifiable bacteriuria. (As there is no urethral disease, the term *abacterial cystitis* is preferred.) It is induced by cold, stress, intercourse, or nylon underwear. Cause: unknown.

Presentation of UTI	Retention of urine	*Pains:* variable
Frequency/dysuria/haematuria	Fever ± D&V	eg suprapubic
Incontinence	Urgency; strangury (p376)	loin; RIF; LIF

Examine for: enlarged bladder, large prostate, renal mass, meatal ulcer, vaginal discharge (p221), loin tenderness, hypertension, signs of CRF (p388).

Bacteria *E coli* >70%—but ≤41% in hospital UTIs; Staphs, Streps, Pseudomonas, Proteus. Klebsiella is rare.

Tests—*Midstream urine (MSU):* Get a clean catch for microscopy (p370). Leukocyte esterase and nitrate dipstick is a quick and reasonably sensitive alternative.[1] Test cultured organisms for sensitivity to a range of antibiotics. MSUs must be fresh. If there are >10⁸ organisms/L (of a pure culture), the result is significant. If there are <10⁸/L ± pyuria (eg >20 WBCs/mm³), the result may still be significant. Repeat the test. *Children:* See OHCS p188.

Consider: Creatinine; blood culture; US; IVU/cystoscopy; PSA (♂ >40yrs) if:
• Recurrent UTI (or first UTI in men) • Overt haematuria • Pyelonephritis
• Persistent microscopic haematuria • Unusual organism • Fever persists

Ultrasound or IVU?[2,3] Ultrasound may miss stones, papillary necrosis, small carcinomas, and clubbed calyces. It is radiation-free, so do it first.

Treatment of simple UTIs[4] (*If pregnant, seek specialist advice.*) Urinate often. Drink plenty: 2 cups/h (even though this ↓antibiotic levels in urine). Double voiding (going again after 5mins) and voiding after intercourse may prevent reinfection. Specific therapy: eg trimethoprim 200mg/12h PO for 3–5 days. Give 10–14 day courses in *males, children, GU malformations, immunosuppression, pyelonephritis, relapses* (2nd UTI, same organism), *reinfections* (2nd UTI, different organism), and *bacterial prostatitis* (eg doxycycline 100mg/24h PO—this is a likely diagnosis if excess pyuria is noted in urine microscoped after prostatic massage, done PR).*

Causes of sterile pyuria	
• Inadequately treated UTI	• Renal TB (▶do 3 early morning urines)
• Appendicitis	• Papillary necrosis from analgesic, p394
• Calculi; prostatitis	• Fastidious culture requirements
• Bladder tumour	• Interstitial nephritis, polycystic kidney
	• Chemical cystitis eg from cytotoxics

1 C Hiscoke 1990 *B J Gen Pr* 40 403 2 J Spencer 1993 *BMJ* i 211 3 M Wilkie 1993 *BMJ* i 211 4 S Hope in *Women's Health*, ed A McPherson OUP *Cranberry juice can help prevent *recurrent* UTI ▣

Renal stones (nephrolithiasis) and renal colic

The Patient Big stones may be symptomless and tiny stones may cause excruciating ureteric spasm. Stones in the *kidney* cause loin pain. Stones in the *ureter* cause renal colic (may radiate from loin to groin but may only be felt in the tip of the penis). *Bladder stones* cause strangury (the distressing desire to pass what will not pass) and *urethral stones* may cause interruption of urine flow. Nausea and vomiting may accompany colic. Pain is often eased by curling up; patients classically cannot lie still.

Other presentations: UTI, haematuria, renal failure.

Signs—*Of the stone:* Little abdominal tenderness; loin tenderness is common. Haematuria (macro or micro). *Of the cause of the stone*, eg corneal opicities from chronic hypercalcaemia (whose cause may itself have signs, eg a parathyroid adenoma ± associated multiple endocrine neoplasia, p546).

Stone prevalence: 0.2%. *Peak age:* 20–50yrs. ♂:♀ ≈ 4:1. *Risk factors:* Low urine output; hypercalciuria, hyperoxaluria; hypocitraturia, hyperuricosuria.

Tests—*MSU:* RBC? UTI? protein? pH? (abnormal crystals usually occur in acid urine; if alkaline, significance is dubious as phosphates crystallize out); if morning urine pH 5.3–6.8, renal tubular acidosis is unlikely.

24h urine for oxalate, Ca^{2+}, creatinine and urate while on usual diet.

Plain abdominal films: ('KUB'—kidneys + ureters + bladder). 90% of renal stones are radio-opaque. Look along the line of the ureters for calcium that may represent a stone.

Blood: U&E, urate, Ca^{2+}, PO_4^{3-}, bicarbonate, and total protein/albumin.

Imaging: IVU; MRI/CT if renal failure precludes IVU.

Management of acute renal colic ►*Beware infection above the stone.*
- Pain relief: diclofenac 75mg IM or 100mg PR or morphine 10mg IM. (NSAIDs are effective and avoid problems with opiate misusers, but they ↓renal blood flow, so monitor renal function while on these drugs.)
- Increase fluid intake.
- Sieve all urine to catch the stone for analysis—or use a chamber pot, Prepare the patient's mind to hear 'the tinkle in the pot like far-away chimes'[1]—triumphantly sounding the vindication of your diagnosis.

Most stones pass spontaneously. If there is any hint of obstruction or infection (fever, pyuria), seek urological help urgently. Procedures include:
- Antegrade nephrostomy (p372) and percutaneous nephrolithotomy (for stones in the kidney or upper half of ureters). These may be combined with lithotripsy (ultrasonic dissolution) if the stone is not too close to a bone.
- Surgical removal is only occasionally required.

Prevention Drink more (>3 litres/24h), especially in summer. Reduce milk intake. For *oxalate* stones: ↓oxalate intake (no chocolate, tea, rhubarb, spinach) and ↓Ca^{2+} excretion, eg with bendrofluazide (=bendroflumethiazide) 5mg/24h PO; pyridoxine (up to 10mg/day PO) if hyperoxaluria. For *calcium phosphate* stones: thiazides, low Ca^{2+} diet. For *triple phosphate (calcium, magnesium, ammonium)* 'staghorn' stones: antibiotics. For *urate* stones: allopurinol, urinary alkalinization (pH >6.5). For *cystine* stones: vigorous hydration, D-penicillamine, urinary alkalinization (eg with sodium bicarbonate 5–10g/24h PO in water).

---

1 Graham Greene 1957 *Under the Garden*, Penguin

When a patient presents you with a stone, ask:

- *What is its composition?* In order of frequency, the likely answer is:
  - —Calcium oxalate stones: these are spiky   (radio-opaque)
  - —Calcium phosphate stones are smooth and big   (radio-opaque)
  - —Triple phosphate staghorn stone: big; horny   (radio-opaque)
    seen with *proteus* UTI with urinary stasis + ↑pH
  - —Urate; xanthine (smooth, brown, and soft)   (radio-lucent)
  - —Cystine stones are yellow and crystalline   (semi-opaque)
- *Why has he or she got this stone now?*
  - —'*What do you eat?*' Chocolate, tea, rhubarb, spinach ↑oxalate levels.
  - —*Is it summer?* Seasonal variations in calcium and oxalate levels are
    thought to be mediated by vitamin D synthesis *via* sunlight on skin.
  - —'*What's your job?*' Can he/she drink freely? ►Is there dehydration?
  - —'*Do you have any predisposing illnesses/drugs?*' In order of likelihood:
    - -Hypercalciuria/hypercalcaemia (p644, eg hyperparathyroidism,
      sarcoid, neoplasia, Addison's, Cushing's, T3↑, Li⁺, vit. D excess)
    - -Medullary sponge kidney
    - -UTI (predisposes to calcium phosphate and staghorn calculi)
    - -Cystinuria
    - -Renal tubular acidosis
    - -Primary or secondary hyperoxaluria
    - -Nephrocalcinosis
    - -Gout and a raised plasma urate (see *OTM* 3e 3254)
    - -Alkali loss from gut, eg with ileostomy (risk of uric acid stones↑)
    - -Aminoacidurias
    - -Syndromes: *Sjögren's*; *Lesch–Nyhan* (IQ↓, motor delay, head banging)
- *Is there a family history?* x-linked nephrolithiasis, or Dent's disease:
  low molecular weight proteinuria, hypercalciuria, nephrocalcinosis?[1]
- *Is there infection above the stone?* Fever? Loin tender? Pyuria?

1 Grand round 1996 *Lancet* **348** 1561

✚ Urinary tract obstruction

▶*Is the bladder palpable?* (See urinary retention, p134.) This is so important, and quite easy to get wrong. If in doubt, ask a colleague, or catheterize the bladder and measure the volume it contains.

▶*Think of urinary tract obstruction whenever renal function worsens.* Always exclude by ultrasound. Beware infection *above* obstruction.

Obstruction may be bilateral if below the level of the ureter or unilateral if ureteric. The latter may remain clinically silent for a long time as long as the other kidney is functioning. Obstructing lesions may be *in the lumen* (eg stones), *in the wall* (eg tumours), or *impinging from outside* (any abdominal mass, or retroperitoneal fibrosis, see below).

Bilateral obstruction *Causes:* Urethral stricture, urethral valves, prostatic hypertrophy, bladder tumours, clots, calculi, pelvic malignancy, retroperitoneal fibrosis (below).
Presentation: Lower abdominal pain (eg with retention), renal impairment, urinary infection, overflow incontinence.

Unilateral obstruction *Causes:* Calculi, tumours, pelvi-ureteric junction (PUJ) obstruction, retroperitoneal fibrosis, compression by lymph nodes, impaction of sloughed papilla.
Presentation: Loin ache, worsened by drinking; a mass; UTI.

Tests Check U&E and creatinine and urine pH (p398). Do ultrasound next. It assesses bladder and kidney size and any hydronephrosis (renal pelvis dilation). IVU is also useful (p372) with plain films for calculi. Antegrade pyelography assesses the site of obstruction and allows sampling of urine and insertion of nephrostomy tubes. Retrograde pyelograms are performed at cystoscopy (risks of introducing infection).

Treatment Relieve obstruction (eg by catheter or nephrostomy tube). Treat the cause. Beware a large diuresis after relief of obstruction—a temporary salt-losing nephropathy may occur involving litres a day. Dehydration and hypokalaemia may occur. Careful monitoring of urine output, weight, and regular electrolytes is necessary.

Retroperitoneal fibrosis (RPF)

In this condition, the ureters are embedded in a dense, fibrous plaque. The term chronic periaortitis is sometimes used as a synonym with RPF, but this seems an unnecessary proliferation of terms.

The Patient is typically a middle-aged man, presenting with backache, fever, malaise, sweating, leg oedema, hypertension, palpable mass, pyuria—or chronic or acute obstructive renal failure. Associated with drugs (methysergide), carcinoma, Crohn's disease, connective tissue diseases, Raynaud's and fibrotic diseases (eg mediastinitis, alveolitis).

Diagnosis IVU showing dilated ureters with medial deviation of the ureters, followed by high-grade retroperitoneal imaging (MRI, CT). Biopsy—periaortic inflammation with lymphocyte and plasma cell infiltrate.

Cause Mostly unknown. Consider lymphoma or drugs (methysergide). Aortic aneurysms may set up a fibrotic inflammatory reaction.

Treatment The options are antegrade nephrostomies to relieve obstruction, plus steroids; or surgery (wrap the ureters in omentum). Consider steroids.

Glomerular disease

Renal disease may be classified by clinical syndrome, pathology, or by cause. The pathology of glomerulonephritis (GN) is complex. Important terms are *focal* (some of the glomeruli affected) versus *diffuse* (all affected), and *segmental* (part of each glomerulus affected) versus *global*. Analysis involves light microscopy (LM), electron microscopy (EM), and immunofluorescence (IF) for immunoglobulin (Ig) and complement.

1 **Minimal change GN** Typically a child presenting with nephrotic syndrome. *Histology:* LM normal; IF negative; EM: fused podocytes. There is a weak association with Hodgkin's disease.

2 **Membranous GN** Accounts for 30% of adult nephrotic syndrome. *Histology:* LM—thickened BM; IF—IgG and C3; EM—subepithelial deposits. There may be underlying malignancy in up to 10% of adults. *Prognosis:* 25% enter remission but ~50% progress to CRF in 10 years.

3 **Focal segmental glomerulosclerosis** *Presentation:* Proteinuria or nephrotic syndrome. *Histology:* focal sclerosis with hyaline deposits; other glomeruli may be normal; IF—IgM and C3. Seen with heroin abuse. *Prognosis:* >50% progress to CRF. Usually steroid resistant.

4 **Membranoproliferative GN (mesangiocapillary)** 50% present as nephrotic syndrome. Some have low C3. *Histology:* LM—cellular expansion of the mesangium. Basement membranes (BM) appear split, producing 'tram-tracks'; EM—2 types: *1* subendothelial deposits and *2* deposits within the basement membrane. Associations: shunt nephritis, endocarditis, mixed essential cryoglobulinaemia, partial lipodystrophy, C3-nephritic factor (a circulating autoantibody), and measles.

5 **Proliferative GN** Classically seen 2 weeks after a *Strep.* infection. ↓C3. *Histology:* LM—proliferation of endothelial and mesangial cells with neutrophils; IF—IgG and C3; EM—subepithelial deposits. *Prognosis:* Excellent.

6 **IgA disease (Berger's disease)** common cause of recurrent haematuria in young men. *Histology:* IF: IgA and C3. Similar picture seen in Henoch–Schönlein purpura (HSP). 30% progress to CRF. See p694.

7 **Rapidly progressive GN—RPGN (=crescentic GN)** *Presentation:* Haematuria, oliguria, hypertension, ARF. *Histology:* Hypercellularity; crescents in >60% of glomeruli; EM and IF variable but typically subepithelial IgG and C3. Vigorous treatment may save renal function: high-dose (pulse) steroids (1g methylprednisolone IV), cyclophosphamide ± plasma exchange. *Associations:* Anti-GBM antibodies, Wegener's, microscopic polyarteritis, Henoch–Schönlein purpura, poststreptococcal infection (rare).

Glomerulonephritis tests ●*Urine microscopy:* RBC casts ± dysmorphic RBC.
●*Urine:* 24h protein excretion and creatinine clearance.
●*Serum:* U&E, FBC, ESR, CRP, albumin, ANA, antineutrophil cytoplasmic antibody (ANCA, p675), DNA-binding, complement (C3, C4), ASO titre, HBsAg.
●*Culture:* Blood, throat, ear if otitis, skin if cellulitis.
●*Radiology:* CXR, renal ultrasound, IVU. ●*Renal biopsy.*

Management Refer *promptly* to renal centre for biopsy and evaluation. ►*Always know the BP. Keep it < 145/90mmHg to minimize progression.* Consider antithrombotic and infection prophylaxis in severe nephrosis. Minimal change usually responds to prednisolone, but may relapse when the dose is reduced. If no response to prednisolone, consider cyclophosphamide or cyclosporin (=ciclosporin, p622). Prognosis in membranous GN is variable. Monitor, and if renal function deteriorates, consider chlorambucil and steroids (Ponticelli regimen). Focal segmental GN is difficult to treat but may respond to steroids, cyclophosphamide, or cyclosporin. GN of any type related to SLE or vasculitis may respond to steroids or immunosuppressants. GN related to infection may respond to treatment of that infection. There is no evidence that specific treatment affects the course of: membranoproliferative GN, proliferative GN, or IgA disease.

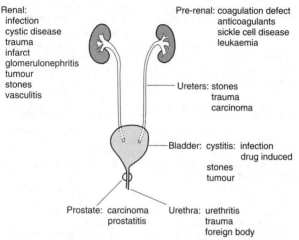

Renal:
infection
cystic disease
trauma
infarct
glomerulonephritis
tumour
stones
vasculitis

Pre-renal: coagulation defect
anticoagulants
sickle cell disease
leukaemia

Ureters: stones
trauma
carcinoma

Bladder: cystitis: infection
drug induced
stones
tumour

Prostate: carcinoma
prostatitis

Urethra: urethritis
trauma
foreign body

Causes of haematuria

The nephrotic syndrome

Essence Proteinuria (>3g/24h) causing hypoalbuminaemia and oedema, often with hypercholesterolaemia. It may be due to loss of –ve charge of the basement membrane ± increased pore size. Nephrotic kidneys retain salt and water—once believed to be from stimulation of the renin-angiotensin-aldosterone system by presumed hypovolaemia caused by capillary leakage (oncotic pressure↓ from hypoalbuminaemia). However, plasma volume may be *increased*, and there is no simple relation between renin concentration and salt retention in many patients.[1]

Presentation Insidious swelling of eyelids, ascites and peripheral oedema. Urine froth due to protein. *Nephrotic crisis:* Unwell, with gross oedema, anorexia, vomiting, pleural effusions and muscle wasting.

Causes 1 Minimal change GN (p380, 90% of children and 30% of adults). 2 Membranous GN. 3 Membranoproliferative GN. 4 Focal segmental glomerulosclerosis. 5 Others: diabetes mellitus, amyloid, neoplasia (<10% of adults with membranous GN) especially lymphoma/carcinoma, endocarditis, PAN, SLE, sickle-cell, malaria, drugs (penicillamine, gold).

Tests *Urine:* 24h specimen for creatinine clearance and protein. Microscopy for RBCs and casts. *Blood:* U&E, albumin, cholesterol, FBC, ESR, CRP, Ig level, protein strip, ANA, DNA-binding, C4, C3, ANCA (p675). *Renal biopsy:* not indicated in a child unless complicated (BP↑ or haematuria) or failure to respond to treatment.

Treatment (For children and the rôle of steroids, see OHCS p282)
- Take time to discuss issues of body-image and the fear of renal failure.
- Bed rest to stimulate diuresis.
- Restrict fluids (1–1.5 L/day). Daily U&E + weight. Aim to lose 1kg/day.
- Monitor BP often. Treat hypertension with conventional regimens (p302).
- Salt-restricted (~50mmol/day) + highish protein diet (unproven benefit—aim for ~1g/kg/24h of mainly first class protein[2]).
- Frusemide (=furosemide) 40–80mg PO + amiloride as K⁺-sparing agent; diuretics relieve oedema but do not treat the underlying disorder. Beware IV diuretics as patients are often volume-depleted and you may precipitate pre-renal failure. Generally give IV diuretics only with IV plasma protein (salt poor), at least till diuresis is established.
- In those refractory to treatment, a 'medical nephrectomy' (using ACE inhibitors and NSAIDs) may need to be considered: for experts only.
- Consider anticoagulation (see below).

Complications 1 Thrombo-embolism (from urinary loss of antithrombin III, low plasma volume, ↑clotting factors II, V, VII, VIII and X). 2 Infection (pneumococcal peritonitis—consider pneumococcal vaccination if nephrotic state persists, p332). 3 Hypercholesterolaemia (atherosclerosis, xanthomata—consider treatment, p654). 4 Hypovolaemia and renal failure. 5 Loss of specific binding proteins (eg transferrin, presenting as iron-resistant hypochromic anaemia).

Renal vein thrombosis This occurs in 15–20% of those with nephrosis, 30% of patients with membranous GN, and acute dehydration.
Presentation: There may be no symptoms or mild abdominal or back pain. Others develop severe pain and loin tenderness. Suspect if there is unexplained loss of renal function with RBC in the urine.
Diagnosis: MRI, Doppler, or renal arteriogram (venous phase).
Treatment: Anticoagulate. Streptokinase may be used to lyse acute thromboses. Pulmonary thrombo-embolism may occur.

---

1 L Baker & J Vande Walle 1995 *Lancet* 346 133 &148 2 *OTM*-3e 1996

✛ Acute renal failure (ARF)—diagnosis

Essence Deterioration in renal function occurring over hours or days. There may be no symptoms or signs, but oliguria (urine volume <400mL/24h) is common. ARF is detected by a rising plasma urea and creatinine. This is a major reason for checking U&Es in an acutely ill person. If both are acutely raised, diagnose ARF: if urea greatly raised out of proportion to creatinine consider dehydration or hypercatabolic state, eg due to fever. ARF kills because of raised potassium, therefore this needs urgent treatment (p386). **Incidence** 180/million/year. ▣

Assessment Although acute tubular necrosis (ATN) is the usual cause, it is vital not to jump to this diagnosis. Systematic assessment is needed:
1. *Is the renal failure acute or chronic?* Suspect chronic renal failure if:
   - Previous blood tests show that abnormalities are not acute (look in notes or contact GP or laboratory's patient database).
   - History of ill health (eg for the last few months).
   - Ultrasound shows small kidneys.

Neither anaemia nor abnormal serum Ca^{2+} and phosphate help distinguish ARF from CRF, as these changes can occur within days of renal failure.

2. *Is there renal tract obstruction?* (Seen in 5% of ARF.) Obstruction must be treated quickly to prevent permanent kidney damage. Obstruction is suggested by haematuria + evidence of stones (renal colic, loin pain, passage of a stone) or 'prostatism' (p52); previous pelvic surgery; or anuria. Examine for a palpable bladder, and an enlarged prostate gland, or any abnormal masses (do vaginal and rectal exam). Do not expect to palpate the kidneys *per abdomen*: they do not enlarge from acute obstruction.

3. *Is there a rare cause of ARF?* Always consider glomerulonephritis (see p380) if there is no history suggesting ATN (see below) or obvious obstruction. A rare cause is more likely if the urine contains protein, blood or casts: here, refer urgently to a renal physician for biopsy and treatment (which may involve steroids and cytotoxic agents).

4. *Now consider acute tubular necrosis (ATN)* Over 80% of ARF is due to ATN. This results from renal ischaemia caused by circulatory compromise, eg frank shock or postural hypotension/dizziness? Risk factors for these are: old age; drugs (NSAIDs, ACE inhibitors, aminoglycosides); sepsis.
On examination: Postural hypotension; JVP↓. Signs are dominated by the disease causing the ATN—with signs of volume depletion (postural hypotension, dehydration) or overload (pulmonary oedema; BP↑). There are no reliable signs or symptoms of renal failure, except perhaps the Kussmaul breathing (p48) of acidosis—if DM has been excluded.

Tests ●Urgent urine microscopy: RBC or RBC casts suggest GN (refer to nephrologist); haem +ve but no RBC suggests myoglobinuria (p394) or haemoglobinuria; lack of casts, cells, and minimal protein suggests pre-renal. ●Urine electrolytes (especially urea). ●Blood: U&E, creatinine, blood cultures, blood gases, FBC; when diagnosis uncertain consider eg C3/C4, ANA, DNA binding (p672), ANCA (p675), ASO titre, Bence Jones protein (p614) in urine. ●ECG. ●CXR. ●Renal ultrasound. ●Daily weight.

Urinary indices distinguishing pre-renal and renal causes of oliguria Causes of ARF are often classified as *pre-renal* (eg volume depletion), *renal* (eg ATN), or *post-renal* (eg urinary tract obstruction). It is often said that pre-renal causes are suggested by a urine osmolality of >500mosmol/kg, and a urine-to-serum creatinine ratio (USCR) of >40 (<350mosmol/kg and USCR <20 for renal causes). This classification is of limited use because pre-renal causes lead to renal causes, and biochemistry is often indeterminant—and the results do not affect management.

⁙ Acute renal failure (ARF)—management

►Seek specialist help earlier rather than later.

1. Treat precipitating cause Treat acute blood loss with blood transfusion, and sepsis with antibiotics (p182). ARF is often associated with other diseases which need more urgent treatment. For example, someone in respiratory failure *and* renal failure may need to be managed on ITU, not a renal unit, to ensure optimum management of the respiratory failure.

2. Treat life-threatening hyperkalaemia The danger is that the heart stops. K^+ >6.5mmol/L will usually need urgent treatment, as will those with ECG changes: tall 'tented' T-waves, decreased P-wave; increased P–R interval, and widening of the QRS complex—leading eventually, and dangerously, to a sinusoidal pattern. Give:
- 10mL calcium gluconate (10%) IV over 2 minutes, repeated as necessary if severe ECG changes. This provides cardio-protection.
- Insulin + glucose. Insulin moves K^+ into cells. Aim for a decrease in serum K^+ of 1–2mmol/L in 30mins, eg: 20u soluble insulin + 50mL of glucose 50% IV.
- Calcium resonium enema to remove K^+ from the body. Prescribe a laxative to prevent constipation.

These are temporary treatments: dialysis may be the only long-term remedy.

3. Treat pulmonary oedema, pericarditis, and tamponade (p768) Urgent dialysis may be needed. If in pulmonary oedema, and no diuresis, consider removing a unit of blood, before dialysis commences.

4. Treat volume depletion if necessary. Resuscitate quickly; then match input to output. Use a large-bore IV line in a large vein (central vein as access is risky in obvious volume depletion).
- Give fluid (blood, colloid, saline, *not* dextrose) as fast as possible until signs of fluid depletion go (JVP visible, no postural BP drop); *then stop fluids.*
- Further fluid depends on urine output (eg output volume + 1 litre/day).

5. Other aspects of care
- Catheterize to assess hourly urine output, and to establish fluid charts.
- If oliguric, 24h fluid maintenance=24h urine output + allowance for any diarrhoea or vomiting + 500mL for insensible losses (more if feverish).
- If oliguric, try frusemide (=furosemide) 40mg–1g IV (slowly; can cause deafness) a 'renal' dose of dopamine (2–5µg/kg/min IVI; SE on p110).
- If clinical suspicion of sepsis, take cultures, then treat vigorously with appropriate antibiotics (p182), doses may need adjusting, see p177–181).
- Do not leave possible sources of sepsis (eg IV lines) *in situ* if not needed.
- Consider H2 agonists (eg ranitidine 150mg/12h PO) as risk of GI bleeding↑.
- Avoid nephrotoxic drugs, eg NSAIDs, ACE inhibitors, care with gentamicin. Check *Data Sheet* for all drugs given.

Further care ●Has obstruction been excluded? ►Examine for masses PR and *per vaginam*; arrange urgent ultrasound; is the bladder palpable? Bilateral nephrostomies relieve obstruction, provide urine for culture, and allow anterograde pyelography to determine the site of obstruction.
- If worsening renal function but dialysis independent, consider renal biopsy.
- Diet: high in calories (2000–4000kcal/day) with adequate high-quality protein. Consider nasogastric feeding or parenteral route if too ill.

Prognosis Depends on cause; (ATN mortality: surgery or trauma—60%, medical illness—30%, pregnancy—10%). Oliguric ARF is worse than non-oliguric—more GI bleeds, sepsis, acidosis and higher mortality.

Urgent dialysis if: ●K^+ persistently high (>6.0mmol/L). ●Acidosis (pH <7.2). ●Pulmonary oedema and no substantial diuresis. ●Pericarditis. (In tamponade (p768), only dialyse *after* pressure on the heart is relieved.) ●High catabolic state with rapidly progressive renal failure.

Acute peritoneal dialysis[1]

Acute peritoneal dialysis is rarely used in richer countries since acute renal failure is treated by haemodialysis. However, it has a place in the treatment of acute renal failure when dialysis is unavailable. Learn the technique from an experienced operator.

The aim is to replace or augment kidney function by using the peritoneal lining as a semipermeable membrane. You put fluid in, and osmosis ensures that 'poisons' flow from high concentrations in the tissues to low concentrations in the fluid that you have put in. There is a run-in time, a time of dwelling, and an outflow time.

Technique The following is an *aide-mémoire*.
- Make sure the bladder is empty. It may be necessary to confirm this by catheterization, or ultrasound.
- Shave lower part of the abdomen; sterile drapes. Don mask and gloves.
- Make sure you have a 1 litre dialysis bag (eg 1.36% dextrose—a higher concentration if there is fluid overload) to hand with an IV cannula and giving set. The fluid must be pre-warmed to 37°C (44°C if the aim is to correct hypothermia).
- Choose the insertion point, usually 2–3cm below the umbilicus in the midline. Clean the skin. Infiltrate down to the peritoneum with 1% lignocaine (=lidocaine). Aspirate as you go. If you aspirate air or bowel fluid you have gone too far. Choose another site.
- Insert an IVI cannula into the peritoneal cavity and use the giving set to run in the dialysis fluid.
- Next insert the peritoneal dialysis catheter though a small vertical skin incision (use a small scalpel). Make sure that the catheter's bend is such that it is not lying up against the anterior abdominal wall. (The direction of the curve is indicated by a mark.) After ~⅔ of the catheter has been inserted, withdraw the obturator, and put in the rest of the catheter (except for the last few cm).
- Use a purse-string suture (3-0 silk) to anchor the catheter. Use tape to ensure that everything is thoroughly secure.
- You are now ready to start exchanging the fluid—eg hourly (⅓ run-in time, ⅓ dwell time, and ⅓ outflow time).
- Monitor TPR and BP every 4h.
- Check plasma glucose and U&E frequently (eg every 12–8h—more frequently, eg hourly, when fluid is being run in and out quickly, as during the treatment of hypothermia).
- If K^+ <3.5mmol/L, add K^+ to dialysis fluid. Aim for plasma K^+ of 4mmol/L.
- Weigh patient daily; weigh bags before attaching them, and on refill.
- At the end of the procedure calculate how much fluid has been retained (½–1 litre is usual).

Complications U&E awry; peritonitis (may respond to intraperitoneal vancomycin + gentamicin or ceftazidime; seek expert help). Take aerobic and anaerobic culture of the exiting dialysis fluid (into blood culture bottles). Antibiotics will need to be continued for ~5 days after the exiting fluid is clear of pus.

1 D Sprigings 1995 *Acute Medicine* 2e, Blackwell Science, ISBN 0-632-03652-4

Chronic renal failure (CRF)

►Why has the patient presented now? Is there anything reversible?

Causes—*Common:* Glomerulonephritis, chronic pyelonephritis, DM, urinary tract obstruction, polycystic kidneys, hypertension.

Others: Amyloid, myeloma, SLE, PAN, gout, Ca^{2+}↑, interstitial nephritis.

Ask about: Family history (polycystic kidneys), *UTIs, drugs,* especially analgesics.

Symptoms Nausea, anorexia, lethargy, itch, nocturia, impotence. *Later*—oedema, dyspnoea, chest pain (from pericarditis), vomiting, confusion, fits, hiccups, neuropathy, coma. **Signs** Pallor, 'lemon-tinge' to skin (rarely uraemic 'frost' on skin), pulmonary or peripheral oedema, pericarditis (± tamponade), pleural effusions, metabolic flap (tremor), hypertension, retinopathy (diabetes mellitus, BP↑), metastatic calcification.

Tests •*Urine:* Microscopy/culture, 24h urinary protein and creatinine clearance (p632). •*Blood:* U&E, glucose, Ca^{2+}↑, PO_4^{3-}↑, PTH↑, urate↑ (may be primary or secondary to CRF), protein, FBC, ESR, protein electrophoresis. •*Radiology:* Renal ultrasound for renal size (typically small; big if: obstructed, DM, polycystic, amyloid or myeloma) and to rule out obstruction. X-ray bones, especially hands, for renal osteodystrophy, ie faulty bone remodelling due to renal failure-induced osteomalacia or osteitis fibrosa from secondary hyperparathyroidism + dihydroxycholecalciferol deficiency (its hallmark is marrow fibrosis with increased osteoclast activity reflected by excess osteoid and non-lamellar bone[ᴹ]). Consider IVU, DMSA, DTPA scan (p734), retrograde pyelography (p372). •*Renal biopsy:* Consider this if renal size is normal.

Treatment Refer to renal unit for early assessment. Dialysis may be needed for symptomatic relief when GFR <5% of normal (p390).
- Treat reversible causes: relieve obstruction, no nephrotoxic drugs (aminoglycosides, cefalosporin with frusemide/furosemide, NSAIDs), treat ↑Ca^{2+}.
- Monitor and treat ↑BP. This may slow decline in renal function.
- Diet advice: adequate calories, vitamins, and iron. Salt restrict (0.5g/kg/day) if ↑BP. Protein restriction may slow progression if proteinuria.
- Preparation of access for dialysis, eg Cimino fistulae or insertion of Tenchkoff catheter, before dialysis required.
- Anaemia due to CRF will respond to erythropoietin (p574) unless sepsis is present. Treat any iron deficiency first. Consider other anaemias.
- Renal bone disease: treat early, as soon as PTH raised. Lower PO_4^{3-} (aim 0.6–1.4mmol/L) by reducing dietary intake (restrict milk, cheese, eggs) and giving phosphate binders (eg calcium carbonate 300–1200mg/8h PO). Avoid aluminium hydroxide as it may cause aluminium accumulation with encephalopathy and osteomalacia-type bone disease. Use vitamin D analogues (alfacalcidol 0.25–1µg/24h PO) and Ca^{2+} supplements *after* PO_4^{3-} lowered to reduce risk of metastatic calcification.
- Pre-transplant work-up: blood group and tissue type. Is there a related donor? Consider pre-transplant immunization.
- Miscellaneous: greatest mortality in CRF is from cardiovascular disease. Treat hypertension (p302) and hyperlipidaemia (p654). Hiccups: try chlorpromazine 25mg/8h PO. Oedema may need high doses of diuretics, eg frusemide (=furosemide) 250mg–2g/day + metolazone 5–10mg/day).

Renoprotection to prevent further loss of renal function Even a small BP drop in a hypertensive patient may save significant renal function.[1] ACE-i (p299) can ↓rate of loss of function even if BP ↔, eg if there is proteinuria (>3g/day). But beware: not *all* patients with nephropathy need ACE-i, and they may be catastrophic in renovascular CRF. If the cause is polycystic disease, or the patient has the DD genotype for the ACE gene, there is little evidence of benefit.[2] How well ACE inhibitors reduce proteinuria in the short-term is a good way of predicting long-term renoprotection.[2]

1 G Navis 1997 *Lancet* 349 1852   2 The REIN study from the GISEN group 1997 *Lancet* 349 1857

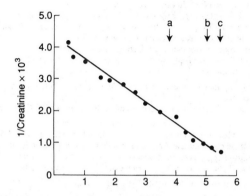

Some patients with CRF lose their renal function (ie GFR) at a constant rate. Creatinine is produced at a fairly constant rate and rises on a hyperbolic curve as renal function declines. The reciprocal creatinine plot is thus a straight line, parallel to the fall in GFR. This is widely used to monitor renal function and to predict when end-stage renal failure requiring dialysis will occur. Rapid decline in renal function greater than that expected may be due to: infection, dehydration, uncontrolled ↑BP, metabolic disturbance (eg Ca^{2+}↑), obstruction, nephrotoxins (injudicious use of drugs). Careful investigation and treatment at this point may delay end-stage renal failure.

Dialysis and transplantation

(See p386–p387 for indications for urgent dialysis, and technique.)

Haemodialysis (HD) Blood flows opposite dialysis fluid and substances are cleared down concentration gradient across a semipermeable membrane.

Problems:
- Infection (HIV, hepatitis, bacteria). ●U&E imbalance. ●BP↓.
- Vascular access (bleeding, thrombi, infection, vascular insufficiency).
- Dialysis arthropathy (amyloid formation especially in shoulders and wrists—due to accumulation of β_2-microglobulin).
- Aluminium toxicity (dementia ± a bone disease similar to osteomalacia, so use aluminium-free dialysis fluid and avoid aluminium-containing phosphate binders. Expense is also a frequent problem.

Out-patient follow-up: Check dietary concordance (p3), including vitamins (iron, B complex, C), general health. Examine dialysis site, BP, JVP, weight, oedema. Check: FBC, U&E, creatinine, Ca^{2+}, albumin, PO_4^{3-}, lipids.

Haemofiltration Used continuously eg in ITU for treatment of acute renal failure. Blood is filtered across a semipermeable membrane allowing removal of small molecules, and replacement fluid equivalent in volume to filtrate is infused (eg 1 litre/h). It is easy to use and causes smaller fluid shifts so fewer hypotensive episodes. Achieves good clearance values.

Intermittent peritoneal dialysis (IPD) See p387.

Continuous ambulatory peritoneal dialysis (CAPD) A permanent catheter is inserted into the peritoneum via a subcutaneous tunnel. Up to 2 litres of dialysate is introduced and kept within the peritoneum at all times. This is exchanged for fresh fluid up to 5 times a day. The patient is not tied to a machine and uraemic anaemia is less than with HD. *Contraindications:* No peritoneal space due to previous abdominal surgery; patient unable to use hands. *Problems:* Peritonitis (usually Staph, Strep, or coliforms—add antibiotics to the dialysate), catheter blockage (adhesions and fibrin—try urokinase into the catheter), weight gain, poor diabetic control, pleural effusion, leakage.

Renal transplantation Usually sited in an iliac fossa and so easy to biopsy. 1 year graft survival: HLA identical: 95%, 1 mismatch: 90–95%, complete mismatch 75–80%. Median cadaveric graft survival is 8y. *Acute graft rejection* (ie in first 3 months) often responds to increased immunosuppression. *Chronic rejection* presents as gradual decrease in graft function; it responds poorly to treatment. *Immunosuppressive drugs:* ●Cyclosporin (ciclosporin), eg 10mg/kg reduce to 4mg/kg after ~2weeks; monitor levels. ●Azathioprine eg 2mg/kg/day ●Steroids ●Antilymphocyte globulin.

Complications:
- Rejection.   ●Obstruction at ureteric anastamosis.
- Persistent hypertension.   ●Cyclosporin-induced nephrotoxicity.
- Atherosclerosis (renal disease and steroids).
- Renal artery stenosis (in the transplant) at 3–9 months post-op.
- Infection from immunosuppression—eg opportunists such as *Pneumocystis carinii* (give prophylactic co-trimoxazole for 6 months), CMV, fungi, bacteria. See p622 for a detailed discussion of immunosuppressives.
- Malignancy from immunosuppressives, eg squamous cell carcinomas; lymphoma.

Urinary tract malignancies

Hypernephroma (*Clear-cell adenocarcinoma* of renal tubular epithelium)
Typical age: 50yrs; ♂:♀≈2:1. *Spread:* Tumour may invade vena cava *via* renal veins; direct spread to nearby tissues and haematogenous to bone, liver and lung where 'cannon ball' secondaries may be seen on CXR: see PLATE 11.

Classical triad: Haematuria, loin pain, abdominal mass. Also: PUO (night sweats), PCV↑ in 2% (the tumour secretes erythropoietin), anaemia, hypercalcaemia and rarely left varicocele as left renal vein compressed.

Tests: Urine RBCs; CXR; ultrasound; CT scan (if contralateral kidney is functioning, IVU is not needed);[1] angiography, if partial nephrectomy (eg if solitary kidneys) or palliative embolization are being considered.[1]

Treatment: Nephrectomy. Progesterone has been tried. Metastatic disease is probably one of the few indications for immunotherapy with interleukin-2 (chemotherapy and radiotherapy are disappointing); SE include rigors (may need IV opiates), myalgia, renal failure, and the vascular leak syndrome which may require colloids and dopamine (interleukin-2 stimulates the release of tumour necrosis factor and cytokines which make vessels leak macromolecules). *Overall 5-yr survival:* 30–50%.

Other GU tumours Transitional cell (renal pelvis) 10%; lymphoma; secondaries; Wilms' nephroblastoma (OHCS p220); bladder tumours p136.

Prostatic carcinoma In 10% it is so indolent that discovery is incidental. The patient is usually elderly but younger men may have a fast-growing anaplastic variety. It is the second most common malignancy of men. Previous vasectomy may be associated with increased risk.

Spread: Bone (sclerotic or lytic lesions); direct to bladder, rectum.

The Patient: Hesitancy, frequency, dribbling; ± flow↓ indicates obstruction (unreliably); bone pain ± weight↓ if metastases. *On PR exam:* No median sulcus between lobes of prostate; nodules; mucosa stuck to prostate.

Risk: Testosterone↑, +ve family history (p684); *not* benign hypertrophy.

Tests: FBC, ESR, U&E, Ca²⁺, prostate specific antigen ≥10nmol/mL (PSA cannot predict reliably if a cancer will cause ill health, see p653; 25% of large benign prostates give PSA up to 10; levels may be influenced by recent ejaculation[3]), transrectal ultrasound, bone x-rays and scintiscan. *Outflow obstruction tests:* bladder ultrasound (residual urine volume); urine flow rates.

Treatment: Transurethral resection if obstruction. If not, and no metastases (PSA <10µg/L, if prostate size ↔; −ve pelvic lymphadenectomy) there is debate about relative merits of radical prostatectomy, radiotherapy, or watchful waiting. Nerve-sparing radical prostatectomy (maintains erectile function) is widely used in the USA;[2] no randomized trials have shown a survival advantage over other options. Monitor with serial PSAs. In metastatic disease, hormonal drugs may give much benefit for 1–2yrs.[4] Testosterone determines prostatic growth, so orchidectomy may slow tumour growth; if unacceptable offer gonadotrophin-releasing analogues, eg 12-weekly goserelin (10.8mg sc as Zoladex LA®) which first stimulates, and then inhibits pituitary gonadotrophin output. Alternatives: cyproterone 100mg/8h PO; flutamide (p556); stilboestrol (=diethylstilbestrol) 1mg/24h PO (DVT risk↑); radiotherapy. Warn that he may become impotent. See p135.

Symptomatic relief: Analgesia and radiotherapy to painful metastases.

Bone secondaries ± cord compression: Rₓ of Ca²⁺↑ (p644) ± decompression.

Prognosis: Very variable. 10% die in 6 months, but 10% live >10yrs.

Screening: PR; PSA (but ↔ in 30% of small cancers); transrectal ultrasound. Do not screen uncritically: there are big problems (OHCS p431).[5]

1 C Dawson 1996 BMJ i 1146 2 1994 NEJM 331 996 3 Bandolier 1998 49 6 4 BMJ 1994 i 780 5 Lancet 1997 349 443

Example of advice to asymptomatic men who ask for a PSA test

The prostate lies below the bladder, and surrounds the tube taking urine out. Prostate cancer is common in older men. Many men over 50 (to whom this advice applies) consider a PSA (prostate specific antigen) test on their blood to detect prostatic cancer. *Is this a good idea?*

- The test is not very accurate, and we cannot say that those having the test will live longer—even if they do turn out to have prostate cancer. This is because the cancer is often very lazy, so that, in most men with prostate cancer, death is from an unrelated cause.
- The test itself has no side-effects, provided you don't mind giving blood and time. But if the test is falsely positive, you may needlessly have more tests, such as sampling the prostate by the back passage (which may cause bleeding and infection in 1–5% of men).
- Only 1 in 3 of those with a high PSA level will have cancer.
- You may also be worried needlessly if later tests put you in the clear.
- Even if a cancer is found, there is nothing we can do to tell you for sure whether it will impinge on your health. Treatment may be recommended—and then you might end up having a bad effect from treatment which was not even needed.
- There is more bad news for those who *do* turn out to have prostate cancer: we do not even know for sure how to treat it! Options are radical surgery to remove the prostate (this treatment may be fatal itself in 0.2–0.5% of patients),[1] radiotherapy, hormones, or simple 'watching and waiting'—which is not so simple (you may become morbidly interested in your prostate, and stop feeling healthy).

Ultimately, you must decide for yourself what you want. In general, the more information we give to men the fewer opt for the test.[2]

1 revdis@york.ac.uk   2 S Woolf 1997 *BMJ* i 989

Acute nephritic syndrome

Presentation Classically 1–3 weeks after a throat, ear, or skin infection with Lancefield Group A β-haemolytic streptococcus, with haematuria (RBC ± cellular casts) +GFR↓ (acute), leading to fluid retention, oliguria, BP↑, and variable uraemia. Proteinuria is present. Common findings are: low C3, circulating mixed cryoglobulins, hypergammaglobulinaemia.

Management Risks are from hypertensive encephalopathy, pulmonary oedema and acute renal failure. Strict bed rest is unnecessary unless severely hypertensive or gross pulmonary oedema. Restrict dietary salt and fluid intake if oliguric. Give diuretics, eg frusemide (=furosemide) PO or IV) and appropriate antihypertensive treatment. Give a course of penicillin to eradicate residual infection. Acute renal failure may require dialysis. Steroids and cytotoxic drugs not indicated. Prognosis is excellent in children. In adults, moderate proteinuria ± urinary sediments may persist. Developing rapidly-progressive glomerulonephritis and chronic renal failure in weeks/months is rare.

Interstitial nephritis

This is an important cause of acute and chronic renal failure. It is associated with inflammatory cell infiltration mostly affecting the renal interstitium and tubules. In acute renal failure, the cause is usually an idiosyncratic reaction to drugs (eg penicillin, NSAIDs, frusemide/furosemide). In chronic renal failure, the cause is usually unknown, but is occasionally: drugs, sickle-cell disease, analgesic nephropathy (see below).

Acute interstitial nephritis is often due to drugs (eg antibiotics, NSAIDs, diuretics) or infections (Staphs, Streps, brucella, leptospira).

Presentation: Renal failure, T°↑, arthralgia, eosinophiluria/eosinophilia.

Diagnosis: This is confirmed by renal biopsy.

Treatment: In ARF: regimen on p386, and corticosteroids. Prognosis: favourable. In CRF: no specific treatment—expect gradual deterioration.

Myoglobinuria

Myoglobin (a muscle protein) can appear in the urine if there is muscle injury or necrosis (rhabdomyolysis), eg crush injury, exercise, trauma, burns, electric shock, coma, sepsis (eg legionella), seizures, ecstasy poisoning (p795), systemic envenoming (p795), or hypokalaemia. Myoglobinuria is often symptomless but can cause acute renal failure (ARF), possibly by tubular damage/blockage. *Diagnosis:* Urine is dark brown. Ward urine tests are +ve for blood but there are no RBCs on microscopy. Look for urine myoglobin in the first 48h. Serum PO_4^{3-}↑↑, urate↑, CK↑, aldolase↑, Ca^{2+}↓ If ARF develops there will be expected biochemical profile (p384) but K^+ and PO_4^{3-} may be ↑↑ if there is massive tissue breakdown. *Treatment:* Mannitol is often recommended (eg 12.5g loading dose then 2g/h IV—but do a smaller test dose first: 200mg/kg slowly IV), and alkalinization of urine with IV bicarbonate. Dialysis or haemofiltration may be required.

Analgesic nephropathy

Prolonged heavy use of analgesics (usually compound) can produce analgesic nephropathy. Incidence has been greatly reduced since phenacetin withdrawal. Other NSAIDs (including aspirin and ibuprofen) may give an interstitial nephritis-like picture. In addition there is an increased incidence of UTI. Frank haematuria should lead one to suspect carcinoma of the renal pelvis, a known association.

Diabetic nephropathy

DM is a common cause of renal failure and ~25% of diabetics diagnosed before age 30yrs develop chronic renal failure. Diabetics are prone to atherosclerosis, UTIs, and papillary necrosis, but glomerular lesions cause
396 most problems, eg from basement membrane thickening and glomerulosclerosis. It may be diffuse or nodular (Kimmelstiel–Wilson lesion). Early on, glomerular filtration rate is elevated (kidney size↑). The principal feature of diabetic nephropathy is proteinuria. This starts slowly with intermittent microalbuminuria (p532), progressing to constant proteinuria and occasionally nephrotic syndrome. Do not pay too much attention to a single test for microalbuminaemia: look for a urine albumin/creatinine ratio >2.5mg/mmol on ≥2 samples. Once proteinuria is established, there is usually a delay before gradual, irreversible ↓in GFR.

Treatment: Scrupulous metabolic control may reduce elevated GFR and microalbuminuria but has little effect on established proteinuria. A low-protein diet may slow the declining GFR. BP↑ worsens diabetic glomerulopathy, and its treatment reduces microalbuminuria, and delays the onset of renal failure—renal failure is predicted by microalbuminuria provided the duration of diabetes mellitus is <15yrs (if >15yrs, microalbuminuria is not predictive). ACE inhibitors (eg enalapril 20mg/day PO, p299) reduce microalbuminuria and may slow progression to CRF even in if normotensive (but be cautious: there may be unsuspected renovascualr disease; watch creatinine). Many will come to dialysis or transplantation and the prognosis is now quite good, but limited if extensive arteriopathy.

Adult polycystic kidney disease

Autosomal dominant condition (genes on chromosome 16 [PKD-1] and 4 [PKD-2, 4q13–q23]) which is a major cause of CRF. Cysts develop anywhere in the kidney, causing gradual decline in renal function. *Prevalence:* 1:1000. *Presentation:* Haematuria, UTI, abdominal mass, lumbar and abdominal pain, hypertension. Associations: aneurysms of intracerebral arteries; subarachnoid haemorrhage; mitral valve prolapse (p306). Examination reveals bilateral, irregular, abdominal masses (~30% may have cysts in the liver or pancreas) and BP↑. Note: PKD-2 type is less severe than PKD-1. *Tests:* Urea↑. Hb↑. Ultrasound (or IVU): large kidneys with multiple cysts. *Treatment* is supportive. Control infection and BP. Some will need dialysis and transplantation. Check family members, although cysts may not be identified with certainty in patients <30 years old.

Infantile polycystic kidney disease (autosomal recessive): OHCS p220.

Medullary sponge kidney

Essence Dilatation of renal collecting tubules. *Presentation* UTIs, nephrolithiasis, gross or microscopic haematuria. Sometimes there is a family history. *Diagnosis* is confirmed by IVU which demonstrates the dilated tubules (1–7.5mm diameter) with contrast medium appearing in the renal papillae. Associated stones may be seen in the renal collecting system but are frequently present within the deformed ducts. *Association with nephrolithiasis:* Medullary sponge kidney has been found to be present in 12% of men and 19% of women presenting with calcium renal stones who do not have predisposing metabolic abnormalities.

Nephrocalcinosis

This is deposition of calcium in the kidney, seen as calcification on plain x-rays. It is usually medullary and may cause symptoms of UTI or stones (p376). Causes of *medullary nephrocalcinosis:* hyperparathyroidism, and distal renal tubular acidosis; rarely medullary sponge kidney, idiopathic calciuria, papillary necrosis, oxalosis. *Cortical calcification* is rare (<5%) and follows serious renal disease eg cortical necrosis or chronic glomerulonephritis.

Vascular disease and renal failure

Renal artery stenosis *Cause:* Atheroma or, in the young, fibromuscular hyperplasia. *Effects:* Hypertension; if bilateral or extensive, renal failure may be caused by dehydration, hypotension or ACE-inhibitors. GFR is maintained by angiotensin II, and renal scanning after captopril shows that GFR is much lowered. *Diagnostic pointers:* Vascular disease elsewhere; severe or drug-resistant hypertension; abdominal bruit; urea↑; proteinuria. *Treatment:* Percutaneous renal angioplasty or bypass surgery.[1]

Haemolytic–uraemic syndrome (HUS) and thrombotic thrombocytopenic purpura (TTP). These may be ends of a spectrum of the same disorder characterized by microangiopathic haemolytic anaemia, platelets↓, and renal failure without the features of DIC (ie no clotting abnormality). In TTP CNS features are prominent including confusion and fits, and skin lesions are seen. Histology shows fibrin and platelets in arterial and glomerular lesions with no immune deposits. HUS is associated with bacterial and viral gastroenteritis (eg *E coli* 0157 toxin via faecally-contaminated hides in abattoirs eg if 'washing' employs static tubs of reused water). *Prognosis:* Mortality: <5%. Haematological and renal features tend to resolve in 2 weeks. *Management:* (Often problematic.) Support on ITU may be needed. Up to 80% need long-term dialysis. TTP is more serious with a very high mortality. Treatment must be prompt and may involve steroids and plasma exchange. Seek expert advice. It may relapse.[2]

Malignant hypertension is associated with rapid renal failure. There is low C3 and microangiopathic haemolytic anaemia. Urinary sediment usually shows dysmorphic RBC and red cell casts. *Treatment:* See p302.

Hypertension in pregnancy (pre-eclampsia) is the association of hypertension, proteinuria and oedema in pregnancy. The kidney shows glomerular endotheliosis with narrowing/obliteration of glomeruli + deposition of fibrin and platelets. Tests show haemolysis, elevated liver enzymes, low platelet counts (=HELLP syndrome). *Treatment: OHCS* p96.

Cholesterol emboli These are seen in association with widespread atherosclerosis and raised cholesterol. *Presentation:* Livedo reticularis, purpura, GI bleeding, renal failure, myalgia, cyanotic peripheries with intact distal pulses. It often follows arterial instrumentation, but may not be seen for months. It is also seen with thrombolysis, anticoagulation, abdominal trauma and spontaneously. *Tests:* ESR↑; eosinophilia; mild proteinuria; inactive urinary sediment; raised urea and creatinine; C3 and C4 normal, and ANCA negative (p675). Diagnosis is confirmed by finding cholesterol clefts in renal biopsy, or colon biopsy (submucosal vessels must be examined). *Prognosis:* Often progressive and fatal; mortality may be from atheroma elsewhere. A few have regained renal function after dialysis.[3,4] Statin drugs have been tried (p654).[5]

Nephronophthisis

This is an inherited medullary cystic disease, which accounts for 20% of childhood renal failure. The kidneys are small and fibrosed. *Synonyms and related diseases:* juvenile nephronophthisis, medullary cystic disease, Senior Loken syndrome. It may exist in association with retinal degeneration, optic atrophy, retinitis pigmentosa (giving tunnel vision), and congenital hepatic fibrosis. *Treatment* is of the associated renal failure (*OHCS* p280).

1 T Kremer Hovinga 1990 *Nephrol Dial Transplant* 5 481 2 Scottish Office Abattoir Inquiry 1997 *BMJ* i 770 3 R Scully 1991 *NEJM* 325 563 4 R Scully 1991 *NEJM* 324 11 5 J Rhodes 1996 *Lancet* 347 1641

Renal tubular disease

Renal tubular acidosis (RTA) The tubules either fail to create an acid urine (type I or 'distal' RTA) or there is bicarbonate wasting and serum bicarbonate falls until the 'filtered load' equals the reduced resorptive capacity and the urine may become acid again (type 2 or 'proximal' RTA): usually occurs with other tubular disorders (Fanconi syndrome, below).

Type I ('distal') RTA: Presentation: In childhood with polyuria, failure to thrive and bone pain; in adults with weakness ($\downarrow K^+$), bone pain (osteo-malacia), constipation, renal calculi (calcium phosphate, struvite, nephrocalcinosis) or renal failure. *Diagnosis:* Urine pH >6 with spontaneous, or ammonium chloride (100mg/kg) induced, acidaemia. Normally urine pH falls below 5.3. (Do not acid load if plasma bicarbonate <19mmol/L.) *Treatment:* bicarbonate replacement (1–3mmol/kg/day) and K^+. Hypokalaemia must be corrected before acidosis to prevent further fall in K^+ and the risk of cardiac arrest. *Prognosis* is variable.

Type 2 ('proximal') RTA: Presentation: In infancy with growth failure, hyperchloraemic acidosis, and alkaline or slightly acid urine. It may be secondary to cystinosis, Fanconi syndrome, or after renal transplant. There is no nephrocalcinosis and the prognosis is good. *Treatment:* Bicarbonate 10mmol/kg/day. (There is no 'type 3' RTA.)

Type 4 RTA: Occurs in disease states associated with aldosterone deficiency, or associated with distal tubular damage. It is seen in Addison's disease, diabetes mellitus (hyporeninaemic hypoaldosteronism), amyloidosis, obstructive uropathy, and drugs (amiloride). If aldosterone deficient, treat with fludrocortisone or a loop diuretic.

When to suspect RTA: ●High urine pH and negative urine culture. ●Hyperchloraemic hypokalaemic acidosis. ●Normal anion gap. ●Hypouricaemia and hypophosphataemia (type 2 RTA). ●Failure of urinary acidification in acidaemia. ●Hyperkalaemia and acid urine, eg in elderly diabetics or obstructive uropathy (type 4 RTA).

Fanconi syndrome entails multiple proximal tubular defects causing glycosuria, aminoaciduria, phosphaturia and RTA. Examples are: ●*Cystinosis* (autosomal recessive; cystine accumulates in lysosomes). It presents from ½–1yrs of age with failure to thrive, polyuria, polydipsia, and rickets. End-stage renal failure develops before 10 years. *Treatment:* Hydration; HCO_3^-, K^+, PO_4^{2-} and calcitrol (*OTM 3e*). Cysteamine bitartrate removes lysosomal cystine, and slows glomerular deterioration. Indomethacin ↓urine volume and ↑appetite/growth (http://www.cystinosisfoundation.ucsd.edu/library.html). ●*Idiopathic adult Fanconi syndrome* is often transient and presents with bone pain, weakness, polyuria, and polydipsia. Treat with replacement of excreted ions and vitamin D. ●*Secondary Fanconi* occurs in myeloma, Wilson's disease (p712), lead toxicity, and drug toxicity (out-of-date tetracycline; ifosfamide).

Alport's syndrome X-linked or autosomal recessive; genes involved: *COL4A5, COL4A3, COL4A4* (*Lancet* 1997 **349** 1770) Nephritis + sensorineural deafness is associated with lens abnormalities, platelet dysfunction and hyperproteinaemia. Does not recur after transplantation. See *OHCS* p742.

Hyperoxaluria Autosomal recessive. May be primary or secondary to gut resection or malabsorption. There are 2 types of primary oxalosis. Type I is more common and calcium oxalate stones are widely distributed throughout the body. It presents as renal stones and nephrocalcinosis in children and 80% are in renal failure by age 20yrs. Pyridoxine may help. Type 2 is more benign with nephrocalcinosis but no renal failure.

Cystinuria The commonest aminoaciduria. Urine: cystine↑, ornithine↑, arginine↑, lysine↑. Cystine stones form. *Treatment:* ↑fluid intake and alkalize urine. (Note: in cells, most cystine is reduced to form cysteine.)

10. Neurology

Other relevant pages: CNS examination (p32); mental state (p34); psychiatry on the wards (p13); facial pain (p46); dementia (p76–8); ►►status epilepticus (p782); ►►coma (p762–764); ►►head injury (p778); ►►rising ICP (p780); ►►cranial arteritis (p674). *Syndromes/diseases* (p694–712): Brown-Séquard; Fabry's; Gilles de la Tourette; ►Guillain–Barré; Huntington's; Jakob–Creutzfeld; Korsakoff (=Korsakov); McArdle; Refsum; Wernicke; Wilson.

Is there a lesion?

There are 4 choices in neurology: •Nothing wrong at all (the hardest diagnosis—you may need to talk in detail to the spouse rather than do an even better scan); •A functional disorder (no structural abnormality—eg pins and needles brought on by over-breathing; •A lesion; or •A general insult, such as a post-ictal state, encephalitis, encephalopathy, or poisoning. A key feature in determining if a lesion is present is lack of symmetry—eg one pupil dilated, or an upgoing plantar response.

Where is the lesion?

The aim is to find a location that can explain *all* the symptoms (only then, if this is not possible, is it necessary to postulate a cause of disseminated CNS lesions, such as multiple sclerosis).

Sensory deficits Map out any deficit separately for each modality (pain, temperature, vibration, two-point discrimination, joint position sense). Look also for LMN or UMN signs as sensory and motor deficits more often occur together than in isolation. Then ask where the lesion is.
Glove and stocking distribution: All modalities or only some ± distal LMN signs. Polyneuropathies produce this pattern (p464).
Complete sensory loss: In all modalities below the level of the lesion occurs with complete section of the cord and is eventually accompanied by LMN signs at the level of the transection and UMN signs below the level—quadriplegia (cervical cord) or paraplegia (thoracic cord).
Dissociated sensory loss: An unequal loss of the sensory modalities. This usually indicates spinal cord disease but is also a feature of some neuropathies. *Brown-Séquard syndrome* (p696) *and* syringomyelia (p476, loss of pain and temperature sensation in a cape distribution, ie neck, shoulders, arms + LMN signs in arms and UMN signs in the lower limbs). *Tabes dorsalis* (a form of neurosyphilis): loss of dorsal column function (vibration and joint position sense) resulting in ataxia and a +ve Romberg's test.

Weakness Where is the lesion? Cerebral cortex, corona radiata, internal capsule, brainstem, spinal cord, peripheral nerve, neuromuscular junction, or muscle? You must first establish what type of weakness is present (upper or lower motor neurone), as described opposite. *How weak is weak?* The British Medical Research Council established a scale for clinicians to use in order to objectify and standardize the recording of muscle power. Though imperfect, it has been accepted worldwide.

Grade 0 No contraction	*Grade 3* Active movement against gravity
Grade 1 Flicker of contraction	*Grade 4* Active movement against resistance
Grade 2 Some active movement	*Grade 5* Normal power

Grade 4 covers the widest range (a subdivision is 4–, 4, and 4+ to describe movement against slight, moderate, and strong resistance). Grade 5 is *normal* in the light of age and build. Some people are not as strong as others but even a 90lb, 95-year-old woman should have Grade 5 strength *for her*. Grade 4 strength is *pathological* and needs to be explained. If your patient is simply not trying due to, for example, excessive sedation, resist the temptation to document 'Strength 4/5 throughout'. This suggests a quadriparesis or severe myopathy. Better to document 'poor effort' and the maximum observed grade for each muscle.

Commonly confused terms used when describing weakness
Mono-	Referring to one limb.
Para-	Referring to both legs.
Hemi-	Referring to an arm and a leg on the same side.
Tetra-	Referring to all four limbs (*quadri-* is an alternative here).
-paresis	(Greek, *relaxation*) Some weakness, but incomplete paralysis.
-plegia	(Greek, *a blow, stroke*) Complete, or severe, paralysis.

Reflexes and their spinal cord level: p33. *Spinal roots for individual muscles:* p408.

Motor neurone lesions *Upper motor neurone* (UMN) lesions occur above the level of the anterior horn cell (eg cerebral cortex, internal capsule, spinal tracts). *Weakness* or *paralysis* is predominantly of upper limb abductors and extensors and lower limb flexors and adductors with little or no muscle wasting. Hypertonia or *spasticity* (especially arm flexors and leg extensors) is manifest as resistance to passive movement that can suddenly be overcome (clasp-knife spasticity). Patients are *hyperreflexic*—reflexes are brisk; *plantars are upgoing* (positive Babinski sign) and *clonus* may be elicited by rapidly dorsiflexing the foot. Up to 3 rhythmic, downward beats of the foot is normal; more is characteristic of an UMN lesion. *Hoffman's reflex* (flicking a finger causes neighbouring digit(s) to flex) may be +ve. UMN weakness always affects muscle groups, never individual muscles.

Lower motor neurone (LMN) lesions are due to loss of function or destruction of cell bodies or axons of anterior horn cells. There is weakness with marked muscle wasting or atrophy. The muscles of affected limbs feel soft and floppy and provide no resistance to passive stretch—*flaccidity*. Muscle tone is reduced—*hypotonia*. The denervated muscle may show fasciculations. Reflexes are reduced or absent (plantars are normal or absent). Flexors and extensors are equally affected.

UMN weakness—where and what is the lesion? *Monoplegia* (one limb): usually a motor cortex lesion (CVA, small tumour) or more rarely a partial internal capsule, brainstem, or cord lesion (eg MS). *Hemiplegia* (leg and arm on same side): Weakness of the leg, arm, and lower face—contralateral motor cortex, corona radiata, or internal capsule, due commonly to CVA but also trauma, tumour, abscess, MS. Crossed paralyses eg ipsilateral larynx, pharynx, tongue, and contralateral arm and leg are typical of brainstem lesions. *Paraplegia* (both legs): Spinal cord (trauma, compression p426, MS p454, infarction, bleed, subacute combined degeneration from low B12, syringomyelia p476). *Tetraplegia or quadriplegia* (all 4 limbs): Cervical cord (same causes as paraplegia plus dislocation of the odontoid peg and repeated CVA).

LMN weakness—where and what is the lesion? If bilateral and most marked distally, think of a polyneuropathy (p464). Is there an associated sensory deficit? This helps identify possible causes. If LMN signs in the upper limbs, check the lower limbs. If there is spastic weakness in the legs, think of spinal cord compression (p426, p468). In the early stages of acute cord damage there will be LMN weakness of upper *and* lower limbs. Spastic weakness below the level of the lesion develops only later. Mixed UMN and LMN weakness with early preservation of reflexes and the invariable presence of muscle fasciculation is typical of motor neurone disease (p466). If weakness is of muscles supplied by a single nerve (p408) suspect a mononeuropathy (p462); if more than one, think of mononeuritis multiplex (p462). Anterior root lesions cause weakness of all muscles supplied by that root (the myotome). *Differential:* Myopathies (p470) may appear similar to LMN weakness. They exhibit no sensory involvement and a predominantly proximal weakness and wasting is seen in most. Associated symptoms and neurophysiology make the diagnosis. Myasthenia gravis is characterized by weakness that worsens with use of the affected muscles (fatigability). There is little wasting and no sensory involvement. See p472 for specific diagnostic tests.

Cerebral artery territories

A basic knowledge of the anatomy of the blood supply of the brain is helpful in the diagnosis and management of cerebrovascular disease (p432–p436). It is important to be able to identify the area of brain that correlates with a patient's symptoms and identify the occluded artery.

Cerebral blood supply The brain is supplied by the two internal carotid arteries and the basilar artery (formed by the joining of the 2 vertebral arteries). These 3 vessels feed into an anastomotic ring at the base of the brain called the circle of Willis (below). This arrangement may serve to mitigate the effects of occlusion of a feeder vessel proximal to the anastomosis by allowing supply from unaffected vessels. The anatomy of the circle of Willis is, however, highly variable and in many people, narrowness of part of the ring means that it cannot provide much protection from ischaemia due to carotid, vertebral or basilar artery occlusion. Retrograde supply from other vessels in the neck may, however, salvage more proximal occlusions of feeder vessels—occlusion of the internal carotid in the neck, for example, may not cause infarction if retrograde flow from the external carotid artery enters the circle of Willis via its anastomosis with the ophthalmic artery.

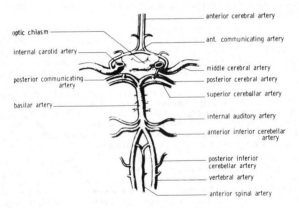

Diagram of the Circle of Willis as seen at the base of the brain

Willis and neurology Thomas Willis (1621-75) is one of those happy Oxford heroes belonging to Christ Church College who hold a bogus DM degree–awarded in 1646 for his Royalist sympathies. He had a busy life inventing terms such as 'neurology' and 'reflex'. Not only has his name been given to his famous circle, but he was the first to describe myasthenia gravis, whooping cough, the sweet taste of diabetic urine, and a variety of small nerves. He was the first person (and few have followed him) who knew the course of the spinal accessory nerve–which he discovered. He is unusual among Oxford neurologists in that, at various times of his life, he developed the practice of giving his lunch away to the poor. He also developed the practice of iatrochemistry: a theory of medicine according to which all morbid conditions of the body can be explained by disturbances in the fermentations and effervescences of its humours.

Arteries and CNS territories

Carotid artery Internal carotid artery occlusion may, at worst, cause total infarction of the anterior ⅔ of the ipsilateral hemisphere and basal ganglia (striate arteries), leading to death. More often, the picture is similar to that of a middle cerebral artery occlusion (below).

The cerebral arteries 3 pairs of arteries leave the circle of Willis to supply the cerebral hemispheres; the anterior, middle and posterior cerebral arteries. The anterior and middle cerebrals are supplied chiefly by the carotid arteries; the posterior cerebral by the basilar artery. Although these arteries are essentially end arteries (there is no significant anastomosis between them), ischaemia due to occlusion of any one of them may be reduced, if not prevented, by retrograde supply from meningeal vessels.

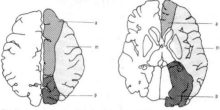

The distribution of supply of the anterior (a), middle (m), and posterior (p) cerebral areries.

Anterior cerebral artery: Supplies the medial aspect of the hemisphere. Occlusion may cause a weak, numb contralateral leg ± similar, if milder, arm symptoms. The face is spared. Bilateral infarction is associated with an akinetic mute state due to damage to the cingulate gyri.

Middle cerebral artery: Supplies the lateral (external) aspect of each hemisphere. Occlusion may cause: contralateral hemiplegia and sensory loss mainly of face and arm; dysphasia and dyspraxia (dominant hemisphere); contralateral neglect (non-dominant hemisphere); sometimes contralateral homonymous hemianopia.

Posterior cerebral artery: Supplies the occipital lobe. Occlusion may cause many effects, including contralateral homonymous hemianopia.

Vertebrobasilar circulation Supplies the cerebellum, brainstem and posterior cerebral artery. Occlusion may cause: hemianopia; cortical blindness; diplopia; vertigo; nystagmus; hemi- or quadriplegia; unilateral or bilateral sensory symptoms; cerebellar symptoms; drop attacks; coma. Infarctions of the brainstem can produce various syndromes, eg the *Lateral medullary syndrome* (occlusion of one vertebral artery or the posterior inferior cerebellar artery). It is due to infarction of the lateral medulla and the inferior surface of the cerebellum causing vertigo with vomiting, dysphagia, nystagmus on looking to the side of the lesion, ipsilateral hypotonia, ataxia, and paralysis of the soft palate, ipsilateral Horner's syndrome, and a dissociated sensory loss (analgesia to pin-prick on ipsilateral face and contralateral trunk and limbs).

Subclavian steal syndrome Stenosis of the subclavian artery proximal to the ipsilateral vertebral artery may cause blood to be *stolen* by retrograde flow from this vertebral artery down into the arm. This results in brainstem ischaemia after arm exertion. A difference in BP of >20mmHg between the arms supports the diagnosis.

Some CNS drugs

The table below contains some of the drugs most commonly used to modify the activity of central nervous system transmitters. When prescribing for the CNS it is important to bear in mind that 1) that the drug must be able to pass through the blood–brain barrier to have an effect—or it must affect other intracrnial structures such as blood vessels; 2) the consequences of any sedative effect; 3) short and long-term side-effects (eg tardive dyskinesia with neuroleptic drugs).

Enhancing	Decreasing
Dopamine	
L-dopa	Major tranquillizers
Bromocriptine (D_2-agonist)	Benzisoxazoles (D_2-blocker)
Selegiline (MAO-B inhibitor)	eg risperidone
Amantadine	Some anti-emetics
Noradrenaline & adrenaline	(=norepinephrine & epinephrine)
Salbutamol (β_2)	Propranolol (β)
Adrenaline (=epinephrine)	Atenolol (β_1)
?Tricyclic antidepressants	Clonidine (α_2 agonist)
MAO inhibitors	Phentolamine (α)
5-HT	
LSD and other hallucinogens	Pizotifen
Sumatriptan	Benzisoxazoles (5-HT_2 blockers)
Some tricyclic antidepressants	eg risperidone
eg trazodone	Clozapine (OHCS p360
Buspirone; lithium	5-HT S_{1C} antagonist[1])
Fluoxetine (OHCS p341)	Mianserin; ondansetron
Acetylcholine	
Carbachol	Atropine
Pilocarpine	Scopolamine
Anticholinesterases	Ipratropium
eg neostigmine	Benzhexol (=trihexyphenidyl)
	Orphenadrine
	Procyclidine
GABA (inhibits CNS activity)	
Baclofen (GABA B)	Alcohol abuse: *acute effects* block
Benzodiazepines	N-methyl-D-aspartate (NMDA) receptors;
Vigabatrin	*with chronic use,* numbers of NMDA
Barbiturates	receptors increase, mediating alcohol
Acamprosate[2] (used in alcohol	withdrawal effects (anxiety, craving)[2]
addiction; derived from taurine)	
Glutamate (*an excitatory amino acid*)	
	Lamotrigine (used in epilepsy)
	Acamprosate ($\downarrow$craving in alcoholics)

1 S Dursun 1993 *BMJ* 307 200 2 *Drug Ther Bul* 1997 35 70

Testing peripheral nerves

Nerve root	Muscle	*Test—by asking the patient to:*
C3,4	trapezius	Shrug shoulder, adduct scapula.
C4,5	rhomboids	Brace shoulder back.
C5,6,7	serratus anterior	Push forward against resistance.
C5,6	pectoralis major (clavicular head)	Adduct arm from above horizontal, and push it forward.
C6,7,8	pectoralis major (sternocostal head)	Adduct arm below horizontal.
C5,6	supraspinatus	Abduct arm the first 15°.
C5,6	infraspinatus	Externally rotate arm, elbow at side.
C6,7,8	latissimus dorsi	Adduct arm from horizontal position.
C5,6	biceps	Flex supinated forearm.
C5,6	deltoid	Abduct arm between 15° and 90°.

Radial nerve

C6,7,8	triceps	Extend elbow against resistance.
C5,6	brachioradialis	Flex elbow with forearm half way between pronation and supination.
C5,6	extensor carpi radialis longus	Extend wrist to radial side with fingers extended.
C6,7	supinator	Arm by side, resist hand pronation.
C7,8	extensor digitorum	Keep fingers extended at MCP joint.
C7,8	extensor carpi ulnaris	Extend wrist to ulnar side.
C7,8	abductor pollicis longus	Abduct thumb at 90° to palm.
C7,8	extensor pollicis brevis	Extend thumb at MCP joint.
C7,8	extensor pollicis longus	Resist thumb flexion at IP joint.

Median nerve

C6,7	pronator teres	Keep arm pronated against resistance.
C6,7	flexor carpi radialis	Flex wrist towards radial side.
C7,8,T1	flexor digitorum sublimis	Resist extension at PIP joint (while you fix his proximal phalanx).
C8,T1	flexor digitorum profundus I & II	Resist extension at the DIP joint of index finger.
C8,T1	flexor pollicis longus	Resist thumb extension at interphalangeal joint (fix proximal phalanx).
C8,T1	abductor pollicis brevis	Abduct thumb (nail at 90° to palm).
C8,T1	opponens pollicis	Thumb touches base of 5th finger-tip nail parallel to palm.
C8,T1	1st & 2nd lumbricals	Extend PIP joint against resistance with MCP joint held hyperextended.

Ulnar nerve

C7,8,T1	flexor carpi ulnaris	Flex wrist towards ulnar side.
C7,C8	flexor digitorum profundus III and IV	Fix middle phalanx of little finger, resist extension of distal phalanx.
C8,T1	dorsal interossei	Abduct fingers (use index finger).
C8,T1	palmar interossei	Adduct fingers (use index finger).
C8,T1	adductor pollicis	Adduct thumb (nail at 90° to palm).
C8,T1	abductor digiti minimi	Abduct little finger.
C8,T1	flexor digiti minimi	Flex the little finger at MCP joint.

The musculocutaneous nerve (C5-6) This may be injured at the brachial plexus, causing weakness of biceps, coracobrachialis and brachialis (see PLATE 4). Forearm flexion is weak. There may be some loss of sensation.

Lower limb

Nerve root Muscle   *Activity to test:*
L**4**,5, S1   gluteus medius &   Internal rotation
              minimus (superior   at hip, hip abduction.
              gluteal nerve)
L5, S1,2   gluteus maximus   Extension at hip (lie prone).
              (inferior gluteal nrv)
L**2**,3,4   adductors   Adduct leg against resistance.
              (obturator nerve)

Femoral nerve
L1,2,3   ilio-psoas   Flex hip with knee flexed and lower
                                        leg supported: patient lies on back.
L2,3   sartorius   Flex knee with hip in external rotation.
L2,3,4   quadriceps femoris   Extend knee against resistance.

Obturator nerve
L2,3,4   hip adductors   Adduct the leg.

Internal gluteal nerve
L5,S1,S2   gluteus maximus   Hip extension.

Superficial gluteal nerve
L4,5,S1   gluteus medius   Abduction and internal rotation of hip.
             gluteus medialis   Abduction and internal rotation of hip.

Sciatic nerve (*and the common peroneal nerve)
L5 **S1**,2   hamstrings   Flex knee against resistance.
L4,5   tibialis posterior   Invert plantarflexed foot.
*L**4**,5   tibialis anterior   Dorsiflex ankle.
*L**5**,S1 extensor digitorum longus Dorsiflex toes against resistance.
*L**5**,S1 extensor hallucis longus Dorsiflex hallux against resistance.
*L**5**,S1 peroneus longus &   Evert foot against resistance.
             brevis
L5,S1   extensor digit. brevis   Dorsiflex hallux (muscle of foot).
S1,2   gastrocnemius   Plantarflex ankle joint.
L5,**S1**,2 flexor digitorum longus Flex terminal joints of toes.
S1,2   small muscles of foot   Make sole of foot into a cup.

Quick screening test for muscle power

Shoulder	Abduction	C5		Hip	Flexion	L1–L2
	Adduction	C5–C7			Extension	L5–S1
Elbow	Flexion	C5–C6		Knee	Flexion	S1
	Extension	C7			Extension	L3–L4
Wrist	Flexion	C7–8		Ankle	Dorsiflexion	L4
	Extension	C7			Plantarflexion	S1–S2
Fingers	Flexion	C7–C8; Extension C7				
	Abduction	T1				

Remember to test proximal muscle power, eg by asking the patient to sit from lying, to pull you towards himself, and to rise from squatting.

NB: Root numbers in bold indicate that that root is more important than its neighbour. Sources vary in ascribing particular nerve roots to muscles–and there is considerable biological variation in individuals. The above is a reasonable compromise, and is based on the MRC guidelines.

Dermatomes

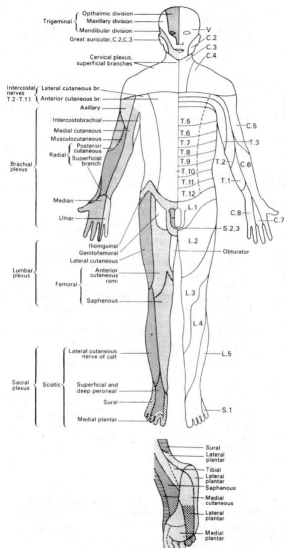

Trigeminal
- Opthalmic division
- Maxillary division
- Mandibular division

Great auricular, C.2, C.3

V
C.2
C.3
C.4

Cervical plexus, superficial branches

Intercostal nerves T.2-T.11
- Lateral cutaneous br.
- Anterior cutaneous br.

Axillary

Intercostobrachial

Medial cutaneous

Musculocutaneous

Radial
- Posterior cutaneous
- Superficial branch

Brachial plexus

Median

Ulnar

Lumbar plexus

Ilioinguinal
Genitofemoral
Lateral cutaneous

Femoral
- Anterior cutaneous rami
- Saphenous

Sacral plexus

Sciatic
- Lateral cutaneous nerve of calf
- Superficial and deep peroneal
- Sural
- Medial plantar

T.5
T.6
T.7
T.8
T.9
T.10
T.11
T.12
L.1
L.2
L.3
L.4
L.5

C.5
T.3
T.2
C.6
T.1
C.8
C.7
S.2,3
Obturator
S.1

Sural
Lateral
Tibial
Lateral plantar
Saphenous
Medial cutaneous
Lateral plantar
Medial plantar

ANTERIOR ASPECT

Dermatomes

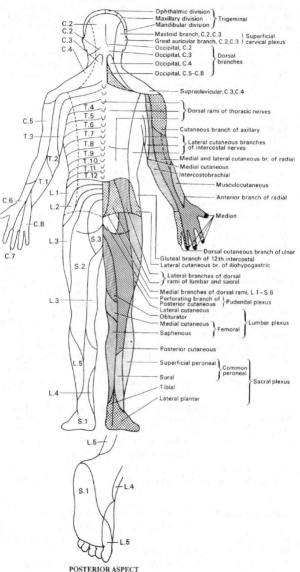

Ophthalmic division ⎫
Maxillary division ⎬ Trigeminal
Mandibular division ⎭

C.2
C.2 — Mastoid branch, C.2, C.3 ⎫ Superficial
C.3 — Great auricular branch, C.2, C.3 ⎭ cervical plexus
C.4
Occipital, C.2
Occipital, C.3 ⎫ Dorsal
Occipital, C.4 ⎬ branches
Occipital, C.5-C.8 ⎭

Supraclavicular, C.3, C.4

C.5
T.3
T.4
T.5
T.6
T.7
T.8
T.9
T.10
T.11
T.12

T.2
T.1

Dorsal rami of thoracic nerves

Cutaneous branch of axillary

Lateral cutaneous branches
of intercostal nerves

Medial and lateral cutaneous br. of radial

Medial cutaneous

Intercostobrachial

Musculocutaneous

Anterior branch of radial

Median

C.6
C.8
C.7

L.1
L.2

L.3

S.3
S.2

L.3

Dorsal cutaneous branch of ulnar

Gluteal branch of 12th intercostal
Lateral cutaneous br. of iliohypogastric

Lateral branches of dorsal ⎫
rami of lumbar and sacral ⎭

Medial branches of dorsal rami, L.1 – S.6
Perforating branch of ⎫ Pudendal plexus
Posterior cutaneous ⎭
Lateral cutaneous
Obturator ⎫ Lumbar plexus
Medial cutaneous ⎬ Femoral
Saphenous ⎭

L.5

Posterior cutaneous

Superficial peroneal ⎫ Common
Sural ⎬ peroneal
Tibial ⎭ Sacral plexus
Lateral plantar

L.4

S.1

L.5
L.4

S.1
L.5

POSTERIOR ASPECT

Lumbar puncture (LP)

Contraindications ●Bleeding diathesis ●Cardiorespiratory compromise ●Infection at site of needle insertion, and most importantly: ● ↑Intracranial pressure (suspect if very severe headache, ↓level of consciousness with falling pulse, rising BP, vomiting, focal signs, or papilloedema), give urgent treatment as needed; discuss urgently with relevant clinician with a view to CT scan. CT is not infallible, so be sure your indication for LP is strong.

Method Explain to the patient *what* sampling CSF entails, *why* it is needed, that *co-operation* is vital, and that he can *communicate with you* at all stages.
●Place the patient on his left side, his back on edge of bed, fully flexed (knees to chin). Avoid allowing the patient to slump.
●Landmarks: plane of iliac crests through L4. In adults, the spinal cord ends at the L1,2 disc. Mark L4, 5 or L3, 4 intervertebral space, eg by a *gentle* indentation of a thumb-nail on the overlying skin (better than a ballpoint pen mark, which might be erased by the sterilizing fluid).
●Wash hands. Don a mask and sterile gloves.
●Sterilize the back with tincture of iodine unless allergic.
●Open the spinal pack. Check manometer fittings. Have 3 plain sterile tubes and 1 fluoride (for glucose) tube ready.
●Inject 0.25–0.5mL 1% lignocaine (=lidocaine) under skin at marked site.
●Wait 1 minute, then insert spinal needle (22G, stilette in place) through the mark aiming towards umbilicus. Feel resistance of spinal ligaments, and then the dura, then a 'give' as the needle enters the subarachnoid space. Note: keep the needle's bevel facing *up*, parallel with dural fibres.
●Withdraw stilette. Wait for CSF.
●Measure CSF pressure with manometer.
●Catch fluid in 3 sequentially numbered bottles (<5–10mL total). Consider taking and privately reserving a labelled sample in case of accident!
●Remove needle and apply dressing. Send CSF promptly for microscopy, culture, protein and glucose (do plasma glucose too). If applicable, also send for: cytology, fungal studies, TB culture, virology (including Herpes PCR), syphilis serology, oligoclonal bands (with serum sample for comparison) if multiple sclerosis suspected. Is there xanthochromia (p438)?
●Advise lying flat for >1h, checking CNS observations and BP regularly. Post-LP headache is partly preventable by reducing CSF leakage by using finer needles shaped to part the dura rather than cut it: see opposite.

CSF **composition** *Normal values:* Lymphocytes <4/mm³; polymorphs 0; protein <0.4g/L; glucose >2.2mmol/L (or about 70% plasma level); pressure <200mmCSF. *In meningitis:* See p442. *In multiple sclerosis:* See p454.

Bloody tap: This is an artefact due to piercing a blood vessel, which is indicated (unreliably) by fewer red cells in successive bottles, and no yellowing of CSF (xanthochromia). To estimate how many white cells (*w*) were in the CSF before the blood was added, use the following:

$$w = CSF\ WCC - [blood\ WCC \times CSF\ RBC \div blood\ RBC]$$

If the patient's blood count is normal, the rule of thumb is to subtract from the total CSF WCC (per μl) one white cell for every 1000 RBCs. To estimate the true protein level subtract 10mg/L for every 1000 RBCs/mm³ (be sure to do the count and protein estimation on the same bottle). Note: high protein levels in CSF make it appear yellow.

Subarachnoid haemorrhage: Yellow CSF (xanthochromia). Red cells in equal numbers in all bottles. The RBCs will excite an inflammatory response (eg CSF WCC raised), most marked after 48h.

Very raised CSF protein: Spinal block; TB; or severe bacterial meningitis.

Raised protein: Meningitis; MS; uraemia; hypothyroidism; DM; Guillain–Barré.

Post-LP headache[1,2]

Incidence: ~30%, typically occurring within 24h of LP, with resolution over hours to 2 weeks (mean: 3–4 days). Patients describe a constant, dull, achy pain bilaterally which is more frontal than occipital. The most characteristic symptom is of *positional exacerbation*—worse when upright and usually pain free when recumbent. There may be mild meningism or nausea. The pathology is thought to be continued leakage of CSF from the puncture site and intracranial *hypotension.*

Prevention: Use the smallest spinal needle that is practical (22G) and keep the bevel aligned as described opposite. *Blunt* needles (more expensive!) can reduce incidence from 30% to 5%—and are recommended[1] (ask an an anaesthetist about supply). Collection of CSF takes too long (>6min) if needles <22G are used.[1]

Treatment: Despite years of anecdotal advice to the contrary *none* of the following have ever been shown to be a risk factor: position during or after the procedure; hydration status before, during, or after; amount of CSF removed; immediate activity or rest post-LP. *Time* is a consistent healer. For severe or prolonged headaches ask an anaesthetist to do a *blood patch*. This is a careful injection of 20mL of autologous venous blood into the epidural space previously punctured. Immediate relief occurs in 95%.

Note: Post-LP brain MRI scans often show diffuse meningeal enhancement with gadolinium. This is thought to be a reflection of increased blood flow secondary to intracranial hypotension. Interpret these scans with caution and in the context of the patient's clinical situation.

1 SA Broadley 1997 *BMJ* ii 1324 2 NH Raskin 1990 *Headache* 30 197

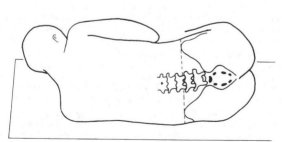

Method of defining the interspace between the 3rd and 4th lumbar vertebrae.

After Vakil and Udwadia *Diagnosis and Management of Medical Emergencies* 2 ed OUP, Delhi.

✝✝✝ Headache

Every day, *thousands* of patients visit doctors complaining of headache; these consultations are rewarding as the chief skill is in interpreting the history—not in *taking* the history, so much as in *allowing* it to unfold. Let the patient tell you about the headache's associations and antecedents: even *who* their headache is. Stress is the usual cause, and referral to a neurologist or lab tests are rarely needed. Some headaches, however, are both disabling and treatable (migraine, cluster headache) while others herald sinister disease (space-occupying lesions) or warrant immediate action (meningitis, subarachnoid haemorrhage, giant cell arteritis). These are the headaches you must recognize. The pattern of pain and associated features help narrow down diagnosis, as summarized below:

Acute single episode

Meningitis	p442, eg + fever, photophobia, stiff neck, rash, coma
Encephalitis	p441, eg + fever, odd behaviour, or consciousness↓
Tropical illness	p188, eg malaria, +ve travel history, 'flu-like illness
Subarachnoid	p438, haemorrhage → *sudden* headache ± stiff neck
Sinusitis	p554 in OHCS, eg + respiratory infection + tender face
Head injury	p778, cuts/bruises, consciousness↓; lucid interval, amnesia

Acute recurrent attacks

Migraine	p416, any pre-attack aura? Seeing spots? Vomiting?
Cluster headache	p415, nightly pain in 1 eye for ~8wks then pain free for 1yr
Glaucoma	p677, red eye; sees haloes, fixed big oval pupil; acuity↓

Subacute onset

Giant cell arteritis p674; eg scalp tenderness; >50yrs old; acuity↓, ESR↑

Chronic headache

Tension headache	'a tight band round my head'; stress at work/home, mood↓
Chronically ↑ICP	eg worse on waking or sneezing, focal signs BP↑, pulse↓
Analgesic headache	p415, rebound headache on stopping taking analgesics
Paget's disease	p646; >40yrs old, bowed (sabre) tibia, alk phos↑↑

Acute single episode

Meningitis, encephalitis, subarachnoid haemorrhage: If the headache is acute in onset, severe, felt over most of the head and accompanied by signs of meningeal irritation (neck stiffness, drowsiness) you must think of meningitis (p442), encephalitis (p441) or subarachnoid haemorrhage (p438). Admit the patient immediately for urgent CT. *LP is contraindicated until CT has excluded mass lesion, haematoma or hydrocephalus.*

After head injury headache is common after minor trauma. It may be at the site of trauma or be more generalized. It lasts ~2 weeks and is often resistant to analgesia. Bear in mind subdural or extradural haemorrhage (p440). Sinister signs are drowsiness, focal signs, and very severe pain.

Sinusitis Presents with dull, constant, aching pain over the affected frontal or maxillary sinus, with tender overlying skin. Ethmoid or sphenoid sinus pain is felt deep in the midline at the root of the nose. Pain is affected by posture eg worsened by bending over. Often accompanied by coryza, the pain lasts only 1–2 weeks. Confirm by imaging (eg CT).

Acute glaucoma: Mostly elderly, long-sighted people. Constant, aching pain develops rapidly around one eye and radiates to the forehead. *Symptoms:* Markedly reduced vision in affected eye, nausea and vomiting. *Signs:* Red, congested eye; cloudy cornea; dilated, non-responsive pupil. Attacks may be precipitated by sitting in the dark eg the cinema, dilating eye-drops or emotional upset. Seek expert help immediately. If delay in treatment of >1h is likely, start IV acetazolamide (500mg over several minutes).

Acute recurrent attacks of headache

Cluster headache (migrainous neuralgia): Thought to be caused by local release of 5-HT close to the superficial temporal artery.[1] Onset: any age but rare in children; $\male$:$\female \geq 5$:1, commoner in smokers. Pain occurs once or twice every 24h, each episode lasting 20–60mins. Clusters last 4–12 weeks and are followed by pain-free periods of months or even 1–2 years before another cluster begins. *The Patient:* Rapid onset severe pain around one eye which may become watery and bloodshot with lid swelling, lacrimation, facial flushing, and rhinorrhoea. Miosis ± ptosis (20% attacks), remaining permanent in 5%. Pain is strictly unilateral and almost always affects the same side. Onset may be remarkably predictable in its timing, often at night and may be triggered by alcohol within a cluster. It may drive the patient to bang his head against a wall, drive his fingernails into his palms or adopt peculiar postures, eg standing on one leg. *Management:* Seek expert help. Prevent with *ergotamine* (unlicensed use) or *sumatriptan* sc 6mg or 100mg po given 1h before expected attack. *Verapamil* given throughout the cluster can help, as may the 5-HT antagonist *methysergide* (has more SEs). O_2 (eg 7–15L/min for 20min) often relieves pain.

Subacute onset

Giant cell arteritis: See p674. **Exclude in all >55 years presenting with a headache that has lasted a few weeks.** Look for tender, thickened, pulseless temporal arteries + ESR >40mm/h. *Ask about:* Jaw claudication during eating. Prompt diagnosis and steroids avoid blindness.

Chronic headache

Tension headache: Associated with stress and anxiety, onset is gradual and once established the headache is typically severe and present all day every day for weeks to years. There is little diurnal variation or fluctuation in severity and sleep is rarely disturbed. The pain is usually bilateral, may be centred on a variety of sites on the cranium and is often described as a tight band around the head. The scalp may be tender. Analgesics and tranquillizers are of limited value, moreover, dependence and analgesic-induced headache can be problematic. Treatment is aimed at reassuring the patient that there is nothing serious wrong and at reducing stress. As lifestyle changes are hard to achieve, massage and other relaxation techniques can help, as may *amitriptyline* 25–50mg/12h PO (~1/3 show signs of depressive illness). 50% of migraine sufferers develop tension headache leaving them with background pain in between migrainous attacks.

Raised intracranial pressure: Here headache is a complaint of ~50% patients. Although variable in nature, headaches are characteristically present on waking or may awaken the patient. They are generally not severe and are worsened by lying down, coughing, or exertion. If accompanied by other signs of ↑ICP such as vomiting, papilloedema, epilepsy, progressive focal neurology, or mental change, admit the patient urgently for diagnostic imaging. *LP is contraindicated.* Any space-occupying lesion (neoplasm, abscess, subdural haematoma) may present in this way, as may benign intracranial hypertension.

Analgesic rebound headache: Persistent headache may be seen in sufferers of tension headache and migraine who overuse analgesics, hypnotics, and tranquillizers.[2] Depression may co-exist. $\female$:$\male \approx 3$:1.

1 P Aubineau 1992 *Lancet* i 1294   2 *Southern Medical Journal* 1993 **86** 1202–5

Migraine

Migraine causes much misery and costs the UK economy £200 million a year in lost production. Its prevalence is 8%. ♀:♂ ≈ 2:1.

Symptoms Classically: •Visual (or other) aura lasting ~15 minutes followed within 1h by unilateral, throbbing headache. Other patterns: •Aura with no headache •Episodic (often premenstrual) severe headaches, typically unilateral, with nausea, vomiting, and sometimes photophobia or phonophobia but no aura (formerly called 'common migraine').

Aura Visual chaos (cascading, distortion, 'melting' and jumbling of print lines, dots, spots, zig-zag fortification spectra); hemianopia, hemiparesis, dysphasia, dysarthria, ataxia (basilar migraine). Mood or appetite change (↑/↓) or ↑sensory awareness (eg to sound) may occur hours before the aura.

Criteria for diagnosis if no aura ≥5 headaches lasting 4–72h with either nausea/vomiting or photophobia/phonophobia *and* ≥2 of these 4 features: •Unilateral •Pulsating •Interferes with normal life •Aggravated by climbing stairs or other routine activity.

Pathogenesis Reduction in cerebral blood flow, possibly due to spreading depression of cortical activity, leading to the aura followed by increased cerebral and extracranial blood flow leading to the headache. Attacks often associated with changes in plasma 5-hydroxytryptamine.

Possible triggers Wine, cheese, chocolate, contraceptive steroids, premenstruation, anxiety, exercise, travel. In many (~50%), no trigger is found, and in only a few does avoiding triggers prevent attacks.

Differential Cluster or tension headache, cervical spondylosis; ↑BP; intracranial pathology, sinusitis, otitis media, caries, TIA. Migraine may be symptomatic of an underlying disorder eg anti-phospholipid syndrome.

Prophylaxis There is no panacea. Stop contraceptive Pill if the migraine produces focal neurology eg hemiplegia (risk of stroke). Use prophylaxis if frequency >twice a month. If one drug doesn't work after 2–3 months, try another. 60% of patients can expect some benefit:
•Pizotifen 500µg/8h PO; or 1.5mg PO at night (a 5-HT *antagonist*). SE: weight gain, ↑effects of alcohol, drowsiness, ↑glaucoma risk.
•Amitriptyline 25–75mg/8h; SE: dry mouth, blurred vision, drowsiness.
•Propranolol 40–80mg/12h PO. •Methysergide (specialist supervision).

Pre-menstrual migraine may respond to diuretics or depot oestrogens.

Treatment of attacks Low-doses may fail as peristalsis is often slow, so try *dispersible* high-dose aspirin 900mg/6h PO after food, or paracetamol 1g/6h PO 10mins after metoclopramide solution (5mg PO, ≤15mg/day; beware extrapyramidal effects) or domperidone. Alternatives:
•Sumatriptan is a 5HT₁ (serotonin-1) *agonist.*[1] Some trials show it may be no better than simple analgesia + metoclopramide; others indicate that the IM form is the best agent of all. Rarely, it may precipitate arrhythmias or angina ± MI—even if no pre-existing risk; CI: previous MI/IHD, coronary vasospasm, uncontrolled ↑BP, recent lithium, SSRIs (p13) or ergot.
•Ergotamine (a 5-HT agonist, constricting cranial arteries) 1mg PO as the headache begins, repeat at 30mins, up to 3mg in a day, and 6mg in a week; or, better, as a suppository (2mg ergotamine + 100mg caffeine) to maximum of 2 in 24h or 4 in one week. Emphasize dangers of ergotamine (gangrene, permanent vascular damage). CI: the Pill (OHCS p64); peripheral vascular disease; ischaemic heart disease; pregnancy; breast-feeding; hemiplegic migraine; Raynaud's; liver or renal impairment; BP↑.
•Breathing into paper bag (raising P_aCO_2) may abort attacks.
•Some people find warm or cold packs to the head helps ease the pain.

---

1 New 5HT₁ agonists (naratriptan, zolmitriptan) are said to offer no clear advantage: *MeReC Bul* 1997 **8** 37

RL.

Trigeminal neuralgia

The patient suffers paroxysms of intense, stabbing pain, lasting only seconds, in the trigeminal nerve distribution. Usually unilateral (96%), affecting the mandibular and maxillary divisions most often, and the ophthalmic division only rarely. The face may screw up with pain (hence *tic doloureux*). Pain may recur many times day and night and can often be precipitated by touching the skin of the affected area, by washing, shaving, eating or talking. Chiefly a condition of those over 50 years old, ♂/♀>1.

Cause Mostly idiopathic. Sensory or motor deficits of the trigeminal nerve cannot usually be demonstrated unless there is a structural cause, eg MS (consider especially in the young), basilar artery aneurysm, or a tumour in the cerebellopontine angle).

Treatment In idiopathic neuralgia aim for pain relief (may need high doses). Spontaneous remission may occur. *Batting order:* Carbamazepine 100–400mg/8h PO; phenytoin 200–400mg/24h PO; baclofen 5–25mg/8h PO. If drugs fail, surgical treatment may be necessary. This may be directed at the peripheral nerve, the trigeminal ganglion or the nerve root. The nerve root may be compressed by tortuous blood vessels as it enters the brainstem and surgical decompression is then useful.

For the differential diagnosis of facial pain, see p46.

✝✝ Blackouts

History It is vital to establish exactly what patients mean by 'blackout'. Do they mean loss of consciousness (LOC)? a fall to the ground without loss of consciousness? a clouding of vision, diplopia, or vertigo? Take a detailed history from the patient *and* a witness (see opposite).

Vaso-vagal syncope[1] Provoked by emotion, pain, fear or standing for too long and due to reflex bradycardia and peripheral vasodilatation. Onset is over seconds (*not* instantaneous), and is often preceded by nausea, pallor, sweating and closing in of visual fields. It cannot occur if lying down. The patient falls to the ground, remaining unconscious for ~2 minutes. Incontinence of urine is rare. There is 'never' incontinence of faeces. Patients may jerk their limbs, but there is no tonic → clonic sequence. After an attack there is no prolonged confusion or amnesia.

Situational syncope *Cough syncope:* Weakness and LOC after a paroxysm of coughing. *Effort syncope:* Syncope on exercise. Cardiac origin eg aortic stenosis, HOCM. *Micturition syncope:* Mostly men, at night, at the end of micturition. *Carotid sinus syncope:* Carotid sinus hypersensitivity in the elderly. Syncope on turning the head or shaving the neck.

Epilepsy presenting as blackout is most likely to be grand mal (LOC) or complex partial (impairment of consciousness). See p448. Attacks vary with the type of seizure, but some features suggest epilepsy as a cause of blackout: attacks when asleep or lying down; aura; identifiable precipitants eg TV; altered breathing, cyanosis, typical movements; urinary and faecal incontinence; tongue-biting (virtually diagnostic); post-attack drowsiness or coma; amnesia; residual paralysis for <24h.

Stokes–Adams attacks Transient arrhythmias (eg bradycardia due to complete heart block) causing ↓cardiac output and LOC. The patient falls to the ground (often with *no* warning except palpitation), pale, with a slow or absent pulse. Recovery is in seconds, the patient flushes, the pulse speeds up and consciousness is regained. Injury is typical of these intermittent arrhythmias. A few clonic jerks may occur if an attack is prolonged. Attacks may happen several times a day and in any posture.

Other causes *TIA:* (p436) Sudden onset focal neurology (motor or sensory symptoms) lasting up to 24 hours. Impaired consciousness if vertebrobasilar territory. *Hypoglycaemia:* Tremor, hunger and perspiration herald lightheadedness or LOC; rare in non-diabetics. *Orthostatic hypotension:* Unsteadiness or LOC on standing from lying in those with inadequate vasomotor reflexes: the elderly; autonomic neuropathy (p463); anti-hypertensive medication; overdiuresis; multisystem atrophy.

Drop attacks Sudden weakness of the legs causes the patient, usually an older woman, to fall to the ground. There is no warning, no LOC and no confusion afterwards. The condition is benign, resolving spontaneously after a number of attacks. Drop attacks also occur in hydrocephalus; these patients, however, may not be able to get up for hours.

Other causes *Anxiety:* Hyperventilation, tremor, sweating, tachycardia and paraesthesiae with lightheadedness, and no LOC suggest a panic attack. *Ménière's disease:* (p420). *Fictitious blackouts* (Münchausen's, p706). ►*Choking:* If a large piece of food blocks the larynx the patient may collapse, turn blue, and be unable to speak. Perform the Heimlich manoeuvre immediately to eject the food.

Examination Cardiovascular, neurological. BP lying and standing.

Tests Investigate fully unless clearly a faint. ECG (heart block, arrhythmia, long Q–T interval), U&E, FBC, glucose. Also EEG, sleep EEG, echo, CT or MRI.

1 MC Petch 1994 *BMJ* i 125

Taking a history of blackouts

During a typical attack
- Does the patient lose consciousness?
- Does the patient injure himself?
- Does the patient move?
- Is the patient incontinent of urine or faeces?
- Does the patient bite his tongue?
- What colour is the patient?
- What is the patient's pulse like?
- Are there associated symptoms (palpitations, chest pain, dyspnoea)?
- How long does the attack last?

Before the attack
- Is there any warning?
- In what circumstances do attacks occur?
- Can the patient prevent attacks?

After the attack
- Is the patient confused or sleepy?
- How much does the patient remember about the attack afterwards?

Dizziness and vertigo

The Patient Complaints of "dizzy spells" are very common and are used by patients to describe many different sensations. The key to making a diagnosis is to find out exactly what the patient means by "dizzy" and then decide whether or not this represents vertigo.

Does the patient have vertigo?
Definition: An illusion of movement, often rotatory, of the patient or his surroundings. In practice, patients rarely describe straightforward spinning—the floor may tilt, sink, or rise or the patient may describe veering sideways on walking or feeling pulled to one side as if by a magnet. *Associated symptoms* include difficulty walking or standing (relief on lying or sitting still); nausea; vomiting; pallor; and perspiration. Attacks may even cause patients to fall suddenly to the ground. Associated hearing loss or tinnitus implies involvement of the labyrinth or eighth nerve and with it vertigo. *What is not vertigo:* Lightheadedness or faintness may be described as dizziness but is often due to anxiety with associated palpitations, tremor, and sweating. Anaemia can cause lightheadedness as can orthostatic hypotension or effort in an emphysematous patient. In all of these, however, there is no illusion of movement or typical associated symptoms. Loss of consciousness during attacks should prompt thoughts of epilepsy or syncope rather than vertigo.

Causes Disorders of the labyrinth, vestibular nerve, vestibular nuclei, or their central connections are responsible for practically all vertigo. Only rarely are other structures implicated (see opposite).

Labyrinthine vertigo *Benign positional vertigo:* (See p422). *Ménière's disease:* Recurrent, spontaneous attacks of vertigo, hearing loss, tinnitus, and a sense of aural fullness caused by endolymphatic hydrops. Vertigo is severe and rotational, lasts 20mins to hours and is often accompanied by nausea and vomiting. Hearing loss is sensorineural, affects primarily low frequencies, fluctuates and is progressive; often to complete deafness of the affected ear. Drop attacks may rarely feature (no loss of consciousness or vertigo). Acute attacks—bed rest and reassurance. An antihistamine (eg cyclizine) is useful if prolonged. Consider surgery or pharmacological ablation of the vestibular organ in very severe cases. *Ototoxicity:* (eg aminoglycosides) may also cause vertigo and deafness.

Vestibular nerve Damage in the petrous temporal bone or cerebellopontine angle often involves the auditory nerve too, causing associated deafness or tinnitus. Causes include trauma and vestibular schwannomas (acoustic neuromas). *Acoustic neuromas* usually present with hearing loss, vertigo coming only later. With progression, ipsilateral cranial nerves V, VII, IX, and X may be affected. Signs of ↑ICP are late. *Vestibular neuronitis:* Abrupt onset of severe vertigo, nausea, and vomiting, with the patient prostrate and immobile. No deafness or tinnitus. Probably due to a virus in the young, a vascular lesion in the elderly. Severe vertigo subsides in days, complete recovery takes 3–4 weeks. Reassure. Sedate. *Herpes zoster:* Herpetic eruption of the external auditory meatus; facial palsy ± deafness, tinnitus, and vertigo (Ramsay–Hunt syndrome).

Brainstem Infarction of the brainstem (vertebrobasilar circulation) produces marked vertigo but other lesions may also be responsible (see opposite). Vertigo is protracted as are the associated nausea, vomiting and nystagmus (p422). It is unusual for vertigo to be the only sign of brainstem disease; multiple cranial nerve palsies and sensory and motor tract defects are commonly also seen. Hearing is spared.

Causes of true vertigo

Vestibular end-organs and vestibular nerve
Ménière's disease
Vestibular neuronitis (acute labyrinthitis)
Benign positional vertigo (*OHCS* p546)
Motion sickness
Trauma
Ototoxicity (aminoglycosides)
Herpes zoster oticus (Ramsay–Hunt syndrome, *OHCS* p756)

Brainstem and cerebellum
MS
Infarction
Haemorrhage
Migraine

Cerebellopontine angle
Vestibular schwannoma (acoustic neuroma)

Cerebral cortex
Vertiginous epilepsy

Alcohol intoxication

Eyes
Ophthalmoplegia with diplopia

Cervical vertigo (controversial)

Nystagmus

(*Nystagmus is tricky: don't worry if you don't grasp all the facts below: you can return to this page later.*) Nystagmus entails involuntary, rhythmic eye oscillation (swivelling). It may be pendular or jerky (commoner). Ask the patient to fix on your finger ~2 feet away then test gaze (up, down, lateral) in both directions. Keep your finger within 30° of the midline to avoid inducing physiological nystagmus. Look for nystagmus especially as the 30° limit is reached. Nystagmus must last for >2 beats to be significant.

Jerk nystagmus may be *horizontal, vertical or rotatory*; it is worse on gaze away from the midline. It has two phases: slow drift of the eye from its resting position (abnormal), and a fast movement or saccade correcting drift whose direction, by convention, defines the direction of the nystagmus. *Causes:* Physiological; lesions of the labyrinth, vestibular apparatus, brainstem or cerebellum; drugs. *Physiological nystagmus* is a normal phenomenon at extremes of lateral gaze or when looking out of a moving train (optokinetic nystagmus). *Drugs:* Intoxication with alcohol, barbiturates, or phenytoin toxicity may produce nystagmus in any direction.

Labyrinthine and vestibular nystagmus (*horizontal, vertical, or oblique*) Tinnitus + hearing↓ suggests disease of the labyrinth (eg Ménière's disease—p420) while vertigo, nausea, vomiting, and a staggering gait may occur in labyrinthine or vestibular lesions (vestibular neuronitis). Occurring only in one direction of gaze (away from the lesion) this type of nystagmus is exacerbated by gaze in that direction (Alexander's law). If visual fixation is removed (Frenzel's glasses or electronystagmography), the nystagmus is made worse. With time the nystagmus often disappears unlike nystagmus of central origin (MS excepted). *Positional nystagmus* is triggered by head movements eg quickly sitting from lying, and is experienced as vertigo. Benign positional vertigo (BPV) is the commonest cause and may follow viral labyrinthitis or head injury. Diagnosis: elicit symptoms and nystagmus by Hallpike's (Bárány's) test: place him quickly supine from sitting with head supported below the bed-head. On turning head to one side: after a few seconds, the patient experiences vertigo, and nystagmus (in one direction) will be seen lasting 10–20sec. If the test is repeated often, the response will adapt (diminish). Unidirectionality, latency, fatigue, and adaptation are not features of central lesions causing positional vertigo, eg posterior fossa masses.

Central *Brainstem:* MS, vertebrobasilar ischaemia. Unidirectional, coarse, gaze-dependent nystagmus that may be horizontal or vertical. Vertigo is rare. Downbeat nystagmus is seen in lesions around the foramen magnum (eg Arnold–Chiari) and in Wernicke's encephalopathy and phenytoin or alcohol toxicity. Upbeat nystagmus is seen in lesions of the floor of the IV ventricle, MS, and Wernicke's encephalopathy. *Cerebellar nystagmus* is the only nystagmus to change direction with the direction of gaze. Nystagmus is, however, most marked towards the side of the lesion. *Internuclear ophthalmoplegia* is due to a medial longitudinal fasciculus lesion and results in gaze palsy (eye on the affected side fails to adduct on lateral gaze although movement of each eye separately is normal) plus nystagmus in the abducting eye. Common causes are MS, brainstem infarction, pontine glioma, Wernicke's, encephalitis, and phenytoin. *See-saw nystagmus:* Seen in parasellar tumours. One eye rises and turns in; the other falls and turns out, accompanied by bitemporal hemianopia.

Pendular nystagmus Eye oscillations of similar size and speed in both directions. They are binocular, in one plane, and may be accompanied by head oscillation. *Causes:* Loss of central vision early in life (eg albinism), prolonged work in the dark—miner's nystagmus, or congenital. Pendular nystagmus is rarely due to demyelination or infarction in the cerebellar pathways. There may be associated palatal myoclonus (a rhythmic elevation of the soft palate and uvula at a rate of 60–100 Hertz).

Deafness (►See OHCS p542)

Simple hearing tests To establish deafness the examiner should whisper a number increasingly loudly in one ear while blocking the other ear with a finger. The patient is asked to repeat the number. Make sure that failure is not from misunderstanding.

Rinne's test Place the base of a vibrating 256 (or 512) Hz tuning fork on the mastoid process. Then move the fork so that the prongs are 4cm from the external acoustic meatus. Normally air conduction (AC) is better than bone conduction (BC). If bone conduction (BC) is better than air conduction (AC) diagnose conductive deafness. If there is hearing loss and AC is better than BC, this suggests sensorineural deafness ie a cause central to the oval window—eg presbyacusis (from ageing or excess noise) or ototoxic drugs or post-meningitis.

Weber's test Place a vibrating tuning fork in the middle of the forehead. Ask which side the patient localizes the sound to—or is it heard in the middle? In unilateral sensorineural deafness the sound is located to the good side. In conduction deafness the sound is located to the bad side (as if the sensitivity of the nerve has been turned up to allow for poor air conduction). Neither of these tests is completely reliable.

Conductive deafness Usually due to wax (remove it under direct vision or by syringing with warm water after prior softening with drops, eg olive oil). Also: otosclerosis, otitis media, glue ear OHCS p538.

Causes of sensorineural deafness Presbyacusis, Ménière's disease (OHCS p546), paroxysmal vertigo, deafness, and tinnitus due to dilatation of the endolymphatic sac. Other causes: meningitis; acute labyrinthitis; head injury; acoustic neuroma; MS; Paget's disease; excessive noise; aminoglycosides; frusemide (furosemide); lead; several rare congenital syndromes OHCS (p540); maternal infections during pregnancy.

Tinnitus (See OHCS p544.)

This is ringing or buzzing in the ears. It is a common phenomenon.

Causes Unknown; hearing loss (20%); wax; viral; presbyacusis; noise (eg gunfire); head injury; suppurative otitis media; post-stapedectomy; Ménière's; head injury; anaemia; hypertension; impacted wisdom teeth. *Drugs:* Aspirin; loop diuretics; aminoglycosides (eg gentamicin). *Psychological associations:* Redundancy, divorce, retirement.

►Investigate unilateral tinnitus fully to exclude a vestibular schwannoma (acoustic neuroma).

Objectively detectable tinnitus: Palatal myoclonus; temporomandibular problems; AV fistulae; bruits; glomus jugulare tumours; (pulsatile tinnitus, OHCS p544).

Treatment *Psychological support* is very important (eg from a hearing therapist). Exclude serious causes; reassure that tinnitus does not mean madness or serious disease and that it often improves in time. Cognitive therapy is recommended.[1] Patient support groups can help greatly.[2]
Drugs are disappointing. Avoid tranquillizers, particularly if the patient is depressed (use nortriptyline here),[1] but hypnotics at night may be helpful. Carbamazepine has been disappointing; betahistine only helps in some of those in whom the cause is Ménière's disease.

Masking may give relief. White noise is given via a noise generator worn like a post-aural hearing aid. Hearing aids may help those with hearing loss by amplifying desirable sound. Section of the cochlear nerve relieves disabling tinnitus in 25% of patients (but deafness results).

1 L Luxon 1993 BMJ i 1490   2 British Tinnitus Association, 105 Gower Street, London W1E 6AH

✚ Acute spinal cord compression

A typical presentation is with weak legs. There are many causes of weak legs (see opposite) but only a few cardinal questions: *was the onset gradual or sudden? Is the weakness progressing? Are the legs spastic or flaccid? Is there sensory loss, in particular a sensory level (a strong indicator of spinal cord disease)? Is there loss of sphincter control (bowels, bladder)?*

Leg weakness of acute onset
▶*Acute cord compression is an emergency.* Hours make a difference—left untreated it may rapidly progress to irreversible loss of muscle power and sensation below the level of the lesion, and a neurogenic bladder and bowel.

The Patient *Symptoms:* Spinal or root pain (p468) usually precedes the development of weak legs, weak arms (often less severe) and sensory loss. Bladder (and anal sphincter) involvement happens late and manifests itself as hesitancy, frequency and later painless retention. *Signs:* Look for a sensory level, commonly a few segments below the myotome level. Initially there will be a flaccid paresis with ↓reflexes in the limbs at *and* below the level of the lesion. Later, UMN signs (↑tone, ↑reflexes, clonus) develop (see p468) below the level of the lesion.

Causes Secondary malignancy (breast, lung, prostate) in the spine is commonest. Rarer: Infection (epidural abscess), disc prolapse, haematoma (warfarin), intrinsic cord tumour, atlanto–axial subluxation.

Differential diagnosis Transverse myelitis; MS; carcinomatous meningitis; Guillain–Barré; cord infarction, eg vasculitis (PAN, syphilis), thrombosis of spinal artery, trauma, compression, dissecting aortic aneurysm.

Tests Do not delay imaging at any cost. MRI is the best choice, but if unavailable, do CT and myelography to show where the lesion is. Biopsy may be needed to identify any mass. Spinal x-ray can help. *Screening blood tests:* FBC, ESR, serum B₁₂, folate, syphilis serology, U&E, LFT, prostate specific antigen. Do a CXR (lung malignancy, lung secondaries, TB). Consider LP.

Treatment Depends on the cause. If malignancy, give dexamethasone IV (4mg 6-hourly) while considering more specific therapy. Options are radiotherapy or chemotherapy with or without decompressive laminectomy; which is most appropriate depends upon the type of tumour, the patient's quality of life and the likely prognosis. Epidural abscesses must be surgically decompressed and antibiotics given.

Lesions of the cauda equina and conus medullaris The main difference between these lesions and those higher up in the cord is that leg weakness is flaccid and areflexic, not spastic and hyperreflexic. *Causes:* as above plus canal stenosis; lumbosacral nerve lesions. *Clinical features:* Cona medullaris lesions show early urinary retention and constipation, back pain; sacral sensory disturbance, impotence ± leg weakness. Cauda equina lesions feature back pain; asymmetrical, atrophic, areflexic paralysis of the legs; sensory loss in a root distribution and sphincter disturbance.

Management of the paralysed patient Irrespective of the cause, paralysed patients need especial care. Avoid pressure sores by frequent inspection of weight-bearing areas and turning. Avoid thrombosis in a weak or paralysed limb by frequent passive movement and elastic stockings. Bladder care is important (catheterization is only one option) and control of incontinence should not be at the expense of fluid intake (OHCS p730). Bowel evacuation may be manual or aided by suppositories—alteration of dietary fibre intake may help. Exercise of unaffected or partially paralysed limbs is important to avoid unnecessary loss of function.

Other causes of leg weakness

●*Chronic spastic paraparesis*
MS; cord compression (eg cervical spondylosis p468); syringomyelia; motor neurone disease; subacute combined degeneration of the cord (vitamin B$_{12}$ deficiency p582); syphilis.

●*Chronic flaccid paraparesis*
Tabes dorsalis; peripheral neuropathies (p464); myopathies (p470).

●*Unilateral foot drop*
DM; stroke; prolapsed disc; MS; common peroneal nerve palsy.

●*Weak legs with no sensory loss*
Motor neurone disease.

●*Absent knee jerks and extensor plantars*
Friedreich's ataxia; taboparesis (syphilis); motor neurone disease; subacute combined degeneration of the cord (but knee jerks more often brisk).

Specific gait disorders (see PLATE 3)

(Even the best professionals have to employ extraordinary tactics simply to *describe* gaits accurately,[1] never mind *diagnose* them accurately.)

●*Spastic:* Stiff, circumduction.

●*Extrapyramidal:* Flexed posture, shuffling feet, slow to start, postural instability. *Example:* Parkinson's disease.

●*Frontal:* Shuffling, difficulty getting feet off the floor ('magnetic'). *Example:* Normal pressure hydrocephalus.

●*Cerebellar:* Wide base, unstable, can't walk heel-to-toe steps. *Examples:* Posterior fossa tumour; alcohol or phenytoin toxicity.

●*Sensory:* Wide base, falls, worse in poor light, ↓joint position and vibration. *Examples:* Cervical spondylosis, tabes dorsalis.

●*Myopathic:* Waddle (hip girdle weakness).

●*Psychogenic:* Wild flinging of arms/legs, usually no falls ('astasia abasia') or overcautious, 'like walking on ice'. *Example:* Depression.

Tests Spinal x-rays. CT ± myelogram; MRI; FBC, ESR, syphilis serology serum B$_{12}$, U&E, LFT, CK/aldolase; PSA (prostate cancer), serum electrophoresis (myeloma), PTT/INR; CXR (TB, Ca bronchus); LP (p412); EMG; muscle biopsy; sural nerve biopsy.

1 'Unda her brella mid piddle med puddle she ninnygoes nannygoes nancing by'—James Joyce, Finnegan's Wake

Abnormal involuntary movements (dyskinesia)

Tremor Rest tremor is rhythmic, present at rest, and abolished on voluntary movement. It occurs in Parkinson's disease (p452), along with other features of the disease. Intention tremor is an irregular, large-amplitude shaking worse on movement eg reaching out for something. It is typical of cerebellar disease. Tremor in anxiety, thyrotoxicosis, benign essential tremor (inherited) and with drugs (eg β–agonists) is abolished at rest, present throughout the whole range of movement and most marked distally. Alcohol and β-blockers may help.

Chorea, athetosis, and hemiballismus *Chorea:* Non-rhythmic, jerky, purposeless movements (esp hands) with voluntary movements possible in between. Causes are Huntington's chorea (choreoathetoid movements), and Sydenham's chorea—a rare complication of streptococcal infection. The anatomical basis of chorea is uncertain although it is often thought of as the pharmacological mirror image of Parkinson's disease (L-dopa worsens chorea). *Hemiballismus:* Large-amplitude, flinging hemichorea (affects proximal muscles) contralateral to a vascular lesion of the subthalamic nucleus (often elderly diabetics). Recovers spontaneously over months. *Athetosis:* Slow, sinuous, confluent, purposeless movements (esp digits, hands, face, tongue), often difficult to distinguish from chorea. Commonest causes are perinatal hypoxia and kernicterus.

Tics Brief, repeated, and stereotyped movements which patients are able to suppress for a while. Tics are common in children, but usually resolve spontaneously. In *Gilles de la Tourette's syndrome* (p698) multiple motor and vocal tics occur. Consider clonazepam or clonidine if tics are severe (haloperidol is more effective but risk of tardive dyskinesia).

Myoclonus Sudden involuntary focal or general jerks arising from cord, brainstem, or cerebral cortex, seen in neurodegenerative disease (eg lysosomal storage enzyme defects), CJD (p702), and myoclonic epilepsies (infantile spasms). *Benign essential myoclonus:* Generalized myoclonus beginning in childhood as muscle twitches. It may be inherited as an autosomal dominant and has no consequences (bar twitches). *Asterixis:* A jerky tremor of outstretched hands (metabolic flap). *Treatment:* Myoclonus may respond to sodium valproate, clonazepam or piracetam.

Dystonia Prolonged muscle contraction producing abnormal postures or repetitive movements due to many causes. *Idiopathic torsion dystonia (ITD)* is the commonest. It presents in early adulthood as a focal dystonia (eg *spasmodic torticollis*—the head is pulled to one side and held there by a contracting sternomastoid). There is no other neurological deficit or history of secondary causes eg Wilson's disease. Patients presenting <40 years old need a therapeutic trial of L-dopa to rule out *Dopa-responsive dystonia* which is rare, but cured by the drug. A few ITD patients respond to benzhexol (=trihexyphenidyl, an anticholinergic). *Blepharospasm* (involuntary contraction of orbicularis oculi) and *writer's cramp* (spasm of hand and forearm muscles only on writing) are other focal dystonias (*OHCS* p522). An *acute dystonia* may occur (especially in young men) soon after starting neuroleptics (head pulled back, eyes drawn upward, trismus). Use anticholinergics (procyclidine 5–10mg IV). Severely disabling focal dystonias may be treated with minute doses of botulinum toxin injected into the muscle (*OHCS* p522) but there may be side-effects.[1]

Tardive dyskinesia Involuntary chewing and grimacing movements due to long-term neuroleptics (including the anti-emetics metoclopramide and prochlorperazine), especially in the elderly. *Treatment:* Withdraw neuroleptic and wait 3–6 months. The dyskinesia may fail to resolve or even worsen. If so, consider tetrabenazine 25–50mg/8h PO.

1 GL Sheean 1995 *Lancet* **346** 154

Dysarthria, dysphasia, and dyspraxia

Dysarthria Difficulty with articulation due to incoordination or weakness of the musculature of speech. Language is normal (see below). *Assessment:* Ask to repeat "British constitution" or "baby hippopotamus".

Cerebellar disease: Ataxia of the muscles of speech causes slurring (patients may seem drunk) and speech irregular in volume and scanning in quality.

Extrapyramidal disease: Soft, indistinct, and monotonous speech.

Pseudo-bulbar palsy: (p466) Spastic dysarthria (*upper motor neurone*). Speech is slow, indistinct and effortful ('Donald Duck'). Due to bilateral hemispheric lesions or motor neurone disease (MND) or severe MS.

Bulbar palsy: Lower motor neurone (eg facial nerve palsy, Guillain–Barré, MND).

Other lesions: Neuromuscular junction (myasthenia; speech is quiet, indistinct, and variable, depending on which muscles are affected). *Palate paralysis:* This produces nasal speech.

Dysphasia (Impairment of language caused by brain damage.) *Assessment:*
1 Is speech fluent, grammatical, meaningful and apt? If so, dysphasia is unlikely.
2 Comprehension: Can the patient follow one, two, and several step commands? (touch your ear, stand up then close the door).
3 Repetition: Can the patient repeat a sentence?
4 Naming: Can he name common and uncommon things (eg parts of a watch)?
5 Reading and writing: Normal? They are usually affected like speech in dysphasia. If normal, the patient is unlikely to be aphasic—is he mute?

Classification: (see opposite):[1] **Broca's (expressive) dysphasia:** Non-fluent speech produced with effort and frustration with mal-formed words, eg "spoot" for "spoon" (or "that thing"). Reading and writing are impaired but comprehension is relatively intact. Patients understand questions and attempt to convey meaningful answers. *Site of lesion: infero-lateral frontal lobe.*

Wernicke's (receptive) dysphasia: Oddly empty but fluent speech, like talking ragtime with phonemic ("flush" for "brush") and semantic ("comb for "brush") paraphasias/neologisms, sometimes mistaken for psychotic speech. He is oblivious of errors. Reading, writing *and* comprehension are impaired, (so replies are inappropriate). *Site of lesion: posterior superior temporal lobe.*

Conduction aphasia: (*Traffic between Broca's and Wernicke's areas is interrupted.*) Repetition is impaired; comprehension and fluency less so.

Transcortical dysphasias: Caused by injury to areas of *cortex surrounding the classical language areas.* Repetition is spared. Naming is affected in all dysphasias, but in anomic aphasia, especially left temporoparietal lesions. Mixed dysphasias are common. Discriminating features of dysphasias take time to emerge after an acute brain injury. Consider speech therapy (variably useful).

Dyspraxia (Impairment performance of complex movements despite preservation of ability to perform their individual components). Motor programmes for skilled movements reside in the dominant hemisphere—disease here causes true dyspraxia. Test for this by asking the patient to copy unfamiliar hand positions; mime the use of objects, eg a comb; and perform familiar gestures, eg salute. The term dyspraxia is used in 3 other ways:
1 *Dressing dyspraxia:* The patient is unsure of the orientation of clothes on his body. Test by pulling one sleeve of a sweater inside out before asking the patient to put it back on (mostly non-dominant hemisphere lesions).
2 *Constructional dyspraxia:* Difficulty in assembling objects or drawing—a 5-pointed star (non-dominant hemisphere lesions, hepatic encephalopathy).
3 *Gait dyspraxia:* Common in the elderly, explaining the presence of a gait disorder even though the individual components involved in walking are unimpaired. Seen with bilateral frontal lesions, lesions in the posterior temporal region, and hydrocephalus.

Classification of aphasias (+ = affected; − = relatively spared)[1]

Type	Fluency	Repetition	Comprehension	Naming	Cause
Global	Non-fluent	+	+	+	Stroke; tumour
Broca's	Non-fluent	+	−	+	Stroke; tumour
Wernicke's	Fluent	+	+	+	Stroke; tumour
Conduction	Fluent	+	−	+	Stroke
Anomic	Fluent	−	−	+	Dementia or head inury

The left hemisphere is dominant (ie controls language) in 99% of right-handed and 60% of left-handed people.

1 Reproduced with permission from *Cognitive Assessment for the Clinician*, 1994 OUP

Stroke: clinical features and investigations

A stroke results either from ischaemic infarction of part of the brain, or from bleeding into the brain. It is manifest by rapid onset (minutes) of focal CNS signs and symptoms. It is the major neurological disease of our times. Incidence is 1.5/1000/year overall, rising rapidly with age to 10/1000/year at 75yrs. Men are at slightly greater risk than women. *Chief causes:* Thrombosis *in-situ*, atherothrombo-embolism (eg from carotids); cardiac emboli (eg AF or post-MI); intracerebral haemorrhage (BP↑, trauma, rupture of aneurysm). *More rarely:* Hypotension (eg sudden drop >40mmHg); vasculitis; thrombophlebitis; venous-sinus thrombosis (p477). *In young patients* suspect thrombophilia (p620), vasculitis, subarachnoid haemorrhage, venous-sinus thrombosis and carotid artery dissection.
►Do not hesitate to get a cardiology, haematology or neurology opinion.

Risk factors BP↑, smoking, DM; heart disease (valvular, ischaemic, AF), peripheral vascular disease, past TIA, ↑PCV, carotid bruit, the Pill in smokers, lipids↑ (statins ↓stroke risk chiefly in those with co-existing heart disease[1]), excess alcohol; clotting↑ (eg ↑plasma fibrinogen, ↓antithrombin III, p620).

The Patient Sudden onset of symptoms, or a step-wise progression over hours (even days) is typical. In theory, focal signs relate to distribution of the affected artery (p404), but collateral supplies cloud the issue. *Cerebral hemisphere infarcts* (50%) may cause: contralateral hemiplegia which is initially flaccid (floppy limb, falls like a dead weight when lifted) then becomes spastic (UMN); contralateral sensory loss; homonymous hemianopia; dysphasia. *Brainstem infarction* (25%): wide range of effects which include quadriplegia, disturbances of gaze and vision, locked-in syndrome (aware, but unable to respond). *Lacunar infarcts* (25%): small infarcts around basal ganglia, internal capsule, thalamus and pons. The patient is conscious. May cause pure motor, pure sensory, mixed motor and sensory signs, or ataxia.

Tests Prompt investigation to confirm diagnosis and avoid further strokes but consider whether results will affect management. Look for:
- *Hypertension:* Look for retinopathy (p676) and a big heart on CXR. Note: acutely raised BP is common in early stroke. In general, don't treat (p434).
- *Cardiac source of emboli: Atrial fibrillation:* (p290) Emboli from the left atrium may have caused the stroke. Look for a large left atrium on CXR and consider echocardiography. *Post-MI:* Mural thrombus is best shown by echocardiography. In stroke due to AF or mural thrombus do CT to exclude a haemorrhagic stroke, then start aspirin; wait before commencing full anticoagulation to avoid bleeds into infarcts. *SBE/IE:* (p312) 20% of those with endocarditis present with CNS signs due to septic emboli from valves. Treat as endocarditis; ask a cardiologist's opinion.
- *Carotid artery stenosis:* In carotid territory (p404) stroke/TIA, two large randomized trials[2] have clearly established the benefit of carotid surgery, so expert bodies now affirm that >70% stenoses (on Doppler screening) merit angiography ± surgery—in fit patients.[2]
- *Hypoglycaemia, hyperglycaemia* and *hyperlipidaemia.*
- *Giant cell arteritis* (p674) eg if ESR↑, or story of headache or tender scalp (not necessarily temporal). Give steroids promptly (p674).
- *Syphilis:* Look for active disease only (p233).
- *Thrombocytopenia* and other bleeding disorders. • *Polycythaemia* (p612)

Minimum tests to exclude preventable causes

Pulse and BP	FBC, platelets	Sickling tests eg in blacks
CXR	ESR/U&E	Blood glucose, lipids
ECG	Lipids (esp. if	Syphilis serology if relevant
Carotid doppler	past angina/MI)[1]	Endocarditis tests (p312)

Then consider: CT scan, echocardiogram, CNS angiogram, clotting tests.

1 *E-BM* 1998 **3** 10 & 41 2 Association of British Neurologists (M Brown) 1992 *BMJ* ii 1071

✚ Stroke: management and prevention

MRI/CT scans Should now be the rule and not the exception but are especially important if: ●Unexpected deterioration after the first 24 hours.
●If unusual features, or diagnosis remains unclear—eg onset slow or not known. Consider especially cerebral tumour and subdural haematoma.
●To distinguish between haemorrhage and ischaemic infarction (do scan within 2 weeks of stroke), eg if considering later anticoagulation.
●Cerebellar stroke—cerebellar haematomas may need urgent surgery.

Differential diagnosis CNS tumour; subdural bleed (p440), Todd's palsy (p710). Consider drug overdose if comatose. The 2 types of stroke are *not* reliably distinguishable clinically but pointers to haemorrhagic stroke are: history of hypertension, meningism, severe headache, and coma within hours. Pointers to ischaemic stroke: carotid bruit, AF, past TIA.

Management (See p432 & p68.) Explain what has happened. Decide on the kindest level of intervention (list below) taking into account quality of life, co-existing conditions and prognosis. Admission to stroke units for nursing/physio saves lives, and is a great motivator. ▶*Communicate fully with patient and relatives.* ●Unless there is strong suspicion of CNS bleeding, acute aspirin (300mg/24h PO) has a small but worthwhile effect.[1]
●Nil by mouth if there is no gag reflex (try water on a teaspoon first).
●Maintain hydration, taking care not to overhydrate (cerebral oedema).
●Turn regularly and keep dry (consider catheter) to stop bed sores.
●Monitor BP; but treating even very high levels may harm (unless there is encephalopathy, or aortic dissection): even a 20% fall in BPs >200/120 mmHg may impair perfusion, as cerebral autoregulation is impaired.[2]
●If cerebral haemorrhage is suspected, consider immediate referral for evacuation (familiarize yourself with local current management).
●Consider *heparin* (p92) for *stroke in evolution,* eg weak arm, then a weak leg.

Mortality 20% at 1 month, 5–10%/year thereafter. **Full recovery** 40%. Drowsiness, head or eye deviation, or hemiplegia suggest prognosis↓.

Sequelae Pneumonia; depression; contractures; constipation; bedsores; 'I'm a prisoner in my own body'; stress in spouse (eg ± alcoholism), only partly relieved by respite admissions.

Prevention ●*Primary:* This means controlling risk factors (p432—eg BP, smoking, DM, and lipids). ▶*Ask the patient to give up smoking.* In middle-aged men (especially if ↑BP), quitting ↓risk of stroke, with the benefits seen within 5yrs. ◄2► (Switching to pipes or cigars achieves little; former heavy smokers retain some excess risk.) Lifelong anticoagulants for those with rheumatic or prosthetic heart valves on left side. Consider anticoagulation in chronic AF especially if there are risk factors for vascular disease. Prevention post-TIA (p436). ●*Secondary:* (ie preventing further strokes) Control risk factors. Consider aspirin (p436) or warfarin if the stroke was embolic, or the patient is in chronic AF (see p290).

The future for ischaemic stroke Randomized trials suggest rapid assessment of 'brain attacks' (like 'heart attacks') and thrombolysis with alteplase (t-PA) *within 3h of onset of symptoms* decreases risk of adverse outcome by 12%.[3] CI: ●Major infarct on CT ●Mild deficits or improvement ●Recent surgery ●Past CNS haemorrhage ●Recent arterial puncture at a non-compressible site ●Seizure at stroke onset ●Anticoagulants or PTT >15sec ●Platelets <100 × 10⁹/L ●Hypertension ●Very high or low glucose. *This treatment cannot be recommended yet,* because the risk of harm has not been fully quantified in patients outside the controlled environment of trials. The position may be different in hospitals which already have CNS thrombolysis teams with a dedicated imaging service on 24-hour call.

1 IST group 1997 *Lancet* 349 1569 ◄2► S Wannamethee 1996 E-BM 1 95   3 E-BM 1996 1 106

Transient ischaemic attacks (TIA)

The sudden-onset of focal CNS signs or symptoms due to temporary occlusion, usually by emboli, of part of the cerebral circulation is termed a TIA if symptoms fully resolve within 24h (TIAs are often much shorter). They are the harbingers of stroke and MI. If they are recognized for what they are, and preventive measures are prompt, disaster may be averted.

The Patient *Symptoms:* Attacks may be single or repetitive—symptoms may be the same or different on subsequent occasions. Ischaemia in the carotid territory (p404): Contralateral weakness, numbness, or paraesthesiae; dysphasia; dysarthria; homonymous hemianopia; amaurosis fugax (one eye's vision is progressively blotted out "like a curtain descending"). *Vertebrobasilar territory:* Hemiparesis; hemisensory loss; bilateral weakness or sensory loss; diplopia; cortical blindness; vertigo; deafness; tinnitus; vomiting; dysarthria; ataxia; drop attacks. *Signs (24h after an attack):* No neurological signs. Listen for carotid bruits (p40) although their absence does not rule out a carotid source of emboli (tight stenoses often have no bruit).[1] Listen for cardiac murmurs suggesting valve disease and identify AF. Fundoscopy during a TIA may reveal retinal artery emboli.

Causes Atherothrombo-embolism from the carotid is commonest. Emboli from the heart (atrial fibrillation, mural thrombus post-MI, valvular disease, prosthetic valves); involvement of more than one cerebral artery territory is suggestive. Haematological disease (polycythaemia, sickle-cell, multiple myeloma) and arterial disease (giant cell arteritis, PAN, SLE, syphilis and many others) are more rarely responsible.

Differential diagnosis of brief focal CNS symptoms: *Migraine* (symptoms spread and intensify over minutes, often with visual scintillations before headache); *focal epilepsy* (symptoms spread over seconds and often include twitching and jerking). Rare: *Malignant hypertension; hypoglycaemia; MS; intracranial lesions; phaeochromocytoma; somatization* (p163).

Tests Aim to find the cause and define vascular risk factors: FBC, ESR, U&E, glucose, lipids, CXR, ECG, syphilis serology (if relevant), carotid Doppler ± angiography, MRI/CT scan (are there existing infarcts?) ± echocardiography (rarely reveals a cardiac cause if no suggestive signs).

Treatment Begin after the first attack—don't wait for another; it could be a stroke. Control risk factors for stroke (p432) and MI (p255, and risk-equation, p740), the commonest mode of death after TIA. *Reversible risk factors:* Hypertension (cautiously lower to 100mmHg diastolic); hyperlipidaemia (p654); help to stop smoking (OHCS p452).
- Give an antiplatelet drug: aspirin if no peptic ulcer (eg 150mg daily PO), *for life*. The dose of aspirin is controversial, but evidence suggests it decreases non-fatal strokes and MI by 25%, and vascular death by 15%.
- Consider oral anti-coagulation in AF, mitral stenosis, recent major septal MI, and if frequent TIAs not controlled by antiplatelet drugs.
- Consider carotid endarterectomy in TIA with carotid distribution if patient is a good operative risk* and >70% stenosis at the origin of the internal carotid artery.[2,3] For benefit to outweigh risk, the team's perioperative stroke/mortality rate must be <5%. Intra-operative transcranial Doppler can monitor middle cerebral artery flow. A patch may be used to reduce the chance of restenosis.[1] Do *not* stop aspirin beforehand.

We do not know what to advise in recurrent TIA with <70% stenosis.

Prognosis The risk of stroke and MI is ~7% per year each (the risk of stroke is 12% in the first year and up to 10% subsequently if carotid stenosis is 70%). Mortality is ~3 times that of a TIA-free matched population.

1 P Morris 1994 *Practitioner* 427 2 ECST 1991 *Lancet* 337 1235 3 C Warlow 1997 *BMJ* ii 1571 *Who is at risk of death/CVA from endarterectomy?* ♀ sex, aged >75, systolic BP↑, occlusion of contralateral artery; stenosis of ipsilateral carotid syphon or external carotid; wide-territory TIAs vs just amaurosis fujax.

Subarachnoid haemorrhage

Spontaneous bleeding into the subarachnoid space is a sudden and frequently catastrophic event. Incidence: 15/100,000; typical age: 35–65yrs.

Cause Rupture of congenital berry aneurysms is the commonest cause (70%) with AVM accounting for 15%. No cause is found in <15%. *Rare associations:* Bleeding disorders, mycotic aneurysm secondary to endocarditis, smoking, hypertension, alcohol, lack of oestrogen (in women). HRT protects, as does being premenopausal (irrespective of age).[1] ♀:♂ >1.

Berry aneurysms Common sites: junction of the posterior communicating with the internal carotid; junction of the anterior communicating with the anterior cerebral; bifurcation of the middle cerebral artery. 15% are multiple. A genetic influence has been suggested. Skin biopsy may demonstrate type 3 collagen deficiency and identify relatives at risk. *Associations:* Polycystic kidneys, Ehlers–Danlos sy, coarctation of the aorta.

The Patient *Symptoms:* Sudden (within a few seconds) devastating headache "*I thought I'd been kicked in the head*", often occipital. Vomiting and collapse with loss of consciousness frequently follow. The patient may remain comatose or drowsy for days. *Signs* Neck stiffness (Kernig's +ve) takes 6h to develop; papilloedema; retinal and subhyaloid (below the lens) haemorrhage. Focal neurology, eg hemiplegia, developing early suggests formation of an intracerebral haematoma, later suggests vasospasm and ischaemia. Presentation may be as coma or seizures.[3]

Differential In general practice, only 25% of patients with severe, sudden headaches have SAH. In most no cause is found and the remainder are diagnosed as meningitis, migraine, glioma, or an intracerebral bleed.

Sentinel headache SAH patients may earlier have experienced a sentinel headache, thought to represent a small warning leak from the offending aneurysm (~6%), but the picture is clouded by recall-bias.[3,4] As corrective surgery is more successful in the least symptomatic, be suspicious of any sudden hemicranial, hemifacial, or periorbital headache, particularly if associated with neck or back pain.[2]

Tests CT shows subarachnoid or ventricular blood but misses 2% of small bleeds. If a –ve scan shows no mass lesion, intracerebral haematoma or hydrocephalus (all contraindications), do an LP, >12h after the onset of headache.[3] The CSF of SAH is uniformly bloody in the early stages of SAH and xanthochromic (yellow) after a few hours. CSF must be spun at once, or else oxyhaemoglobin forms in vitro.[3] *If there is no blood in the CSF the patient has not had a SAH.* A traumatic tap can confuse (don't rely on there being fewer CSF RBCs in each successive bottle).

Management ▶Get a neurosurgical opinion (immediately if ↓level of consciousness, progressive focal deficit or cerebellar haematoma suspected).
●Bed-rest + chart of BP, pupils, coma level. ?Repeat CT if deteriorating.
●Stool softeners to reduce need to strain. ●Re-examine CNS often.
●*Surgery* to clip off the aneurysm is aimed at preventing rebleeding and is most beneficial in those with few or no symptoms (≤ grade II). If surgery is a possibility, do angiography promptly.[2] Consider evacuation.
●*Medical:* Cautiously control *severe* hypertension; analgesia for headache; bed rest ± sedation for ~4 weeks. Keep properly hydrated (running 'dry' out of respect for ICP↑, worsens vasospasm). *Vasospasm:* Nimodipine (60mg/4h PO for 2–3 weeks, or 1mg/h IVI) is a Ca^{2+}antagonist that improves outcome.

Rebleeding is a common mode of death in those who have had a subarachnoid. Rebleeding occurs in 30% of patients, often in the first few days—or around the 12th day. **Vascular spasm** follows a bleed, often causing ischaemia and permanent neurological deficit. If this happens surgery is not helpful at the time but may be so later.

Mortality in subarachnoid haemorrhage

Grade:	Signs:	Mortality:
I	None	0%
II	Neck stiffness and cranial nerve palsies	11%
III	Drowsiness	37%
IV	Drowsy with hemiplegia	71%
V	Prolonged coma	100%

Almost all the mortality occurs in the first month. Of those who survive the first month, 90% survive a year or more.

1 WT Longstreth 1994 *Ann Int Med* **121** 168   2 J Ostergaard 1990 *BMJ* ii 190
3 J van Gijn 1997 *Lancet* **249** 1491   4 F Linn 1994 *Lancet* **344** 590

⁝⁝⁝ Subdural haemorrhage

▶*Consider this very treatable condition in all whose conscious level fluctuates, and also in those who seem to have a slowly evolving stroke.* Bleeding is from bridging veins between cortex and venous sinuses, resulting in accumulation of haematoma between dura and arachnoid. This causes a gradually increasing ICP, shift of midline structures away from the side of the clot and, if left untreated, eventual tentorial herniation and coning.

Most subdurals are secondary to trauma but they can occur without. *The trauma may have been so minor or have happened so long ago that it is not recalled.* The elderly are particularly susceptible, as brain shrinkage makes bridging veins more vulnerable. Others at risk are those prone to falls (epileptics, alcoholics) and those on long-term anticoagulation.

Symptoms Development of a subdural haemorrhage may be insidious so be alerted by a fluctuating level of consciousness (present in 35%). Typical complaints are of physical and intellectual slowing, sleepiness, headache, personality change and unsteadiness.

Signs ↑ICP (780). Localizing neurological symptoms (eg unequal pupils, hemiparesis) occur late and often long after the injury (63 days average).

Tests CT will show the presence of clot.

Differential Evolving stroke, cerebral tumour, dementia.

Treatment Evacuation via burr holes may lead to complete recovery.

▶▶Extradural haemorrhage

▶*Suspect this if, after head injury, conscious level falls or is slow to improve.* Extradural bleeds are commonly due to a fractured temporal or parietal bone causing laceration of the middle meningeal artery and vein, typically after trauma to a temple just lateral to the eye. Any tear in a dural venous sinus will also result in an extradural bleed. Blood accumulates beween bone and dura.

Symptoms and signs Look out for a deterioration of consciousness after any head injury that initially produced no loss of consciousness or after initial drowsiness post-injury seems to have resolved. This 'lucid interval' pattern is typical of extradural bleeds. It may last a few hours to a few days before a bleed declares itself by a deteriorating level of consciousness caused by a rising ICP. Increasingly severe headache, vomiting, confusion and fits can follow, accompanied by a hemiparesis with brisk reflexes and an upgoing plantar. If bleeding continues, coma deepens, a bilateral spastic paraparesis develops, and breathing becomes deep and irregular. Death follows a period of coma and is due to respiratory arrest. Bradycardia is common, accompanied by raised blood pressure. Ipsilateral pupil dilatation is a late sign.

Investigation CT shows a haematoma which is often lens-shaped. Skull x-ray may be normal or show fracture lines crossing the course of the middle meningeal vessels. *Lumbar puncture is contraindicated.*

Management Urgent evacuation of the clot through multiple burr holes may be necessary *before* transfer to a neurosurgical centre, so any surgeon should be prepared to release a clot. Prompt improvement follows, as haematoma exudes from the burr holes (OTS 21.51). Definitive surgery involves identification and ligation of the bleeding vessel.

Prognosis Excellent if diagnosis and operation early. Poor if coma, bilateral spastic paresis or decerebrate rigidity are present pre-op.

Encephalitis

► *Herpes simplex encephalitis needs urgent treatment with aciclovir (p203).*

Encephalitis is inflammation of brain parenchyma and is only distinguished from meningitis by the relative involvement of meninges and
brain. There is usually some degree of inflammation of the parenchyma
in meningitis and of the meninges in encephalitis.

Cause Viruses are the commonest cause (Herpes simplex, HSV,
Japanese (B) encephalitis, HIV, coxsackie virus, ECHO virus, rabies). Think
also of CMV in the immunocompromised. Measles may also cause *subacute
sclerosing panencephalitis* (SSPE) and rubella *progressive rubella panencephalitis. Other causes:* Neurosyphilis; *Borrelia burgdorferi* (p232); *Staph aureus*
(p222) and other bacteria originating from pus elsewhere (eg frontal
sinus) may reach the brain where they may cause abscesses. In the
immunocompromised also consider *Listeria* (p223) and toxoplasmosis.

The Patient Presentation varies to some degree with the organism
responsible. Typically there is fever; the symptoms and signs of meningitis (p442) and raised ICP (p780); altered consciousness; convulsions and
sometimes focal neurological signs or psychiatric symptoms. Patients
with HSV encephalitis may also experience olfactory or gustatory hallucinations, temporal lobe seizures, and amnesia. SSPE presents ~6 years after
the original infection with a slow deterioration featuring personality
change, dementia, myoclonic seizures, and ataxia, eventually leading to
death. Progressive rubella panencephalitis is similar.

Diagnosis is made from knowledge of epidemics and knowledge of
whether the patient is immunocompetent; unreliable clinical signs (eg
temporal lobe signs ± temporal lobe swelling seen on CT or MRI ± periodic complexes on EEG in HSV encephalitis); associated infection (eg
mumps); and demonstration of virus in CSF (culture, serology or PCR—
the quickest), throat swabs or stool culture.

Management Get expert help early and admit to ITU for supportive
care. In an ill patient, it may be necessary to treat blind with drugs covering several treatable causes of encephalitis. Most important is to realize that any fulminant acute encephalitis could be due to HSV and should
therefore be treated immediately with aciclovir. Ceftriaxone, benzylpenicillin + thiamine (in case of *Wernicke's encephalopathy* p712)[1] are
other reasonable empirical treatments to use until the agent responsible
is identified (this may never happen).

Post-infectious encephalomyelitis (acute disseminated encephalomyelitis) may occur after measles, varicella zoster, rubella, mumps or
influenza virus infection, or after vaccinia or nervous tissue-derived
rabies vaccinations. Clinically similar to encephalitis, it typically presents
with convulsions, coma, fever, or pareses about 2 weeks after the initial
infection. Involuntary movements, cranial nerve lesions, nystagmus, and
ataxia are also common.

1 CYW Tong 1997 *Lancet* **349** 470

✝✝✝ Meningitis

Meningitis is inflammation of the pia mater and arachnoid, most commonly caused by bacterial, viral, fungal, or other infection. ▶▶Bacterial meningitis is a killer, and can kill *very* quickly. Emergency treatment: p444.

The Patient Rapid onset (<48h) of signs and symptoms of:
- *Meningism:* Headache; photophobia; stiff neck; Kernig's sign +ve (pain and resistance on passive knee extension with hips fully flexed). Brudzinski's sign +ve (hips flex on bending head forward); opisthotonus.
- ↑ICP: Headache; irritability; drowsiness; vomiting; fits; ↓pulse; ↑BP; ↓consciousness/coma; irregular respiration; papilloedema (late sign).
- *Septicaemia:* Malaise; fever; arthritis; odd behaviour; rash (petechiae suggest meningococcus); DIC (bleeding); ↓BP; ↑pulse; tachypnoea.

Tests *Lumbar puncture* is critical to diagnosis. Perform at once provided there are no signs of ↑ICP (↓consciousness, *very* bad headache, frequent seizures) or focal neurology,[1] in which case do a CT scan first to rule out a mass lesion or hydrocephalus. Send 3 bottles of CSF for Gram stain, Ziehl–Nielsen stain (tuberculosis), cytology, virology, glucose, protein, culture and india ink for cryptococcus. CSF may be normal (p412 & p443) early on so repeat the LP if symptoms and signs persist. *CSF in meningitis* See opposite. Neutrophils >1180/mL predict bacterial meningitis with >99% certainty. Gram stains of CSF are +ve in 60–90% of bacterial meningitis (~40% if antibiotics have already been given). *Other tests:* Blood cultures (preferably before antibiotics); blood glucose (to compare with CSF); FBC; U&E; CXR (lung abscess?); culture urine, nasal swabs and stool (virology); skull x-ray if history of head injury.

Risk factors *Place:* Overcrowded closed communities, schools, day centres. *Head injury:* Especially basal skull fractures or cranial or spinal surgery. *Septic site:* Distant (pneumonia) or near (sinusitis; mastoiditis; otitis media). *Host factors:* Complement or antibody deficiency, OHCS p210; old or young. *Immunosuppression:* Carcinoma; AIDS; no effective spleen; sickle-cell disease; hypogammaglobulinaemia; DM. *Foreign body:* CSF shunts.

Aseptic meningitis CSF has cells but is Gram-stain –ve and no bacteria can be cultured on standard media. *Infective:* Virus (echovirus, mumps, coxsackie, herpes simplex and zoster, HIV, measles, 'flu); partly treated bacterial meningitis; fungi; atypical TB; syphilis; Lyme disease; parameningeal infection; leptospirosis; listeria; brucella. *Non-infective:* Below.

Non-infective meningitis Meningeal inflammation can be caused by meningeal infiltration by malignant cells (leukaemia, lymphoma, other tumours); chemical meningitis (intrathecal drugs, contrast, LP contaminants); drugs (NSAIDS, trimethoprim); sarcoidosis; SLE; Behçet's disease.

Differential diagnosis Any acute infection; local infections causing neck stiffness (eg of cervical lymph nodes); tetanus (CSF normal in all of these). Acute encephalitis (generalized CNS damage more marked than meningism); subarachnoid haemorrhage (p438, blood in CSF).

Prognosis and sequelae Acute bacterial meningitis has a mortality of 70–100% untreated; *Neisseria meningitidis* meningitis has an overall mortality in the West of ~15%. Survivors are at risk of permanent neurological deficits including mental retardation, sensorineural deafness (up to 40% although many do recover), and cranial nerve palsies. Viral meningitis is self-limiting, has a good prognosis, and no long-term sequelae.

Recurrent meningitis Is there access to the subarachnoid space *via* occult spina bifida or skull fractures, or one of the above risk factors, or an associated disease, eg SLE, sarcoid, Behçet's (p694), or benign recurrent aseptic Mollaret's meningitis (PCR suggests it is from *Herpes simplex*)?

1 M Anderson 1993 *JNNP* 56 1243–58

Typical CSF in meningitis (There are no hard-and-fast rules.)

	Pyogenic	Tuberculous	Viral ('aseptic')
Appearance	often turbid	often fibrin web	usually clear
Predominant cell*	polymorphs	mononuclear	mononuclear
Cell count/mm^3	<90–1000	10–350/mm^3	50–1500/mm^3
Glucose	< $^2/_3$ plasma	< $^2/_3$ plasma	> $^2/_3$ plasma
Protein (g/L)	>1.5	1–5	<1
Organisms	in smear and culture	often absent in smear	not in smear or culture

*≤5 lymphocytes/mm^3 may be normal, so long as there are no neutrophils. Normal protein: 0.15-0.45g/L. Normal CSF glucose: 2.8-4.2mmol/L (↓by: bacterial, fungal, mumps or carcinomatous meningitis, herpes encephalitis, hypoglycaemia, sarcoid, CNS vasculitides—*OTM* 3e 4055).

The predominant cell type may be lymphocytes in listerial and cryptococcal meningitis. Normal opening pressure: 7-18cmCSF; in meningitis it may be >40 (typically 14-30cmCSF).

⚕ Meningitis treatment ►*Prompt antibiotics save life.*

If you suspect your patient has meningitis and are outside hospital, *nothing* must delay blind therapy with IV/IM benzylpenicillin 1.2g while awaiting transport. If possible, do blood culture first. In hospital, LP (p412), blood cultures, and blood glucose are essential for accurate diagnosis but *must not* delay empirical antibiotic therapy. Do *not* wait for the ward round, expert advice, or test results: delay may be fatal. *Act now and don't worry about future criticism*: you may end up with a live patient on your side.

Empirical therapy What is the most likely organism? This depends on the patient's age; whether the disease is community or hospital-acquired; knowledge of local outbreaks; and whether the patient is immunocompromised, has a shunt or CSF leak. Select antibiotics to cover the likely possibilities while waiting for identification and antibiotic sensitivities.

Which antibiotic?[1] *See below + p177–9 for doses (alternatives in brackets).*
Pneumococcus: Cefotaxime (ceftriaxone) ± vancomycin.
Meningococcus: Benzylpenicillin (cefotaxime, ceftriaxone).
H influenzae: Cefotaxime (ceftriaxone, chloramphenicol; up to >50% may be chloramphenicol-resistant); give rifampicin (20mg/kg/12h PO if >3mths old; max 600mg) for 4 days pre-discharge in type b infection.[1]
E coli: Cefotaxime (ceftriaxone).
Staph aureus: Cloxacillin (p177); for resistant staphs, see MRSA (p222).
Listeria monocytogenes: Gentamicin + ampicillin (penicillin G, p223).
M tuberculosis: Rifampicin, ethambutol, isoniazid, *and* pyrazinamide.
Cryptococcus neoformans: Amphotericin B + flucytosine (p340, p244).

Treating pyogenic meningitis[1] (See *OHCS* for children's doses.)
Send blood glucose, cultures, and CSF before treating unless there is evidence of meningococcal meningitis (benzylpenicillin 1.2g then comes first) or LP is contraindicated by CT (p442). Involve senior support and a microbiologist early. Nurse patient in ITU and and insert a central line.
- Set up IVI. Give chosen empiric antibiotic. Dose examples:
  Cefotaxime 2–4g/8h IVI; ↓doses in renal failure; see p178 + *Data sheet*.
  Ceftriaxone 2g/12h IVI; halved if GFR <10mL/min, p179; give over 30min.
  Benzylpenicillin 2.4g/4h slowly IV.
  Ampicillin 1–2g/4h IV.
- Treat shock with plasma IVI until BP >80mmHg systolic and urine flows (p766). If ↑ICP, ask a neurosurgeon's advice about whether dexamethasone indicated?[1] Relieve *severe* pain (eg parenteral morphine 5–10mg per 4h). For nausea, try domperidone (60mg/8h PR).
- Once the organism and its sensitivities are known, change empiric therapy if necessary (discuss with microbiologist).
- Continue parenteral antibiotics for 10 days. Follow with rifampicin to eliminate nasal carriage.
- Look out for complications: cerebral oedema; cranial nerve lesions; deafness; cerebral venous-sinus thrombosis (p477).
- For novel biological treatments for meningococcaemia, see p710.

Meningococcal prophylaxis *Talk to your consultant in community disease control.* Offer prophylaxis to: ●Household/nursery contacts (ie within droplet range). ●Those who have kissed the patient's mouth. ●Yourself (rarely necessary). Give rifampicin (600mg/12h PO for 2 days; (Meningi >1yr 10mg/kg/12h; <1yr 5mg/kg/12h) or ciprofloxacin (500mg vae—adults only). Neither is guaranteed in pregnancy, but such school contacts is unlikely to harm and is recommended. Vaccination is from group A and C strains and may be used for ... or for travellers to endemic areas.

Most frequent causative organisms of community-acquired meningitis by age of patient[2]

Neonates:
  E coli
  β-haemolytic *streptococci*
  Listeria monocytogenes
Children <14 years:
  Haemophilus influenzae if <4yrs and unvaccinated
  Meningococcus (Neisseria meningitidis)
  Streptococcus pneumoniae
  TB (endemic areas)
Adults:
  Meningococcus
  Pneumococcus (Streptococcus pneumoniae)
Elderly and immunocompromised:
  Pneumococcus
  Listeria monocytogenes
  TB
  Gram negative organisms
  Cryptococcus

Hospital acquired (nosocomial) and post-traumatic meningitis

(May often be multi-drug-resistant)
  Klebsiella pneumoniae
  E coli
  Pseudomonas aeruginosa
  Staphylococcus aureus

Meningitis in special situations

Patients with CSF shunts are at especial risk of meningitis (eg staphylococcal), as are those patients having spinal procedures (eg spinal anaesthetics) where *Pseudomonas* species may be the culprit.

1 A Tunkel 1995 *Lancet* 346 1675 2 A Goldman 1997 *Lancet* 349 466

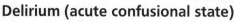

⫶⫶ Delirium (acute confusional state)

▶ *Common in hospitalized patients (5–15% patients in general medical or surgical wards) so consider any unexplained behaviour change in a hospital patient as possible delirium and look for an organic cause.*

The Patient 1 *Consciousness* is impaired with onset over hours or days. Impaired consciousness is difficult to describe but when you talk to the patient you have the sense that they aren't really with you. This has been described more formally as a mild impairment of thinking, attending, perceiving and remembering—or more simply as a mild global impairment of cognitive processes associated with a reduced awareness of the environment. Conscious level fluctuates throughout the day with confusion typically worsening in the late afternoon and at night. 2 *Disorientation* in time (does not know time, day or year) and place (often more marked) is the rule. 3 *Behaviour:* Inactivity, quietness, reduced speech and perseveration or else hyperactivity, noisiness and irritability (these patients can be very disruptive). 4 *Thinking:* Slow and muddled, commonly with ideas of reference or delusions (eg accusing staff of plotting against them). 5 *Perception:* Disturbed, often with illusions and hallucinations, especially visual but also auditory and tactile. 6 *Mood:* Lability, anxiety, perplexion, fear, agitation, or depression. 7 *Memory:* Impaired during delirium and on recovery, amnesia is usual.

Differential diagnosis If agitated, consider anxiety (check conscious level). If delusions or hallucinations, consider primary mental illness (eg schizophrenia) but remember that in hospitalised, ill patients with no psychiatric history, mental illness is rare and delirium is common.

Causes
- Systemic infection: pneumonia, UTI, surgical wound; IV lines
- Drugs: eg opiates, anticonvulsants, L-dopa, sedatives, recreational
- Alcohol withdrawal (2–5 days post-admission; ↑LFT + ↑MCV; history of alcohol abuse), also drug withdrawal
- Metabolic: hypoglycaemia, uraemia, liver failure, electrolyte imbalance
- Hypoxia: respiratory or cardiac failure
- Vascular: stroke, myocardial infarction
- Intracranial infection: encephalitis, meningitis
- Raised intracranial pressure/space occupying lesions
- Epilepsy: Status epilepticus, post-ictal states
- Head injury: especially subdural haematoma
- Nutritional: thiamine, nicotinic acid, or B_{12} deficiency

Management
1 Identify and treat the underlying cause.
2 Reduce distress and prevent accidents.
3 Nurse in a *moderately lit,* quiet room with the *same* staff in attendance (minimizes confusion) where the patient can be watched closely. Repeated reassurance and orientation to time and place is helpful.
4 Minimize medication, especially if sedative. If the patient becomes agitated and disruptive, however, some sedation may be necessary. Use a major tranquillizer—haloperidol 0.5–2mg IM/PO, p13—or chlorpromazine 50–100mg IM/PO (but not in the elderly, in whom it is liable to cause cardiac side-effects and hypotension). Wait 20 minutes to judge effect—further doses can be given if needed. Benzodiazepines may be used for night-time sedation. *Note:* In alcohol withdrawal do *not* use chlorpromazine, use diazepam instead (p524).

Epilepsy: diagnosis

Epilepsy is a tendency to spontaneous, intermittent, abnormal electrical activity in part of the brain, manifest as *seizures*. These may take many forms: for a given patient they tend to be stereotyped. *Convulsions* are the motor signs of electrical discharges. Many of us would have seizures in abnormal metabolic circumstances—eg Na⁺↓, hypoxia (reflex anoxic seizures in faints): we would not normally be said to have epilepsy. In deciding if an event is epileptic, don't pay *too* much attention to associated incontinence and abnormal movement (not everything that twitches is epilepsy): but tongue-biting is very suggestive. Prevalence of active epilepsy is ~1%.

The Patient There may be a *prodrome* lasting hours or days preceding the seizure. This is not part of the seizure itself. The patient or friends may notice a change in mood or behaviour. An *aura*, which is itself part of the seizure, may precede its other manifestations. The aura may be a strange feeling in the gut, or a sensation or an experience such as *déjà vu* (a disturbing sense of familiarity), or strange smells or flashing lights. It implies a partial seizure (it is a focal event), often, but not necessarily, temporal lobe epilepsy (TLE). After a partial seizure involving the motor cortex (Jacksonian convulsion) there may be temporary weakness of the affected limb(s) (Todd's palsy). After a generalized seizure the patient may feel awful with headache, myalgia, confusion, and a sore tongue.

Diagnosis Decide first: is this epilepsy? (Differential on p418) A detailed description from a witness of the fit is vital. Try hard not to diagnose epilepsy in error—therapy has significant side-effects, the diagnosis is stigmatizing and has implications for employment, insurance and driving. Decide next what type of epilepsy it is. The onset of the attack is the key to the major question: partial or generalized? If the fit begins with focal features, it is a partial seizure, however rapidly it is generalized. Ask next: what if anything brings it on (eg flickering light (TV) or alcohol)? Can this be avoided? TV-induced seizures—almost always generalized—rarely require drugs. Then decide what the best drug is. Start at low dose. Gradually (eg over 8 weeks) build up until fits controlled. Persist until drug at maximum dose before considering a change of therapy (p450).

Classification

1 *Partial seizures:* Features are referrable to a part of one hemisphere suggesting structural disease. (a) *Elementary symptoms* (consciousness not impaired eg focal motor seizures); (b) *Complex symptoms* (consciousness impaired eg olfactory aura followed by automatism). Usually TLE; (c) *Secondary generalized:* Evidence of focal origin before generalized seizure.

2 *Generalized seizures:* No features referrable to only one hemisphere. (a) *Absences (petit mal):* Brief (10sec) pauses, eg suddenly stops talking in mid-sentence, then carries on where left off. Presents in childhood. (b) *Tonic–clonic (classical grand mal).* Sudden onset, loss of consciousness, limbs stiffen (tonic) then jerk (clonic); may have one without the other. Drowsy afterwards. (c) *Myoclonic jerk* (eg thrown suddenly to ground, or a violently disobedient limb: one patient described it as "my flying-saucer epilepsy", as crockery which happened to be in the hand would take off). (d) *Atonic* (becomes flaccid). (e) *Akinetic.* Note also *infantile spasms.*

Causes of seizures (Often none is found) *Physical:* Trauma, space-occupying lesions, stroke, raised BP, tuberous sclerosis, SLE, PAN, sarcoid, and vascular malformations. *Metabolic causes:* Alcohol withdrawal, hypoglycaemia, hyperglycaemia, hypoxia (including cardiac eg bradyarrhythmias), uraemia, hypo- and hypernatraemia, hypocalcaemia, liver disease, and drugs (eg phenothiazines, tricyclics, cocaine or withdrawal of benzodiazepines). *Infections:* Encephalitis, syphilis, cysticercosis, HIV.

Evaluation of an adult who has just had a first-ever seizure

►For status epilepticus see p782.

● Obtain as much history as possible from patient and witnesses. Try to form an opinion as to whether the witness is reliable. In the heat of the moment many witnesses may report twitching when none in fact took place (perhaps they want to please you by seeming to be observant and they 'helpfully fill in the gaps in reality'—so, *beware*).

● You must attempt to establish a cause. Adult seizures are almost always 'symptomatic', ie secondary to another pathology.

● Clues from the history may point to an obvious illness or other toxic/metabolic cause for the seizure. If not, then these tests may help:

● U&E/LFT ● Ca^{2+}, Mg^{2+}, PO_4^{3-} ● FBC + INR/PTT ● Serum & urine toxic screens.

● Blood levels of medications. ● Consider lumbar puncture.

● Neuroimaging CT/MRI (± IV contrast; ± angiography).

● Emergency EEG only if concerned about non-convulsive status (p782).

● Admission for ~24h is often indicated for investigations and observation. Urgent treatment may be needed if seizures recur.

● You must give advice against driving and document your discussion.

►*Involve patients in all decisions.* Compliance depends on communication and doctor-patient concordance issues (p3). Living with epilepsy creates many problems (eg cannot drive, or operate machinery) and fears (eg of sudden death), and drug issues. A problem is that neurologists haven't got much time to explore these issues as each will have 1500 people with epilepsy on their books (in the UK). Each general practice will only have ~50 patients, but GPs may have no special interest in epilepsy. One way forward is a yearly visit to a GP-based epilepsy nurse, to monitor drugs, address employment, leisure, and reproductive issues—and, after ~4 fit-free years, to see if drugs can be carefully withdrawn.[1]

Investigation of a first seizure◈ If onset is focal or there are focal signs on examination, a CT scan is warranted—and, possibly, EEG. Childhood seizures warrant an EEG (to identify 3-per-second spike and wave activity—this is common and is treated with sodium valproate). If no suggestion of focus, opinions differ as to how far to take investigations. Consider: EEG, FBC, ESR, U&E, Ca^{2+}, LFT, CXR, plasma glucose, syphilis serology, ECG. ►*Exclude cardiac causes of unexplained CNS events.* Also, do not assume that if one CT scan is normal, there is no structural lesion. If the epilepsy worsens, further imaging may be needed (MRI is getting increasingly sophisticated in identifying small areas of cortical dysgenesis).

Therapy Treat with *one* drug (with *one* doctor in charge) only. Slowly build up doses (over 2–3 months) until seizures are controlled, or toxic effects are manifest, or maximum plasma level (p751) or drug dosage reached. Beware drug interactions (consult formulary). Most specialists would not recommend treatment after one fit but would start treatment after two. ►Discuss options with the patient. If he has only one fit every 2 years, he may accept the risk (particularly if there is no need to drive or operate machinery) rather than have to take drugs every day.

Generalized: Try sodium valproate as first-line, then carbamazepine.

Partial: Carbamazepine is first-line, then try sodium valproate. Ethosuximide for absence seizures.

Commonly used drugs
Carbamazepine: Start with 100mg/12h PO. A slow-release form is available,[2] which is useful if intermittent side-effects experienced when dose peaks. Toxic effects: rash, nausea, diplopia, dizziness, fluid retention, hyponatraemia, blood dyscrasias.

Sodium valproate: Start with 200mg/12h, PO max 30mg/kg/24h. Monitor LFTs. Give after food. Toxic effects: sedation, tremor, weight gain, hair thinning, ankle swelling, hyperammonaemia (causing encephalopathy), liver failure. Monitoring of drug levels is not needed.

Phenytoin: No longer first line for generalized or partial epilepsy due to toxicity: nystagmus, diplopia, tremor, dysarthria, ataxia. Side-effects: intellect↓, depression, impaired drive, polyneuropathy, acne, coarsening of facial features, gum hypertrophy, and blood dyscrasias. Furthermore, dosage is difficult and requires continual monitoring (p751).

Other drugs Phenobarbitone; benzodiazepines; the newer anticonvulsants (see opposite).

Changing from one drug to another Indications: on inappropriate drug; side-effects unacceptable; treatment failure. Introduce new drug at its starting dose; slowly increase to middle of its therapeutic range. Only then start to withdraw the old drug over about 6 weeks.

Uncontrolled epilepsy

Review the diagnosis. Ask a neurologist to help. If epilepsy, decide which type. Is the drug appropriate? Has the top dose been tried? If not, introduce appropriate drug slowly and remove other drugs slowly (as above). The patient should be on only one drug. If seizures not controlled change to second most appropriate drug. Only consider maintenance on 2 drugs if all appropriate drugs tried singly at maximum dose. Consider *vigabatrin* as an add-on in partial seizures. There are few interactions, but it may cause depression or aggression—so avoid if a history of these. Dose example: two 500mg tabs/24h PO; max 4g/day. Lower the dose in renal failure, and in the elderly. *Lamotrigine* is an alternative (licensed as monotherapy or add-on). It may help most types of epilepsy. It is not particularly sedating. Blood dyscrasias and hepatotoxicity may occur during initiation: monitor FBC, INR and LFT. Withdrawal if rash or flu-like symptoms. Dose with valproate: start with 25mg on alternate days for 2 weeks; work up to 50mg/12h PO over 4 weeks; max 100mg/12h. Dose without valproate is ~double this; elderly: not recommended. *Gabapentin* is an easier anticonvulsant to use. It is still new and like topiramate, the newest of all, is licensed as an add-on. Try it in refractory partial seizures. *Surgery* has a place in some refractory epilepsy.

Stopping anticonvulsants

80% of patients who develop epilepsy will enter prolonged remission with drug therapy—and there is no sure way of finding out for how long treatment is needed. Unnecessary use of anticonvulsants is a problem because of their many side-effects. Impaired cognition and memory are very real problems[3] as is teratogenic in pregnancy. Against this is the risk to employment and driving prospects if seizures return. A key question, therefore, is whether or when to withdraw drugs. ►Discuss the risks and benefits with patients to enable them to make an informed choice.

At 2-year follow-up in the large (N=1013) Medical Research Council (UK) randomized study of withdrawal of anticonvulsants in those who had had no fits for 2 years, 59% of those who stopped remained seizure-free, compared with 78% in those who continued.[4] In this study, the 3 main predictors of remission were: ●Longer seizure-free periods ●Previous use of only one anti-epileptic drug ●Absence of tonic–clonic seizures. In general, prognosis for remission from seizures is better in patients with less severe epilepsy who lack evidence of structural CNS abnormalities on examination or investigation (EEG and CT scan).

The best way to withdraw anticonvulsants in adults is unknown; the Medical Research Council used decrements every 4 weeks as follows:

phenobarbitone	30mg
phenytoin	50mg
carbamazepine	100mg
valproate	200mg
primidone	125mg
ethosuximide	250mg

(For children, see electronic version.▣)

Driving and jobs (OHCS p468). Epilepsy in pregnancy (OHCS p161).

1 L Ridsdale 1995 *BMJ* i 1219   2 S Ryan 1990 *Arch Dis Chi* 65 930–5
3 JS Duncan 1990 *Epilepsia* 31 584–91   4 *Lancet* 1991 i 1176

Parkinsonism and Parkinson's disease

Parkinsonism is a syndrome of *tremor, rigidity, bradykinesis (slowness)*, and difficulty in stopping and starting walking. *Prevalence:* 1 : 200 if >65 yrs old. *Tremor:* 4–6Hz (cycles per sec). It is most marked at rest and coarser than cerebellar tremor. It is typically a 'pill rolling' of thumb over fingers. *Rigidity:* Limbs resist passive extension throughout movement (*lead-pipe rigidity*, not spasticity which is clasp-knife rigidity). *Cogwheel rigidity:* Juddering on passive extension of the flexed forearm, or pronation/ supination. Thought to be combined rigidity and tremor. *Bradykinesis:* Slow movement; monotonous speech (± dysarthria). Expressionless face. Dribbling. Short shuffling steps with flexed trunk as if forever a step behind one's centre of gravity (*festinant gait*). Feet as if frozen to the ground. Peristalsis↓. Blink rate↓. Fidgeting↓. Micrographia.

Parkinson's disease (PD) is one cause of parkinsonism (due to degeneration of substantia nigra dopaminergic neurones; the pathological hallmark is Lewy bodies in this area, p76). Degeneration may be related to observed mutations in mitochondrial DNA, with local inability to produce ATP. There is interest in toxins (MPTP, a toxin related to heroin, can cause parkinsonism). Symptoms usually start between 60 and 70yrs old. *Management:* Assess disability and cognition regularly and objectively (eg time how long to walk 20 yards; can he/she dress alone, and turn over in bed?). Choose the lowest dose of drug giving adequate symptom relief, without troublesome side-effects. Avoid Zimmer frames (flow of movement is spoilt) unless fitted with wheels and a handbrake.[1] *Drugs:*

1 *L-dopa:* Deciding when to start this is difficult because its effects wear off over time. Ask the patient what he/she thinks, and get the opinion of someone with an interest in Parkinson's disease (geriatrician, GP, or neurologist). Start with 100mg/12h PO, soon increasing to 100mg/8h. Slowly ↑dose to ≤1000mg/24h. Give enough peripheral dopa-decarboxylase inhibitor (≥25mg/100mg L-dopa). Balance L-dopa's side-effects (eg unwanted movements, nausea) with improved mobility.

2 *Selegiline* 10mg/24h PO *may* avert L-dopa's end of dose deterioration. Not everyone agrees on its benefits. Mortality may be↑ (unconfirmed).[2]

3 Over the years therapy may become less effective and patients tend to switch between periods of immobility and periods of exaggerated involuntary movements ('on–off effect'). This problem may be ameliorated by: *slow-release L-dopa* (opposite); frequent (every 2h) small doses of L-dopa; and dopaminergic agonists such as *bromocriptine*.

4 Watch for dementia (in >20%) and depression (~50%; antidepressants may worsen Parkinson's; *nortriptyline* may be least problematic here).

5 Anticholinergics (ie antimuscarinics—see below) may help tremor.

6 Subcutaneous *apomorphine* (an injectable D_1 and D_2 dopamine agonist) may help patients with severe on–off effects. Injections or continuous infusion may be required. Liaise with a special PD centre.[3]

7 Neural transplants may be a drug delivery system in the future.

At all stages *help carers*[4] (p478); assess *speech therapy / physiotherapy* needs.

Causes of parkinsonism Neurodegeneration; *neuroleptics* (eg metoclopramide, prochlorperazine); *arteriosclerosis.* Rarely *postencephalitis; supranuclear palsy* (Steel–Richardson–Olszewski syndrome with absent vertical gaze, both upward and downward, and dementia); *multisystem atrophy* (formerly Shy–Drager syndrome) (orthostatic BP↓, atonic bladder); *carbon monoxide poisoning; Wilson's disease; communicating hydrocephalus.*

Treatment of drug-induced parkinsonism It may be unwise to reduce or stop the drug (eg in schizophrenia where relapse could spell catastrophe), so try an antimuscarinic (eg procyclidine 2.5mg/8h PO).

Drugs combining L-dopa and dopa-decarboxylase inhibitors

Trade name	L-dopa content	Benserazide	Carbidopa
Madopar 62.5®	50mg	12.5mg	
Madopar 125®**	100mg	25mg	
Madopar 250®	200mg	50mg	
*Sinemet-110®	100mg		10mg
*Sinemet-275®	250mg		25mg
Sinemet-plus®	100mg		25mg
Sinemet ʟs®	50mg		12.5mg
Half sinemet cʀ®	100mg		50mg

*The proportion of carbidopa may be suboptimal.
**This proportion is available in a slow-release form (Madopar cʀ®).

Generics: Madopar® is co-beneldopa (1 part benserazide to 4 parts levodopa). Sinemet® is co-careldopa (carbidopa with levodopa). Doses are expressed as co-careldopa x/y where x and y are strengths in mg of carbidopa and levodopa respectively. For example, Sinemet-275® = co-careldopa 25/250 = 25mg carbidopa + 250mg levodopa.

1 J Pearce 1992 *Parkinson's Disease. . .*, OUP 2 A Lees 1995 BMJ ii 1602 3 *Drug Ther Bul* 1995 33 49
4 UK Parkinson's Disease Society, 22 Upper Woburn Place, London WC1H ORA, tel. 0171 383
3513 See also C Marsden 1994 *Journal of Neurol Neurosurg Psych* 57 672-681

Multiple sclerosis (MS)

This chronic, relapsing/remitting disorder is characterized by formation of plaques of demyelination (+ axon loss[a]) at sites throughout the CNS (but not peripheral nerves). Pathogenesis involves focal disruption of the blood-brain barrier with associated immune response and myelin damage.

Epidemiology Commoner in temperate areas, but prevalence is very variable: England 40/100,000; Orkney and Shetland 120/100,000; rarer in Black Africa and Asia. Lifetime UK risk: ~1:1000. Adult travellers take their risk with them; children acquire the risk of the natives they settle amongst. Female preponderance; mean age of onset 30 years.

The Patient *Presentation:* First presentations are usually monosymptomatic: unilateral optic neuritis (pain on eye movement and rapid deterioration in central vision); numbness or tingling in the limbs; leg weakness or brainstem or cerebellar symptoms such as diplopia or ataxia. Less often there may be more than one symptom. Other manifestations are listed opposite. Symptoms may be worsened by heat (eg a hot bath) or exercise. *Progression:* The early picture is usually one of relapses followed by remissions with full functional recovery. With time, remissions become incomplete causing accumulation of progressive disability. Steady progression of disability from the outset also occurs, while some patients experience no progressive disablement at all.

Examination Look carefully for neurological deficits other than the presenting problem. Lhermitte's* sign (paraesthesiae in limbs on flexing neck) may be positive (also in cervical spondylosis or B_{12} deficiency).

Diagnosis This is clinical, requiring demonstration of lesions disseminated in time and space, unattributable to other causes. Isolated neurological deficits are never diagnostic, but may become so if a careful history reveals previous epsiodes (such as unexplained blindness for a week or two). Investigations may support but not make the diagnosis.

Tests None is pathognomonic. CSF: lymphocytosis, ↑protein (but < 1g/L). Oligoclonal bands of IgG on CSF electrophoresis (95%). Delayed visual, auditory, and somatosensory evoked potentials. MRI is sensitive but not specific for plaque detection and useful for showing other causes, eg cord compression. Correlation of MRI picture with clinical condition is poor.

Treatment There is no cure, but increasing dietary *polyunsaturated fats* may help (↑plasma linoleic acid, up-regulating anti-inflammatory cytokines).
- *Methylprednisolone* 1g/24h IV shortens relapses, but use sparingly (not more than twice a year) in view of steroid side-effects. It does not alter the overall course of the disease.
- *β-interferon 1b* can ↓relapse rate by ⅓; it reduces lesion accumulation on MRI, and *may* slow the accumulation of disability.[1] Licensed for use by neurologists in relapsing-remitting disease, it is expensive (£806/month) with side-effects ('flu-like symptoms, depression, abortion). CI: Depression, active liver disease, pregnancy/lactation, uncontrolled epilepsy.
- *Palliation:* Spasticity—use *baclofen* 15–100mg/day PO or *diazepam* 2–15mg/24h PO (beware dependence). Bladder dysfunction—intermittent clean self-catheterization can help. Otherwise aim to help the patient live with their disability (p66).
- *Check benefits eligibility*—advice eg from Disabled Living Foundation and MS Society (p756); many aids are available eg for incontinence (p74).

Prognosis At 5yrs 70% are still employed (35% at 20yrs) and 20% are dead from complications. Relapses last a few months while remissions may last many years, especially if the first sign is optic neuritis, when remission may outlive the patient (45–80% go on to MS after 15 years).

---

1 *Lancet* 1998 **351** 573 & *Neurology* 1993 **43** 653 (β-interferon 1a is also made) *Jean Lhermitte, Paris, 1877–1959

Clinical features of multiple sclerosis
- Depression*
- Fatigue
- Motor
  - Weakness
  - Spasticity
- Altered sensation
  - Numbness
  - Paraesthesiae
- Pain
  - Paroxysmal, eg trigeminal neuralgia
  - Dysaesthetic
- Bladder
  - Frequency, urgency, incontinence (common)
  - Hesitancy (less common)
- Bowel
  - Constipation
- Sexual dysfunction
  - Impotence
- Swallowing disorders
- Eyes
  - Visual defects on exercise or ↑T° (Uhthoff's sign)
  - Optic neuritis
  - Diplopia
  - Nystagmus
- Cerebellum
  - Ataxia
  - Intention tremor
- Cognitive impairment, eg
  - Memory impairment
  - Euphoria
  - Dementia
- Vertigo

Rarities
- Epilepsy
- Aphasia
- Extra-pyramidal disorder

∗ ▶Depression is common, severe, and treatable: fluoxetine may be better than desipramine as anticholinergic effects limit dose. Avoid electroconvulsive therapy if MRI shows contrast-enhancing lesions: *See* A Feinstein 1997 BMJ ii 692 + OHCS p388 for psychological treatment.

Space-occupying lesions

The Patient He or she may show features of ↑intracranial pressure, evolving focal neurology, seizures, false localizing signs, odd behaviour, local effects (skull-base masses). *Raised intracranial pressure (p780):* Headache (p414), vomiting, papilloedema (only in 50% of tumours), altered consciousness. *Seizures:* Seen in ~50% of tumours. Suspect in all adult-onset seizures, especially if focal, or with a localizing aura. *Evolving focal neurology:* Depends on the site (see opposite for localizing signs). Ask first *where* the mass is then *what* it is. Frontal lobe masses present late. *False localizing signs:* These are caused by ↑ICP. VI nerve palsy is commonest (p33) due to its long intracranial course. *Subtle personality change:* Irritability, lack of application to tasks, lack of initiative, socially inappropriate behaviour. *Local effects:* (skull-base masses) proptosis, epistaxis.

Types Tumour (primary or secondary), aneurysm, abscess (25% multiple); chronic subdural haematoma, granuloma (eg tuberculoma), cyst (eg cysticercosis). *Histology:* 30% secondaries (breast, lung, melanoma; 50% multiple). Primaries include: Astrocytomas, glioblastoma multiforme, oligodendrogliomas, ependymomas (all <50% 5yr survival), cerebellar haemangioblastomas (40% 20yr survival); meningiomas (♀:♂ ≈ 2:1).

Differential diagnosis Stroke, head injury, vasculitis (SLE, syphilis, PAN, giant cell arteritis), MS, encephalitis, post-ictal (Todd's palsy p710), metabolic or electrolyte disturbances. Also colloid cyst of the third ventricle and benign intracranial hypertension (see below).

Tests CT scan, MRI (good for posterior fossa masses). Consider biopsy of deep-seated masses. Avoid lumbar puncture.

Tumour management *Benign:* Complete removal if possible but some may be inaccessible. *Malignant:* Complete removal of gliomas is difficult as resection margins are rarely clear, but surgery does give a tissue diagnosis and debulking pre-radiotherapy. If a tumour is inaccessible but causing hydrocephalus, a ventriculo-peritoneal shunt can help. Radiotherapy is used post-op for gliomas or metastases and as sole therapy for some tumours when surgery is not an option. Adjuvant chemotherapy is used in gliomas (of uncertain value). Prophylaxis for epilepsy is an important issue, but frequently fails. Treat headache with codeine phosphate 60mg/4h PO. Dexamethasone 4mg/8h PO for cerebral oedema. Mannitol if ↑ICP acutely, p780. Meticulous palliative treatment (p688).

Prognosis Complete removal of a benign tumour achieves cure but the prognosis of those with malignant tumours is poor.

Colloid cyst of the third ventricle These congenital cysts declare themselves in adult life with memory loss, headaches (often positional), obtundation, incontinence, dim vision, bilateral paraesthesiae, weak legs, and drop attacks with no loss of consciousness. *Tests:* CT scan/MRI. The condition responds to ventriculo-peritoneal shunting: ►so remember this whenever confronted by a patient with dementia and falls or gait problems.

Benign intracranial hypertension (Pseudotumour cerebri) Think of this condition in those who present as if with a mass (headache, ↑ICP and papilloedema)—and *when none is found.* It typically affects young, obese women. Diplopia and visual blurring may occur and on examination, VI nerve palsy and enlargement of the blind spot may be seen. Consciousness and intellectual function are preserved. *Cause:* Not usually found. *Treatment:* Repeated LP; thiazides (p302; they may not prevent visual loss); dexamethasone (more SE than thiazides);[1] consider shunting, advise ↓weight. *Prognosis:* Usually resolves spontaneously. Permanent significant visual loss in 10% (ie not so benign). Recurrence in 10%.

1 S Yusuf 1996 *Lancet* 347 1738   http://www.tbts.org/

Localizing signs

Temporal lobe
Seizures; hallucinations (smell, taste, sound, *déjà vu*); complex partial with automatisms; dysphasia; field defect (contralateral upper ¼); forgetfulness; fugue; functional psychosis; fear/rage; hypersexuality.

Frontal lobe
Hemiparesis; fits (contralateral movement); personality changes (indecent; indolent; indiscreet); grasp reflex (fingers drawn across palm are grasped) significant only if unilateral; dysphasia (Broca's area p430); loss of smell unilaterally.

Parietal lobe
Hemisensory loss; ↓two-point discrimination; ↓stereognosis (ability to recognize object in hand by touch alone); sensory inattention; dysphasia (p430); Gerstmann's syndrome (p698).

Occipital lobe
Contralateral visual field defects (hemianopia).

Cerebellum
Intention tremor; past-pointing; dysdiadochokinesis (impaired *rapid* movements, eg pronation–supination); nystagmus (p422); truncal ataxia (*if worse when eyes closed then lesion is of dorsal columns; not cerebellum*).

Cerebellopontine angle (usually vestibular schwannoma)
Ipsilateral deafness; nystagmus; reduced corneal reflex, VII and V nerve palsies; ipsilateral cerebellar signs.

Corpus callosum
Usually severe rapid intellectual deterioration with focal signs of adjacent lobes; signs of loss of communication between lobes (eg left hand unable to carry out verbal commands).

Midbrain
Unequal pupils; inability to direct eyes up or down; amnesia for recent events with confabulation; somnolence.

Cranial nerve lesions

Approach to cranial nerve lesions

Where is the lesion? Try to think systematically. Is it muscle (eg a dystrophy)? Neuromuscular junction (eg myasthenia)? Cranial nerve outside the brainstem (eg compression)? Within the brainstem (eg MS)? Cranial nerves may be affected singly or in groups and knowledge of which nerves are involved helps locate the lesion. Causes of cranial nerve lesions are given below. See p32 for how to test cranial nerves.

Any cranial nerve may be affected by diabetes mellitus; MS; tumours; sarcoid; vasculitis, eg polyarteritis nodosa; SLE (p672); syphilis.

I Trauma; frontal lobe tumour; meningitis.

II *Field defects* start as small areas of visual loss (scotomas). *Monocular blindness:* Lesions of one eye or optic nerve eg MS, giant cell arteritis. *Bilateral blindness:* Methyl alcohol, tobacco amblyopia; neurosyphilis. Field defects—*Bitemporal hemianopia:* Optic chiasm compression eg pituitary adenoma, craniopharyngioma, internal carotid artery aneurysm. *Homonymous hemianopia:* Affects half the visual field contralateral to the lesion in each eye. Lesions lie beyond the optic chiasm in the tracts, radiation or occipital cortex eg stroke, abscess, tumour.
Optic neuritis (pain on moving eye, loss of central vision, afferent pupillary defect, papilloedema). Causes: demyelination; rarely sinusitis, syphilis, collagen vascular disorders.
Optic atrophy (pale optic discs and reduced acuity): MS; frontal tumours; Friedreich's ataxia; retinitis pigmentosa; syphilis; glaucoma; Leber's optic atrophy; optic nerve compression.
Papilloedema (swollen discs): (1) ↑ICP (tumour, abscess, encephalitis, hydrocephalus, benign intracranial hypertension); (2) retro-orbital lesion (eg cavernous sinus thrombosis p477); (3) inflammation (eg optic neuritis); (4) ischaemia (eg accelerated hypertension).

III alone Diabetes mellitus; giant cell arteritis; syphilis; posterior communicating artery aneurysm; idiopathic; ↑ICP if causes uncal herniation through the tentorium—this compresses the nerve. Third nerve palsies without a dilated pupil are due to diabetes mellitus or another vascular cause. Early dilatation of a pupil implies a compressive lesion. Diplopia from a third nerve lesion may cause nystagmus (p422).

IV alone Rare and due to trauma to the orbit.

VI alone MS, pontine CVA, false localizing sign in ↑ICP.

V *Sensory:* Trigeminal neuralgia (p415), *Herpes zoster*, nasopharyngeal carcinoma. *Motor:* Bulbar palsy, acoustic neuroma.

VII *LMN:* Bell's palsy (p460); polio, otitis media, skull fracture, cerebellopontine angle tumours, parotid tumours, *Herpes zoster* (Ramsay–Hunt syndrome *OHCS* p756). *UMN:* (spares the forehead—bilateral innervation) Stroke, tumour.

VIII (p420, 424) Noise, Paget's disease, Ménière's disease, *Herpes zoster*, acoustic neuroma, brainstem CVA, drugs (eg aminoglycosides).

IX, X, XII Trauma, brainstem lesions, neck tumours.

XI Rare. Polio, syringomyelia, tumours near jugular foramen, stroke, bulbar palsy, polio, trauma, TB.

Groups of cranial nerves VII, VIII, then V and sometimes IX: cerebellopontine angle tumours. V, VI (Gradenigo's syndrome): lesions within the petrous temporal bone. III, IV, VI: stroke, tumours, Wernicke's encephalopathy, aneurysms, MS, myasthenia gravis, muscular dystrophy, myotonic dystrophy, cavernous sinus thrombosis.

Bell's palsy MNO

An *idiopathic palsy* of the facial nerve (VII) resulting in a usually unilateral facial weakness or paralysis. Other causes of a facial palsy must be excluded before a diagnosis of Bell's palsy is made (see opposite). Many feel that Bell's is a viral neuropathy—HSV-1 has been implicated.[1]

The Patient The onset of facial weakness is rapid and may be associated with or preceded by an ache below the ear. Weakness worsens for 1–2 days before stabilizing and pain resolves within a few days. Symptoms and signs are usually unilateral. If bilateral, consider another diagnosis.

Symptoms: The mouth sags and is drawn towards the normal side on smiling producing a grimace; food gets trapped between gum and cheek; drinks and saliva escape from the side of the mouth; dysarthria; taste impairment; intolerance of loud or high-pitched sound (hyperacusis) due to paralysis of stapedius. Failure of eye closure often results in an excessively watery or dry eye, ectropion (sagging and turning-out of the lower lid), conjunctivitis or injury from foreign bodies..*Signs:* Inability to wrinkle up the forehead, close the eyes forcefully, whistle or blow out the cheek. Wide palpebral fissure.

Natural history Patients with an incomplete paralysis and no axonal degeneration typically recover completely within a few weeks. Those with complete paralysis nearly all fully recover too but ~15% have axonal degeneration. In these patients, recovery frequently begins only after 3 months, may be incomplete, fail to happen at all, or else be complicated by the formation of aberrant reconnections. These produce synkinesis: eg eye blinking is accompanied by synchronous upturning of the mouth. Misconnection of parasympathetic fibres can produce so-called crocodile tears when eating stimulates unilateral lacrimation. Cutting the tympanic branch of IX solves this problem (rarely needed).

Management If presentation is within a few days of onset, high-dose prednisolone (0.5mg/kg/12h PO for 5 days) is given by most in an effort to prevent weakness becoming paralysis by reducing nerve oedema.[2] Evidence for the value of prednisolone is, however, not universally acknowledged; it must not be given in Ramsay Hunt syndrome. Electrodiagnostic studies at one week can help predict delayed recovery by identifying axonal degeneration. Protect the eye with dark glasses and the instillation of artificial tears if there is any evidence of drying. If ectropion is severe, lateral tarsorrhaphy can be helpful. If recovery fails in the long term (wait at least 9 months), surgical correction of the drooping face can be attempted although results are rarely satisfactory.

1 S Murakami 1996 *Ann Intern Med* **124** 27 2 Many neurologists give steroids "to reduce oedema in the nerve" particularly to those seen within 6 days of onset. One helpful study is that by TS Shafshak (1994 *J Laryng & Otology* **108** 940-3 & *Bandolier* 1995 2/11 3) showing that the extra benefit of steroids may be confined to those treated within 24h of onset. Spontaneous recovery is good in any case (85%). For every 3 persons treated with steroids within 24h, 1 extra had a good recovery compared with no treatment; for ethical reasons, this study was not randomized. Older randomized studies have been inconclusive, but did not look specifically at early treatment. A recent meta-analysis supports the use of steroids (IG Williamson 1996 *Br J Gen Pract* (Dec) 743-7 & E-BM 1997 **2** 79.)

Other causes of a VII nerve palsy[1]

Infection
Ramsay Hunt syndrome (cephalic *Herpes zoster* OHCS p756)
Lyme disease*
HIV
Meningitis
Polio
TB

Brainstem lesions
Brainstem tumour
Stroke
MS

Cerebello-pontine angle lesions
Acoustic neuroma

Systemic disease
Diabetes mellitus
Sarcoid*
Guillain–Barré*

Miscellaneous
Orofacial granulomatosis
Parotid tumours
Cholesteatoma
Otitis media
Trauma to skull base
Underwater barotrauma
Pregnancy

*Common causes of a bilateral facial palsy

1 DG James 1996 *J R Soc Med* **89** 184–87

Mononeuropathies

These are lesions of individual peripheral (including cranial) nerves.

Causes Trauma; compression; leprosy; diabetes. If several peripheral nerves are affected, the term *mononeuritis multiplex* is used. *Causes:* Diabetes mellitus; leprosy; sarcoid; amyloid; PAN; cancer.

Median nerve C5–T1 *Lesions at the elbow:* Inability to flex the interphalangeal joints of the index finger (Ochner's test—ask the patient to clasp his hands together, the affected index finger will protrude); inability to flex the terminal phalanx of the thumb and loss of sensation over the lateral 3½ digits and palm. *Lesions at the wrist:* Common due to lacerations sustained by accident with the hands outstretched or suicide attempts. The commonest cause, however, is compression at the wrist.

Carpal tunnel syndrome: Compression of the median nerve within the carpal tunnel (commoner in women). *Cause:* Usually idiopathic or due to repeated occupational trauma but also to soft tissue swelling: pregnancy, menopause, gout, acromegaly, rheumatoid arthritis, myxoedema, amyloidosis. *The Patient:* aching pain in the hand and arm, (especially at night), and paraesthesiae in the thumb, index and middle fingers, all relieved by dangling the hand over the edge of the bed and shaking it. There may be sensory loss and weakness of abductor pollicis brevis with associated wasting of the thenar eminence. Light touch, two-point discrimination, and sweating may be impaired. *Tests:* Neurophysiology to find the level of the lesion and assess axonal degeneration (and the likelihood of improvement after surgery) is vital. Maximal flexion of the wrist for 1 min (Phalen's test) may elicit symptoms. Tapping over the nerve at the wrist induces tingling (Tinel's test). *Treatment:* Splinting, local hydrocortisone injection (*OHCS* p658) ± surgical decompression.

Ulnar nerve C7–T1 Vulnerable to trauma or compression at the elbow. The result is weakness and wasting of the medial wrist flexors; weakness and wasting of the interossei and medial two lumbricals which produces a claw hand deformity; wasting of the hypothenar eminence which abolishes finger abduction and mild sensory loss over the medial 1½ fingers and the ulnar side of the hand. Flexion of the 4th and 5th fingers is weak. Consider surgical release. With lesions at the wrist (digitorum profundus intact), claw hand will be more marked.

Radial nerve C5–T1 This nerve opens the fist. It may be damaged by compression against the humerus. Test for wrist and finger drop with elbow flexed and arm pronated. Sensory loss is variable, but always includes the dorsal aspect of the root of the thumb.

Sciatic nerve L4–S2 Damaged by pelvic tumours or fractures to pelvis or femur. Lesions affect the hamstrings and all muscles below the knee (foot drop), with loss of sensation below the knee laterally.

Common peroneal nerve L4–S2 Frequently damaged as it winds round the fibular head by trauma or even prolonged sitting cross-legged. Lesions lead to inability to dorsiflex the foot (foot drop), evert the foot, extend the toes and sensory loss over dorsum of foot.

Tibial nerve S1–3 Lesions lead to an inability to stand on tiptoe (plantarflexion), invert the foot, or flex the toes. Sensory loss over the sole.

Autonomic neuropathy

Dysfunction of the autonomic nervous system may be classified as primary or secondary autonomic failure, a side-effect of drug treatment, part of a polyneuropathy, or the result of ageing.

The Patient may suffer from postural hypotension (dizziness or syncope on standing, after exercise, or a large meal), impotence, inability to sweat (noticed in hot climates), diarrhoea (especially nocturnal) or constipation, urinary retention or incontinence, and Horner's syndrome (p700).

Tests of autonomic function Measure BP lying and standing; postural drop of ≥30/15mmHg is abnormal.
- Quantify the variation in heart rate during respiration by taking an ECG during quiet breathing. A variation of <10 bpm is abnormal.
- Pressure studies of the bladder (cystometry).
- Pupil. Instil 0.1% adrenaline (ie epinephrine; this dilates if post ganglionic sympathetic denervation, not if normal); 2.5% cocaine (dilates if normal; not if sympathetic denervation); 2.5% methacholine (constricts if parasympathetic denervation, not if normal).

Ageing Postural hypotension is common in the elderly (25% >74 yrs). Review medications (see below) and discourage unnecessarily prolonged bed-rest. Elderly people often have disordered thermoregulation and so are particularly vulnerable to hypothermia (and more rarely hyperthermia). While autonomic dysfunction may be simply due to ageing, other diagnoses (eg DM or multisystem atrophy) should be considered.

Drugs The following drugs may be responsible for autonomic dysfunction: antihypertensives (esp thiazides), diuretics (over-diuresis), L-Dopa, tricyclic antidepressants, phenothiazines, benzodiazepines.

Polyneuropathies (p464) An autonomic neuropathy may occur as part of diabetic neuropathy, Guillain–Barré syndrome, chronic inflammatory demyelinating polyneuropathy, alcoholic/nutritional neuropathies, and amyloidosis. *Diabetic polyneuropathy:* Autonomic involvement may be marked with dysphagia and vomiting due to upper GI atonia; diarrhoea (especially nocturnal); bladder atonia (difficulty voiding with overflow incontinence); impotence; and postural hypotension. Pupils may be constricted with a reduced response to light.

Primary autonomic failure (no known cause) occurs alone, as part of multisystem atrophy (MSA) or (rarely) associated with classical Parkinson's. Middle-aged or elderly men are most affected. Onset is insidious (symptoms as above) and slow progression for several years is typical. Extrapyramidal symptoms (p452) may precede those of autonomic failure in MSA although the condition may be unmasked by a sudden worsening of mild postural hypotension when presumed classical Parkinson's is treated with L-dopa. Patients rarely survive more than 10 years after a diagnosis of pure autonomic failure or MSA.

Secondary failure Craniopharyngioma, vascular lesions; spinal cord lesion; tabes dorsalis; Chagas' disease; HIV; familial dysautonomia.

Treatment Treat any underlying cause. In symptomatic postural hypotension, advise to stand slowly. Head-up tilt of the bed at night increases renin release, reducing fluid loss and raising standing BP. Patients with post-prandial dizziness should be advised to eat little and often, and to reduce carbohydrate and alcohol intake. Reserve fluid-retaining drugs (fludrocortisone 0.1mg/24h PO increasing as needed) for severely affected people. Refer to a specialist if symptoms fail to respond.

Polyneuropathies

Polyneuropathies are generalized disorders of peripheral nerves (including cranial nerves) whose distribution is usually bilaterally symmetrical and widespread—eg sensory, and involving the forearm and lower legs (known as 'glove and stocking anaesthesia'). They may be classified by time course (acute or chronic); by the functions disturbed (motor, sensory, autonomic, mixed); or by the underlying pathology (demyelination, axonal degeneration or both). Guillain–Barré syndrome, for example is an acute, predominantly motor, demyelinating neuropathy whereas chronic alcohol abuse leads to a chronic, initially sensory then mixed, axonal neuropathy. The causes of polyneuropathies are given opposite.

Mostly motor	Mostly sensory
Guillain–Barré syndrome	Diabetes mellitus
Lead poisoning	Uraemia
Charcot–Marie–Tooth syndrome	Leprosy

The Patient *Sensory neuropathy:* Numbness; "feels funny"; tingling or burning sensations often affecting the extremities first ('glove and stocking' distribution). There may be difficulty handling small objects such as a needle. *Motor neuropathy:* Often progressive (may be rapid) weakness or clumsiness of the hands; difficulty walking with falls or stumbles; respiratory difficulty. Signs are those of a LMN lesion: Wasting and weakness most marked in the distal muscles of hands and feet (foot or wrist drop). Reflexes are reduced or absent. Involvement of the respiratory muscles may be shown by a ↓vital capacity. *Cranial nerves:* Difficulties swallowing; talking; double vision. *Autonomic neuropathy:* See p463.

Diagnosis The history is vital; make sure you are clear about the time course of the illness; the precise nature of the symptoms; any preceding or associated symptoms (eg diarrhoea prior to Guillain–Barré syndrome; weight loss in cancer; arthralgia due to a connective tissue disease); travel; sexual history (infections); alcohol use; medications; and family history. Pain is typical of neuropathies due to DM or alcohol. *Examination:* Do a careful neurological examination looking particularly for lower motor signs (weakness, wasting, reduced or absent reflexes) and sensory loss which should be carefully mapped out for each modality. Do not forget to assess the autonomic system (p463) and cranial nerves (p458). Look also for signs of excessive trauma (eg burns on the fingers) indicating reduced sensation. Scuff marks on shoes suggest foot drop. If there is nerve thickening think of leprosy or Charcot–Marie–Tooth. Examine other systems for clues to the cause, eg signs of alcoholic liver disease.

Investigations FBC, ESR, glucose, U&E, LFT, thyroid function tests, plasma B₁₂, protein electrophoresis, syphilis serology, ANCA (p675), ANA, CXR, urinalysis and consider an LP. Consider also specific tests for inherited neuropathies (eg porphyria), lead levels and anti-ganglioside antibodies. Nerve-conduction studies ± biopsy may be valuable.

Treatment Treat the cause if possible (eg withdraw precipitating drug). Involve physiotherapists and occupational therapists. Care of the feet (and careful choice of shoes) is important in sensory neuropathies to minimize trauma and subsequent disability. In Guillain–Barré syndrome, p702, IV immunoglobulin is beneficial.

Causes of polyneuropathies

Inflammatory
Guillain–Barré, chronic inflammatory demyelinating polyneuropathy (CIDP), sarcoidosis

Metabolic
Diabetes mellitus, renal failure, hypothyroidism, hypoglycaemia, mitochondrial disorders

Vasculitides
Polyarteritis nodosa, rheumatoid arthritis, Wegener's granulomatosis

Malignancy
Paraneoplastic syndromes (esp small cell lung cancer), polycythaemia rubra vera

Infections
Leprosy, syphilis, Lyme disease, HIV

Vitamin deficiencies and excesses
Lack of B_1, B_6, B_{12} (eg alcoholic); also excess vit B_6 (eg 100mg/day)

Inherited
Refsum's syndrome (p708); Charcot–Marie–Tooth syndrome (p696), porphyria, leucodystrophies (and many more)

Toxins
Lead, arsenic

Drugs
Alcohol, cisplatin, isoniazid, vincristine, nitrofurantoin. Less frequently: metronidazole, phenytoin

Others
Paraproteinaemias eg multiple myeloma, amyloidosis

Bulbar palsy

This is palsy of the <u>tongue</u>, muscles of <u>chewing/swallowing</u>, and facial muscles due to loss of function of brainstem motor nuclei. Signs are of a *lower motor neurone* lesion; eg <u>flaccid, fasciculating</u> tongue (p33, like a sack of worms); <u>jaw jerk is normal or absent</u>, <u>speech is quiet, hoarse, or nasal</u>.

Causes: **MND** (below); <u>Guillain–Barré; polio</u>; <u>syringobulbia</u> (p476); <u>brainstem tumours</u>; also as part of *central pontine myelinolysis* (in malnourished alcoholics), and in carcinoma or <u>hyponatraemia</u>. Pontine <u>demyelination</u> causes progressive quadriparesis and bulbar palsy, which is often fatal.

Pseudobulbar palsy An <u>upper motor neurone lesion</u> involving muscles of eating, swallowing, and talking <u>due to bilateral lesions above the midpons</u>. The <u>tongue is spastic</u>, the <u>jaw jerk increased</u>, and speech like <u>Donald Duck</u>. <u>Emotions may be labile</u> (eg giggling during the examination). *Causes:* <u>Pseudobulbar palsy is more common than bulbar palsy</u> and is caused by <u>strokes affecting the corticobulbar pathways bilaterally</u>, *MS*, and *MND*.

Motor neurone disease (MND)

MND is caused by degeneration of neurons in motor cortex, cranial nerve nuclei, and anterior horn cells. Upper and lower motor neurones may be affected but there is *no* sensory loss—so distinguishing MND from multiple sclerosis and polyneuropathies. MND never affects external ocular movements (cranial nerves III, IV, and VI) which distinguishes it from myasthenia gravis (p472). The cause is unknown, but as MND is rather like polio, viruses have been suggested. 3 patterns of MND are distinguished:
- *Amyotrophic lateral sclerosis (ALS)* (50% of patients) Combined LMN wasting and UMN hyperreflexia contribute to weakness. If familial, suspect a mutation in the gene for copper/zinc superoxide dismutase (SOD-1).
- *Progressive muscular atrophy* (25%) Anterior horn cell lesion, affecting distal muscles before proximal. Better prognosis than ALS (see above).
- *Bulbar palsy* This accounts for about 25% of patients.

Prevalence 7/10,000. ♂:♀ ≈ 3:2. ≤10% are autosomal dominant.

►Think of MND in those >40 with stumbling (spastic gait, foot-drop), weak grip (door-handles are difficult), or aspiration pneumonia. Look for UMN signs: weakness; spasticity; brisk reflexes; plantars↑; and LMN signs: weakness; wasting; fasciculation of tongue, chest, abdomen, back, thigh. Is speech or swallowing affected? The diagnosis is strongly supported by a combination of progressive upper and lower motor neurone signs with involvement of at least 2 limbs, or a limb and bulbar muscles. Fasciculations are not enough on their own to diagnose an LMN lesion: look for weakness or atrophy too. MRI of brain and cord serves to exclude structural causes; lumbar puncture helps to exclude inflammatory ones, and neurophysiology can detect subclinical denervation and help exclude motor neuropathies.

Prognosis MND is incurable, and usually fatal within 5yrs. Median age at death is 60yrs. In India, patients are younger (10–30yrs), and the course more benign, eg with only one limb affected (monomelic amyotrophy).▣

Treatment Kindness is more helpful than expert neurological advice. Aim to help patients overcome problems (p66), and relieve symptoms.
Spasticity: As for multiple sclerosis (p454).
Drooling: Propantheline 15–30mg/8h PO; amitriptyline 25–50mg/8h PO.
Dysphagia: Blend food; would he or she like a nasogastric tube, or percutaneous catheter gastrostomy?—or would this prolong death?
Joint pains and distress: Consider large doses of narcotics.
Respiratory failure: Tracheostomy and ventilation may not be kind or wise, but can allow some patients to fulfil wishes to go home.
Antiglutamate drugs: Riluzole is licensed in MND. It appears to prolong life (but probably not its quality) by a few months; it is costly.▣

Cervical spondylosis

This is a degenerative condition of the lower cervical spine that causes compression of the spinal cord or its roots. Degeneration of the annulus fibrosus of the intervertebral disc causes the formation of bony spurs or osteophytes around the joint which narrow the spinal canal. As the neck moves into full flexion or extension, the cord is damaged as it is dragged over the protruding osteophytes anteriorly and indented by a thickened ligamentum flavum posteriorly.

The Patient with cord compression This may present with:
1 Neck pain and stiffness
2 Brachialgia (arm pain)
3 Spastic leg weakness ± ataxia.

Crepitus (palpable creaking), restricted neck movement and neck pain without neurological complaint are common in people over 50yrs so ask about other symptoms. Brachialgia is felt as stabbing pain in the pre- or post-axial borders of the upper limb, or as a constant, dull ache in forearm or wrist. Hands may be weak and clumsy and numbness or paraesthesiae may be experienced in part of the hand or forearm. Weakness in one leg and unsteadiness in walking are typical of myelopathy. The leg feels heavy and stiff and the toe often scrapes the floor. Progression results in bilateral, worsening weakness. Numbness and tingling of the feet and ankles are common. Bladder involvement occurs late (hesitancy or precipitancy); incontinence is uncommon.

Signs: Limited, painful neck movement ± crepitus—be careful! Neck flexion may produce tingling down the spine—a positive Lhermitte's sign.

Arm: Lower motor neurone signs at the level of the compressed cord and upper motor neurone signs below. Atrophy of hand and forearm muscles may be visible. Sensory loss, especially pain and temperature.

Leg: Spasticity is evident, weakness less so. Reflexes may be brisk ± plantars extensor. Position and vibration sense↓. Use the latter to establish a sensory level, often several segments below level of cord compression.

Root compression Pain in arms and fingers and diminished reflexes, dermatomal sensory disturbance (numbness, tingling), lower motor neurone weakness and eventual wasting of muscles innervated by the affected root. *The intervertebral joints involved* in ↓order of frequency are:

C5/C6	Thumb sensation, biceps muscle
C7/C8/T1	Little finger sensation, flexor carpi ulnaris
C6/C7	Middle finger sensation, latissimus dorsi, triceps reflex
C4/C5	Elbow sensation, supraspinatus.

Investigations MRI is the investigation of choice to identify and localize cord and root compression (myelography if MRI is not available). Plain film views of the neck can also be of value.

Differential diagnosis Multiple sclerosis, neurofibroma of the nerve root, subacute combined degeneration of the cord (from B_{12} deficiency).

Treatment A soft neck collar restricts anterior–posterior movements of the neck and may thereby relieve pain, but patients don't like them. Do not automatically dismiss a patient with chronic root pain in the arm as suffering simply from 'wear and tear' spondylosis in the neck as they may benefit considerably from surgical root or cord decompression. Consider this if there is objective evidence of a root lesion or myelopathy and especially if the history is short, myelopathy is progressing, or pain is unrelenting. Progression may be halted and leg weakness may even improve. Operative risks are, however, significant.

Primary disorders of muscle

Signs and symptoms: **Muscle weakness** Rapid onset suggests inflammatory or metabolic cause. **Fatigability** (weakness increases with exercise) suggests myasthenia (p472). **Myotonia** (delayed muscular relaxation after contraction, eg on shaking hands) is characteristic of myotonic disorders. Spontaneous **pain** at rest occurs in inflammatory disease as does local tenderness. Pain on exercise suggests ischaemia or metabolic myopathy. **Oddly firm** muscles (due to infiltrations with fat or connective tissue) suggest pseudohypertrophic muscular dystrophies. Muscle **tumours** are rare; common causes of **lumps** are herniation of muscle through fascia; haematoma, and tendon rupture. **Fasciculation** (spontaneous, irregular and brief contractions of part of a muscle) suggest LMN disease. Look carefully for evidence of systemic disease.

Investigations: Consider electromyography and muscle biopsy; and investigations relevant to systemic causes (eg T_3).

1 *Muscular dystrophies* are a group of genetic diseases with a progressive degeneration of some muscle groups. The primary abnormality may be in the muscle membrane. The secondary effects are marked variation in the sizes of individual fibres and the deposition of fat and connective tissue. The main symptom is progressive weakness of the muscle groups involved. The commonest type is **Duchenne's** (pseudohypertrophic), inherited as sex-linked recessive (30% due to spontaneous mutation) and is (almost always) confined to boys. The Duchenne gene is on the short arm of the X chromosome (Xp21), and its product, dystrophin, is absent (or present in only very low levels) in Duchenne's muscular dystrophy. The serum creatine kinase is raised at least 40-fold. It presents at about age 4yrs with increasingly clumsy walking progressing to difficulty in standing up. Few survive to age 20 years. There is no specific treatment (p66). Genetic counselling is important.

2 *Myotonic disorders* are characterized by myotonia (tonic spasm of muscle). Muscle histology shows long chains of central nuclei within the fibres. The most important disorder is *Dystrophia myotonica*—inherited as an autosomal dominant. The onset is usually 20–30yrs with weakness (hands and legs) and myotonia. Muscle wasting and weakness in the face gives a long, haggard appearance. Additional features include: cataract; frontal baldness (in men); atrophy of testes or ovaries; cardiomyopathy; mild endocrine abnormalities (eg diabetes mellitus); and mental impairment. Most patients die in middle age of intercurrent illness. Procainamide hydrochloride may help the myotonia. Genetic counselling is important.

3 *Acquired myopathies of late onset* are often a manifestation of systemic disease. Look carefully for evidence of: carcinoma; thyroid disease (especially hyperthyroidism); Cushing's disease.

4 *Polymyositis* (p670).

5 *Myasthenia gravis* (p472).

6 *Toxic myopathies:* Alcohol; labetolol; cholesterol-lowering drugs; steroids; chloroquine; colchicine; procainamide; zidovudine; vincristine; ciclosporin; hypervitaminosis E; cocaine; heroin; phencyclidine (PCP).

✝ Myasthenia gravis (MG)

Essence An antibody-mediated, autoimmune disease with too few functioning muscle acetylcholine receptors, leading to muscle weakness. Anti-acetylcholine receptor antibodies are detectable in 90% of patients, and cause depletion of functioning post-synaptic receptor sites.

Presentation Usually in young adults with easy muscle fatigability. It may progress to permanent weakness. Muscle groups commonly affected (most likely first): extraocular; bulbar; neck; limb girdle; distal limbs; trunk. Look especially for: ptosis; diplopia; 'myasthenic snarl' on smiling. On counting aloud to 50 the voice weakens. Reflexes are often brisk. Weakness may be exacerbated by pregnancy, $K^+\downarrow$, infection, overtreatment, change of climate, emotion, exercise, gentamicin, opiates, tetracycline, quinine, quinidine, procainamide, β-blockers. ♀:♂ ≈ 2:1. *Associations:* Thymic tumour; hyperthyroidism; rheumatoid arthritis; SLE.

Tests

1 Tensilon® test (only do if resuscitation facilities and atropine to hand). Prepare 2 syringes—1 with 10mg edrophonium and 1 with 0.9% saline. Give first 20% of each separately IV as test dose. Ask independent observer to comment on effect of each. Wait 30sec before giving rest of each syringe. The test is +ve if edrophonium injection improves muscle power. This test is not always as dramatic as is often stated.
2 Anti-acetylcholine receptor antibody (raised in MG).
3 Neurophysiology to show a decremental response in muscle to repetitive nerve stimulation ± increased 'jitter' in single-fibre studies.
4 CT of thymus gland.

Treatment options

1 Symptomatic control with anticholinesterase, eg *pyridostigmine* 60–600mg/24h PO taken through the day; SE: diarrhoea, colic, controllable by propantheline 15mg/8h PO; signs of cholinergic toxicity: hypersalivation, lachrymation, sweats, vomiting, miosis.
2 Immunosuppression with *prednisolone*, using a single-dose alternate day regimen. Starting dose 5mg, increased by 5mg/week up to 1mg/kg on each treatment day.[1] Remission (may take months) prompts a dose reduction. SE: weakness (hence the low starting dose). If no remission, and weakness is severe, try *azathioprine* 2.5mg/kg/day (do FBC and LFT weekly for 8 weeks, then every 3 months) or weekly methotrexate.
3 Thymectomy (if thymoma and if early onset with troublesome symptoms) gives remission in 30% and worthwhile benefit in another 40%.[1]
4 Plasmapheresis, emergency or pre-thymectomy, gives 4 weeks' benefit.

Prognosis Relapsing or slow progression. If thymoma, 5-yr survival 30%.

Myasthenic syndrome

This typically occurs in association with bronchial small cell carcinoma (known as Eaton–Lambert syndrome) or rarely with other autoimmune diseases. Unlike true MG it: ●Affects especially proximal limbs and trunk ●Autonomic involvement is common ●There is **hypo**reflexia ●Only a slight response to edrophonium ●Repeated muscle contraction may lead to *increased* muscle strength and reflexes ●It is the presynaptic membrane which is affected (the carcinoma appears to provoke production of antibody to calcium channels). Treatment (by expert only): 3,4-diaminopyridine. ►Do regular chest x-rays as symptoms may predate lung cancer by 4 years or more.

Other causes of muscle fatigability Polymyositis; SLE; botulism.

1 J Newsom-Davis 1993 *Prescribers' J* 33 205

Neurofibromatosis[1]

Type I neurofibromatosis (NF1, von Recklinghausen's disease) Incidence 1 in 2500, ♀:♂ ≈ 1:1; no racial predilection. Inheritance is autosomal dominant, the gene is on chromosome 17. Expression of type 1 neurofibromatosis (NF1) is variable, even within a family.

The Patient *Café-au-lait spots* are flat, coffee-coloured patches of skin seen in the first year of life (clearest in UV light), increasing in size and number with age. Adults have 6 or more >15mm across. They do *not* predispose to skin cancer. *Freckling* occurs in axillae, groin, neck base and submammary area (♀) and is usually present by age 10. *Dermal neurofibromas* appear at puberty and are small, violaceous nodules, gelatinous in texture. They may become papillomatous. They are not painful but may itch. Numbers increase over time. *Nodular neurofibromas* arise from nerve trunks. Firm and clearly demarcated, they can give rise to paraesthesiae if pressed. *Lisch nodules* are hamartomas on the iris which cannot be seen with the naked eye (use a slit lamp). They develop in early childhood and are harmless. Short stature and macrocephaly are also seen.

Complications These occur in ~1/3 of NF1 patients. Mild learning disabilities are common. *Local effects of neurofibromas:* Nerve roots—compression; gut—bleeds, obstruction; bone—cystic lesions, pseudarthrosis, scoliosis. Hypertension (6%) due to renal artery stenosis or phaeochromocytoma. Plexiform neurofibromas (large, subcutaneous swellings). Malignancy (5% patients with NF1): optic glioma, sarcomatous change in a neurofibroma. Epilepsy (slight↑).

Management By a multidisciplinary team including clinical geneticist, neurologist, and surgeon. Yearly measurement of BP and cutaneous survey is advised. Dermal neurofibromas are unsightly, and catch on clothing; if troublesome, lesions can be removed surgically, but removal of all lesions is unrealistic. Genetic counselling is important (*OHCS* p212).

Type 2 neurofibromatosis (NF2)
Autosomal dominant inheritance. Much rarer than NF1 with an incidence of only 1 in 35,000. The gene responsible is on chromosome 22.

The Patient *Bilateral vestibular schwannomas* (acoustic neuromas) become symptomatic in the teens or twenties when sensorineural hearing loss is the first sign. There may be tinnitus and vertigo. The rate of tumour growth is unpredictable and variable. The tumours are benign but cause problems by pressing on local structures and by ↑ICP. *Café-au-lait spots* are fewer than in NF1. *Juvenile posterior subcapsular lenticular opacity* (a form of cataract) occurs before other manifestations and can be useful in screening those at risk.

Complications Schwannomas of other cranial nerves, dorsal nerve roots, or peripheral nerves. Meningiomas (45% NF2) which may be multiple. Glial tumours also but less commonly. Consider NF2 in any young person presenting with one of these tumours in isolation.

Management Screening hearing tests yearly from puberty with brain MRI only if abnormalities detected. A negative MRI in the late teens is helpful in assessing risk to any offspring. A clear scan at 30 years (unless a family history of late onset) indicates that the gene has not been inherited. Treatment of vestibular schwannomas is neurosurgical and complicated by hearing loss/deterioration and facial palsy. Mean survival from diagnosis has been reported at 15 years[2] and best practice is still unclear.

1 S Huson 1994 *The Neurofibromatoses* Chapman & Hall 2 DGR Evans 1992 *Q J Med* **304** 603–18

Diagnostic criteria for neurofibromatosis[1]

Neurofibromatosis type 1 (von Recklinghausen's disease)
Diagnosis is made if 2 of the below are found:
1 Six or more café-au-lait macules >5mm (prepubertal) or >15mm (post-pubertal)
2 Two or more neurofibromas of any type or one plexiform
3 Freckling in the axillary or inguinal regions
4 Optic glioma
5 Two or more Lisch nodules
6 Distinctive osseous lesion typical of NF1, eg sphenoid dysplasia
7 First-degree relative with NF1 according to the above criteria

Differential: McCune–Albright, multiple lentigenes, urticaria pigmentosa

Neurofibromatosis type 2
Diagnosis is made if either of the below are found:
1 Bilateral vestibular schwannomas seen on MRI or CT
2 First degree relative with NF2 and either:
  a) Unilateral vestibular schwannoma
  b) One of the following:
    Neurofibroma
    Meningioma
    Glioma
    Schwannoma
    Juvenile cataract (NF2 type)

Differential: NF1

1 NIH Consensus Statement 1988: *Diagnostic Criteria for NF1 and NF2* (modified 1992)

Syringomyelia

Syrinx was one of those versatile virgins of Arcadia who, on being pursued by Pan to the banks of the river Ladon, turned herself into a reed—from which Pan made his pipes, and, in so doing, she gave her name to all manner of tubular structures, eg syringes—and syrinxes, which are tubular or slit-like cavities which form for unknown reasons in or close to the central canal of the cervical spinal cord.

Pathogenesis As the syrinx enlarges it expands into adjacent grey and white matter, compressing decussating spinothalamic fibres anteriorly, the ventral horns which contain the anterior horn cells, and the descending corticospinal fibres. Extension into the brainstem is called *syringobulbia*. Spinal cord injury patients must be followed closely because they are at risk of developing a syrinx many years after their injury.

Cause Obscure. A developmental anomaly is suggested by an association with the Arnold–Chiari malformation (p694) in which the cerebellum extends through the foramen magnum and down the spinal cord.

Cardinal signs Wasting and weakness of the hands and arms, with loss of pain and temperature sensation (dissociated sensory loss) over the trunk and arms, eg in a cape distribution (suspended sensory loss)—reflecting early involvement of fibres conveying pain and temperature sensation which decussate anteriorly in the cord, and of cervical anterior horn cells. Sensory loss may lead to painless burns and Charcot's joints. *Other features:* Horner's syndrome (cervical sympathetics) and upper motor neurone signs in the legs. There may be body asymmetry, limb hemihypertrophy, or podomegaly/chiromegaly (unilaterally enlarged hands or feet, perhaps from release of trophic factors via the anterior horn cells). *Charcot's joints:* On losing sensation, joints are destroyed by too great a range of movement. They are swollen and mobile. Causes: syringomyelia (eg shoulder), tabes dorsalis (eg knee), diabetes, and leprosy.

Investigations CT or MRI scan.

Natural history The symptoms may be mild and unchanging for years, but there then may be a rapid deterioration.

Treatment Surgical decompression at the foramen magnum may be tried if there is a Chiari malformation. It aims to promote free flow of CSF through the foramen magnum, preventing syrinx dilation. These procedures may relieve pain, and prevent progression of symptoms.

Tropical spastic paraplegia

There is spastic paraplegia, with paraesthesiae, sensory loss, and disorders of micturition which progresses over weeks or months, and becomes disabling. It is caused by sexually acquired human T-cell lymphotropic virus type I (HTLV-I) retrovirus infection (endemic in Japan, the Caribbean, Africa, S America, and the southern USA).

Cerebral venous/sinus thrombosis

Isolated sagittal sinus thrombosis—Presentation Headache, vomiting, papilloedema. Headaches are severe and migraine-like or else of a 'thunderclap'-type[1] reminiscent of that of subarachnoid haemorrhage (ie sudden and severe, sometimes with an ominous snapping). There may be preliminary headache worsened by coughing. If venous infarction supervenes, focal neurology will be seen, eg hemiplegia. Sagittal sinus thrombosis is usually accompanied by thrombosis of other sinuses eg lateral sinus thrombosis (6th and 7th cranial nerve palsies, fits, field defect, ear pain), cavernous sinus thrombosis (central retinal vein thrombosis, grossly oedematous eyelids, chemosis), sigmoid sinus thrombosis (cerebellar signs, lower cranial nerve palsies), inferior petrosal sinus (5th and 6th cranial nerve palsies—Gradenigo's syndrome).

Predisposing factors
Venous sinus thrombosis is associated with the conditions listed below,[2] but in one-third of patients no cause is found. Previously reports were dominated by post-partum cases but it is now believed that $\male : \female \approx 1:1$.

Systemic diseases	Infections	Drugs
Dehydration	Meningitis	The Pill
Heart failure	Cerebral abscess	Androgens
Diabetes	Septicaemia	Antifibrinolytics
Renal disease	Fungal infections	
Hyperviscosity (p618)	Otitis media	Post-partum
Crohn's/uc (p514)		

Differential Thunderclap headaches also occur in migraine, dissection of a carotid or vertebral artery, as well as in *benign thunderclap headache*.

Tests Angiography is the gold standard (1 Corkscrew collaterals 2 ↓Veins/capillaries in infarcted area 3 Filling defect itself visualized). MRI reveals filling defect. CT may be normal at first then at ~1 week develops the delta sign where transversely cut sinus shows filling defect (dark). CSF: RBC and bilirubin↑; opening pressure↑.

Management Seek expert help. One small randomized study shows that heparin saves lives and improves outcome in survivors. Heparin must be given even if imaging suggests haemorrhagic infarcts have developed. Intracranial haemorrhage is not an automatic contraindication.[3]

Prognosis In one unpublished series of 110 cases from India, mortality was reported at 14.4%.

1 S de Bruijn 1996 *Lancet* 358 1623 2 OTM 3e pp3956-7 3 K Einhäupl 1991 *Lancet* 338 597

Living with neurological illness

This page is dedicated to the carers who, by various accidents, find themselves responsible for a friend or relative who has a chronic neurological illness—the diagnosis could be stroke, Parkinson's disease, Alzheimer's disease, or motor neurone disease. It is worthwhile, as a thought-experiment, to spend a morning imagining that you are such a carer—for example trying to expunge the smell of soiled sheets from your clothes, while awaiting a relief visit from your neighbour, who said she would "sit with him" so you can catch the bus into town, and, like a guilty hedonist, play truant from your rôle as nurse for a few sanity-giving hours of normal life. You wait. No one comes. You stop bothering about the smell on your clothes, and turn towards your husband, about to say something to make light of this little lapse in neighbourliness, but when your eyes meet his, you realize he does not recognize you—and you keep your thoughts to yourself. Knuckles whiten as you grasp his collar to lift him forward on the commode, and you seem to hear a mocking voice over your left shoulder saying: " . . . so I see we're getting angry with him today, are we?" The ceaseless round from mouth to anus, from bed to chair, from twilight to twilight, continues, *ad infinitum*.

It's all we can do to spend *two minutes* on this thought-experiment, let alone a whole morning—or the rest of our lives. As professionals we need to be aware of the strategies we may adopt to avoid full-frontal involvement with the naked truth of the shattered lives which, like a tragic subplot, stand behind the farce of morning surgery or outpatients in which we hear ourselves forever saying in tones of plummy complacency: "And how are *you* today Mrs Salt—your husband, I know . . . just the same: marvellous how you manage. You are a real support to each other. Let me know if I can do anything." We pretend to be busy, we ensure that we *are* busy, we surround ourselves with students, with white coats, and a miasma of technical expertise—we surround ourselves with *anything* to ensure that there is no chink through which Mrs Salt can shine her rays of darkness. Poor Mrs Salt. Poor us—to be frightened of the darkness, panicking at the thought that we might not have anything to offer, or that we might be called on to offer up our equanimity as a sacrifice to Mrs Salt. How dare one little grain upset our carefully contrived universe?

Respite care, meals on wheels, laundry services, physiotherapy, transport, day care centres, membership of clubs for carers, and visits from the district nurse or from a nurse specializing in chronic neurological diseases, will go some way to mitigate Mrs Salt's problems. As ever, the only way forward is by taking time to listen, and communicating. Carers' needs are different at different times. First there is uncertainty, and the need for help in handling this. Next comes the moment of diagnosis, with the numbness, denial, and anger that may follow. Then there may be a time of adjusting to reality, characterized by either a frenzied searching for information and advice, or a careful titration by the carer of how much information he or she can handle at any one time. Issues of driving, mobility, finance, and employment are likely to occur throughout the illness, and advice will need to be constantly tailored to suit individual circumstances. But the best thing you can ever offer these carers is the unwritten contract, that, come what may, you will be there, available, ineffectual as usual, but incapable of being alienated by whatever the carer may disclose to you.

See R Pinder 1990 *The Management of Chronic Illness: Patient and Doctor Perspectives on Parkinson's Disease*. Macmillan, London, and L Ridsdale 1995 *Brit J Gen Prac* **45** 226

Diet:

Relevant pages in other chapters:
Signs and symptoms: Abdominal distension (p38); epigastric pain (p46); flatulence (p46); guarding (p46); heartburn (p48); hepatomegaly (p48); LIF and LUQ pain (p50); palmar erythema (p52); rebound tenderness (p56); regurgitation (p56); RIF pain (p56); RUQ pain (p56); skin discolouration (p56); splenomegaly (p152); tenesmus (p58); vomiting (p60); waterbrash (p60); weight loss (p60).

Surgical topics: Contents to *Surgery* (p80). *Other topics:* Hepatitis (p210).

Healthy, enjoyable eating[1]

There are no good or bad *foods*, only good or bad *diets* for individuals in specified circumstances. Eating should be a pleasure; it can also be healthy. Evidence concerning diet and disease is weaker than that eg relating smoking to lung cancer. Dietary advice[1] has changed much over the years: the following embodies principles consistent with current practice. Perhaps even this advice needs to be taken with a (small) pinch of salt.

1 Body mass index *Weight /(height)*^{2} In general, aim for ~20–25 (p502).

2 Reduce saturated fats (We do not know if unsaturated fats should also be reduced in those of normal weight.[2]) Select lean meat; remove obvious fat and poultry skin. Eat fish (30g/day or 1–2 fish dishes/wk probably offers some protection from heart disease[3]), pulses, nuts. Choose low-fat dairy products (eg Edam or cottage cheese) and unsaturated fats for cooking (olive, rape seed, or sunflower oil). Avoid high-fat foods (eg shop-bought pastries, cakes, most biscuits and crisps, sausages, salami, meat pies, taramasalata, chips, chocolate). Oily fish rich in omega-3 fatty acid (eg mackerel, herring, pilchards, salmon) particularly helps those with hyperlipidaemia. If tinned fish, avoid those in unspecified oils. Nuts are also valuable here: walnuts lower total cholesterol and have one of the highest ratios of polyunsaturates to saturates (7:1).[4] Soya protein lowers cholesterol, low-density lipoproteins, and triglycerides.

3 Reduce refined sugar (it can cause dental caries, obesity, diabetes, and, by replacing unrefined food, diverticulosis.) Use fruit to add sweetness. Have low-sugar drinks. Don't add sugar to drinks or cereals. (In a thin, elderly, normoglycaemic person, sugar may be no great evil.)

4 Eat plenty of fruit and fibre—eg >5 different pieces of fruit[5] (ideally with skins) or 5 portions of pulses, beans or lightly cooked greens each day. The term *fibre* is imprecise. Most is *non-starch polysaccharides* (NSP, the preferred term). Wholemeal bread, potatoes, pasta, rice, oats, and high-fibre breakfast cereals are helpful. Note: More fluid is needed with high NSP diet. ●Aim for 8 cups daily (≈2½ pints). ●Warn about bulky stools. ●NSP can inhibit absorption of elements (Ca^{2+}, iron), so it may be wise to restrict main intake to 1 meal a day. For vit. E, see p529.

5 Reduce salt Use spices (and herbs) to add variety to life.

6 Enjoy moderate alcohol use ♀: <15u/week; ♂: <20u/week (higher levels are controversial)—taken regularly with food, not in binges. This may be the key to the 'French paradox': while the French have a lipid profile similar to their neighbours, and eat *more* dairy fat, their death rate from heart disease is ⅓ that of their neighbours. We know that alcohol inhibits platelet aggregation: one reason why it is one of the best cardioprotective agents known. There is no evidence that spirits or beer drinkers should switch to wine. There is evidence that the benefit accrues *only* to those whose LDL cholesterol is >~5.25mmol/L.[6]

▶*Avoid this diet if:* ●<5yrs old ●Need for low residue (Crohn's, UC, p516) or special diet (coeliac disease, p522) ●If weight *loss* expected (eg HIV+ve). Different parts of the diet merit emphasis in: hyperlipidaemia (p654); diabetes (p530); obesity (p502); constipation (p488); liver failure (p504); cirrhosis (p506); chronic pancreatitis (p522); renal failure.

Difficulties It is an imposition to ask us to change our diet (children often refuse point-blank); a more subtle approach is to take a meal we enjoy (eg crisps and Coke®) and make it healthier, eg caffeine-free Diet Coke®, and crisps made from jacket potatoes, fried in sunflower oil (poly+mono-unsaturates:saturates ≈7:1; sodium 2%; fibre >5%[a]).

1 HMSO 1991 *Health & Social Subjects* 41 2 J Mann 1990 *BMJ* i 1297 3 D Kromhout 1993 *Proc Nut Soc* 52 437 4 J Sabate 1993 *NEJM* **328** 603 5 S Zino 1997 *BMJ* i 1787 ◄6► E Rim 1996 *BMJ* i 312[a]

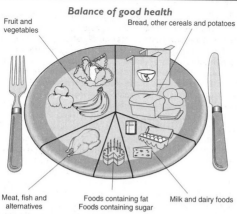

Balance of good health

Fruit and vegetables

Bread, other cereals and potatoes

Meat, fish and alternatives

Foods containing fat
Foods containing sugar

Milk and dairy foods

This food model has been developed nationally to communicate current recommendations for healthy eating.[1,2] It is nicely summarized by the so-called plate model above, which shows rough proportions of the various food groups that should make up each meal.

Starchy foods: Bread, rice, pasta, potatoes and other starch should form the main energy source. Both wholemeal (high in non-starch polysaccharide or fibre) and white cereals should be encouraged. It is food model has been developed nationally to communicate current recommendations for healthy eating.[1,2] It is nicely summarized by the so-called plate model above, which shows rough proportions of the various food groups that should make up each meal.

Starchy foods: Bread, rice, pasta, potatoes and other starch should form the main energy source. Both wholemeal (high in non-starch polysaccharide or fibre) and white cereals should be encouraged. It is important to increase fluid intake with a diet high in non-starch polysaccharide. The target should be 8 cups (1–2½ pints) daily.

Fruit and vegetables: 5 portions should be eaten daily. 1 portion is equal to a piece of fresh fruit or glass of fruit juice, 1 serving of cooked vegetables, or a small salad.

Meat and alternatives: Meat should be lean and cooked without additional fat. Portions should be small. Lower fat alternatives such as white meat (without the skin), white fish, and vegetable protein sources (eg pulses, soya) should be encouraged.

Dairy foods: Low-fat choices should be made, eg semi-skimmed milk; edam or cottage cheese; low-fat yoghurts.

Fat and sugary foods: Patients should avoid using extra fat for cooking so grilling, boiling, steaming, or baking should be encouraged. Fatty spreads (eg butter) should be kept to a minimum and snack foods such as crisps, sweets, biscuits, or cake should also be avoided. Excess sugar in the diet causes obesity and dental caries but no further disease associations have been proven.

1 DoH 1995 *Nutritional Aspects of Cardiovascular Disease: Report on Health & Social Subjects* no. 46
2 Committee on Medical Aspects of Food Policy 1994 *Diet and Heart Disease*, HMSO

Jaundice (icterus) refers to a yellow pigmentation of skin, sclerae and mucosa due to a raised plasma bilirubin (visible at >35μmol/L). Examine the sclerae in good light. Jaundice may be classified by the type of circulating bilirubin as conjugated or unconjugated or by the site of the problem as pre-hepatic, hepatocellular, or obstructive—this is rather an oversimplification as some jaundice does not fit neatly into one category.

484

Bilirubin is formed from the breakdown of haemoglobin. It is conjugated with glucuronic acid by hepatocytes making it water soluble. If there is excess bilirubin (eg haemolysis) or an inborn failure of uptake (Gilbert's syndrome, p698) or conjugation (Crigler–Najjar syndrome), unconjugated bilirubin enters the blood. As it is water insoluble, it does not enter urine. This is *unconjugated* (=acholuric) hyperbilirubinaemia. Conjugated bilirubin flows out into the gut, where bacteria convert it to urobilinogen. Some is reabsorbed and appears in urine. The rest is converted to stercobilin, colouring faeces brown. If the common bile duct is blocked, conjugated bilirubin overspills into the blood. Being water soluble, some is excreted in urine, making it dark. Less conjugated bilirubin enters the bowel, therefore, the faeces become pale. This is *obstructive* or *cholestatic* hyperbilirubinaemia. Obstruction is rarely complete. *Hepatocellular jaundice* implies ↓hepatocyte function ± varying degrees of cholestasis. The result is a mixed conjugated *and* unconjugated jaundice.

Causes *Drugs—↑Transaminases:* Halothane, isoniazid, paracetamol excess. *Cholestasis:* The Pill, co-amoxiclav. *Mixed:* Chlorpromazine, erythromycin.

Pre-hepatic: Haemolysis; ineffective erythropoiesis; Crigler–Najjar syndrome (rare) and Gilbert's syndrome (common).

Hepatocellular: Viruses (hepatitis A, B, C, E, Epstein–Barr virus); leptospirosis; autoimmune diseases (eg chronic hepatitis, p512); rare syndromes (Rotor, Dubin–Johnson, Wilson's disease); cirrhosis.

Cholestatic: Intrahepatic: primary biliary cirrhosis, primary sclerosing cholangitis, cholangiocarcinoma; sepsis; hepatocellular disease. Extrahepatic: gallstones; bile duct, head of pancreas, or periampullary carcinoma; benign stricture of common bile duct; enlarged porta hepatis (eg lymphoma).

At the bedside Ask about recreational drugs, transfusions, injections, piercing, tattooing, sexual activity, travel, jaundiced contacts, family history, alcohol, and *all* medications (tablets, injections, anaesthetics—find all drug charts if an in-patient). Look for hepatomegaly, splenomegaly (see p152, eg infection, portal hypertension, haemolysis), and signs of chronic liver disease (p678). ▶Examine the urine and stools.

Tests *Urine:* Bilirubin, urobilinogen—sensitive tests for unconjugated jaundice (no urinary bilirubin) and biliary obstruction (↑urinary bilirubin, absent or ↓urobilinogen). *Blood:* Take precautions—hepatitis risk: LFTs, γGT, bilirubin (cholestasis: ↑bilirubin, ↑γGT, ↑alk phos, mildly ↑transaminases. Hepatocellular picture: ↑AST and ↑ALT); prothrombin time and serum albumin (best markers of degree of hepatocyte damage); U&E, creatinine, glucose, ethanol, FBC, reticulocytes, EBV + CMV serology, hepatitis A, B and C serology. Consider Wilson's (copper, caeruloplasmin) α₁-antitrypsin deficiency (p650) or haemochromatosis (iron, total iron-binding capacity).

Imaging: Is the common bile duct dilated? If it is, there is extrahepatic cholestasis (dilation may take days to develop). Do ultrasound first (non-invasive). If the bile ducts are dilated, do ERCP (p498) or percutaneous transhepatic cholangiography (mortality <1%; SE: biliary peritonitis; haemorrhage; cholangitis). Consider CT scan. If the bile ducts are not dilated, the next step is liver biopsy (p506).

✴ Diarrhoea and rectal bleeding

Diarrhoea is the passage of liquid stool or the frequent passage of normal stool. Common causes are self-limiting gastroenteritis and drug side-effect; but diarrhoea may signify serious disease—colon cancer, inflammatory bowel disease, ischaemia, pseudomembranous colitis. The history gives the best clue to diagnosis. *Here are the chief areas to focus on:*

- *Is the diarrhoea acute or chronic?* Acute: suspect infection. Travel abroad? Anyone else affected? Unusual diet? Ulcerative colitis may present acutely. Chronic, intermittent diarrhoea alternating with constipation suggests irritable bowel syndrome (IBS, p518). Weight loss, anorexia, anaemia, and diarrhoea at night all suggest an organic cause.
- *Is there blood, mucus or pus?* See below for causes of bloody diarrhoea. *Irritable bowel syndrome (IBS):* Mucus but 'never' blood. *Polyps:* Blood or mucus or both. Pus suggests *inflammatory bowel disease or diverticulitis.*
- *Is the large or small bowel to blame?* Large bowel: watery stool ± mucus or blood; pelvic pain relieved by defecation ± tenesmus, urgency. Small bowel: periumbilical (or RIF) pain, not relieved by defecation; watery or pale, fatty, smelly stools (steatorrhoea p522).
- *Could there be a non-GI cause?* Think of thyrotoxicosis; autonomic neuropathy (p463; eg from DM); drugs (antibiotics, cimetidine, propranolol, chemotherapeutic agents, digoxin, excess alcohol, laxative abuse).

Tests ►Do a PR: feel for a rectal mass (rectal carcinoma); impacted faeces (overflow diarrhoea); test for faecal occult blood. FBC (anaemia). If large bowel, do stool microscopy (pathogens, cysts, ova). If steatorrhoea check faecal fats. Do rigid sigmoidoscopy + biopsies on all with chronic diarrhoea of large bowel origin to identify IBD or melanosis coli (laxative abuse) not visible macroscopically. If normal but symptoms continue, consider double-contrast barium enema (may reveal a polyp or colonic tumour beyond the reach of the sigmoidoscope). Colonoscopy is the gold standard. Suspected infectious diarrhoea? See opposite.

Bloody diarrhoea *Infection:* Campylobacter—which may also cause peritonism, *Shigella, Salmonella, E coli,* amoebiasis. *Inflammatory bowel disease:* Ulcerative colitis, Crohn's disease. *Other:* Colorectal cancer; pseudomembranous and ischaemic colitis (p126); diverticulitis.

Rectal bleeding (± diarrhoea): Diverticulitis, colorectal cancer, polyps, haemorrhoids, radiation proctitis, trauma, fissure-in-ano, angiodysplasia (AVM common in the elderly).

Pseudomembranous colitis is caused by overgrowth of *Clostridium difficile,* following any antibiotic therapy.[1] *Treatment:* Vancomycin 125mg/6h PO or metronidazole 400mg/8h PO (cheaper; more palatable). Liaise with a microbiologist.

Functional diarrhoea is chronic diarrhoea without other symptoms of irritable bowel syndrome (IBS p518) in the absence of an identifiable organic cause. Like IBS it is a diagnosis of exclusion and IBD, pancreatic insufficiency, coeliac disease, and infection must all be first ruled out.

Cryptosporidium parvum A fungal infection of the immunocompromised causing diarrhoea in 10–50% of AIDS patients. It may be self-limiting if CD4 count is not too low. Quantify oocyst excretion. If treatment is needed, talk with a microbiologist. Paromomycin 1g/12h PO has been successful. In infants, encourage breastfeeding.[1] Water purification does not remove *all* cysts, the HIV +ve should probably use bottled water. ▣

Managing diarrhoea Treat causes. Give clear fluids PO. If dehydrated or elderly, check U&E. 0.9% saline (eg with ≥20mmol K⁺/L) IVI if shocked. If it is essential to reduce symptoms, try codeine phosphate 30mg/6h PO.

1 NJ Beeching 1994 *Current Opinion in Infectious Diseases* 7 685-91

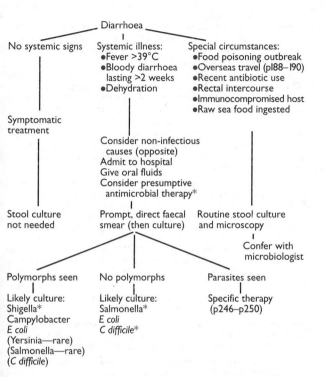

Diarrhoea

No systemic signs | Systemic illness:
●Fever >39°C
●Bloody diarrhoea lasting >2 weeks
●Dehydration | Special circumstances:
●Food poisoning outbreak
●Overseas travel (pl88–190)
●Recent antibiotic use
●Rectal intercourse
●Immunocompromised host
●Raw sea food ingested

Symptomatic treatment

Consider non-infectious causes (opposite)
Admit to hospital
Give oral fluids
Consider presumptive antimicrobial therapy*

Stool culture not needed | Prompt, direct faecal smear (then culture) | Routine stool culture and microscopy

Confer with microbiologist

Polymorphs seen | No polymorphs | Parasites seen

Likely culture:
Shigella*
Campylobacter
E coli
(Yersinia—rare)
(Salmonella—rare)
(C difficile) | Likely culture:
Salmonella*
E coli
C difficile* | Specific therapy (p246–p250)

* Prompt, specific treatment (p238 & p486—eg ciproflocacin) may be needed before sensitivities are known. Be guided by likely diagnosis following the direct smear.

✛ Constipation

▶Always ask a patient exactly what he means by 'constipation'. There are various formal (and different) definitions of constipation but the infrequent passage of stool (< 3 times weekly) or difficulty in defecation 488 is a reasonably practical working definition. It is often hard to know whether one is dealing with slow colonic transit, pelvic floor dysfunction or anal sphincter problems. ◁1▷

To the patient, constipation may mean passing stools less often than is normal for them or for 'inner cleanliness'; that their faeces are too hard; that defecation hurts or even that they have diarrhoea. These patient-defined symptoms are what you have to tackle!

Tests Most constipation does not need investigation, especially in mildly affected younger patients. In older patients it is important to rule out colorectal cancer (p140), particularly if constipation is of recent onset or is associated with rectal bleeding, mucous discharge, or tenesmus.

Treatment Treat the cause (see opposite). Encourage mobilization if necessary and advise a diet rich in fibre (p482) with adequate fluid intake—unless the cause is GI obstruction, megacolon, or colonic iner-tia/hypotonia.[2] ▶Consider drugs only if these measures fail, and try to use them for short periods only.

Bulk producers: Act to retain water and ↑microbial growth. 1) Bran 10–30g/day doubles faecal output, increases frequency of defecation and, speeds gut transit. SE: intolerance; uncooked bran has a high phy-tate content (so ↓calcium, iron and zinc availability). 2) Mucilaginous polysaccharides which arise in seeds and gums eg sterculia 62% granules in 5mL sachets, one sachet/12h PO after food, taken unchewed with plenty of water. 3) Ispaghula granules 10mL in plenty of water once or twice daily with meals (halve the dose in children). 4) Methylcellulose (3–6 500mg tablets/day with plenty of water).

Stool softeners: Liquid paraffin—do not use regularly (SE: anal seepage, lipoid pneumonia, malabsorption of fat-soluble vitamins).

Osmotic agents: ▶Take with plenty of water. Epsom salts; magnesium hydroxide mixture (25–50mL/24h PO); lactulose solution (3.35g/5mL), adult dose is 15mL/12h PO adjusted to produce 2–3 soft stools/day. Children <1yr 2.5mL/12h; 1–4yrs 5mL/12h; 5–10yrs 10mL/12h.

Stimulants: Senna (15–60mg/day); bisacodyl tablets (5–10mg at night) or suppositories (5 or 10mg in the mornings—use the lower dose in chil-dren <10yrs); co-danthrusate, ie 50mg danthron (=dantron) with 60mg ducosate. Danthron (dantron) is associated with colonic and liver tumours in animals so reserve its use for the very elderly and terminally ill. As a general rule, patients should not be put on stimulant laxatives longterm—the bowel becomes habituated to them (but there are no good, longterm follow up studies).[1] Exhaust other categories first and if you must use them, do so only in the short-term.

Phosphate enemas and *glycerine suppositories* may be useful additional agents. Excessive use of soapy tap water enemas may lead to water intoxication.

Cost *Cheap:* Bran, bisacodyl. *Moderate:* Magnesium hydroxide, methyl-cellulose, ispagula, sterculia. *Expensive:* Lactulose.

Inadequate evidence exists to determine differences in efficacy between classes of laxatives. ◁1▷

◁1▷ SM Tramonte 1997 E-BM **2** 147   2 *Medicines Resource Centre Bulletin* 1994 **5** 21

Causes of constipation

Hospitals and other adverse environments
  Being forced to use a bed pan
  Immobility (or just lack of exercise)
  Lack of privacy
  Unable or unwilling to obey calls to stool
  Dehydration
  Diet deficient in roughage

Pain on defecating
  Anal fissure
  Post-operative pain on straining

Obstruction
  Stricture (eg due to Crohn's)
  Colorectal carcinoma
  Pelvic mass (eg fetus, fibroids)
  Diverticulosis
  Congenital abnormalities
  Rectocoele

Metabolic / endocrine
  Myxoedema
  Hypercalcaemia

Drugs
  Narcotic analgesics (eg morphine, codeine)
  Anticholinergics (tricyclics, phenothiazines)
  Iron

Neuromuscular
  Spinal or pelvic nerve injury
  Hirschsprung's disease
  Systemic sclerosis
  Diabetic neuropathy
  Chronic pseudo-obstruction

Other causes
  Irritable bowel syndrome
  Old age
  Idiopathic megarectum/colon

Peptic ulceration and gastritis

Peptic ulceration includes either duodenal or gastric ulceration—2 distinct entities. It may also occur in Barrett's oesophagus (p491) or rarely in a Meckel's diverticulum. Dyspepsia (p44) is often the presenting complaint.

Duodenal ulcers *Causes:* ~90% are *Helicobacter pylori* +ve; most of the rest are NSAID-associated. DU is associated with ↑gastric acid secretion and rapid gastric emptying. The rôle of stress is controversial. *The Patient:* Epigastric pain, gnawing or burning, relieved by eating (weight↑) and worse at night ("I get up and drink milk"); waterbrash (saliva fills the mouth). Nausea and vomiting are rare in uncomplicated DU. 50% are asymptomatic, the rest experience spontaneous remissions and relapses. *Diagnosis:* Upper GI endoscopy (omit anti-ulcer drugs 1 week pre-op). Test for *H pylori* (serology, histology or ^{13}C test, see p11 and p40). Unless ulceration is very severe or ectopic or there is persistent diarrhoea or a family history suggesting Zollinger–Ellison (rare, p712), measuring gastrin is unnecessary. *Differential diagnosis:* Duodenal Crohn's disease; lymphoma; TB; pancreatic cancer eroding into the duodenum; non-ulcer dyspepsia (p44).

Gastric ulceration Most often the lesser curvature where acid-secreting and antral mucosae meet, but can be anywhere. Benign gastric ulcers are *not* premalignant. *Causes:* Unclear but 80% are *H pylori* +ve; NSAID use ↑risk 3–4 fold; reflux of duodenal contents (↑by smoking); delayed gastic emptying. *The Patient:* May be asymptomatic. Epigastric pain (can't distinguish from other causes; eg DU) that is usually *worsened* by food. Weight loss if pain is severe. *Diagnosis:* Gastric cancer may present this way, and its prognosis is better if caught early, so *all* suspected GU must be endoscoped. Take multiple biopsies from around the ulcer, its rim and base (histology and *H pylori*), and take brushings for cytology.

Treatment Avoid any food that worsens symptoms, eat little and often, and avoid eating before bed (↑acid secretion overnight). Stop smoking as it ↑relapse rates in DU and slows healing rates in GU. *Ulcer healing:* 1) Eradicate any *Helicobacter pylori*: eg 1 week's omeprazole* 20mg/12h PO + amoxicillin 1g/12h PO + clarithromycin 500mg/12h PO. Trials are underway of blind eradication therapy in dyspepsia. Note: *H pylori* has not yet fulfilled Koch's postulates (p171).[1,2] 2) Acid suppression with H_2-receptor antagonists (cimetidine 800mg PO *nocte* or ranitidine 300mg PO *nocte*) for 8 weeks. Some use a PPI (proton-pump inhibitor, eg omeprazole* 20mg/24h) as first-line. If symptoms persist, re-endoscope, recheck for *H pylori*, and reconsider the differential. If you are persistent (and it is persistent) DU, re-eradicate if necessary and start a PPI, eg omeprazole* 20–40mg/24h for 4–8 weeks.

Maintenance: 1) Stop NSAIDs; if not possible, give prophylactic misoprostol (200µg/6h with NSAID, CI: pregnancy). 2) Consider lifelong cimetidine 400mg or ranitidine 150mg PO *nocte* in: aggressive ulceration; those who've perforated or bled or might not survive these again (frail elderly, concomitant disease eg renal). 3) Consider elective surgery (p166).

Complications Haemorrhage (may be catastrophic, leading to haematemesis, melaena, shock; chronic leading to anaemia); perforation (p166); pyloric stenosis (nausea, projectile vomiting, weight loss); penetration through serosa (eg into head of pancreas for a DU).

Gastritis Mucosal damage with no ulcer. *Type A*: the entire stomach (associated with pernicious anaemia; may progress to gastric atrophy or cancer); *Type B*: the antrum (± duodenum), associated with *Helicobacter pylori*; *Type C*: due to irritants, eg NSAIDs, alcohol, bile reflux. *Exacerbators:* Stress, smoking, alcohol, NSAIDs, steroids—if on NSAIDs.[3]

---

1 *BNF* 1998 examples (p35) 2 JR Graham 1995 *Lancet* 345 1095 3 M Guslandi 1992 *BMJ* i 655
* Consumes 5% of UK drug costs; new PPIs (lanzoprazole, pantoprazole) are cheaper and may be as good

Gastro-oesophageal reflux disease & hiatus hernia

Brief periods of relaxation of the lower oesophageal sphincter are responsible for the gastro-oesophageal reflux of acid. This is a normal occurrence but if reflux is prolonged or excessive it may cause inflammation of the oesophagus (oesophagitis) known as gastro-oesophageal reflux disease (GORD). This is common with a prevalence of 5%.

491

The Patient *Symptoms:* Heartburn—a burning, retrosternal discomfort felt anywhere from epigastrium to the throat that characteristically worsens with stooping, lying, and hot drinks and is relieved by antacids; waterbrash (mouth fills with saliva); nocturnal cough, or wheeze.

Causes Smoking, alcohol, fat, coffee; pregnancy, obesity, tight clothes, big meals; surgery in achalasia, hiatus hernia; drugs (tricyclics, anticholinergics, nitrates); systemic sclerosis.

Tests Barium swallow may show hiatus hernia (this doesn't prove oesophagitis); 24h pH monitoring (do symptoms coincide with acid in the oesophagus?); oesophageal manometry. To help exclude cancer, investigate if: >45yrs old; weight↓; dysphagia; prolonged symptoms; or if lifestyle changes don't help. *Differential diagnosis:* Oesophagitis from swallowed corrosives (drugs included eg NSAIDS); or infection, especially in the immunocompromised (CMV, herpes, candida); GU; DU; GI cancers; non-ulcer dyspepsia.

Complications Oesophagitis/ulcer, anaemia, benign stricture (p492), Barrett's oesophagus (p694; premalignant ectopic gastric mucosa).

Management *Lifestyle:* ↓Intra-abdominal pressure (braces not belts; no corsets; lose weight). Raise bed head by >10cm (gravitation helps). Help gastric emptying by: small, low-fat meals, and no food <3h before bed. *Is his medication to blame (eg alendronate, p646)?*

Drugs: Try magnesium trisilicate mixture, 10mL/6h PO; alginates (Gaviscon®, 10–20mL/8h PO after food) coat the oesophagus and form a floating raft on gastric contents (∴reflux↓). H₂ antagonists reduce acid. If symptoms are resistant or severe, consider a proton pump inhibitor (eg omeprazole 20–40mg/24h PO). Effects of long-term suppression of acid secretion on gastric cancer incidence is unknown (it may be↑). Cisapride (10mg/8h PO ½h before food; 5mg/8h if <60kg, or <19yrs old, eg for 12 weeks; SE: arrhythmias, fits, LFTs↑) helps gastric emptying, ie is 'prokinetic'. If symptoms persist for >4 weeks, do gastroscopy. *Fundoplication:* p166.

Hiatus hernia Proximal stomach herniates through the diaphragmatic hiatus into the thorax. Most (80%) are sliding hernias where the gastro-oesophageal junction slides up into the chest. The rest are para-oesophageal or rolling hernias where the gastro-oesophageal junction remains in the abdomen but a bulge of stomach herniates up into the chest alongside the oesophagus. Hiatus hernia is common (30% if >50 years) and 50% have symptomatic gastro-oesophageal reflux. Obesity is a risk factor. A barium swallow is the best diagnostic test. Advise weight loss and treat reflux symptoms as above. Surgery (Nissen's fundoplication, p166) may be indicated if symptoms are intractable, there is recurrent stricturing, or Barrett's oesophagus has been demonstrated (p694).

✚ Dysphagia

Dysphagia is difficulty in swallowing. It is a serious symptom, and, unless short-lived, requires investigation to exclude neoplasia (start with endoscopy). If the patient experiences a lump in the throat *when they are not swallowing*, the diagnosis is likely to be anxiety (globus hystericus). Dysphagia may lead to malnutrition and nutritional support is often needed.

Causes

Mechanical block
Malignant stricture
  Oesophageal cancer
  Gastric cancer
  Pharyngeal cancer*
Benign strictures
  Oesophageal web or ring
  Peptic stricture
Extrinsic pressure
  Lung cancer
  Retrosternal goitre
  Mediastinal cancers
Pharyngeal pouch*

Motility disorders
Achalasia
Diffuse oesophageal spasm
Systemic sclerosis
Bulbar palsy (p466)
Pseudobulbar palsy
Myasthenia gravis
Syringomyelia (p476)

Others
Oesophagitis
  Infection (Candida, herpes)
  Reflux oesophagitis

Differential diagnosis There are 5 key questions to ask:
1 Did you have difficulty swallowing fluids *and* solids from the start?
  Yes: Think of motility disorders (achalasia, neurological causes).
  No: Suspect a stricture (benign or malignant).
2 Is it difficult to make the swallowing movement?
  Yes: Suspect bulbar palsy, especially if he coughs on swallowing.
3 Is swallowing painful (odynophagia)?
  Yes: Suspect a malignant stricture or oesophagitis.
4 Is the dysphagia intermittent or is it constant and getting worse?
  Intermittent: Suspect oesophageal spasm.
  Constant and worsening: Suspect malignant stricture.
5 Does the neck bulge or gurgle on drinking?
  Yes: Suspect a pharyngeal pouch (food may be regurgitated).

Investigations Barium swallow; endoscopy with biopsy; oesophageal manometry (this requires swallowing a pressure transducer); FBC; ESR. *Whenever dysphagia is reported as being high up, get an ENT opinion.

Diffuse oesophageal spasm Intermittent dysphagia for solids and liquids and chest pain. Barium swallow demonstrates the abnormal contractions which revel in names such as corkscrew oesophagus.

Achalasia Failure of oesophageal peristalsis and of relaxation of the lower oesophageal sphincter due to loss of ganglia from Auerbach's plexus. Dysphagia to both liquids and solids, chest pain and regurgitation of old food. On barium swallow, there is a grossly expanded oesophagus tapering to a tight lower sphincter. CXR: air/fluid level behind the heart, and double right heart border produced by the expanded oesophagus. *Treatment:* Nitrates or hydralazine may help in the short-term. Cure is achieved by cardiomyotomy in ~75%. Balloon dilatation may also work.

Benign oesophageal stricture *Causes:* oesophageal reflux; corrosives; trauma. *Treatment:* Endoscopic dilatation ± bougies.

Oesophageal carcinoma (p142) Associated with achalasia, Barrett's oesophagus (p491), tylosis (rare; inherited; hyperkeratosis of the palms; 40% get oesophageal cancer), Plummer–Vinson syndrome and smoking.

Plummer–Vinson (Paterson–Brown–Kelly) syndrome There is an oesophageal web + iron-deficiency anaemia, and oesophageal cancer.

Haematemesis is the vomiting of blood. *Melaena* is altered blood (black and tarry) passed PR. It implies bleeding proximal to the splenic flexure. Both are typical signs of an upper GI bleed.

494

Causes *Common:* ●Gastric/duodenal ulcer ●Gastritis ●Mallory–Weiss tear (oesophageal tear due to vomiting) ●Oesophageal varices ●Portal hypertensive gastropathy ●Drugs: NSAIDs, steroids, thrombolytics, anticoagulants. *Rarer:* ●Haemobilia ●Nose bleeds (swallowed blood); oesophageal/gastric malignancy ●Oesophagitis ●Angiodysplasia ●Haemangiomas ●Ehlers–Danlos or Peutz–Jeghers' syndrome (p706) ●Bleeding disorders ●Aorto–enteric fistula (in those with an aortic graft[1]).

Assessment Swift, relevant history and examination. *History:* "Do you feel faint when you sit up?" If "Yes" put up an IVI before continuing. Ask about drugs (NSAIDs; steroids; anticoagulants); alcohol abuse; previous GI bleed; peptic ulcer or its symptoms (p490); retching/vomiting; liver disease; dysphagia. Does the patient have serious concomitant disease, eg cardiovascular disease, respiratory disease, hepatic impairment, renal impairment, or malignancy? *Examination:* Document vital signs—pulse, blood pressure lying and standing/sitting, JVP, urine output. Look for signs of chronic liver disease (p506); telangiectasia or purpura; jaundice (biliary colic + jaundice + melaena suggests haemobilia). *Rockall risk score:* Calculating the risk score (opposite) may help stratify risk.

Assess whether patient is in shock:
●Cool and clammy to touch (especially nose, toes, fingers)
●Pulse >100bpm
●JVP <1cm H_2O
●Systolic BP <100mmHg
●Postural drop
●Urine output <30mL/h

Immediate management if shocked (See also p766–7.)
●Protect airway; insert 2 large-bore 'drips'; send bloods. Give high-flow O_2.
●Give IV colloid quickly then blood (ORh–ve until cross-match done).
●Correct clotting abnormalities (vitamin K, FFP, platelet concentrate).
●Set up CVP line to guide fluid replacement. Aim for >5cm H_2O. CVP may mislead if there is ascites or CCF. A Swan–Ganz catheter may help.
●Catheterize and monitor urine output.
●Urgent diagnostic endoscopy. Notify surgeons of all severe bleeds.

Endoscopy Within 4h if you suspect variceal bleeding; within 12–24h if shocked on admission or significant co-morbidity. Endoscopy can identify the site of bleeding, estimate the risk of rebleeding (rebleeding doubles mortality) and can be used to administer treatment. *Risk of rebleeding:* Active arterial bleeding seen (90% risk); visible vessel (70% risk); adherent clot/black dots (30% risk). *No site of bleeding identified:* Bleeding site missed on endoscopy; bleeding site has healed (Mallory–Weiss tear or Dieulafoy lesion); nose bleed (swallowed blood); site distal to 3rd part of the duodenum (Meckel's diverticulum, colonic site).

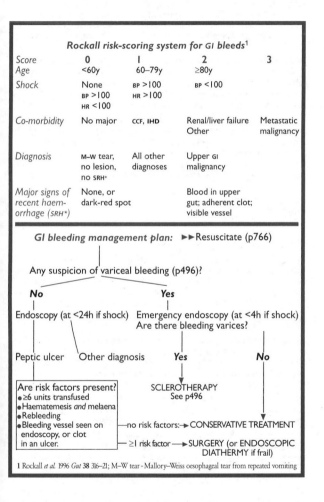

Rockall risk-scoring system for GI bleeds[1]

Score	0	1	2	3
Age	<60y	60–79y	≥80y	
Shock	None BP >100 HR <100	BP >100 HR >100	BP <100	
Co-morbidity	No major	CCF, IHD	Renal/liver failure Other	Metastatic malignancy
Diagnosis	M–W tear, no lesion, no SRH*	All other diagnoses	Upper GI malignancy	
Major signs of recent haemorrhage (SRH*)	None, or dark-red spot		Blood in upper gut; adherent clot; visible vessel	

GI bleeding management plan: ►►Resuscitate (p766)

Any suspicion of variceal bleeding (p496)?

No — Endoscopy (at <24h if shock)

Peptic ulcer   Other diagnosis

Yes — Emergency endoscopy (at <4h if shock)
Are there bleeding varices?

Yes — SCLEROTHERAPY See p496

No — CONSERVATIVE TREATMENT

Are risk factors present?
- ≥6 units transfused
- Haematemesis *and* melaena
- Rebleeding
- Bleeding vessel seen on endoscopy, or clot in an ulcer.

— no risk factors:→ CONSERVATIVE TREATMENT

— ≥1 risk factor —→ SURGERY (or ENDOSCOPIC DIATHERMY if frail)

1 Rockall *et al.* 1996 *Gut* 38 316–21; M–W tear = Mallory–Weiss oesophageal tear from repeated vomiting

Management of variceal bleeding Resuscitate then proceed to urgent endoscopy. Give octreotide 50µg/h ɪᴠɪ for 2–5 days.[1] After identifying bleeding varices check for bleeding elsewhere (~30%) before proceeding to sclerotherapy or banding.[2] If bleeding continues, pass a Sengstaken–Blakemore tube (see opposite). A bleed is the equivalent of a large protein meal so start treatment to avoid hepatic encephalopathy (p505). Give sucralfate 1g 6-hourly to protect against stress ulceration. *Prognosis:* Worse if jaundice, ascites, hypoalbuminaemia, encephalopathy.

Medical management of all upper ɢɪ bleeds
While waiting for endoscopy or if not indicated (nil by mouth until ᴏɢᴅ): 1) Decide if a central line is indicated (shock; significant co-morbidity; rebleed; poor peripheral access). 2) Monitor vital signs hourly until stable, then 4 hourly—you are watching for a rebleed (see below). 3) Daily ᴜ&ᴇ; clotting studies if >4units blood needed (keep 2 units in reserve).

Rebleeds A rebleed is a serious event: 40% of patients who rebleed will die and of patients with upper ɢɪ bleeding who died, 50% rebled. Be aware of those patients who are at risk and maintain a high index of suspicion—some will vomit blood and leave you in little doubt, others will not. If the patient is rebleeding, check vital signs every 15 minutes and call in the cavalry (your senior cover and the on-call surgical registrar).

How to identify a rebleed:
●Rising pulse rate.
●Falling ᴊᴠᴘ.
●Decreasing hourly urine output.
●Haematemesis or melaena.
●Fall in ʙᴘ (a late and sinister finding).

Indications for surgery Severe bleeding, Rockall score (p495) >6, rebleeding, active bleeding during ᴏɢᴅ, continuing bleeding after transfusion (if >60yrs, 6 units; if <60yrs, 8 units). *Varices:* ●Oesophageal transection with gun stapler re-anastomosis ●Transthoracic transoesophageal ligation. *Gastric ulcer:* ●Under-running ●Excision ●Partial gastrectomy.

Portal hypertension

Blood from the gut bypasses the liver, returning to the heart via collateral veins at the oesophago–gastric junction. These veins dilate to form thin-walled varices, which may bleed catastrophically. Worldwide, hepatic fibrosis from schistosomiasis is the main cause.

Causes *Pre-hepatic:* Portal vein thrombosis; pancreatic tumour/pseudocyst. *Intrahepatic:* Cirrhosis; Hodgkin's; myelofibrosis; alcoholic hepatitis; schistosomiasis; sarcoid. *Post-hepatic:* Budd–Chiari (p696); right heart failure; constrictive pericarditis; veno-occlusive disease.

The Patient Signs of chronic liver disease (p506); splenomegaly; abnormal collateral abdominal veins (caput medusae, p30).

Management Propranolol or nadolol 40–160mg/24h ᴘᴏ (aim to ↓pulse by 20%) reduces 1° and 2° bleeding and mortality; adding isosorbide mononitrate 10–40mg/12h ᴘᴏ augments the β-blocker-induced fall in portal pressure, and reduces bleeding rates.[3,4] Intensive sclerotherapy regimens can also substantially reduce the risk of rebleeding, but have not consistently improved survival (sᴇ: mucosal necrosis, ulceration, stricture). Shunts (splenorenal or portal vein to vena cava) do not save lives.

1 M Woodley 1992 *Manual of Medical Therapeutics* 27e 288 2 JJ Sung 1995 *Lancet* 346 1666
3 C Hayes 1990 *Lancet* 336 1666 4 Villanueva 1996 *NEJM* 334 1624

Passing a Sengstaken tube

In life-threatening variceal bleeding, this can buy time while arranging a definitive oesophageal procedure (eg transection). It uses balloons to compress stomach and oesophageal varices.

- Before insertion, inflate the balloons with a measured volume (eg 120–300mL) of air giving pressures of 60mmHg (check with a sphygmomanometer).
- Deflate, and clamp exits.
- Pass the lubricated tube (try to avoid sedation) and inflate the gastric balloon with the predetermined volume of air.
- Inflate the oesophageal balloon. Check pressures. They should be 20–30mmHg greater than on the trial run.
- Tape to patient's forehead to ensure the gastric balloon impacts gently on the gastro-oesophageal junction.
- Place the oesophageal aspiration channel on continuous low suction and arrange for the gastric channel to drain freely.
- Leave *in situ* until bleeding stops. Remove after <24h.

Various other techniques of insertion may be used, and tubes vary in detailed structure. So don't worry about exact details of placing these tubes, which, in practice, are rarely necessary, and may cause problems such as inhalation during insertion and mucosal ulcers. *Don't try to pass one yourself if you have no or little experience:* ask an expert; if none is available, transfer urgently to a liver centre.

Endoscopy

Upper GI endoscopy may be *diagnostic* or *therapeutic* (marked •). A flexible endoscope is swallowed after local anaesthetic has been sprayed onto the back of the mouth. Sedation may be given (midazolam 2.5–7.5mg IV; less in the elderly; titrate against level of sedation and monitor O_2 saturation with a pulse oximeter). The airway must be protected and there must be continuous suction to prevent aspiration. *Pre-op care:* Fast from 8h (but water up to 90 min pre-op may be OK); consent; warn not to drive till ~24h post-op; arrange follow-up. If cardiac ischaemia is likely to be a problem (pulse↑ during procedure), consider metoprolol 100mg PO 2h pre-op.[1] *Mortality:* 1:2000. *Morbidity:* 1:200.

Diagnostic indications

Symptoms:	*Suspected:*	*Suspicious findings on:*
Haematemesis/melaena	Peptic ulcer	Barium meal
Dyspepsia (esp. if >40yr, or weight↓; see p44)	Pyloric stenosis	
	H pylori	
Dysphagia	Coeliac disease	
Post-gastrectomy	Upper GI malignancy	
Ingested foreign body		

Therapy
- Diathermy of bleeding ulcers.
- Sclerotherapy for varices (eg with ethanolamine oleate).
- Dilating benign strictures.
- Placement of stents through obstructing growths.
- Laser palliation of oesophageal carcinoma or treatment of bleeding from angiodysplasia or other vascular anomalies.

Endoscopic retrograde cholangiopancreatography (ERCP) uses a side-viewing duodenoscope. Mortality is <0.2% overall, but rises to 0.4–0.6% with stone removal. A catheter is advanced from the endoscope through the ampulla into the common bile duct. X-rays after injection of contrast medium show lesions within the biliary tree and pancreatic ducts. *Before the procedure:* Obtain formal consent and check clotting as for liver biopsy (p507); give antibiotic prophylaxis (eg ciprofloxacin 750mg PO) 2h before; morphine eg 5mg IM 1h before; and give high-flow O_2 by mask for 5 minutes before passing the endoscope to prevent hypoxia. MRI is a non-invasive alternative in some cases.

Therapeutic manoeuvres:
- Sphincterotomy with gallstone removal.
- Dilatation of benign biliary strictures.
- Palliation of malignant bile duct obstruction with stents.

Complications: (~1%) Pancreatitis; bleeding; cholangitis; perforation.

Sigmoidoscopy allows examination of the rectum. It should precede barium enema in suspected cancer. Flexible instruments gain better access than rigid ones (but still miss ~25% of colon cancers[2]). Do a biopsy, as macroscopic appearances may be normal in many conditions eg inflammatory bowel disease or amyloidosis.

Colonoscopy *Indications:* Suspected colon cancer, with normal radiology; biopsy when radiology suggests malignancy or Crohn's; estimation of extent of UC; surveillance for cancer in UC; investigating lower GI bleeding; *S bovis* endocarditis (p312). *Preparation:* Sodium picosulfate (Picolax®) 1 sachet morning and afternoon the day before or if urgent, rapid preparation with 2 hypertonic phosphate enemas (CI: severe constipation, diarrhoea, diverticulosis). *Therapy:* • Polypectomy using a diathermy snare • Diathermy to angiodysplasia • Treatment of volvulus.

1 J Rosenberg 1996 *BMJ* ii 258   2 JP Dinning 1994 *Arch Int Med* 154 853

The mouth

▶Diagnoses come out of your patient's mouth: so open it, and inspect it with a bright light. If the patient wears false teeth, ask him to take them out so you can get a proper look. Most oral cancers start as odd red painless spots. Don't hesitate to refer to an oral surgeon if uncertain.[1]

Ulceration *Apthous:* Shallow, painful ulcers (single or in crops) on the tongue or buccal mucosa that heal without scarring and are found in 20% of the healthy population. They are associated with Crohn's and coeliac disease and Behçet's syndrome (p694). Treatment is difficult, and often not needed. Hydrocortisone 2.5mg lozenges held on the ulcer may help, as may tetracycline mouthbath (125mg/5mL), 10mL/8h held in the mouth for 3mins, for ≤3 days. *Other causes:* Trauma (eg false teeth), lichen planus, erythema multiforme, pemphigus, pemphigoid, infections (viral, syphilis, Vincent's angina, p710). ▶Biopsy any ulcer which does not heal after 3 weeks to exclude malignancy: typical features of a rolled edge and induration may be absent.

Oral candidiasis (thrush) causes creamy-white patches on the mucosa, surrounded by a thin margin of erythema. Patches are hard to remove and bleed if scraped. Those at risk: very young or old, DM, the immunosuppressed (cytotoxics; steroids; haematological malignancy; AIDS). ▶Finding oral candidiasis in an apparently fit young man (not using steroid inhalers) suggests AIDS. *Differential:* Lichen planus (lacy appearance). *Treatment:* Nystatin pastilles (100,000u) sucked slowly every 6h PO, or amphotericin lozenges (10mg) sucked every 3–6h. Systemic candidaemia is a rare complication. Treat with IV amphotericin (p340).

Leucoplakia White thickening of the tongue or oral mucosa (also vulva, larynx, anus). It is a premalignant condition. ▶Frank malignancy may co-exist with leucoplakia. *Causes:* Poor dental hygiene, smoking, sepsis, syphilis. *Hairy leucoplakia* is a shaggy white patch on the side of the tongue due to EBV which is seen in HIV; it is not premalignant.[2]

Oral pigmentation Dark-brown blotches anywhere in the mouth suggests Addison's or drugs (eg anti-malarials). A dark line below the gingival lining suggests lead or bismuth poisoning. Brown spots on the lips characterize Peutz–Jeghers' syndrome (p706). Tiny yellow spots may be *Fordyce spots* (sebaceous glands). Telangiectasia may signify Osler–Weber–Rendu syndrome (p706).

Gingivitis Gum inflammation ± hypertrophy may occur with poor oral hygiene; ciclosporin; nifedipine; phenytoin; in pregnancy; scurvy (p520); acute myeloid leukaemia (typically M4 p602); Vincent's angina (p710).

The tongue may be *furred* or *dry* (dehydration, Sjögren's syndrome); *black* due to overgrowth of papillae or *Aspergillus niger* infection after antibiotics; or smooth and red (*glossitis*), due to iron, folate or B12 deficiency. Loss of patches of papillae gives rise to *geographic tongue;* red rings and lines whose outlines change with time. This usually has no significance but may be associated with riboflavin (vitamin B₂) deficiency.

Tongue cancer typically appears on its edge as a raised ulcer with firm edges and indurated environs. Examine underneath of tongue and ask patient to deviate his extended tongue sideways. Spread: the anterior ⅓ of the tongue drains to the submental nodes; the middle ⅓ to the submandibular nodes, and the posterior ⅓ to the deep cervical nodes. Treatment: surgery or radiotherapy. 5-yr survival (early disease): 80%.

A ranula is a bluish salivary retention cyst to one side of the frenulum, named after the bulging vocal pouch of frogs' throats (genus *Rana*).

1 Screening is futile; see our electronic version & *Euro J Cancer* 1995 31B 202 2 *Lancet* Ed 1989 ii 1194

Altered body mass index

Those who are thin are often aggressively or subtly punishing to the obese. The thin doctor is in danger of abusing his authority by using it as a weapon with which to attack the already vulnerable obese patient. Because if we starve we lose weight, we falsely suppose that our weight is simply under our control. It is not. The control is most complex and includes genetic and physiological factors. Attempts to reduce weight may be resisted by the body's altered metabolism, which, like a thermostat, varies in such a way as to maintain weight around a 'setpoint'. An obese person who diets to maintain an average weight experiences the same unpleasantness as does a thin person who is starving himself. So be cautious in telling your obese patient that he cannot have his gall bladder removed unless he first loses 4 stone in weight.

Obesity is rarely caused by disease, so avoid costly tests for Cushing's, hypothyroidism or hypothalamic disorders, unless there are other signs of these conditions. Obesity is associated with excess mortality from diabetes mellitus, heart disease, stroke, pneumonia and accidents.

Body mass index (BMI) classification[1] BMI=weight/(height)^2, weight in kg, height in metres. The normal range is 20–25. Grade 1 obesity is defined as a BMI = 25–30. Grade 2 as BMI = 30–40, and grade 3 as BMI >40.

Management Weight loss for all grades of obesity (see opposite) should be slow. An average of 0.5–1.0kg weight loss per week is desirable. Rapid weight loss due to a large calorie deficit results in loss of water, glycogen and lean body mass rather than loss of fat. The result is rapid weight gain after the ferocious diet is over. Note that there is no good evidence that losing weight saves lives once patients are overweight. We should concentrate on *preventing* obesity, not treating it.

The process of change A useful model to use when tackling obesity has come from work done in stop smoking programmes (opposite). It depicts the changes involved in any lifestyle change and takes account of a patient's motivation and confidence in their ability to lose weight. Both are needed if the patient is to succeed. Techniques vary depending on where the patient fits into the model. Non-confrontational, motivational interviewing; joint doctor/patient problem-solving; practical healthy eating advice (p482); reinforcement and encouragement as well as suggestions on coping with relapse or failure are all helpful at different stages. *Self-help books* can be both a useful resource and a motivation for change.[1]

Be aware of the seasoned dieter overwhelmed with guilt about food, feelings of loss of control, inadequacy, and low self-esteem. After individual assessment, referral to a psychologist or psychiatrist may be sensible. Many dieticians now use behavioural techniques to help patients lose weight—such a referral may be more acceptable to the patient.

It is clear that the prescriptive appproach used by many doctors in the past is ineffective in obesity. A more considered and enlightened approach is overdue. Self-help groups can be useful in all grades of obesity. Gastric restriction surgery for the severest forms of obesity is an option if all the above methods have failed. (Appetite suppressants such as fenfluramine are not used: they cause heart valve problems and psychosis.)

Obese patients in hospital Obese patients can be malnourished. Don't start obese patients on a reducing diet if they are acutely ill or have leg ulcers or pressure sores. Under physiological stress they will lose protein from muscle, liver, and muscle. (A greatly reduced body mass index, eg BMI <20, is also common in hospital and may require nutritional support.)

1 G Butler 1995 *Manage Your Mind*, OUP, ISBN 0-19-262383-4

Managing obesity: the process of change

The process of change

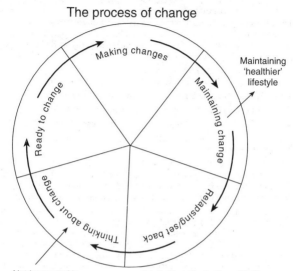

Adapted from Prochaska and Dr Clemente

✠ Acute liver failure

Liver failure causes 5 chief problems: **1)** Hypoglycaemia **2)** Hepatic encephalopathy **3)** Haemorrhage **4)** Ascites **5)** Infection. It also causes jaundice (but this is not itself a big problem). It may occur suddenly in the previously healthy—acute liver failure—or more often as decompensation of chronic liver disease. Decompensation may be precipitated by infection (especially spontaneous bacterial peritonitis), sedation, GI bleeds, diuretics, alcoholic binges, constipation or electrolyte imbalance. Encephalopathy occurring within 8 weeks of the first signs of liver failure is termed fulminant liver failure and encephalopathy at 8–24 weeks is late-onset liver failure. The prognosis of fulminant liver failure is poor.

Causes of acute liver failure in the previously well

Viral hepatitis: Any type (delta virus and hepatitis B ↑risk), Weil's disease.

Drugs: Paracetamol excess, halothane, idiosyncratic reactions.

Toxins: Amanita phalloides mushrooms, carbon tetrachloride.

Vascular: Budd–Chiari (p696), veno-occlusive disease, heatstroke (p766).

Others: Acute fatty liver of pregnancy, Wilson's disease, Reye's syndrome, malignant infiltration.

The Patient Look for signs of chronic liver disease (p506) ± hepato(spleno)megaly and ascites (less to the fore in *acute* failure). Other features: fetor hepaticus (a characteristic sweet smell on the breath), fever, nausea, vomiting, hypertension, hypoglycaemia, encephalopathy.

Hepatic encephalopathy Grade I: Untidiness, irritability, slow thinking, euphoria, inverted sleep rhythm. Grade II: Increasing drowsiness, lethargy, inappropriate behaviour, incontinence, confusion, slurred speech. Grade III: Stupor from which patients may be roused, incoherence, restlessness, significant confusion. Grade IV: Coma. Diagnosis is clinical backed up by blood tests consistent with hepatic failure. Test for constructional apraxia by asking patients to draw a 5-pointed star. Serial attempts can easily be compared. EEG may show high-voltage slow waveforms. *Cause:* Uncertain, but excess ammonia produced by gut flora, mercaptans, and the generation of false transmitters are all implicated.

Diagnosis of acute liver failure depends upon the presence of a conjugated jaundice, raised transaminases (indicating hepatocellular damage) and a prolonged prothrombin time associated with acute liver disease.

Tests: PT, FBC, U&E, glucose, paracetamol level, blood cultures, urine microscopy, cytology/culture of ascites, viral serology, LFTS, CXR.

Complications (Seek expert help!) *Bleeding:* Treat with vit K 10mg/day IV for 2–3 days with platelets, fresh frozen plasma, and blood as needed.

Serious infection: Until sensitivities are known, give ceftriaxone 1–2g/24h IV. Avoid gentamicin (↑risk of renal failure). *Ascites:* See p506.

Hypoglycaemia: Check blood glucose regularly. Give IV glucose (eg 50g) if levels fall below 2mmol/L. Watch plasma K^+.

Cerebral oedema: Happens in most with Grade IV encephalopathy (ankle clonus, decerebrate posture, dilated pupils). Give mannitol. Hyperventilate.

Hepatorenal syndrome: Albumin IV, haemodialysis.

Pain: Low-dose paracetamol is least problematic. Avoid NSAIDS (risk of GI bleeds). Opiates are ok in low, well-spaced doses titrated against pain.

Liver transplantation If this is going to be undertaken, do before irreversible CNS damage occurs. Immunosuppression with tacrolimus improves results.

Management of coma in acute liver failure

Fulminant liver failure is assumed to be potentially reversible and treatment is designed to buy time for the patient's liver to regenerate.

- Seek expert help. Do they advise transfer to a liver unit?
- Nurse with a 20° head-up tilt in ITU.
- Treat the cause if known (eg paracetamol overdose, p796).
- Caution with secretions and blood if hepatitis B is suspected.
- Check blood glucose 1–4 hourly and give 50mL 50% dextrose IV if <3.5 mmol/L. Give 10% dextrose IV, 1L/12h to avoid hypoglycaemia.
- NGT to avoid aspiration and remove any blood (bleeding varices) from stomach. Protect the airway with an endotracheal tube.
- Monitor temperature; pulse; RR; BP; pupils; urine output; blood glucose; INR; U&E; LFTs; EEG. Do daily weights (ascites) and blood cultures.
- Minimize absorption of nitrogenous substances and worsening of coma by restricting protein and emptying the bowel with lactulose and magnesium sulfate enemas. Aim for 2 soft stools/day.
- Give neomycin 1g/6h PO to reduce numbers of bowel organisms.
- Consider haemodialysis if water overload develops.
- Reduce acid secretion and risk of gastric stress ulcers, eg with cimetidine 200mg/8h IV or a proton pump inhibitor (p490).
- Avoid sedatives (but diazepam is used for seizures), or other drugs with hepatic metabolism (see BNF).

Note: attempts to correct acid–base balance are often harmful.

✝ Cirrhosis

Essence The architecture of the liver is irreversibly destroyed by fibrosis and regenerating nodules of hepatocytes.

Causes Unknown (30%), alcohol (25%), hepatitis B or C. *Others:* Chronic active hepatitis (p512), Wilson's disease (p712), Budd–Chiari syndrome (p696), haemochromatosis (p509), biliary cirrhosis (p508), drugs (methotrexate), α_1-antitrypsin deficiency (rare, autosomal recessive, due to lack of an enzyme which antagonizes trypsin, p650.)

The Patient There may be no symptoms or signs. In compensated disease there may be Dupuytren's contracture, parotid enlargement (alcohol abuse, not cirrhosis *per se*), hepatomegaly (but a small, hard liver in advanced cirrhosis), palmar erythema, gynaecomastia, testicular atrophy (all attributed to ↑oestrogen levels), clubbing, xanthelasmata, xanthomata, and spider naevi. These consist of a central arteriole with leg-like branches which blanch on central pressure and are usually confined to skin drained by the superior vena cava (face, neck, upper chest and back). *Portal hypertension:* Ascites (shifting dullness, p31); abnormal abdominal veins; bleeding varices; splenomegaly. *Decompensated cirrhosis:* the above plus jaundice; scratch marks; hepatic encephalopathy (eg hepatic flap) and if there is hypoalbuminaemia, leuconychia and pitting oedema. Altered vitamin D metabolism may cause osteomalacia.

Diagnosis Liver biopsy and blood tests: *Biochemistry* may be normal or show raised plasma transaminases (AST, ALT) and alkaline phosphatase. Later, when the synthetic capability of the liver is affected there may be ↓albumin, ↑PT (↓synthesis of clotting factors), ↑bilirubin, ↓glucose, ↓Na⁺. Hepatitis serology and iron biochemistry (haemochromatosis) may be needed to establish a cause. Severity may be graded as opposite.

Complications Portal hypertension (± variceal bleeding p494, hepatic encephalopathy p504), hepatocellular carcinoma, ascites, renal failure.

Management Treat the cause; prevent further liver damage; avoid or treat complications. Nutritional support if malnourished (p104), abstinence from alcohol (alcoholic cirrhosis), care if other causes, and avoid drugs metabolized by the liver (see p9 and *BNF*). *Ascites:* Fluid cytology to exclude other causes (eg malignancy, TB). Bed-rest; salt restriction 40–100mmol/24h depending on severity of ascites; fluid restriction (<1.5 litre/day). Check U&E and plasma creatinine eg every other day and chart daily weight and urine output. If hyponatraemic give albumin IV. Give spironolactone 100mg/24h PO increasing the dose every 2 days up to 400mg/24h. Aim for a daily weight loss of ≤½ kg/day (to prevent uraemia). If response is poor, use frusemide (=furosemide), ≤120mg/24h PO. Beware hypokalaemia. Over diuresis causes dehydration, uraemia and hyponatraemia and can precipitate encephalopathy or hepatorenal failure. If encephalopathy develops or creatinine >160µmol/L with Na⁺ <128mmol/L, stop diuretics. Paracentesis with concomitant albumin infusion (6–8g per litre fluid removed) is safe in those with good renal function and normal Na⁺. *Spontaneous bacterial peritonitis* complicates up to 25% of ascites; it may be fatal. Prophylaxis: ciprofloxacin 250mg PO or co-trimoxazole 960mg PO on weekdays.◁1▷ *Encephalopathy:* p504. *Bleeding varices:* p496. *Pruritus:* Cholestyramine 4g/8h PO, 1h after other drugs.

Prognosis Highly variable depending upon the cause and stage of disease. Overall 5-year survival is ~50%. Poor prognostic indicators are: any complication (see above), plasma Na⁺ <110mmol/L, albumin <25g/L, ↑PT, continuing drinking in alcoholic cirrhosis.

◁1▷ N Singh 1995 *Ann Int Med* **122** 595 & *E-BM* 1995 **1** 20

Grade	Serum bilirubin	Serum albumin	Ascites or encephalopathy	Operative mortality
A	Normal	≥35g/L	none	2%
B	20–50μmol/L	30–35g/L	mild	10%
C	>50μmol/L	<30g/L	severe, uncontrolled	50%

Child's grading of liver disease in portal hypertension

Liver biopsy

Liver biopsy has a mortality of 0.01–0.1% that is not clearly reduced by using ultrasound guidance.[1] You must get the patient's formal consent, and arrange for FBC, platelets, PT, and LFTs to be taken and group and save blood prior to the procedure. Percutaneous biopsy is not safe if the PT is prolonged (in such patients a transjugular biopsy is an option). After the biopsy the patient should lie on his or her right side for 2h then spend the next 22 hours in bed. Vital signs must be monitored regularly (eg every ¼h at first). Look out for the tachycardia that signals a bleed. Next day check for signs of pneumothorax (CXR) and blood or bile leaks. The patient should avoid strenuous exercise for the next week. 1 G Vautier 1994 BMJ ii 1455

Primary biliary cirrhosis (PBC)

This is a slowly progressive non-suppurative cholangiohepatitis, with destruction of the small interlobular bile ducts, cholestasis, fibrosis and eventual hepatic cirrhosis. The cause is unknown (putatively autoimmune). Women make up 90% of patients and the peak age at presentation is 45 years old. The spectrum of disease is very variable—in some surveys, 50% of newly diagnosed patients are symptom-free.

The Patient may be asymptomatic. Early on, fatigue and pruritus are the dominant features. Later, jaundice (cholestatic with pale stools and dark urine), hepatosplenomegaly and melanotic skin pigmentation may be seen. Patients may present with catastrophic bleeding from oesophageal varices secondary to portal hypertension, or in frank liver failure (encephalopathy, ascites). *Other features:* Clubbing, xanthomata, xanthelasmata, arthralgia, osteoporosis, osteomalacia, hirsutism.

Associated disease Thyroid disease, Sjögren's syndrome (70%), pancreatic hyposecretion, CREST syndrome (p670), coeliac disease, extrahepatic malignancy, hepatocellular carcinoma.

Tests LFTs: ↑Alk phos (↔in 14%); ↑γGT; mildly↑ AST/ALT. Bilirubin: often normal initially, rising as disease worsens. Albumin and PT: normal until end-stage disease. TSH: Often↑. *Imaging:* Ultrasound and ERCP exclude extrahepatic cholestasis. Liver biopsy confirms diagnosis and, histology allows disease staging (below). *Immunology:* 95% are AMA+ve (antimitochondrial antibody, directed against pyruvate kinase); titres >1:80 are highly suggestive. If AMA –ve look for anti-M2, a subtype of AMA. Normal people, or those with thyroid disease may rarely be AMA +ve. Other autoantibodies are often present in low titres, eg antinuclear, antithyroid, and anticentromere antibodies. Immunoglobulins are↑, especially IgM.

Staging

I Destruction of interlobular ducts	II Ductal proliferation
III Fibrosis and	IV Frank cirrhosis.

Differential Autoimmune hepatitis, reaction to phenothiazines, sarcoid.

Treatment *Symptomatic therapy:* Pruritus is treated with cholestyramine 4g/6–12h PO. If this fails, consider UV light treatment or plasmapheresis (p618, this also ↓xanthomata). Intractable itch is an indication for liver transplantation. Malabsorption can be helped by eating little and often and avoiding saturated fats. Carbohydrate and medium-chain triglyceride supplements can be given to maintain energy intake. Vitamin D as calciferol 250µg PO (up to 4/day; beware hypercalcaemia) may be needed for osteomalacia. Vitamin A (=retinol) 100,000 units/month IM and vitamin K 10mg/month may also be needed. See p494 for management of bleeding oesophageal varices. *Specific therapy:* Ursodeoxycholic acid (UDCA, ursodiol) ↑hepatic secretion of bile acids (which otherwise harm hepatocyte membranes), reduces production of cytokines and interleukin 2, 4, and 6, and may reduce itch.[1,2] Long-term follow-up (open trials) suggests that it may reduce the need for transplantation, but this has not been confirmed by randomized trials. SE: diarrhoea.

Liver transplantation is indicated when quality of life becomes poor (eg serum bilirubin >100–150µmol/L); it may cure (PBC is a major indication for transplantation). Recurrence in the graft can occur[3] but appears not influence graft success. 1-yr survival post-op is ~90%, and then it approximates to that of healthy persons matched for age and sex.

Prognosis Median survival: 7–10yrs.[4] If asymptomatic, symptoms are likely to develop over 2–4yrs, but ⅓ stay symptom-free for many years.

1 N LaRusso 1997 *Lancet* 350 1046 2 A Lim 1994 *BMJ* ii 491 3 M Knoop 1996 *Transpl Int* 9 supl s115-9 4 M Kaplan 1996 *NEJM* 335 1570

Primary haemochromatosis (HC)

▶A not uncommon, and a *treatable* condition: so think of it! It is an inherited disorder of iron metabolism in which there is inappropriate, excess absorption of iron from the small bowel and resultant iron loading of the liver, heart, pancreas, joints, and pituitary. It is complicated by hepatic cirrhosis, diabetes mellitus, cardiomyopathy, hypogonadism, hepatocellular carcinoma, and arthropathy and if left untreated is life-shortening. HC is common, easily treatable, and if diagnosed early enough, complications can be avoided and life expectancy returned to that of the normal population.

Genetics Inheritance: autosomal recessive. The carrier rate is high at 1 in 8 to 1 in 10 (more than cystic fibrosis). Between 1 in 200 and 1 in 2000 people are homozygous in the West. The gene (HLA-H) has recently been identified on chromosome 6[1] and is responsible for almost all HC. Expression of the disease is highly variable. ♂ ≫ ♀ and women with the disease tend to present ~10 years later. This is due to slower iron accumulation because of increased physiological blood loss (pregnancy, menstruation). Homozygotes in the developing world (hookworm, iron-deficient diet) are also less likely to develop symptoms of the disease.

The Patient Asymptomatic or nonspecific tiredness and arthralgia (especially the 2nd and 3rd MCP joints) early on. As iron accumulates, more symptoms become evident by late middle age: arthritis in other joints, impotence and testicular atrophy, hepatomegaly ± signs of cirrhosis, diabetes, cardiomyopathy, and a slatey-grey skin pigmentation.

Tests Liver biopsy (the gold standard) allows estimation of degree of iron loading (normal hepatic iron index (HII) $\leq$ 1.1, raised in HC)[2] and identification of cirrhosis. *Blood tests:* Serum ferritin is a good measure of iron stores (if there is no concomitant inflammation as it is an acute phase protein) and is often significantly raised; ↑serum iron; transferrin saturation >70%; ↓total iron-binding capacity. Check blood glucose (diabetes) and ECG.

Management Regular venesection (usually a unit 1–2 times weekly) until mildly iron deficient which may take months. Iron will continue to accumulate so maintenance venesection (~5 units a year) is needed *for life*. Monitor serum ferritin and rebleed at levels >100μg/L.

Prognosis Venesection returns the life-expectancy of non-cirrhotic and non-diabetic patients to normal. Fatigue and lethargy are relieved, cardiomyopathy may be reversed, liver function tests normalize, and the liver returns to a normal size. Gonadal failure, however, is irreversible while arthropathy may improve, remain the same, or worsen. The risk of hepatocellular carcinoma remains in those with cirrhosis and screening with α-fetoprotein should be considered.

Screening Siblings should have their serum ferritin tested; genetic testing is likely to be readily available soon. Given the high carrier rate, the chance of a carrier marrying a homozygote is also quite high: children should also be tested. Population screening is a possibility in the future.

Secondary haemochromatosis is iron overload eg from frequent transfusions, eg for haemolysis. Venesection is *not* a treatment option. Desferrioxamine (=deferoxamine) by SC infusion pump (1–3g over 12h) with ascorbic acid, 200mg/day PO, can ↑urinary excretion of iron to >50mg/day.

1 J Feder 1996 *Nature Genetics* 13 399 2 HII = [Fe] (μmol/g dry weight of liver)/age (yrs). It is the best way (short of genetic testing) to identify homozygous patients; >1.9 is diagnostic of haemochromatosis.

Neoplasia and the liver

Primary hepatic tumours arise in the liver while secondary tumours (30 times commoner) are metastases from primary tumours elsewhere.

Hepatocellular carcinoma (HCC) A tumour of liver parenchymal cells. Rare in the West (1–2/100,000/year) but a million deaths/year worldwide and a major cause of malignancy in Africa and South-east Asia. *Causes:* Chronic hepatitis B; cirrhosis (eg hepatitis C, alcohol, haemochromatosis); long-standing ulcerative colitis ± primary sclerosing cholangitis; aflatoxin; parasites (eg *Clonorchis sinensis*). Contraceptive steroids >8 yrs may ↑risk ~4-fold. *Management:* Chemotherapy, selective tumour embolization, and transplantation are disappointing. Surgical resection of single tumours <3cm diameter gives a 3-year survival rate of 59% (base-line 3-year survival rate is 13%).[1] *Prognosis:* Death is usually within 6 months. Fibrolamellar HCC, which occurs in younger people with non-cirrhotic livers, has a somewhat better prognosis.

Cholangiocarcinoma develops from the intra- or extrahepatic biliary tree. It is rare, comprising only ~10% of hepatic malignancy (more in the Far East) and is most common between 50–70 years. *Causes:* Thorotrast (contrast agent previously used in neuroradiology); infestation with *Clonorchis sinensis*; congenital biliary tree cystic disease; long-standing ulcerative colitis. *Management:* Hilar tumours may, rarely, be resectable but response to chemotherapy is poor. Palliative stenting of an obstructed extrahepatic biliary tree either percutaneously or via ERCP can improve quality of life. *Prognosis:* 4–6 months on average.

Metastases in the liver signal advanced disease. Treatment and prognosis vary with the type of primary tumour and the extent of liver involvement. Chemotherapy may be appropriate and lone metastases may be resected, but in most cases, the aim should be palliation.

The Patient Presentation varies with the type of tumour. Secondaries, HCC, and intrahepatic cholangiocarcinoma: malaise, weight loss and anorexia. Jaundice tends to occur late. Extensive tumour may stretch the liver capsule causing right hypochondrial pain. Extrahepatic cholangiocarcinoma: painless jaundice early, cachexia (p40) and abdominal pain later. Benign tumours are often asymptomatic but any hepatic tumour may rupture into the peritoneum causing bleeding and an acute abdomen. *Signs:* A hard, enlarged and knobbly liver is typical of metastases but also cirrhosis (usually a small liver), syphilitic gumma, cysts, abscesses and primary tumours (the last four are rare in the UK). Look for abdominal masses, ascites, jaundice and signs of chronic liver disease (p31). There may be an arterial bruit over the liver in HCC.

Investigations *Imaging:* Ultrasound and/or CT both for identification of lesions and to guide liver biopsy which is needed for definitive diagnosis. Do an ERCP if extrahepatic cholangiocarcinoma is suspected. *Differential of cystic lesions:* Congenital cysts, polycystic liver, hydatid cysts (p248), pyogenic or amoebic abscess (fever and ↑WCC). If secondary malignancy is identified, a search should be made for the primary (CXR, mammography, upper and lower GI endoscopy). Tailor these investigations to the patient; playing an exhaustive game of hunt the primary in the terminally ill is both pointless and cruel. *Blood tests:* Hepatitis B and C serology. Plasma α-fetoprotein is raised in 80% of HCC (and germ-cell tumours, fulminant hepatic failure, chronic hepatitis) and normal in cholangiocarcinoma and metastatic disease. Seriously deranged LFTs imply a poorer prognosis and a cholestatic picture is typical of cholangiocarcinoma.

1 T Ezaki 1992 *BMJ* i 196

Primary liver tumours

Malignant
Hepatocellular carcinoma
  Fibrolamellar variant
Cholangiocarcinoma
Angiosarcoma
Hepatoblastoma (in children)
Fibrosarcoma, leiomyosarcoma

Benign
Hepatic adenoma
Haemangioma
Focal nodular hyperplasia
Fibroma, leiomyoma, lipoma

Origin of secondary liver tumours

Males	*Females*	*Rare (either sex)*
Stomach	Breast	Pancreas
Lung	Colon	Leukaemia
Coion	Stomach	Lymphoma
	Uterus	Carcinoid tumours

Chronic and autoimmune hepatitis

Chronic hepatitis is defined as any hepatitis lasting >6 months. There may be no symptoms or signs or there may be fatigue, RUQ pain, arthralgia, complications of cirrhosis, jaundice, or signs of chronic liver disease.

Causes (Typically alcohol, idiopathic/autoimmune, or viral.)

Viruses	Metabolic	Cholestasis	Drugs
Hep B	Wilson's disease	PBC	Nitrofurantoin
Hep C	α_1-antitrypsin (p650)	Sarcoidosis	Methyldopa
Hep D(δ)	Haemochromatosis	Autoimmune cholangitis	Isoniazid

Diagnosis and investigations Detailed history (travel, transfusions, sex, IV drugs, family history, medications), and examination. Liver biopsy confirms diagnosis, but not always cause, so do blood tests: Hepatitis B and C serology, autoantibodies (ANA, SMA, anti-liver-kidney-microsomal, anti-soluble liver antigen, and anti-mitochondrial antibodies), α_1-antitrypsin, iron biochemistry (p509), caeruloplasmin (p712), copper, LFTs.

Classification Traditionally divided by its histology into *chronic persistent* (CPH) and *chronic active* hepatitis (CAH). In CPH, the limiting plate between hepatocytes is intact; in CAH it is breached and there is piecemeal necrosis and in more severe cases, bridging necrosis. This division is of decreasing value as histology correlates poorly with outcome.

Chronic hepatitis B develops in 3% of UK patients infected and affects 300 million people worldwide. It is commoner in neonates, those with poor cellular immunity, hypogammaglobulinaemia, and men. There is often no obvious acute hepatitis. It is slowly progressive but may eventually lead to cirrhosis and hepatocellular carcinoma (300 X excess risk if HBsAg +ve). *Histology:* May be almost normal, CAH or CPH with CPH more common. *Treatment:* α-Interferon if HBsAg +ve with circulating HBeAg (p211);[1] dose: 5–10 million units SC or IM 3 times a week for 16 weeks. ~40% respond (loss of e antigen).This is more likely if HIV–ve, with severe inflammation on biopsy. SE: fever, rigors, headaches, myalgia, malaise, alopecia, depression, marrow suppression—so give the first few injections in hospital. Paracetamol may help fevers and myalgia. Contraindicated in decompensated disease. Transplantation is done but there may be HBV recurrence (lamivudine *may* suppress this, eg 100mg/day for 1yr, starting 4 weeks pre-transplantation).

Chronic hepatitis C Develops in ~75% of those infected (0.7/1000 UK) and may lead to cirrhosis and hepatocellular carcinoma. *Poor prognosis:* long duration; ♂; ↑age; excess alchohol; Hep B or HIV; cirrhosis. *Treatment:* α-interferon. Use 3–6 million units twice weekly IM or SC for 6 months. Transaminases return to normal in ~50% but many will relapse on discontinuation. 10–25% achieve clearance of virus and resolution of liver inflammation. Ribavirin plus α-interferon is being trialled.

Autoimmune CAH Type I presents (typically in young women) with anorexia; malaise; few signs of liver disease (palmar erythema, spider naevi) and associated autoimmune disease or a family history of such (eg rheumatoid arthritis, vitiligo, Hashimoto's thyroiditis). Also Cushingoid features or jaundice. *Diagnosis:* Liver biopsy, autoantibodies (vary with type), LFTS (↑transaminases, ↑bilirubin), hypergammaglobulinaemia. *Treatment:* Prednisolone ~50mg/24h PO. Taper after a few weeks to a maintenance dose of ~10mg/24h PO. Azathioprine (1.5–2mg/kg/day PO) may be used in addition to steroid. Continue for 2yrs then try to withdraw. At least 75% will relapse and require ongoing treatment.

▶Liver transplants are considered in patients with CAH/CPH if liver failure supervenes. Patient selection is rigorous and timing critical.

Prevention of hepatitis B and hepatitis B-associated cirrhosis, chronic hepatitis, and hepatic neoplasia

Use hepatitis B vaccine (Engerix B®). Dose: 1mL into deltoid, repeated at 1 and 6 months (child: 0.5mL × 3—into anterolateral thigh). *Indications:* Everyone (the WHO recommendation, even in areas of 'low' endemicity). This strategy is expensive, but not as expensive as trying to rely on the ultimately unsuccessful strategy of vaccinating at-risk groups—health workers (including GPs, dentists, nurses etc), IV drug abusers, homosexuals, those on haemodialysis, and the sexual partners of known hepatitis Be antigen-positive carriers.[2] The immuno-compromised (and others) may need further doses. Serology helps time boosters and to identify poor or non-responders—correlates with older age, smoking and ♂ sex. ►*Know your own antibody level!*

Anti-HBs	Actions and comments: (UK advice: USA advice is different[3])
>1000iu/L	Good level of immunity; retest in ~4 years.
100–1000	Good level of immunity; if level approaches 100, retest in 1y.
<100	Inadequate; give booster dose and retest.
<10	Non-responder; give booster and retest; if <10, get consent to check hepatitis B status: HBsAg+ve means chronic infection; Anti-HB core +ve represents past infection and immunity.

CI: any severe febrile infection. Antibody production may be checked one month after the last dose (but the value of this labour-intensive regimen is unproven[4]). Note: protective immunity begins about 6 weeks after the first immunizing dose, so it is inappropriate for those who have had recent exposure; here, specific antihepatitis B immun-oglobulin is the best option if not previously immunized.

1 M Bartholemew 1997 *Lancet* 349 20 2 P Van Damme 1997 BMJ i 1033 3 A Tilzey 1995 *Lancet* 354 1000
4 R Chapman 1995 *Prescribers' J* 35 133

ulcerative colitis (UC)

Ulcerative colitis and Crohn's disease (p516) are together known as inflammatory bowel disease. uc is the commoner; it is defined as a recurrent inflammatory disease of the large bowel which always involves the rectum and spreads in continuity proximally to involve a variable amount of the colon. It never spreads beyond the ileocaecal valve although there may be backwash ileitis. Outside the Tropics it is the commonest cause of prolonged bloody diarrhoea. uc is more common in *non-smokers* than smokers by 2–6 times (the reverse is true in Crohn's) and ♀:♂>1. *Cause:* Unknown. There is some degree of genetic susceptibility but no evidence for involvement of an infectious agent.

▶Suspect uc whenever bloody diarrhoea lasts more than 7 days.

The Patient *Symptoms:* (Sometimes none) Typically gradual onset (or acute) of rectal bleeding, diarrhoea, and abdominal pain, mimicking GI infection. If only the rectum is involved (proctitis), constipation with blood on the stool is typical. If more extensive and serious, there is severe diarrhoea (>8 motions/day, eg nocturnal, and accompanied by urgency and tenesmus) with weight↓, fever, and symptoms of hypoproteinaemia or anaemia. In fulminant colitis, stool is liquid and mixed with blood and pus. There may be extra-intestinal features (see p516). *Signs:* Few if chronic, eg clubbing. If fulminant: fever, tachycardia, hypotension, weight loss, dehydration, tender colon, extra-intestinal manifestations.

Diagnosis *Sigmoidoscopy:* Red, raw mucosa; contact bleeding; inflammatory 'pseudopolyps' due to confluent ulcers. *Rectal biopsy:* Inflammatory infiltrate; mucosal ulcers; crypt abscesses. *Abdominal x-ray:* Colonic dilatation (± perforation) in fulminant disease; absent faeces implies involvement. *Barium enema:* Fuzzy mucosal margins, pseudopolyps, ulceration, (colon shortening and loss of haustrae if chronic). *Never do a barium enema if severe* (risks perforation). *Exclude infectious causes* (stool culture, microscopy). *Differential:* Crohn's, ischaemic colitis, infection (pseudomembranous colitis, amoebiasis, *Shigella, Campylobacter, E Coli*; also *cryptosporidium* and others if immuncompromised).

Complications Haemorrhage; dehydration; toxic dilatation and perforation; colon cancer (↑risk with ↑duration and extent; risk 11% at 26yrs). *Surveillance:* Frequent biopsies reveal occult cancers in ~1 in 400 colonoscopies—do colonoscopy ~8yrs after presentation, and repeat only if symptoms warrant it;[1] liver involvement, eg fatty liver; hepatitis; PSC*.

Medical management This consists of *managing acute relapses* (opposite) and *maintaining remissions*—eg with sulfasalazine (5-ASA linked to a sulfapyridine molecule) 1g/12h PO lowers relapse rate by 65%. SE: rash, male infertility—monitor FBC (agranulocytosis, folate deficiency). Mesalazine (5-ASA alone) 400–800mg/8h PO is as effective but lacks sulfonamide SE; likewise olsalazine (two 5-ASA moieties). Long-term (eg 6 months) azathioprine may reduce need for steroids.

Surgery Proctocolectomy and ileostomy; ileorectal anastomosis; pouch formation. *Indications:* Failed medical therapy or complications.

---

*Primary sclerosing cholangitis (PSC) causes inflammatory fibrosis and stricture of intra- and extrahepatic bile ducts. Chronic biliary obstruction and secondary biliary cirrhosis progress to liver failure and death (or transplantation) over ~10yrs.

The cause of PSC is unknown. Immunological mechanisms are suspected (50–60% have HLA-DR 3). Patients with uc have a 10–20 fold ↑risk of developing PSC (3–10%). Those with more extensive uc are most at risk. PSC occurs in <1% of patients with Crohn's disease and only then if there is colitis.

Signs: jaundice; pruritus; weight↓; RUQ pain; fatigue; hepatosplenomegaly. Alk phos monitoring is recommended in all uc patients (↑in 3%); if there are no bony metastases, Paget's, or osteomalacia, PSC is the probable cause).

Diagnosis: 1 On cholangiography: generalized bleeding and stenosis of biliary tree ('beaded' appearance of the bile ducts is characteristic). 2 Gallstones are absent and there has been no bile duct surgery. 3 Cholangiocarcinoma has been excluded by extended follow-up. Biochemistry: Alk phos rises first; a full-blown cholestatic picture is common later with fluctuating bilirubin. Hypergammaglobulinaemia may be present; ANCA (p675), SMA & ANA may be +ve, but AMA (p508) is –ve.

Complications: 10–30% will develop cholangiocarcinoma (p510) for which Ca1-9-9 is a useful marker. There is an increased incidence of colonic dysplasia and cancer. Bacterial cholangitis may also occur.

There is no cure (colectomy has no effect). Treat pruritus with cholestyramine; bacterial cholangitis with antibiotics. Ursodeoxycholic acid improves symptoms and LFTs—any effect on prognosis is unproven. Some extrahepatic strictures may be amenable to excision or stenting at ERCP. Liver transplant is the best option if young with advanced disease. Recurrence in the new liver is not a big problem. 4-year survival is said to be 80–90%. 1 AT Axon Gut 1994 35 587

Acute management of active ulcerative colitis

In mild UC, (<5 motions daily and well) give oral prednisolone, 20mg/day in divided doses, along with daily steroid enemas (eg Colifoam®) for 4 weeks. If symptoms improve, reduce steroids gradually. If not, ↑dose. In those passing >8 motions each day who are otherwise well, give steroid enemas and start oral prednisolone at 40mg/day for a week then reduce weekly to 30mg then 20mg which is given for a further 4 weeks before reduction is attempted. If patients are systemically unwell and passing >8 motions daily, admit to hospital and follow the 5-day regimen below. Cyclosporin (=cyclosporin) may also be useful (watch renal function though).

5-day regimen for severe colitis

- Get expert help. Inform surgeons.
- Nil by mouth. Set up IVI (eg 1 litre 0.9% saline + 2 litres dextrose-saline/24h, + 20mmol K⁺/litre—less if elderly). Chart: TPR, BP.
- Twice-daily physical examination. Record stool frequency/character.
- Daily: FBC, U&E, plain films, abdominal girth.
- Hydrocortisone 100mg/6h IV plus two 125mg hydrocortisone acetate foam enemas/day (~50% will be absorbed systemically).
- Consider the need for IV nutrition. Give IM vitamins (p524).
- If the patient's condition has improved at 5 days, transfer onto oral prednisolone 40mg OD (reduce at 6 weeks) plus sulfasalazine to maintain remission (see main text).
- *Colectomy indications:* Deteriorating colitis after 5 days; 'toxic' dilatation of colon (megacolon); perforation. 'Toxic' means the patient is worsening. Total surgical mortality: 2–7%; with perforation, 50%.

✝ Crohn's disease

A chronic inflammatory disease affecting any part of the gut from mouth to anus but favouring the terminal ileum and ileocaecal region. Unlike ulcerative colitis (uc), there is unaffected bowel between areas of active disease (skip lesions). *Pathology:* The bowel wall is thickened and oedematous with a red, ulcerated mucosa ± deep, serpiginous fissures. Inflammation is transmural with an infiltrate of macrophages, lymphocytes and plasma cells and there may be granulomas in the walls of small blood vessels or lymphatics. *Cause:* Unknown. There is a genetic element; smoking ↑risk 3–4 fold and Crohn's patients have diets higher in refined sugar and lower in fibre than healthy controls. One hypothesis suggests immune hyperreactivity (↑lymphocyte activity) of the gut with excessive vulnerability to antigens. ▣

The Patient *Symptoms:* Diarrhoea ± malabsorption; cramping abdominal pain; rectal bleeding; weight loss; fever; failure to thrive in children; extra-intestinal manifestations (see opposite). Rectal involvement and rectal bleeding is less common than in uc, fever and abdominal pain more so. *Signs:* Anal and perianal lesions (pendulous skin tags, abscesses, fistulae); clubbing; signs of weight loss, anaemia or hypoproteinaemia; aphthous ulceration of the mouth; abdominal tenderness (eg right side).

Complications Strictures causing subacute/acute GI obstruction; fistulae between loops of bowel and other bowel, bladder or vagina; renal disease (secondary to obstruction of the right ureter by ileocaecal disease); iron, folate and B_{12} deficiency; malignancy. Prolonged illness (15–20 years) predisposes to large and small bowel cancer (5% at 10 years).

Tests Sigmoidoscopy + rectal biopsy ± imaging of small and large bowel with barium (instillation into small bowel and enema respectively). These may reveal strictures, 'rose thorn' ulcers and a 'cobblestone' mucosa. ▶Look for associated carcinoma. Do stool microscopy and culture to exclude an infective cause and look for fat globules (malabsorption). *Markers of activity:* ESR; CRP; serum α_1 glycoproteins.

Treatment Use doses as for uc (less effective). *Prednisolone* relieves symptoms, but does not alter prognosis. *Budesonide* may have fewer side-effects (p620).[1] Treat rectal disease with *hydrocortisone acetate foam enemas*, 1 applicatorful (125mg)/12–24h PR, for 1–2 weeks, then on alternate days. *Metronidazole* 400mg/8h PO helps, especially in perianal or colonic disease (?by reducing antigen load), but use for ≤3 months (risk of neuropathies). *Azathioprine* (2mg/kg/day PO) may allow withdrawal of steroids (SE: marrow suppression—do regular FBC). *Sulfasalazine* can help colonic disease but has no rôle in maintenance therapy. If bile salt malabsorption causes diarrhoea, *cholestyramine* 4–8g/8h PO may be helpful. If intensive treatment fails, seek expert advice. ▶Drugs must not be used to delay surgery. *Pregnancy:* Steroids and sulfasalazine are permitted. Avoid metronidazole and azathioprine.

Nutrition If steatorrhoea, try a low-fat diet; if lactose intolerant, a lactose-free diet; if strictures, a low fibre diet. Elemental diets (eg E028)[1] ▣ are as good as steroids in active disease but are unpalatable and relapse is more common. Gradual re-introduction of foods maintains improvement and makes the diet more interesting.[2] Consider TPN if oral/NGT fluids impossible (eg obstructed). Enteric-coated fish oil has prevented some relapses (3 × 500mg caps/day), but it is too early to advocate general use.[3]

Surgery Most patients will need at least one operation in their life for strictures, abscesses, fistulae, or intractable, severe symptoms. Surgery is never curative. Pouch surgery is *not* done in Crohn's disease.

1 N Wright 1997 *BMJ* i 454   2 AM Riordan 1993 *Lancet* ii 1131   3 A Belluzzi 1996 *E-BM* 1 214

Inflammatory bowel disease: extra-intestinal manifestations

Related to disease activity
Erythema nodosum
Pyoderma gangrenosum**
Arthropathy (asymmetrical)
Conjunctivitis
Episcleritis
Uveitis
Thrombo-embolic disease
Gallstones (not in uc)
Amyloidosis

Unrelated to disease activity
Sacroiliitis
Ankylosing spondylitis
Primary sclerosing cholangitis (p514)**

* more common in ulcerative colitis than Crohn's disease

Irritable bowel syndrome (IBS)

Irritable bowel syndrome is characterized by troublesome gastrointestinal symptoms experienced in the absence of any organic pathology. The disease is one of negatives: there is no structural pathology, no test is diagnostic, and there is no cure. This is unfortunate given that IBS is the commonest diagnosis made in GI clinics. In fact, the lifetime prevalence of IBS is ≥20%; luckily most sufferers choose not to go to a doctor.

The Patient Usually 30–40 years but IBS may present in the elderly or as a continuation of toddler's diarrhoea. $♀:♂ ≈ 2.5:1$. *Symptoms:*

1 Abdominal pain or discomfort, commonly felt in one or both iliac fossae, often relieved by defecation or passage of flatus.
2 A sensation of abdominal distention or 'bloating'.
3 Disordered bowel habit, continuous or intermittent. This may be predominantly diarrhoea, predominantly constipation, or both.[1] A 'morning rush' is common—patients feel the urgent need to defecate several times on getting up, during and after breakfast.

Less discriminating symptoms include a sense of incomplete rectal emptying and the passage of mucus. *The presence of blood in the stool must never be ascribed to IBS—an organic cause must be sought.* Upper GI symptoms may include nausea, dysphagia, and early satiety. In women, gynaecological symptoms such as dyspareunia, urinary frequency, and urgency are common. *Signs:* Few and nonspecific (eg tender, palpable colon). Symptoms are chronic, with remissions interrupted by relapses precipitated by stress, gastroenteritis, or changes in bowel flora produced by antibiotics.

Causes These are unknown. Psychological factors, prior gastroenteritis, food intolerance and bile acid malabsorption have all been implicated. Whatever the cause, much of IBS may be explained by abnormal smooth muscle activity and a greater awareness of the bowel.

Diagnosis is by exclusion of other possible causes of the symptoms (most are features of various organic disorders). How far to investigate probable IBS is a judgment call—a balance must be struck between costly over-investigation (and exposure of the patient to unnecessary risks) and under-investigation with resultant failure to rule out serious and possibly curable organic disease. In young people with a classical history, sigmoidoscopy, FBC and ESR is probably adequate. In those >40 with a recent change in bowel habit, colonic cancer must be excluded (FOB, double contrast barium enema and/or colonoscopy). In those with severe diarrhoea consider infection (stool culture); IBD (rectal biopsy) and malabsorption (faecal fats) before diagnosing IBS.

Differential diagnosis Colonic cancer, inflammatory bowel disease, coeliac disease, gastrointestinal infection, thyrotoxicosis, pelvic inflammatory disease, endometriosis.

Treatment Rarely entirely successful so be pragmatic. Reassurance and explanation are vital. If food intolerance is suspected, try an exclusion diet. If troublesome diarrhoea: consider a bulking agent plus loperamide. If predominant constipation: try a bulking agent plus lactulose or magnesium hydroxide. Fibre is *not* a panacea—it may actually worsen pain and bloating in some IBS. Antispasmodics (mebeverine 135mg/8h PO) may reduce colic and bloating (avoid anti-cholinergic anti-spasmodics—many side-effects). Tranquillizers (eg diazepam) should be used only if symptoms are clearly stress-related and short-term to tide patients over particularly stressful periods. Cognitive therapy also helps.

Prognosis Over 50% continue to have symptoms at 5 years.

Carcinoma of the pancreas

This accounts for 1–2% of all malignancies and some 6500 deaths a year in the UK. Most are ductal adenocarcinomas although a tiny minority arise from exocrine or endocrine cells and these have a better prognosis. 60% arise from the head of the pancreas, 15% the tail, and 25% the body. Ductal pancreatic cancer metastasizes early—by the time of presentation most patients have disseminated disease. *Risk factors:* Smoking, previous gastric resection and possibly diabetes. Acute and chronic pancreatitis are not risk factors.

The Patient *Symptoms:* Epigastric abdominal pain that is intractable, severe, gnawing, worse at night, radiates to the back and may be relieved by sitting forward; dramatic weight loss; dyspepsia; pruritus is uncommon. *Signs:* Obstructive jaundice, cachexia (p40); fever; enlarged gall bladder—remember Courvoisier's law: *If in painless jaundice the gall bladder is palpable, the cause will not be gallstones*—the reason is that stones excite a fibrotic reaction in the gall bladder, which then shrinks down. *Rarer presentations:* Thrombophlebitis migrans (seen in 10%) or marantic (ie associated with wasting) endocarditis (both may cause embolism); gastric outlet obstruction; diabetes mellitus (usually enough β-cells remain to allow normoglycaemia); pancreatitis due to duct obstruction; hepatomegaly due to metastases.

Tests Ultrasound demonstrates a dilated biliary tree and masses in the pancreas and liver; ERCP delineates the anatomy of the biliary tree and localizes the site of obstruction (p498); CT allows a better assessment of the resectability of the tumour, eg presence of hepatic metastases, degree of local invasion; CT-guided needle biopsy allows differentiation of adenocarcinoma from other cell types with a better prognosis.

Treatment Only 13% are suitable for resection by Whipple's operation (partial gastrectomy/duodenectomy + partial pancreatectomy ± cholecystectomy ± distal choledochectomy). Others may benefit from palliative surgery designed to bypass the various obstructions, eg gastrojejunostomy bypasses duodenal obstruction; cholecysto-jejunostomy bypasses obstructed common bile duct and jejuno-jejunostomy diverts food away from the biliary tree. Simpler percutaneous or ERCP stent insertion can be used to relieve obstructive jaundice. Disabling pain may be relieved by percutaneous blockade of the coeliac ganglion.

Survival Due to high operative mortality (5–20% depending on the surgeon's experience[1]) and low 5-year survival even after a successful resection, Whipple's procedure should itself be considered as palliative. Median survival after bypass surgery is 24 weeks (9 weeks without surgery) and after Whipple's is 40 weeks. Patients with the rarer *nonductal* tumours, however, survive much longer—this is why all patients with suspected pancreatic cancer need skilled surgical assessment.[2,3]

1 J Cameron 1993 *Ann Surg* **17** 430   2 J Kingham 1995 *Lancet* **346** 986   3 R Charnley 1994 *BMJ* **i** 1715
See the Johns Hopkins pancreas cancer web http://128.220.85.41/PANCREAS_WHATS_NEW

Carcinoid tumours

A diverse group of tumours of argentaffin cell origin, by definition capable of producing 5-HT. Common site: appendix (25%) and rectum. They also occur elsewhere in the GI tract, and in the ovary, testis, and bronchi.

Tumours may be benign but 80% >2cm across metastasize. Symptoms and signs are initially few. GI tumours can cause appendicitis, intussusception or obstruction. Hepatic metastases may cause RUQ pain. Carcinoid tumours may secrete ACTH resulting in Cushing's syndrome and can be part of MEN-1 syndrome. Carcinoid syndrome occurs in ~10%.

Carcinoid syndrome usually implies hepatic involvement. Signs: paroxysmal flushing (± migrating wheals) eg with D&V, abdominal pain, ± CCF (tricuspid incompetence and pulmonary stenosis). *Carcinoid crisis:* When the tumour outgrows its blood supply, large amounts of mediators are released. Symptoms worsen dramatically and may be life-threatening.

Diagnosis 24h urine 5-hydroxyindoleacetic acid↑ (=5HIAA, a 5-HT metabolite; levels change also with drugs and diet: discuss with lab). If liver metastases are not found, localization of the primary (CXR, CT chest, pelvis) may be attempted as curative resection may be possible.

Treatment of carcinoid syndrome Mainly palliative. Octreotide (a somatostatin analogue) blocks release of tumour mediators and counters their peripheral effects. Effects lessen over time, so other tacks may be needed (loperamide or cyproheptadine for diarrhoea; ketanserin for flushing; interferon α). Surgical debulking (eg enucleating) or embolization of hepatic metastases can help reduce symptoms. These must be done with octreotide cover to avoid precipitating a massive carcinoid crisis. Crisis is treated with high-dose octreotide and careful management of fluid balance (central line needed). *Median survival:* 5–8 years; 38 months if metastases are present, but may be *much* longer (~20 years); so beware of giving up too easily, even if metastases are present.

Nutritional disorders

Scurvy This is due to lack of vitamin C in the diet. ►*Is the patient poor, pregnant, or on an odd diet?* Signs: 1 Listlessness, anorexia, cachexia (p40). 2 Gingivitis, loose teeth, and foul-smelling breath (halitosis). 3 Bleeding from gums, nose, hair follicles, or into joints, bladder, gut. *Diagnosis:* No test is completely satisfactory. WBC ascorbic acid ↓. *Treatment:* Dietary education, ascorbic acid 250mg/24h PO.

Beriberi There is heart failure with general oedema (wet beriberi) or neuropathies (dry beriberi) due to lack of vitamin B₁ (thiamine). For treatment and diagnostic tests, see Wernicke's encephalopathy (p712).

Pellagra This is due to lack of nicotinic acid. Other nutritional deficiencies are likely to be present. The classical triad of signs is: diarrhoea, dementia and dermatitis. Others: neuropathy, depression, tremor, rigidity, ataxia, fits. Pellagra may occur in the carcinoid syndrome. *Treatment:* education, electrolyte replacement, nicotinamide 500mg/24h PO.

Xerophthalmia This vitamin A deficiency is a major cause of blindness in the Tropics. Conjunctivae become dry and develop oval or triangular spots (Bitôt's spots). Corneas become cloudy and soft. See OHCS p512. Give vitamin A 200,000 IU stat PO, repeat in 24h and a week later (halve dose if <1yr old; quarter if <6 months old); get special help if pregnant; vitamin A embryopathy must be avoided.[1] Re-educate, and monitor diet.

Lathyrism This is an acute spastic paralysis occurring in lathyrus pea eaters (due to a toxin). Treatment is unsatisfactory.

Favism There is sudden severe haemolysis in those with certain types of G6PD deficiency on eating broad beans or inhaling their pollen.

1 A Potter 1997 *BMJ* i 317

Gastrointestinal malabsorption

The Patient Diarrhoea; ↓weight; steatorrhoea. Signs of deficiencies: anaemia (↓Fe, ↓B₁₂, ↓folate); bleeding (↓vitamin K); oedema (↓protein). Common UK causes are coeliac disease, Crohn's, chronic pancreatitis.

Causes *Biliary insufficiency:* Primary biliary cirrhosis; ileal resection; biliary obstruction; cholestyramine.

Pancreatic insufficiency: Chronic pancreatitis; pancreatic carcinoma; cystic fibrosis.

Small bowel mucosa: Coeliac and Whipple's disease (p712); tropical sprue; radiation enteritis; small bowel resection; brush border enzyme deficiencies (eg lactase insufficiency); drugs (metformin, neomycin, alcohol); amyloid (p616).

Bacterial overgrowth: Spontaneous; in diverticula; post-op blind loops. Try metronidazole (400mg/8h PO) or oxytetracycline (250mg/6h PO).

Infection: Giardiasis; diphyllobothriasis (B₁₂ malabsorption); strongyloidiasis.

Intestinal hurry: Post-gastrectomy dumping; post-vagotomy; gastrojejunostomy.

Tests FBC (MCV↓, macrocytosis); ↓Ca²⁺ (↓vit. D due to fat malabsorption); ↓Fe; ↓folate; ↑PT (↓vitamin K). *Stool:* Sudan stain for fat globules; stool microscopy for infestation. *Barium follow-through:* Diverticula; Crohn's; radiation enteritis. *Hydrogen breath hydrogen test:* (bacterial overgrowth) Take samples of end-expired air; give glucose; take more samples at ½h intervals. If there is overgrowth there is ↑exhaled hydrogen. *Small bowel biopsy:* Use endoscopy. *ERCP:* Biliary obstruction; chronic pancreatitis.

Tropical sprue Villous atrophy and malabsorption occurring in the Far and Middle East and Caribbean (not Africa). *Cause:* Unknown. Tetracycline 250mg/6h PO + folic acid 15mg/24h PO may help.

Coeliac disease Prolamin (alcohol-soluble proteins in wheat, barley, rye ± oats) intolerance causes villous atrophy and malabsorption. *Associations:* HLA B8 (~80%) and DQw2; autoimmune disease; dermatitis herpetiformis.

The Patient: Steatorrhoea; abdominal pain; bloating; nausea, vomiting; aphthous ulcers, angular stomatitis; weight↓; fatigue; weakness; osteomalacia; failure to thrive (children). ⅓ are asymptomatic. Occurs at any age but peaks at 0–5y and 50–60y, ♀:♂>1. *Diagnosis:* Anti-endomyseal, anti-reticulin, α-gliadin antibodies. Jejunal biopsy: villous atrophy. This must reverse on a gluten-free diet along with a reduction of symptoms and α-gliadin antibody levels all of which should recur on gluten challenge.

Treatment: Lifelong gluten-free diet. Rice, maize, soya, potatoes (sometimes oats), and sugar are OK. Gluten-free biscuits, flour, bread and pasta are prescribable in the UK. Check compliance by α-gliadin antibodies.

Complications: Anaemia; 2° lactose-intolerance; GI T-cell lymphoma (suspect if worsening despite diet); malignancy (gastric, oesophageal, bladder, breast, brain); myopathies; neuropathies; hyposplenism.

Chronic pancreatitis Epigastric pain 'bores' through to back (eg relived by sitting forward or hot water bottles on epigastrium/back: look for *erythema ab igne's* dusky greyness here);[1] bloating; steatorrhoea; ↓weight; diabetes.

Causes: Alcohol; rarely: familial; cystic fibrosis; haemochromatosis; pancreatic duct obstruction (stones or pancreatic cancer); hyperparathyroidism.[2]

Tests: Ultrasound (dilated biliary tree; stones); if normal[3] consider CT/ERCP (p498); plain film: speckled pancreatic calcification; blood glucose.

Drugs: ●Give analgesia (± coeliac-plexus block[2]). ●Lipase, eg enteric-coated capsules (Nutrizym GR® 1–4 caps PO with meals) ●Fat-soluble vitamins (eg Multivite pellets®). *Diet:* Low-fat (+ no alcohol) may help. Medium-chain triglycerides (MCT oil®) may be tried (no lipase needed for absorption, but diarrhoea may be worsened).[2] *Surgery:* For unremitting pain; narcotic abuse (beware this); weight↓: pancreatectomy or pancreaticojejunostomy.

1 A Ala 1998 *Lancet* 351 67 2 K Mergener 1997 *Lancet* 350 1379 3 V Moreira 1998 *Lancet* 351 67

Alcoholism[1]

An alcoholic is one whose repeated drinking leads to harm in his work or social life. ▶Denial is the leading feature of alcoholism, so be sure to question relatives. Screening tests: MCV↑; gamma-GT↑. (note that alcohol can do you good in low doses, eg <21u/week in men, see p482.[2])

Probing questions [Useful mnemonic: **control**] Can you always control your drinking? Has alcohol ever led you to neglect your family or your work? What time do you start drinking? Do you sometimes start before this? Do friends comment on how much you drink or ask you to reduce intake? Do you ever drink in the mornings to overcome a hangover? Go through an average day's alcohol, leaving nothing out.

Organs affected by alcohol ●*The liver:* (Normal in 50% of alcoholics.)
Fatty liver: Acute and reversible, but may progress to cirrhosis if drinking continues (also seen in obesity, diabetes mellitus and with amiodarone).
Hepatitis: (Fever, jaundice and vomiting)—80% progress to cirrhosis (hepatic failure in 10%). Biopsy: Mallory bodies ± neutrophil infiltrate.
Cirrhosis (p506): 5yr survival is 48% if drinking continues (if not, 77%).
●*CNS:* Poor memory/cognition: ▶multiple high-potency vitamins IM may reverse it; cortical atrophy; retrobulbar neuropathy; fits; falls; wide-based gait (PLATE 3) neuropathy; Korsakoff's ± Wernicke's encephalopathy, p702-12.

●*Gut:* Obesity, diarrhoea; gastric erosions; peptic ulcers; varices (p496); pancreatitis (acute and chronic).

●*Blood:* MCV↑; anaemia from: marrow depression, GI bleeds, alcoholism-associated folate deficiency, haemolysis, sideroblastic anaemia.

●*Heart:* Arrhythmias; BP↑; cardiomyopathy; sudden death in binge drinkers.[2]

Withdrawal signs Pulse↑; BP↓; tremor; fits; hallucinations (*delirium tremens*)—may be visual or tactile, eg of animals crawling all over one.

Alcohol contraindications Driving; hepatitis; cirrhosis; peptic ulcer; drugs (eg antihistamines); carcinoid; pregnancy (fetal alcohol syndrome—IQ↓, short palpebral fissure, absent filtrum and small eyes).

Management *Alcohol withdrawal:* Admit; do BP + TPR/4h. Beware BP↓. For first 3 days give generous diazepam, eg 10mg/6h PO or PR if vomiting (in seizures, see p782), then ↓diazepam (eg 10mg/8h PO for days 4–6, then 5mg/12h for 2 more days). The once-preferred chlormethiazole (=clormethiazole) readily causes addiction + respiratory depression (it is said[1●]); phenothiazines are problematic too. ●Vitamins may be needed (p712).
Prevention (OHCS p454): Alcohol-free beers; alcohol-free pubs; low-risk drinking, eg ≤20u/week if ♂; ≤15u/week if ♀—there are no absolutes—risk is a continuum. (higher limits are controversial[2▣]). 1u is 9g ethanol, ie 1 measure of spirits, 1 glass of wine, or ½ pint of beer.
Treatment of the established alcoholic may be rewarding, particularly if he really wants to change. If so, group therapy or self-help (eg 'Alcoholics Anonymous') may be useful. Encourage the will to change. Think about graceful ways of declining a drink, eg "I'm seeing what it's like to go without for a bit." Suggest the patient does not buy him or herself a drink when it is his turn. Suggest: "Don't lift your glass to your lips until after the slowest drinker in your group takes a drink. Sip, don't gulp." Give follow-up and encouragement. *Anxiety, insomnia, and craving* may be mitigated by acamprosate (p406); CI: pregnancy, severe liver failure, creatinine >120µmol/L; SE: D&V, libido fluctuation; dose example: 666mg/8h PO if >60kg and <65yrs old.[6] *Reducing pleasure that alcohol brings* (and withdrawal craving) with naltrexone 50mg/24h PO can halve relapse rates.[4] SE: vomiting, drowsiness, dizziness, cramps, arthralgia. CI: hepatitis, liver failure. It is costly. Confer with experts if drugs are to be used.

1 BMJ 1997 i 1499 2 *Lancet* 1995 i 1643 3 1997 BMJ ii 846 4 BMJ 1995 ii 3 5 *Lancet* 1995 i 456 6 *Drug Th Bul* 1997 35 70

12. Endocrinology

Relevant pages in other chapters:
Diabetic emergencies (p784); the diabetic patient undergoing surgery (p108); the eye in diabetes (*OHCS* p508); thyroid emergencies (p786); thyroid lumps (p150); Addison's disease, thyroid disease, and surgery (p110); Addisonian crisis and hypopituitary coma (p788); phaeochromocytoma emergencies (p788); hyperlipidaemia (p654).

Endocrinology and pregnancy: Thyroid disease in pregnancy (*OHCS* p157); diabetes in pregnancy (*OHCS* p156).

The essence of endocrinology

- Define a clinical syndrome.
- Match it to a gland malfunction.
- Measure the gland's output to the peripheral blood. Is release diurnal? What other variabilities are there? Define clinical syndromes associated with too much or too little secretion (*hyper-* and *hypo-* syndromes, respectively; *eu-* means normal, neither ↑ nor ↓ , as in *euthyroid*).
- Find a radiological technique to image the gland.
- Characterize any internal bioassays which nature is kind enough to provide you with. For example you could regard thyroid stimulating hormone (TSH) as a convenient bioassay of thyroid gland function: the same is true for HbA1c in diabetes mellitus (p532).
- Find ways of stimulating the gland, defining variations from the norm.
- Find ways of inhibiting the gland. Measure intermediate metabolites to further define pathophysiology and guide treatment.

✝✝✝ Diabetes mellitus: classification & diagnosis

Definition Diabetes mellitus (DM) is a syndrome caused by the lack of, or diminished, effectiveness (see opposite) of endogenous insulin and is characterized by hyperglycaemia and deranged metabolism.

528

Type 1 (insulin-dependent DM, IDDM) Usually juvenile onset but may be *any* age and associated with other autoimmune diseases (+HLA DR3 & DR4 & islet cell antibodies around the time of diagnosis). There is insulin deficiency. Concordance is >30% in identical twins. 4 genes are thought to be important—one (6q) determines islet sensitivity to damage (eg from viruses or cross-reactivity from cows' milk-induced antibodies). Patients *always need insulin*, and are prone to ketoacidosis and weight loss.

Type 2 (non-insulin-dependent DM=NIDDM=maturity onset DM) Older age group and often obese. ~100% concordance in identical twins. Due to impaired insulin secretion or insulin resistance. *Note:* NIDDM may eventually require insulin: *this does not mean the patient now has IDDM.* Insulin is likely to be needed in those with ketonuria, glucose >25mmol/L, sudden onset, weight↓, dehydration. If ketoacidosis, then IDDM exists.

Causes of secondary diabetes *Drugs* (steroids and thiazides), *pancreatic disease* (pancreatitis, surgery in which >90% pancreas is removed, haemochromatosis, cystic fibrosis, pancreatic cancer), *other endocrine disease* (Cushing's disease, acromegaly, phaeochromocytoma, thyrotoxicosis), *others* (acanthosis nigricans, congenital lipodystrophy with insulin receptor antibodies, and glycogen storage diseases).

Presentation of DM Patients may be asymptomatic. *Acute:* Ketoacidosis (p784)—unwell, hyperventilation, ketones on breath, weight loss, polyuria and polydipsia. *Subacute:* History as above but longer and in addition lethargy, infection (pruritus vulvae, boils). *Complications* may be the presenting feature: infections, neuropathy, retinopathy, arterial disease (eg myocardial infarction or claudication).

Diagnosis 1 Fasting venous plasma glucose >7.8mmol/L* or random >11.1 on two occasions. 2 Glucose tolerance test (GTT): fasting glucose >7.8 and/or 2h glucose ≥11.1mmol/L. 3 Glycosuria: requires further investigation even if symptomless (sensitivity 32%, specificity 99%[1]). *Note:*
- If 2 fasting glucose levels >6 but <8mmol/L, give dietary advice (as for NIDDM, p482) and repeat glucose in 6 months. Do not label as having diabetes mellitus (because of insurance implications).
- Screening for glycosuria is easy but is not a cost-effective way of screening entire populations of symptomless people.[2] ~1% of the population have low renal threshold for glucose; simultaneous blood and urine glucose measurements can be used for diagnosis.
- Impaired glucose tolerance progresses to frank DM in ~5%.

WHO diagnostic criteria for diabetes (on two fasting glucose estimations)

<6mmol/L	DM excluded
>6mmol/L but <7.8 mmol/L	Impaired glucose tolerance (IGT)
>7.8 mmol/L	Diabetes mellitus

2-hour oral glucose tolerance test ●**Fast** overnight and give **75g of glucose** in **300mL water** to drink. ●Do venous **plasma glucose before** and **2h after** drink. DM **diagnosed if fasting glucose >7.8mmol/L** and/or 2h glucose ≥11.1mmol/L. *Impaired glucose tolerance* implies fasting glucose ≥6 but <7.8 and/or 2h glucose >7.8l and <11.1mmol/L (and risk of death from MI ↑ × 2).

Can a single HbA1c (p532) test replace the OGTT? If >7%, DM is likely (specificity 99.6%; sensitivity 99%), and risk of microvascular complications occurs.[3]

*The USA Diabetic Ass^n proposes a fasting glucose >7mmol/L as the cut-off point for diagnosing DM (if 6-7mmol/L, diagnose 'impaired fasting glucose'); see *Diabetes Care* 1997 **20** 1859
1 J Yudkin 1990 *BMJ* i 1463 2 D Mant 1990 *BMJ* i 1053 3 M Stewart 1997 *Lancet* 349 223

The insulin resistance syndrome ('syndrome X')

This is the association of insulin resistance in tissues, with hyperinsulinaemia (fasting insulin >89.4pmol/L), central obesity, hypertension, hyperglycaemia, coronary artery disease, ↑plasma triglyceride level, ↓HDL (p564), ↑plasminogen activator, ± ↑risk of Alzheimer's disease,[1] perhaps due to glycation end-products found in CNS plaques.

Causes of insulin resistance Obesity   Pregnancy   Asian origin
Acute and chronic renal failure* Acromegaly   Isoniazid   Rifampicin
Sympathetic tone†[2]   Cystic fibrosis Werner's syn, *OHCS* p759
Polycystic ovaries (p556)   Ataxia telangiectasia

Mechanism of insulin resistance Obesity probably causes insulin resistance by the associated ↑rate of release of non-esterified fatty acids causing post-receptor defects in insulin's action. *Other mechanisms:* ●Mutation of the gene encoding insulin receptor ●Circulating autoantibodies to the extracellular domain of the insulin receptor.

Management Advise weight loss and exercise; manage hyperglycaemia, with drugs or insulin. *Future prospects:* Vitamin E improves insulin sensitivity and delays oxidation of LDL (the postulated common factor in development of atheroma, hypertension, hypercholesterolaemia, and diabetes: this LDL down-regulates nitric oxide production which is required for healthy endothelium).[3] We do not know if vitamin E saves lives. Drugs to ↑insulin sensitivity are under development: one, troglitazone, was withdrawn (voluntarily) due to hepatic toxicity.

1 J Kuusito 1997 *BMJ* ii 1045 2 Effects may be partly reversed by selective imidazoline-I₁-receptor agonists (A Krentz 1998 *Lancet* **351** 152) 3 A Gazis 1997 *BMJ* i 1846 *Effect of insulin resistance in renal failure is offset unpredictably by ↓renal catabolism of insulin, so diabetes may be hard to control at this time.

Not done anymore.

╫╫╫ The newly diagnosed diabetic

►*Patient motivation and education are the keys to success.*

530

The aim of treatment is the avoidance of complications. Aim for nor-moglycaemia, but if life on the verge of hypoglycaemia is intolerable, this aim may be modified. In type 2 diabetes mellitus (IDDM), strict plasma glucose control *does* reduce renal, CNS and retinal damage, but the price is, on average, one hypoglycaemic coma a year, and a lifestyle compromised by frequent blood glucose tests. ◁1▷ Discuss this with your patient.

Initial treatment need not include hospitals—even in IDDM. If there is ketonuria or he/she is ill or dehydrated, do admit. Children are liable to get ketotic rapidly, so prompt paediatric referral is a must (*OHCS* p262–265). If pregnant, share care with an interested obstetrician (*OHCS* p156). Stress the need for special pre-conception counselling (*OHCS* p94).

Education/negotiation is crucial on drugs, diet, and the issues below:
● Monitoring blood or urine glucose and *adapting treatment accordingly.*
● Explain that when all *more*, not less, insulin is needed. Consider exposing to a 'hypo'; show how to abort it with sugar/sweets (►carry them always).
● Introduce to a specialist *nurse/dietician, chiropodist,* and *diabetic association.*
● *Regular* follow-up and *regular* exercise (↓insulin resistance and ↓risk of MI).
● Patients must inform their *driving licence authority* (*OHCS* p468 for restrictions).
● *Healthy eating:* p482 (saturated fats↓, sugar↓, starch-carbohydrate↑, moderate protein) adapted tastes and needs (eg to prevent obesity). It may be important to ensure that some starchy carbohydrate (bread, potato, pasta) is taken at each meal. If any hint of renal failure (creatinine↑, microalbuminuria, p396) restrict protein, and consider ACE↓ (p299).

Insulin Strength: 100u/mL. Formulations of different durations: soluble insulin is short-acting (peak 2–4h, lasting ~8h). Longer-acting suspensions have onset of action of 1–2h, peak 4–12h and duration 16–35h. The hierarchy of increasing lengths of action is: isophane insulin, IZS (amorphous), IZS (mixed), IZS (crystalline), protamine zinc insulin. Tailor the insulin regimen to the individual by checking control at different times of the day (see p531). Note: IZS = insulin zinc suspension.

Oral hypoglycaemics: *Sulfonylureas* ↑insulin secretion. *Tolbutamide* is short-acting; useful in elderly (hypoglycaemia unlikely). Dose 0.5–1g/12h. *Glibenclamide's* action is intermediate. Beware pre-lunch hypoglycaemia. Dose: 2.5–15mg/24h with breakfast. *Chlorpropamide* is long-acting and can be given once a day—avoid in renal impairment and in the elderly (risk of hypoglycaemia). Dose: 100–500mg/24h PO with breakfast (no alcohol: it may cause flushes); other SE: headache, photosensitivity, Na⁺↓. *Gliclazide* is also given once a day (40–160mg with breakfast); hypoglycaemic risk is low.

Metformin (a biguanide) Action: insulin sensitivity↑; hepatic gluconeogenesis↓. SE: anorexia; D&V; B_{12} absorption↓; *not* hypoglycaemia (so HGV drivers may use it). It may be best suited to obese subjects as an adjunct. Avoid in hepatic and renal impairment. *Dose:* 500mg/8h PO after food.

Acarbose (α-glucosidase inhibitor, ↓breakdown of starch to sugar**)** It is an adjunct to oral hypoglycaemics. It (in practice effects can disappoint).[2] Dose: 50mg chewed at start of each meal (start with a once-daily dose; max 200mg/8h). SE: wind (can be terrible; less if *slow* dose build-up), abdominal distension/pain, diarrhoea. CI: ●Pregnancy ●GI obstruction ●Hernias ●Crohn's and UC ●Past laparotomy ●Hepatic or *severe* renal failure.

◁1▷ Diabetes control & complications trial research group 1993 *NEJM* **329** 977 & 1995 *An Int Med* **122** 561 & E-BM 1995 **1** 9   2 *Drug Ther Bul* 1994 **32** 51

Some commonly used insulin regimens

1 A single dose of very long acting insulin (Ultralente®) with 3 doses of short-acting insulin (15–30 minutes before each meal). This tends to be favoured by younger subjects (it offers greater flexibility in lifestyle). Also may be of value in those with erratic control.

2 A mixture of short- and medium-acting insulin (eg soluble and Lente) at 7AM and 6PM (ie ½h before meal). Give ⅔ of total insulin in the morning and ⅔ as Lente. To improve control before breakfast, adjust evening Lente; before lunch—morning soluble; before supper—morning Lente; before bed—evening soluble.

3 Single dose of soluble and Lente may be sufficient in the elderly.

4 'Pen' devices (eg NovoPen II®) are popular because of their ease of use (eg during parties). Short-acting insulin is given 15–30mins before each meal, with basal insulin requirements being provided by a conventional evening dose of long-acting insulin; mixed soluble (short) and isophane preparations (medium) are also available (eg PenMix® 10/90, 20/80, 30/70, 40/60, 50/50).

5 If meal times are random, or postprandial glucose↑, very rapidly absorbed, genetically engineered human insulin *lispro* (*Humalog®*) can be injected *just before eating*. It helps iron-out glucose variability and can ↓tendency to pre-lunch hypoglycaemia.[1] It can be mixed with Ultralente (needed at night if lispro injections separated by >5h).[2]

Encourage regular home blood glucose monitoring in all patients, but it is particularly critical with hypoglycaemic unawareness (consider also relaxing control). Discuss the pros and cons with your patient.

Begin with at least 8u of soluble insulin before meals, monitoring blood glucose; transfer to one of the above when control is achieved.

1 *BNF & Drug Ther Bul* 1997 **35** 57   2 J Nancy *Postgrad Med* 1997 **101** (2)

⚕ Assessment of the established diabetic

Continuing assessment of the diabetic patient has 3 main aims: **1** To educate. **2** To find out what problems the patient is having with the diabetes (glycaemic control and morale). **3** To find or pre-empt complications.

Assess glycaemic control from: **1** Home fingerstick glucose records.

2 History of hypoglycaemic attacks (and whether symptomatic).

3 Glycated (glycosylated) haemoglobin (=HbA1c)—levels relate to mean glucose level over previous 8 weeks (ie RBC half-life). Aim is to keep at or *just* above normal range (≈2.3–6.5%). Complications increase in frequency with increasing HbA1c in NIDDM (and probably IDDM though data are still being collected). Note that *fructosamine* (glycated plasma protein) levels relate to control over previous 1–3 weeks. May be useful in pregnancy to assess shorter-term control, also if there is a condition interfering with HbA1c measurement (eg some haemoglobinopathies).

Assessment of complications

● Check injection sites for infection, lipoatrophy, or lipohypertrophy.

● *Vascular disease:* Look for evidence of cerebrovascular, cardiovascular and peripheral vascular disease. MI is 3–5 times more common in DM and is more likely to be 'silent' (ie without classic symptoms). Stroke is twice as common. Women are at particular relative risk—DM removes the cardiovascular advantage conferred by female gender. Reduce other risk factors (see p255). Treat hypertension vigorously with close attention to drug effects in DM, eg high-dose thiazides ↑blood glucose and lipids; ACE-inhibitors slow progression of renal disease (p396), so are a good first choice. Treat lipid disorders: good glycaemic control will help. Fibrates are useful for ↑triglycerides and ↓HDL. HMG CoA reductase inhibitors (eg simvastatin) are useful if LDL is raised too. An aspirin a day may ↓risk of MI in diabetics as in non-diabetics (no significant risk to eye).

● *Kidneys* (p396): Check urine regularly. If dipstick is +ve for protein, collect 24h urine for creatinine clearance and for quantifying albuminuria. Measuring microalbuminuria (p394) helps detect early renal disease. Control BP with ACE inhibitor if tolerated (cautions and CI: see p299).

● *Diabetic retinopathy:* (Visible after dilating pupils with 0.5% tropicamide.) Blindness is *not* rare (≤20% of IDDM) but *is* preventable. *Arrange regular fundoscopy for all patients,* eg by retinal photography. Refer if maculopathy from visible hard exudates. ►Pre-symptomatic screening enables laser photocoagulation to be used. *Pathogenesis:* Capillary endothelial change → vascular leakage → microaneurysms. Capillary occlusion → hypoxia + ischaemia → new vessel formation. High retinal blood flow caused by hyperglycaemia (and BP↑ and pregnancy) triggers these events, and causes capillary pericyte damage.

Microvascular occlusion causes *cotton-wool spots*; there may be *blot haemorrhages* at interfaces with perfused retina. *New vessels* form on disc or ischaemic areas, proliferate, fibrose, and can detach the retina.

1) *Background:* Microaneurysms (dots), microhaemorrhages (blots) and hard exudates. Refer to specialist if near the macula.

2) *Pre-proliferative retinopathy:* cotton-wool exudates (small retinal infarcts) and extensive microhaemorrhages.

3) *Proliferative retinopathy:* New vessels form. Needs *urgent* referral.

4) *Maculopathy:* More common in NIDDM. Suspect if visual acuity↓.

● *Cataracts:* These occur earlier in DM (senile and juvenile 'snowflake' cataracts). The osmotic changes in the lens induced in acute hyperglycaemia reverse after normoglycaemia (so wait before buying glasses).

● *Rubeosis iridis:* Iris new vessels. It occurs late and can lead to glaucoma.

● *Metabolic complications:* p784. *Diabetic feet:* p534. *Neuropathy:* p534.

✚ Diabetic neuropathy and the diabetic foot

▶Amputation is preventable: good care saves legs.

The feet of all patients with DM should be examined regularly. Feet are affected by a *combination* of peripheral neuropathy and peripheral vascular disease, though one or other may predominate.

Symptoms Numbness, tingling, and burning, often worse at night.

Signs Sensation↓ (especially vibration) in 'stocking' distribution; absent ankle jerks; deformity (pes cavus, claw toes, loss of transverse arch, rocker-bottom sole). Neuropathy is patchy, so examine all areas. If the foot pulses cannot be felt, consider Doppler pressure measurement.

Any evidence of neuropathy or vascular disease puts the patient at high risk of foot ulceration. Educate (daily foot inspection, comfortable shoes—ie very soft leather, increased depth, cushioning insoles, weight-distributing cradles, extra cushioning—no barefoot walking, no corn-plasters). Regular chiropody. Treat fungal infections (p244).

Foot ulceration Usually painless, punched-out ulcer in an area of thick callous ± superadded infection, pus, oedema, erythema, crepitus, odour.

Assess degree of: 1 Neuropathy (clinical). 2 Ischaemia (clinical and Dopplers; consider angiography—even elderly patients may benefit from angioplasty). 3 Bony deformity eg Charcot joint (clinical, x-ray). 4 Infection (do swabs, blood culture, x-ray; probe ulcer to assess depth).

Management: Regular chiropody (ie at least weekly) initially to debride the lesion. Relieve high-pressure areas with bed rest and special footwear. If there is cellulitis, admission is mandatory for IV antibiotics: start with benzylpenicillin 600mg/6h IV and flucloxacillin 500mg/6h IV ± metronidazole 500mg/8h IV, refined when microbiology results are known. Seek surgical opinion early. Good glycaemic control is beneficial.[1]

Absolute indications for surgery
- Abscess or deep infection
- Spreading anaerobic infection
- Osteomyelitis
- Severe ischaemia—gangrene/rest pain
- Suppurative arthritis

The degree of peripheral vascular disease, patient's general health, and patient request will determine whether local excision and drainage, vascular reconstruction, and/or amputation (and how much) is appropriate.

Other aspects of diabetic neuropathy The cause of neuropathy is unknown, but its consequences potentially severe—loss of legs. ◁1▷ Altered cellular Na^+ permeability has been suggested as a mechanism.

Somatic neuropathy:
1 Symmetric sensory polyneuropathy—distal numbness, tingling, and visceral pain, eg worse at night. Consider aspirin, paracetamol, or a tricyclic drug (± a low-dose phenothiazine or carbamazepine,[2] p450).
2 Mononeuritis multiplex—especially III and VI cranial nerves.
3 Amyotrophy—painful wasting of quadriceps; reversible.

Autonomic neuropathy: (see p463 for biology) Postural BP↓; urine retention; impotence; diarrhoea at night. The latter may respond to 3 doses of tetracycline 250mg PO or long-term codeine phosphate[2] (the lowest dose which controls symptoms, eg 15mg/8h PO). Vomiting associated with *gastroparesis* may respond to anti-emetics or cisapride (p491). Postural hypotension may respond to fludrocortisone 0.1mg–0.3mg/24h PO (SE oedema). Consider poldine methylsulfate for gustatory sweating, and ephedrine hydrochloride 30–60mg/8h PO for neuropathic oedema.[2]

▶In all patients, optimize diabetic control.

1 Diabetes control & complications trial research group 1995 *An Int Med* **122** 561 & ▶E-BM 1995 1 9
2 BNF 1998 *see also* D Neale 1989 *Common Foot Disorders*, Churchill Livingstone

Diabetic patients with intercurrent illness

The stress of illness often increases basal insulin requirement. If calorie intake↓ (if vomiting) then increase long-acting insulin (by ~20%); reducing short-acting in proportion to meal size. Check blood sugar often.

1 **Insulin-treated; mild illness** (eg gastroenteritis). Maintain calorie intake with oral fluids (lemonade etc.). Continue normal insulin. Test blood glucose and urine ketones regularly (eg twice daily). Increase insulin if blood glucose consistently >10mmol/L.

2 **Insulin-treated; moderate illness** (eg pneumonia). Normal insulin and supplementary sliding scale of rapid-acting insulin (p109), four times daily (before meals and bedtime snack).

3 **Insulin-treated; severe illness** (eg MI, severe trauma). IV soluble insulin by pump and IV dextrose (p109).

4 **Diet and tablet treated; moderate/severe illness** If on metformin, stop. If on sulfonylureas and illness likely to be self-limiting, keep on tablets, supplement with sc insulin, and sliding scale or IV infusion (p109). Tail off insulin as patient recovers.

Hypoglycaemia

►This is the commonest endocrine emergency. Prompt diagnosis and treatment is essential. See p784 for emergency management.

Definition Plasma glucose <2.5mmol/L. Threshold for symptoms varies.

Symptoms *Autonomic*—Sweating; hunger; tremor.
Neuroglycopenic—Drowsiness; personality change; fits; rarely focal symptoms, eg transient hemiplegia, loss of consciousness.

Two types:

●**Fasting hypoglycaemia** (requires full investigation if documented).
Causes: By far the commonest cause is insulin or sulfonylurea treatment in the known diabetic. In the non-diabetic subject with fasting hypoglycaemia the following mnemonic is useful: EXPLAIN.

Ex Exogenous drugs, eg insulin or chlorpropamide (p530; it's long-acting).
Does he have access to these, eg as a (para)medic? Is there a diabetic in the family? *Alcohol,* eg alcoholic on a binge with no food. Also: *atorvastatin; aminoglutethimide; 4-quinolones; pentamidine; ACE-i,* if DM: see *EBM* 1998 61.

P Pituitary insufficiency.

L Liver failure plus some rare inherited enzyme defects.

A Addison's disease.

I Islet cell tumours (insulinoma) and immune hypoglycaemia (eg anti-insulin receptor antibodies in Hodgkin's disease).

N Non-pancreatic neoplasms (especially retroperitoneal fibrosarcomas and haemangiopericytomas).

In addition: *malaria, especially with quinine administration.*

Diagnosis and investigations

1 Document hypoglycaemia by the patient taking finger-prick samples on filter-paper (at home for later analysis) during attack, or in hospital.

2 Exclude liver failure and malaria.

3 Admit for overnight fast. Take two separate samples for glucose, insulin, beta-hydroxybutyrate, and C-peptide.

Interpretation of results

1 Hypoglycaemia with high or normal insulin and no elevated ketones. *Causes:* insulinoma; sulfonylurea administration; insulin administration (no detectable C-peptide); insulin autoantibodies.

2 Insulin low or undetectable, no excess ketones. *Causes:* Non-pancreatic neoplasm; anti-insulin receptor antibodies.

3 Insulin low or undetectable, ketones high. *Causes:* Alcohol; pituitary or adrenal failure.

Note: if insulinoma suspected, confirm with a suppressive test: eg infuse IV insulin and measure C-peptide. Normally insulin suppresses C-peptide, but this suppression does not occur in patients with insulinomas. Localize the insulinoma using CT scanning. If none is visible, sophisticated techniques (eg intra-operative pancreatic vein sampling) may be needed.

●**Post-prandial hypoglycaemia** This occurs particularly after gastric surgery ('dumping', p164), and in those with mild type II diabetes.

Investigation: Prolonged OGTT (5h, p528).

Treatment ►►See p784. Treat with oral sugar, and a long-acting starch (eg toast); if coma, glucose 25–50g IV or glucagon 0.5–1mg SC (± a repeat after 20mins; *follow with carbohydrate*). If episodes frequent, advise many small meals high in starch. If post-prandial glucose↓, have slowly absorbed carbohydrate (high fibre, complex carbohydrates). Insulinomas: surgical removal if possible; diazoxide and a thiazide diuretic.

Basic thyroid function tests

Thyroid hormone abnormalities are usually due to a problem with the thyroid gland itself. Primary abnormalities of thyroid-stimulating hormone (TSH) and thyrotrophin-releasing hormone (TRH) are very rare.

Physiology The hypothalamus secretes TRH, a tripeptide, which stimulates the production of TSH, a polypeptide, from the anterior pituitary. TSH increases the production and release of thyroxine (T4) and triiodothyronine (T3) from the thyroid, which exert negative feedback on TSH production (the basis of the TRH test p540). The thyroid produces mainly T4, which is 5 times less active thanT3. T3 is mainly formed from the peripheral conversion of T4 (85% of T3 is produced this way). Most T3 and T4 in plasma is protein bound, mainly to thyroxine-binding globulin (TBG). The *unbound* portion is the active moiety. T3 and T4 increase cell metabolism, via nuclear receptors, and are thus vital for normal growth and mental development. They also enhance catecholamine effects.

Basic tests Write why you want the test. Different labs do different tests. In general, if you expect *hyperthyroidism* the most sensitive test is plasma T3 (which is raised): if you expect *hypothyroidism* the most sensitive tests are *plasma T4* (lowered) and TSH (raised).

1—Plasma T4 (total T4, ie total thyroxine)
Method: Collect any time, uncuffed. *Problems of interpretation: False high* (as bound, as well as free T4 measured): pregnant; oestrogens; hereditary thyroid binding globulin excess. *Euthyroid hyperthyroxinaemia* may be familial, or due to amiodarone (p544), or thyroid hormone resistance.

False low: Salicylates; NSAID; phenytoin; corticosteroids; carbamazepine; thyroid-binding globulin deficiency.

2—Plasma total T3 *Method:* As for T4.
Problems of interpretation: (For amiodarone see p544.)

False high: Pregnancy; oestrogens.

False low: Severe infection; post-surgery; post-myocardial infarct; chronic liver disease; chronic renal failure; propranolol; phenytoin; salicylates; NSAID; carbamazepine.

3—Plasma basal thyroid-stimulating hormone (TSH)
Indications: Suspected hypothyroidism, risk of hypothyroidism.

Method: Collect blood at any time of day.

Problems of interpretation: Normal TSH is <5.7mu/L (some lab variation). >5.7mu/L with normal T4 indicates *partial thyroid failure* caused by: Hashimoto's, drugs (lithium, antithyroids, excess iodine, eg expectorants), hyperthyroidism treatment, autoimmune disease (IDDM, pernicious anaemia, Addison's), iodine deficiency, dyshormonogenesis.

Immunometric assays (IMA) of TSH are now replacing radioimmunoassays and these are so sensitive that low TSHs may be quantified—so TRH tests are not now needed (p540) when borderline raised thyroid hormone levels suggest hyperthyroidism. A TSH IMA level <~0.5u/L suggests hyperthyroidism. The normal range of TSH widens in the elderly (eg add 1mu/decade over 40yrs to the upper limit). It is sensible to measure T3 when a patient on T4 replacement for hypothyroidism only feels right when you are apparently over-treating him or her, as suggested by finding undetectable TSH levels. If the T3 is normal in these circumstances you may not be over-treating your patient.

If T3 and T4 are low, but TSH is not raised, then diagnose *secondary* hypothyroidism (p544). Look for pituitary failure (p558).

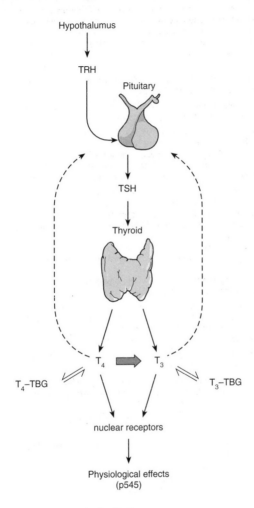

Special thyroid function tests

1—Free T4 and free T3 may be useful when a false low or high T4 or T3 is suspected (p538). They are expensive. If unavailable consider: free thyroxine index which is an estimate of free T4 derived from measuring unoccupied thyroxine binding sites on thyroxine binding globulin (TGB). Occasionally, low TSH may be due to non-thyroidal illness, and finding a high free T4 level (>25pmol/L) may be helpful in indicating that there really is thyroid disease.

2—The TRH test

Indications: Suspected hyperthyroidism (and other tests equivocal); T3 marginally raised; suspected Graves' disease.

Method: Measure plasma TSH before, and 20 minutes and 60 minutes after, injection of 200µg TRH (protirelin).

Interpretation: If the rise in TSH is >2mu/L after TRH, hyperthyroidism is excluded. If it is ≤2mu/L then the reason is:
- Hyperthyroidism
- Euthyroid Graves' disease
- Multinodular goitre
- Solitary autonomous thyroid nodule
- Thyroxine replacement
- The first 8 weeks of hyperthyroid treatment.

Other tests of thyroid anatomy and pathology

1—Thyroid isotope scanning *is indicated:*
- If there is an area of thyroid enlargement.
- If hyperthyroid without thyroid enlargement (is there diffuse uptake or a solitary nodule?).
- If hyperthyroid with one nodule (solitary nodule or multinodule?).
- To determine the extent of retrosternal goitre; to detect ectopic thyroid tissue.
- To detect thyroid metastases (whole-body CT).
- If subacute thyroiditis is a possibility.

Interpretation: The main question is: has the enlarged area increased (hot), or decreased (cold), or the same (neutral) uptake of pertechnetate as remaining thyroid? 20% of cold nodules are malignant. Few neutral and almost no hot nodules are malignant.

2—Ultrasound distinguishes cystic (usually benign) from solid (possibly malignant) 'cold' nodules.

3—Thyroid autoantibodies (antithyroid globulin; antithyroid microsomal) raised in Hashimoto's and some Graves' (if positive there is increased risk of later hypothyroidism).

Thyroid-stimulating immunoglobulins (against TSH receptor) may be raised in Graves' (this test is not widely available).

Serum thyroglobulin is useful in monitoring the treatment of carcinoma.

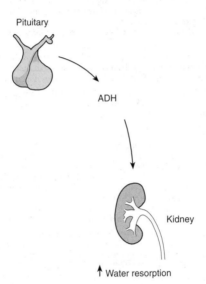

Pituitary

ADH

Kidney

↑ Water resorption

⚕ Hyperthyroidism (thyrotoxicosis)

Symptoms Weight↓ despite appetite↑, frequent stools, tremor, irritability, frenetic activity, emotional lability, dislike of hot weather, sweating, itch, oligomenorrhoea. Infertility may be the presenting problem.

Signs Tachycardia (even sleeping); AF; warm peripheries; fine tremor; thyroid enlargement, or nodules; thyroid bruit, myopathy. If BP↑ consider phaeochromocytoma. *Additional signs in Graves' disease:* Bulging eyes (exophthalmos, p543); lid lag (eyelid lags behind eye's descent as patient watches your finger descend slowly); ophthalmoplegia; vitiligo; pretibial 'myxoedema' (oedematous swellings above lateral malleoli: the term *myxoedema* is confusing here); thyroid acropachy (like clubbing).

Tests TSH ↓; free T4 and free T3 ↑ (p538–40). Consider ultrasound if goitre is present, or thyroid scan if subacute thyroiditis suspected; thyroid autoantibodies. If ophthalmopathy, test visual fields, acuity and eye movements. Can the lids close fully? If not, there is a risk of keratopathy.

Causes—*Graves' disease:* Common, especially women aged 30–50yrs. Genetic influence. ♀:♂ ≈ 9:1. The disease probably results from antibodies against TSH-receptors. Signs as above, with diffuse thyroid enlargement. It may cause normochromic normocytic anaemia, ESR↑, calcium↑, abnormal LFTs. Associated with: IDDM and pernicious anaemia. Patients are usually hyperthyroid, but may be or become, hypo- or euthyroid.
Toxic adenoma: ie a nodule producing T3 and T4. On scanning, the nodule is 'hot' (p540) and the rest of the gland is suppressed.
Subacute thyroiditis: Usually post-partum. Goitre (often painful). ESR↑. Probably viral cause. Usually self-limiting. On scans, no radioiodine uptake.
Other causes: Toxic multinodular goitre; self-medication (detected by raised T4, low T3); follicular carcinoma of thyroid; choriocarcinoma; struma ovarii (ovarian teratoma containing thyroid tissue).

Treatment Options are drugs (carbimazole, propylthiouracil), partial thyroidectomy, and radioactive iodine. *Carbimazole* may be given at ~40mg/24h PO for 4 weeks, then gradually reduced according to TFTs every 1–2 months. Maintain on ~15mg/24h for 12–18 months then withdraw. >50% relapse. (Warn to seek advice if rashes, sore throat or fevers occur, as 0.03% on carbimazole get agranulocytosis: do FBC, eg every 2 weeks for 3 months;[1●] other SE: headache, alopecia, pruritus, and jaundice.
Immediate symptomatic control is achievable with propranolol 40mg/6h PO.
As relapse is common with the above 'low-dose' carbimazole regimen, some people are now receiving the *block-and-replace regimen*[1]—eg carbimazole 40mg/24h PO until hypersecretion has stopped, then T4 is added in (eg 50–150μg/24h PO); this two-drug regimen is continued for about 1 year. About half of those with Graves' disease will have a lasting remission. Monitor by measuring free T4. The advantages of 'block-and-replace' is that hypersecretion is better controlled, and follow-up is less onerous for patients.[2] Don't use in pregnancy. *Partial thyroidectomy* carries risk of damage to recurrent laryngeal nerves and parathyroids. Furthermore, patient may be hypo- or hyperthyroid after surgery. *Radioiodine*(^{131}I) can be repeated until euthyroid but the patient will almost always ultimately become hypothyroid. Decisions on treatment rest on local expertise and the patient preference. Youth is no longer a contraindication to radioiodine in women.

Ophthalmopathy: (p543) Control hyperthyroidism; steroids if ophthalmoplegia or gross oedema. *Consult eye surgeon early* (eg papilloedema, vision↓).

Atrial fibrillation: p290. Control hyperthyroidism.

Complications Heart failure, angina, osteoporosis, gynaecomastia.

In pregnancy and in infancy Get expert help. See OHCS p157.

1 *Drug Ther Bul* 1997 **37** 88 2 AM McGregor 1996 *Oxford Textbook of Medicine*, OUP, 1612 (12.4)

Thyroid eye disease

Thyroid eye disease is a clinical diagnosis which may be made in the presence or absence of thyroid autoantibodies. It occurs when there is retro-orbital inflammation and lymphocyte infiltration which causes swelling of the contents of the orbit. At the time of presentation, the patient may be euthyroid, hypothyroid or hyperthyroid.

History Double vision, discomfort or protrusion and sometimes decreased acuity. ▶Decreasing acuity or loss of colour vision may mean optic nerve compression: *Seek expert advice immediately as decompression may be needed.* Nerve damage does not necessarily go hand-in-hand with protrusion. Indeed, if the eye cannot protrude for anatomical reasons, optic nerve compression is all the more likely—a paradox!

Signs Exophthalmos—appearance of protruding eye; proptosis—eyes protrude beyond the orbit (look from above in the same plane as the forehead); conjunctival oedema; corneal ulceration; papilloedema; loss of colour vision. Ophthalmoplegia (especially of upward gaze) also occurs due to muscle swelling and fibrosis.

Investigations Rose Bengal eye-drops may stain the upper cornea, indicating superior limbic keratitis, while CT or MRI scanning of the orbits will reveal enlarged eye muscles.

Management Hypromellose eye-drops 0.25% for lubrication as often as is needed. There is no upper limit to dose frequency or volume instilled. Eyelids can be stitched together at their outer corners (lateral tarsorraphy) or else may be taped closed. Medical decompression may be achieved with high-dose systemic steroids. Lid retraction may be reduced by 5% guanethidine eye-drops but these are rarely tolerated for long. Surgical decompression uses space in the ethmoidal, sphenoidal, and maxillary sinuses, via a medio-inferior approach. Orbital radiotherapy, cytotoxic drugs, and plasmapheresis (p618) have proved unreliable. Diplopia may be managed with a Fresnel prism stuck to one lens of a spectacle, so allowing for reasonably easy changing as the exophthalmos changes.

Eye disease may pre-date other signs of Graves' disease, and does not always respond to treatment of thyroid status. Furthermore, it may develop for the first time following treatment of hyperthyroidism.

♦♦♦ Thyroid hormone lack (hypothyroidism; myxoedema)

This is common and easy to treat. ►As it is insidious both the patient and the doctor may not realize anything is wrong, so we must all be alert to subtle and nonspecific symptoms, particularly in women over 40 years old.

Symptoms Unhappy, no twinkle in the eye, weight↑, constipation, dislike of cold, menorrhagia, hoarse voice, lethargy, depression, dementia.

Signs Bradycardia, dry skin and hair, goitre, slowly relaxing reflexes, CCF, non-pitting oedema (eg eyelids, hands, feet) ± 'toad-like face'.

Diagnosis TSH (↑in thyroid failure, ↓in rare secondary hypothyroidism due to TSH lack from the pituitary, p558). T4↓. Fasting cholesterol and triglyceride may be↑. FBC: eg normochromic macrocytic anaemia. CK, AST and LDH may be↑ due to abnormal muscle membranes. See also p540.

Causes of primary hypothyroidism

Spontaneous primary atrophic hypothyroidism: Common, autoimmune disease which is essentially Hashimoto's without the goitre and is associated with IDDM, Addison's disease, or pernicious anaemia. ♀:♂ ≈ 6:1.

After thyroidectomy or radioiodine treatment.

Drug-induced: Antithyroid drugs; amiodarone, below; lithium; iodine in expectorants; para-aminosalicylic acid. Treat by stopping drug or as below.

Iodine deficiency: If dietary insufficiency.

Dyshormonogenesis: Autosomal recessive eg from peroxidase deficiency. Look for ↑radioimmune gland uptake displaced by potassium perchlorate.

Rare associations:[1] Cystic fibrosis, primary biliary cirrhosis, POEMS syndrome (**p**olyneuropathy, **o**rganomegaly, **e**ndocrinopathy, **M**-protein band from a plasmacytoma + **s**kin pigmentation/tethering).

Screen for hypothyroidism if:[2] ●Hypothermia ●Congenital hypothyroidism ●On carbimazole ●After neck irradiation ●On amiodarone or Li⁺

Also consider in: ●Post post-partum thyroiditis ●Hypercholesterolaemia ●Infertility ●Dementia or depression ●Antepartum+type I DM ●Obesity ●Autoimmunity (eg Addison's) ●Turner's syndrome
Do *not* screen ill 'on take' patients if no reason to suspect hypothyroidism.

Treatment *If healthy/young:* Thyroxine (=levothyroxine), ~150µg/24h PO. Review in 12wks. Adjust dose according to clinical state and to keep TSH <5mu/L. Lifelong therapy is needed. *Once dose is stable and TSH no longer↑, you do not need to monitor TSH routinely. If pre-existing heart disease (eg the elderly)* (►thyroxine may precipitate angina) start with 25µg/24h; ↑dose eg every 4 weeks. Thyroxine's half-life is ~7 days, so any change in dosage will take ~4 weeks to be assessed accurately by a TSH test (but note that TSH itself has a half-life of only ~1h).[3] *If also ischaemic heart disease:* give propranolol 40mg/6h PO and start with 25µg/24h of thyroxine.

Causes of goitre+hypothyroidism *Hashimoto's thyroiditis:* Autoimmune disease in which there is lymphocyte and plasma cell infiltration. Usually in women aged 60–70yrs. Often euthyroid. Autoantibody titres high. Treat as above if hypothyroid or to reduce goitre if TSH high. *Drugs:* As above.

The effects of amiodarone on the thyroid are complex and variable. It commonly causes a rise in free T4, and a fall in free T3, but clinically the patient may remain euthyroid. 2% of patients have clinically significant changes—which may be hyperthyroidism or hypothyroidism. Be guided more by clinical state than tests. Seek expert help. Note that t₁/₂ is long (40–100 days), so problems persist after withdrawal.

Secondary hypothyroidism (from pituitary failure, p558) is very rare.

How to withdraw thyroxine If T4 was started but the diagnosis is now in doubt, stop for 6 weeks, then measure T4 and TSH to make diagnosis.

Thyroid disease in pregnancy and neonates See OHCS p157.

Why symptoms of hypothyroidism are so many, so various and so subtle
Almost all our cell nuclei have receptors showing a high affinity for T_3: that known as TRα-1 is abundant in muscle and fat; TRα-2 is abundant in brain; and TRβ-1 is abundant in brain, liver, and kidney. These receptors, via their influence on various enzymes, affect the following processes:
- The metabolism of substrates, vitamins and minerals.
- Modulation of all other hormones and their target-tissue responses.
- Stimulation of O_2 consumption and generation of metabolic heat.
- Regulation of protein synthesis, and carbohydrate and lipid metabolism.
- Stimulation of demand for co-enzymes and related vitamins. (OTM 3e 1607.)

If tests suggest subclinical hypothyroidism . . .
(TSH↑ but T_4 & T_3 ↔, and no obvious symptoms)

The context may be follow-up after partial thyroidectomy or [131]iodine therapy, or the test may have been for questionable reasons: here slightly high TSHs are common (~10% have TSH 3.5–20mU/L if >55yrs old).

- Recheck the history: if any non-specific features (eg depression) (p544) discuss benefits of treating with the patient: she may simply feel better, without realising that she was not functioning optimally. Also, atheroma and hypercholesterolaemia *may* improve marginally.[4]

- Risks from well-managed treatment of subclinical hypothyroidism are small (theoretical ↑risk of atrial fibrillation and osteoporosis).[4]

- *Factors biasing towards treatment:* Past Graves' disease
Positive thyroid autoantibodies
Organ-specific autoimmunity (type I DM,
myasthenia, pernicious anaemia, vitiligo)

If the patient does not fall into any of these categories, one option is only to treat if TSH >10mU/L. Monitor others yearly. Progress to overt hypothyroidism is more likely with higher TSHs, or if >60yrs or ♂.

1 R Beauwens 1997 *Lancet* 349 1023 2 A Weetman 1997 *BMJ* i 1175 3 R Lindsay 1997 *Lancet* 349 413+1023 4 *Drug Ther Bul* 1998 36 1 & *Lancet* 1997 349 413

Hyperparathyroidism

This is excess parathyroid hormone (PTH, p642, the hormone which $\uparrow Ca^{2+}$).

Primary hyperparathyroidism Plasma PTH is inappropriately high with a correspondingly high plasma Ca^{2+}. *Presentation:* Most commonly as $Ca^{2+}\uparrow$ on routine tests. Any symptoms are usually due to: bone pain/fracture; renal stones; constipation; abdominal pain, duodenal ulcer, pancreatitis; depression. Hence mnemonic: 'bones, stones, abdominal groans and psychic moans'. Other presentations:

- Dehydration and confusion
- BP↑
- Walking problems
- Thirst, nocturia, anorexia (∵ $Ca^{2+}\uparrow$)
- Stiff joints
- Myopathy

Thirst may be very bad. Hyperparathyroidism must pass through your mind whenever a patient says "I always take a jug of water to bed".[1]

Associations: BP↑; multiple endocrine neoplasia: *MEN type I* (pancreatic islet cell tumour and pituitary adenoma), and: *MEN type IIa* (phaeochromocytoma and medullary carcinoma of thyroid).

Causes: Single (90%) or multiple adenoma; carcinoma; hyperplasia.

Tests: Plasma $Ca^{2+}\uparrow$, phosphate ↓ (unless renal failure), alk phos↑, plasma PTH ↑ or ↔ (this is technically difficult, consult lab first). Is there radiographic evidence bone reabsorption ie *osteitis fibrosa et cystica* (brown tumours) and subperiosteal resorption (especially on hand x-ray)? Also do CXR, SXR ('pepper-pot skull') and pelvic x-ray.

Treatment—if required—is surgery—neck exploration with removal of adenoma if present, or of most of gland if hyperplasia. Venous sampling or ultrasound is used to locate source of PTH if initial surgery is unsuccessful. Do plasma Ca^{2+} daily for ≥14 days' post-surgery (danger is $Ca^{2+}\downarrow$). Mild symptoms may not merit surgery—advise a high fluid intake to prevent stone formation; review every 6 months.

Parathyroid-related protein (PTHrP) This is produced by some tumours, and causes some of the hypercalcaemia seen in malignancy. It increases osteoclast activity and tubular resorption of urinary calcium.

Secondary hyperparathyroidism (PTH↑ as appropriate for a low calcium). Causes: chronic renal failure; dietary deficiency of vitamin D. See renal osteodystrophy, p388.

Tertiary hyperparathyroidism is the continued secretion of large amounts of PTH after prolonged secondary hyperparathyroidism: the original cause of the secondary hyperparathyroidism (hypocalcaemia) has gone, but the parathyroids now act autonomously and cause hypercalcaemia. Treatment is as for primary hyperparathyroidism.

Hypoparathyroidism

Primary hypoparathyroidism PTH secretion↓, eg after neck surgery, causing $Ca^{2+}\downarrow$ with normal or raised phosphate and normal alk phos. For signs and symptoms of hypocalcaemia, see p642. Associations: pernicious anaemia; Addison's; hypothyroidism; hypogonadism. Treatment is with alfacalcidol (p642). Lifelong follow-up.

Pseudohypoparathyroidism (failure of target cell response to PTH). Signs: Round face, short metacarpals and metatarsals. Symptoms and treatment as for 1° hypoparathyroidism. Plasma PTH and alk phos ↔ or ↑.

Pseudopseudohypoparathyroidism The morphological features of pseudohypoparathyroidism, but normal biochemistry.

1 A Churcher 1995 *Lancet* 346 915

Adrenal cortex and Cushing's syndrome

Physiology The adrenal cortex produces: *glucocorticoids* (eg cortisol) which affect metabolic functions (carbohydrate, lipid and protein metabolism), *mineralocorticoids* (eg aldosterone, p636), androgens, and *oestrogens*. Corticotrophin-releasing factor (CRF) from the hypothalamus stimulates ACTH (from pituitary) which stimulates cortisol production by the adrenal cortex. Cortisol is excreted as urinary free cortisol and as various 17-oxogenic steroids (17OGS). Metyrapone inhibits a step in cortisol synthesis, resulting normally in loss of negative feedback, raised ACTH, and raised steroids excreted as 17OGS.

Cushing's syndrome is due to chronic glucocorticoid excess, either exogenous or endogenous (adrenal or pituitary neoplasm, or ectopic ACTH secretion). Signs: (PLATE 8) Tissue wasting, myopathy, thin skin, purple abdominal striae, easy bruising, osteoporosis, water retenion, neck (*buffalo-hump*, supraclavicular fat pad), predisposition to infection, bad wound healing, hirsutism. Amenorrhoea. Hyperglycaemia (30%).

Tests: See p550. First, confirm the diagnosis. Then, localize the source on the basis of laboratory testing (below). Do not order imaging studies until biochemical studies have suggested a likely source. *Note:* adrenal 'incidentalomas' occur on 1% or more of CTs, so identification of an adrenal tumour does *not* prove adrenal source of cortisol excess. Pituitary incidentalomas also are not infrequent. Order abdominal CT if adrenal source is suspected; pituitary MRI (and consider petrosal sinus sampling) if pituitary source (Cushing's disease) is suspected (p560).

Causes and treatment:

1 *Corticosteroid (and ACTH) administration:* Reduce dose as much as possible. In asthma, consider inhaled rather than oral steroids.

2 *Adrenal gland adenoma:* Surgical removal of tumour.

3 *Adrenal carcinoma:* Surgical removal of tumour and medical therapy (ketoconazole, aminoglutethimide) for residual glucocorticoid excess.

4 *Cushing's disease* (adrenal hyperplasia due to excess ACTH from pituitary tumour. Commoner in women. Peak age: 30–50yrs). The treatment of choice is surgical: selective removal of the pituitary adenoma via a trans-sphenoidal or trans-frontal approach. Radiotherapy is also used.

   Other approaches if pituitary surgery is not possible (or unsuccessful) include medical treatment (as above) or bilateral adrenalectomy (but this may be complicated by *Nelson's syndrome* with development of enlarging pituitary tumour and hyperpigmentation).

5 *Ectopic ACTH production:* Especially small cell carcinoma of the lung and carcinoid.

Prognosis: Untreated: 50% dead within 5yrs. Treat the underlying disease. If unresectable, treat with medication to block adrenal cortisol production (eg ketoconazole which inhibits adrenal steroid synthesis).

Assessment of suspected Cushing's

Screening tests

- The best screening test is *24h urinary free cortisol* (normal is <280nmol/24h).

- The *dexamethasone suppression test* is an alternative.
  Give dexamethasone 1mg PO at midnight, check serum cortisol before, and at 8am (normal 450–700nmol/L).
- False positives are seen with depression, obesity, and drugs that affect metabolism of dexamethasone (eg phenytoin, phenobarbitone)—'pseudocushing's'.

Further investigations—for positive screening tests

- *Low-dose dexamethasone suppression test*—Give dexamethasone 0.5mg/6h PO for 2 days.
  —Measure: •Morning serum cortisol at 48 hours
  •24h urinary free cortisol during day 2 of test
  •Creatinine during day 2 of test.
- *High-dose dexamethasone suppression test*
  Indications: 1) If low-dose dexamethasone suppression test is positive,
  2) Cushing's is clinically obvious with high 24h urinary free cortisol.
  —Give dexamethasone 2mg/6h PO for 2 days.
  —Measure: same as above.
- *Simultaneous ACTH and cortisol level.*

Interpreting the results

Cushing's disease: There is some, but not normal, suppression of plasma cortisol with high-dose dexamethasone. Plasma ACTH is high–normal but rarely >250ng/L.

Adrenal tumour: Usually no suppression of cortisol with high-dose dexamethasone. Plasma ACTH is undetectable.

Ectopic ACTH secretion: No suppression of cortisol with high-dose dexamethasone. Plasma ACTH generally >250ng/L. Hypokalaemic alkalosis is common.

1 A Levy 1994 *BMJ* i 1087

Addison's disease

This adrenal gland disease leads to <u>primary adrenocortical insufficiency</u>. Its signs are capricious; as diagnosis may only be made at necropsy it's called *the unforgiving master of <u>nonspecificity</u> and disguise.*[1] Symptoms include:

- Weakness
- <u>Abdominal pain</u>
- Depression
- 'Viral illness'
- Anorexia
- D&V (or nausea)
- Arthralgia
- Myalgia
- Weight loss
- Confusion
- Constipation
- Dizziness

Signs <u>Hyperpigmentation (palmar creases, buccal mucosa)</u>, <u>vitiligo</u>, <u>postural hypotension</u>. Critical deterioration (p788) is indicated by <u>tachycardia, fever, shock, and coma</u>.

Tests—*General:* <u>Hyperkalaemia, hyponatremia, hypoglycaemia</u> (may be symptomatic), <u>uraemia</u>, mild acidosis, <u>hypercalcaemia</u>, eosinophilia, neutropenia, lymphocytosis, normocytic anaemia, abnormal LFTs.

Specific: Short <u>ACTH stimulation test</u> (Synacthen® test): Do <u>plasma cortisol before and ½h after tetracosactrin</u> (=tetracosactide, Synacthen®) 250µg IM. Exclude Addison's if initial cortisol >140nmol/L, and 2nd cortisol is both >500nmol/L and >200nmol/L above first. If not excluded proceed to:

Prolonged ACTH stimulation test: Measure plasma cortisol before and 6h after tetracosactrin depot (zinc phosphate complex) 1mg IM. Do this on 3 successive days. Addison's is diagnosed if plasma cortisol is <690nmol/L, 6h after 3rd injection. Steroid drugs may interfere with this assay: check with your local laboratory.

Measurement of ACTH and cortisol: Take blood for ACTH and cortisol at 09.00h and 22.00h. Diagnose Addison's if low cortisol with ACTH >300ng/L.

Adrenal antibodies, AXR and CXR (signs of previous TB eg calcification).

Causes <u>80% idiopathic in</u> UK. Probably <u>autoimmune</u> (adrenal antibodies raised). <u>Associated with Graves', Hashimoto's</u>, IDDM, pernicious anaemia, hypoparathyroidism, vitiligo. *Other causes:* TB; metastases (adrenal insufficiency only after >90% involvement of both adrenals); AIDS (CMV, *Mycobacterium avium intracellulare*, other opportunistic adrenal infections).

Treatment Treat cause. <u>Replace steroids: *hydrocortisone*</u> 20mg in morning, 10mg at bedtime PO. Adjust dose by measuring plasma cortisol at 0.5, 1, 2, 3h after morning dose. Aim for peak 700–850nmol/L. Evening dose is half morning dose. *Fludrocortisone* PO 0.05mg every 2nd day to 0.15mg daily. Adjust on clinical grounds. If postural hypotension: increase. If hypertension, headache, oedema, hypokalaemia, alkalosis: decrease.

Addison's is often associated with other autoimmune disease—even at the time of diagnosis. Hyperthyroidism should be looked for, particularly if there is difficulty in maintaining adequate cortisol levels on treatment.

Warn against abruptly discontinuing treatment. Patients should have syringes at home (+ in-date parenteral hydrocortisone) for IM use in case vomiting prevents oral intake. Emphasize that any doctor or dentist giving treatment must know that the patient is taking steroids. Counsel about the need to take more in intercurrent illness. Give *steroid card*. Advise about wearing a bracelet declaring that steroids are taken. For dental treatment double morning hydrocortisone. If severe URTI double morning and evening hydrocortisone while ill. If vomiting, replace hydrocortisone with hydrocortisone sodium succinate 100mg IM; IV fluids if dehydrated.

Follow-up 6-monthly.

Prognosis Normal lifespan if treated.

---

1 CM Brosnan 1996 *BMJ* i 1085

Hyperaldosteronism

Primary hyperaldosteronism is excess production of aldosterone independent of the renin-angiotensin system. Consider this diagnosis when the following features are present: hypertension, hypokalaemia, alkalosis in someone not on diuretics. Sodium tends to be mildly raised or normal.

Causes: >50% due to unilateral adrenocortical adenoma (*Conn's syndrome*). Also: bilateral adrenocortical hyperplasia; adrenal carcinoma (rare); glucocorticoid-remediable aldosteronism (GRA). In GRA there is a genetic enzyme defect (eg fusion of 2 nearby genes on chromosome 8q) leading to excess adrenal 18-oxocortisol and 18-hydroxycortisol with overproduction of mineralocorticoids.

Tests: Do 3 K^+ measurements on salt replete diet (no diuretics, hypotensives, steroids, potassium, laxatives, metoclopramide for 4 weeks). If 1 or more measure is <3.7mmol/L, do plasma samples for: aldosterone and renin. Normal or high renin excludes the diagnosis. If ↓renin and ↑aldosterone, provocative testing is useful (saline infusion to see if aldosterone is suppressible; posture study to see if renin can be stimulated). If consistent with primary hyperaldosteronism (non-suppressible aldosterone with suppressed renin) do abdo CT or MRI to localize tumour. Seek expert assistance. For GRA (suspect particularly if family history of early hypertension) a genetic test is available. *Note:* renal artery stenosis is a more common cause of refractory ↑BP and ↓K^+. Evaluate with renal scan, MRI angiography, or contrast angiogram (the gold standard).

Treatment: Conn's: Surgery; spironolactone 300mg/24h PO for 4 wks pre-op. Hyperplasia: Spironolactone or amiloride. If GRA is suspected: dexamethasone 1mg/24h PO for 4 wks. If BP still↑, give spironolactone; stop dexamethasone.

Secondary hyperaldosteronism Due to a high renin (eg from renal artery stenosis, accelerated hypertension, diuretics, CCF, hepatic failure).

Bartter's syndrome (primary hyper-reninaemia) is recessively inherited and presents as failure to thrive, polyuria, and polydipsia. BP is *normal* and there is no oedema. The chief feature is hypokalaemia with increased urinary K^+ excretion and hypochloraemic metabolic alkalosis. Urinary chloride is elevated. Plasma renin↑.

Treatments include K^+ replacement, NSAIDs, amiloride, captopril.

Phaeochromocytoma

This is a rare, but treatable cause of hypertension. It is usually (90%) a benign tumour producing catecholamines, usually (90%) in the adrenal medulla, and these are usually (90%) unilateral. Inheritance: sometimes autosomal dominant. Association: multiple endocrine neoplasia (MEN type I, p546). Tumours in the medulla may be in paraganglia (=phaeochrome bodies, ie collections of epinephrine-secreting chromaffin cells)—typically by the aortic bifurcation (organ of Zuckerkandl).

The Patient: Episodic hypertension, chest tightness, restlessness, anxiety, and weakness. He or she may have been labelled 'neurotic', or have extensive investigations for CCF/cardiomyopathy, or terminal haematuria (with bladder phaeos). For other features, see opposite.

Tests: Glycosuria during attacks in 30%. Screening: 24h urine collection for 4-OH-3-methoxymandelate (HMMA, VMA) or total (or free) metadrenalines. Full investigation: consult specialist centre: consider MIBG scan (metiodobenzylguanidine) or pentolinium suppression test + abdomen CT/MRI scan.

Treatment: Surgery. Careful BP control for 2 weeks pre-op: α-blocker (phenoxybenzamine p788) *before* β-blockers (propranolol). Consult anaesthetist. Post-op, collect 24h urine as above ; monitor BP (risk of BP↓↓).

Emergency treatment: p788. Prognosis: Normal life if surgery successful.

The clinical features of phaeochromocytoma

Although phaeochromocytomas are rare we must constantly keep these *episodic* features in the back of our minds so that when patients start telling us the diagnosis, as they always do, albeit obliquely, we can hear the silent ticking of the time-bomb inside them, muffled, as it always is, by seemingly benign complaints such as nausea, restlessness, weakness, headaches, anxiety, and heat intolerance ("No bedclothes for me tonight, dear"). Other episodic features include:

- Chest tightness
- 'Spots before the eyes'
- Pins and needles
- Hemianopia
- Pulsatile scotomas

- Skin mottling
- Weight loss
- Dyspnoea
- Purpura
- Sweating

- Abdominal pain
- Tremor
- Cold feet
- Vomiting
- Faints (postural BP drop)

- Palpitations
- Flushing
- Claudication
- Pallor

Symptoms are precipitated by stretching, sneezing, stress, sex, smoking, surgery, or parturition—or by agents such as cheese, alcohol, or the tricyclic you so kindly prescribed, thinking that the patient's bizarre symptoms were only explicable by depression.

These crises may last for a few minutes or a week. Suddenly the patient may feel "as if about to die"—and then they get better, or go on to stroke or cardiovascular collapse. On examination, there may be no signs, or hypertension (± signs of cardiomyopathy or heart failure) and thyroid swelling (episodic) and glycosuria during an attack—or terminal haematuria from a bladder phaeochromocytoma.

If you get the diagnosis right (and surgery is successful) life-span is normal, but follow urine catecholamines yearly for many years (phaeochromocytomas can recur or prove metastatic).

Hirsutism, virilism, gynaecomastia, impotence

Hirsutism is common (10% of women) and usually benign. It implies increased hair growth in women, in the male pattern. If menstruation is normal there is almost certainly no increased testosterone production. Treatment: local removal of unwanted hair. If menstruation is abnormal the cause is usually *polycystic ovary syndrome* (Stein–Leventhal syndrome): bilateral polycystic ovaries; secondary oligomenorrhoea; infertility; obesity; hirsutism. The cause is androgen hypersecretion. Tests: ultrasound; plasma LH:FSH ratio↑, and less consistently, ↑testosterone and ↓oestradiol (*OHCS* p756). Oligomenorrhoea and infertility are treated with clomifene.

Another cause of hirsutism with irregular menses is *late-onset congenital adrenal hyperplasia*—most often due to deficiency of the 21-hydroxylase enzyme in the adrenal gland. *Ovarian tumours* are a rare cause.

Management: ●Do not abandon the patient once you have ascertained that there is no serious illness. Find out what her expectations are.
●Explain that she is not turning into a man.
●Has she tried depilation with wax or creams, or electrolysis (which is expensive, and time-consuming, but *does* work)?
●Has she tried bleaching the area with 1:10 hydrogen peroxide?
●Would she be prepared to shave regularly?
●Oestrogens help by increasing serum sex-hormone-binding globulin— but always combine with a progesterone (= 'the Pill') to prevent excess risk of uterine neoplasia. Marvelon® contains desogestrel, a fairly non-androgenic progestagen, but there is ↑risk of DVT and PE (*OHCS* p66). Dianette® contains 2mg cyproterone acetate (an anti-androgen) with ethinylestradiol 35μg, so also gives contraceptive cover. An expensive alternative is flutamide▪—a potent inhibitor of androgen uptake ± nuclear binding in target tissues; LFTs must be monitored continuously.

Virilism is rare. It is characterized by: amenorrhoea, clitoromegaly; deep voice; temporal hair recession; hirsutism. This condition needs investigation for androgen-secreting adrenal and ovarian tumours.

Gynaecomastia implies an abnormal amount of breast tissue in males (it may occur in normal puberty). It is due to an increase in the oestrogen/androgen ratio. It is seen in syndromes of androgen deficiency (eg Klinefelter's, Kallman's). It may result from liver disease or testicular tumours (oestrogens↑), or accompany hyperthyroidism. The commonest causes are drugs: oestrogens, especially stilboestrol (=diethylstilbestrol); spironolactone; cimetidine; digoxin; testosterone; marijuana.

Impotence Failure in adult male to sustain adequate erection for vaginal penetration. It is common in old age. Psychological causes are common and are more likely if impotence occurs only in some situations, if there is a clear stress to account for the onset of the impotence, and if early morning erections occur (although these may persist at the onset of organic disease). Psychological causes may exacerbate organic causes. The major organic cause is *diabetes*. Other organic causes are:
Drug causes: Antihypertensives (including diuretics and β-blockers), major tranquillizers, alcohol, oestrogens, antidepressants, cimetidine.
Pathological causes: Hyperthyroidism, hypogonadism, MS, autonomic neuropathy, atheroma, bladder-neck surgery, prolactin↑, cirrhosis, cancer.
Tests: U&E; LFTs; glucose; TFTs; cholesterol; testosterone (eg if libido↓). Nocturnal tumescence studies are not usually needed. If alprostadil does not induce erection, the cause is probably vascular. Doppler may show ↓blood flow, but is rarely needed as vascular reconstruction is difficult.
Treatment: Manage underlying causes. Offer counselling ± vacuum aids, implants, or alprostadil, ie prostaglandin E1, transurethrally as MUSE®, or, more reliably,[1] as intracavernosal self-injection (technique: see *Mentor*▪).

1 P Werthman 1997 *Urology* **50** 809 (MUSE–medicated urethral system for erection; SE: faints, pain, priapism)

Hypopituitarism

The 6 anterior pituitary hormones commonly measured are: adrenocorticotrophic hormone (ACTH), growth hormone (GH), follicle-stimulating hormone (FSH), luteinizing hormone (LH), thyroid-stimulating hormone (TSH), and prolactin (PRL). Pituitary opioids are not usually measured.

Causes of hypopituitarism Hypophysectomy, pituitary irradiation, pituitary adenoma (either non-functional or functional causing eg Cushing's or acromegaly with hyposecretion of other hormones). Other causes include: craniopharyngioma, sphenoid meningioma, Sheehan's syndrome (pituitary necrosis after post-partum haemorrhage), TB.

Symptoms Insidious onset—often elderly, afternoon tiredness, pallor, anorexia, libido↓, impotence, amenorrhoea, headache, depression, dyspareunia, symptoms of hypothyroidism (p544).

Signs Atrophy of breasts, small testes (reduced ejaculate)—hypogonadism, ↓muscle:fat ratio, reduction of all hair, thin flaky wrinkled skin (*monkey face*), postural hypotension, visual field defect.

Incidental findings: Hypotension, hyponatraemia, a low T4 without the expectedly high TSH.[1]

Tests Lateral SXR (pituitary tumour), CT/MRI scan, assessment of visual fields, basal T4, TSH, PRL (5mL clotted blood, consult lab), testosterone. U&E (dilutional hyponatraemia), FBC (normochromic, normocytic anaemia).

Triple stimulation test: (can be done in out-patients). *Contraindications:* Epilepsy, heart disease. Test done in morning (water only taken from 22.00h the night before). Have 50% glucose to hand and IV line open. Be alert throughout to hypoglycaemia. Discard first 3mL of blood samples (they will contain citrate) and flush cannula after. Consult lab.

- Insert IV cannula with 3-way tap (citrate, samples, injection).
- Attach 20mL syringe filled with citrate for flushing. Take samples for T4, TSH, oestradiol/testosterone, FSH, LH, PRL, cortisol, glucose, GH.
- Inject insulin IV 0.15u/kg (0.3u/kg if acromegaly or Cushing's; 0.05u/kg if marked hypopituitarism).
- Flush and inject IV 200µg TRH and 50µg gonadotrophin-releasing hormone (GnRH). Use same syringe. Flush.
- Collect blood samples as follows: FSH, LH, TSH at 20mins and 60mins. GH, cortisol, glucose at 30, 60, 90, and 120mins. Finally, give a good breakfast.

Interpretation of triple stimulation test: Glucose must fall below 2.2mmol/L. Normal values are: GH >20mu/L, peak cortisol >550mmol/L, TSH at 20mins 3.9–30mu/L, TSH at 60mins 3.0–24mu/L. Values less than these indicate some pituitary deficiency. Note: it has been commented that as the overnight metyrapone test (p550) gives similar information on hypothalamic-pituitary axis integrity, it may be safer and preferable.[2]

Treatment Hydrocortisone as for Addison's disease (p552). Thyroxine (=levothyroxine) as for hypothyroidism (p544, but TSH levels are not helpful). For men, testosterone enanthate 250mg IM every 3 weeks or *transdermal Andropatch®*—applied to clean, dry, unbroken skin on back, upper arm, thigh, or abdomen for 24h (don't use the same site within 7 days); those over 130kg may need 3 patches/day; adjust according to plasma testosterone level. Oestrogen (for pre-menopausal women) eg in contraceptive steroids. Some patients may need growth hormone.

Other causes of hypogonadism Trauma, post-orchitis (mumps, brucellosis, leprosy), chemotherapy or irradiation, cirrhosis, alcohol (toxic to Leydig cells), cystic fibrosis; various syndromes: Kleinfelter's (commonest), Laurence–Moon–Biedl (*OHCS* p752), dystrophica myotonica, Prader–Willi (*OHCS* p756) and Kallman's syndrome (hypogonadism + colour blindness + nerve deafness + cleft lip + anosmia).

1 C Chan 1997 *Lancet* **349** 26 & 576   2 TM Fiad 1994 *Clinical Endocrinology* **40** 603

Hormone	Effect on pituitary		Peripheral effect
Insulin	→ ACTH↑	→ → →	Cortisol↑
	→ Growth hormone↑		
	→ → → →	→ → →	Glucose↓
Thyrotrophin-releasing hormone	→ TSH	→ → →	T4↑
Growth hormone releasing hormone	→ LH↑	→ → →	Effects on fertility
	→ FSH↑	→ → →	Effects on fertility

Pituitary tumours

▶Symptoms are caused by local pressure, hormone secretion, or hypopituitarism (p558).

Pituitary tumours (almost always benign adenomas) account for 10% of intracranial tumours.

Histological classification There are 3 types.

1 *Chromophobe*—70%. Some are non-secretory, but cause hypopituitarism. Local pressure effect in 30%. Half produce prolactin (PRL); a few produce ACTH or growth hormone (GH).

2 *Acidophil*—15%. Secrete GH or PRL. Local pressure effect in 10%.

3 *Basophil*—15%. Secrete ACTH. Local pressure effect rare.

Classification by hormone secreted

PRL only	—35%	ACTH	—7%
GH only	—20%	LH/FSH/TSH	—1%
PRL and GH	—7%		
No obvious hormone	—30%*		

*Many produce alpha-subunit which may serve as a tumour marker.

Clinical features of local pressure effect Headache; visual field defects (bilateral hemianopia, initially of superior quadrants); palsy of cranial nerves III, IV, VI; occasionally disturbance of temperature, sleep, feeding and erosion through floor of sella leading to CSF rhinorrhoea. Diabetes insipidus (p566) is a very rare result of pituitary tumour: it is more likely to result from hypothalamic disease.

Investigations Pituitary MRI; accurate assessment of visual fields; prolactin, baseline TFTs, morning plasma cortisol, alpha subunit if no clinical evidence of hormone excess; triple stimulation test (p558); water deprivation test if diabetes insipidus is suspected (p566).

Treatment Start hormone replacement as indicated by triple stimulation test before surgery.
Surgery: If intrasellar tumour, remove by trans-sphenoidal approach. Suprasellar extension of tumour may need transfrontal approach.
Medical treatment: Bromocriptine is the treatment of choice for most prolactin-secreting tumours (lowers PRL and can shrink tumour). Surgery is not indicated routinely for these. It may also work for some GH-secreting tumours (p562) and also 'non-functional tumours' (some making alpha subunit); use higher doses—eg 20–40mg PO daily.
Radiotherapy: Following surgery if complete removal of tumour has not been possible. Used less often now as side-effects (necrosis) prominent.

Peri-operative care Check with anaesthetist/surgeon. One regimen is: Hydrocortisone sodium succinate 100mg IM, with pre-med, then every 4h for 72h. Then hydrocortisone 20mg PO in the morning. Retest pituitary function after a few weeks (p558) to assess replacement needed.

Pituitary apoplexy Rapid expansion of a pituitary tumour due to infarction or haemorrhage may cause sudden local pressure effect. Suspect if sudden onset of headache in someone with a known tumour, or if there is sudden headache and loss of consciousness (ie may present like subarachnoid haemorrhage). *Treatment* is urgent surgery under steroid cover.

Craniopharingioma This is not, strictly speaking, a pituitary tumour as it originates from Rathke's pouch and is situated between pituitary and floor of third ventricle. 50% present with local pressure effects in childhood. *Investigations:* CT scan, lateral SXR (calcification). *Treatment:* Surgery; irradiation; post-operative triple stimulation test (p558).

Infarction or haemorrhage may cause sudden local pressure effect.

Hyperprolactinaemia

This is the most common biochemical disturbance of the pituitary. It tends to present early in women (amenorrhoea) but late in men.

Symptoms[1] Women: libido↓, weight gain, apathy, vaginal dryness, menstrual disturbance (amenorrhoea; infertility; galactorrhoea). Men may present with impotence and reduced facial hair. Local pressure effects may occur (p560).

Causes of raised basal plasma prolactin (>390mu/L)

Physiological: Pregnancy; breastfeeding; stress; sleep.

Drugs and other chemicals: Phenothiazines (including metoclopramide); haloperidol; α-methyldopa; oestrogens; TRH.

Disease: Pituitary disease; chronic renal failure; hypothyroid; sarcoidosis.

Investigations Basal plasma prolactin: non-stressful venepuncture between 09.00–16.00h. CT/MRI scan of the pituitary fossa. Lateral SXR.

Management This depends in part on local surgical expertise. A reasonable approach is as follows:

Microprolactinomas—tumour <10mm diameter on MRI. If post-menopausal, follow PRL levels. If pre-menopausal, give bromocriptine 1.25mg PO at 22.00 with food; increase weekly by 1.25–2.5mg/day until ~2.5mg/12h. Rarely, patients may require >10mg daily. Follow PRL. Usually hyperprolactinaemia due to a microadenoma does not progress significantly over time but here is a *rationale for treatment*:
- Fertility is restored to women. Bromocriptine should be stopped as soon as a pregnancy test is positive (check immediately if menses are late). This minimizes risk to developing fetus—teratogenicity has been reported but there are no large studies to quantify risk. PRL will rise during pregnancy, there is no need to follow it. If there is headache or visual loss though, check fields and consider neuroimaging.
- Complications of oestrogen deficiency associated with high PRL are avoided. An alternative approach is to treat with a combined OCP (the Pill). A theoretical concern is that oestrogen may stimulate growth of prolactinoma, but it is generally safe with microadenomas. Follow PRL.
- Surgery is generally not indicated. Microprolactinomas rarely progress to macroadenoma, they rarely expand in pregnancy, and they may recur after surgery.

Macroprolactinomas (>10mm diameter): Try treating with bromocriptine for these also but if there are visual symptoms, pressure effects, or if pregnancy is contemplated (~25% of macroadenomas will expand during pregnancy) then surgery is generally indicated. Usually a trans-sphenoidal approach is used. Follow-up with serial PRL and MRI. Bromocriptine, and in some cases radiation therapy, may be required post-op because complete surgical resection is uncommon.

1 A Levy 1994 *BMJ* i 1087

Acromegaly ®

This rare disease is due to hypersecretion of growth hormone (GH) from a pituitary tumour. It usually presents between the ages of 30–50yrs.

Incidence 3/million/year.

Symptoms Insidious onset (look at old photos). Most features are due to growth of soft tissues. Coarse, oily skin, large tongue, prominent supraorbital ridge, prognathism, teeth spacing increased, as is shoe size, thick spade-like hands, deepening voice, arthralgia, kyphosis, proximal muscle weakness, paraesthesiae (due to carpal tunnel syndrome—p462), progressive heart failure, goitre. Features of a pituitary tumour—hypopituitarism, and local mass effect may occur (p560). Sweating and headache are also common.

Complications DM; BP↑; cardiomyopathy; large bowel tumours (benign or malignant).

Investigations

- Isolated GH measurement may show raised secretion, but levels vary with the time of day and other factors so random measurements are not diagnostic.
- Serum IGF-1 (insulin-like growth factor-1) is the best screening test for acromegaly. Levels provide a measure of GH secretion over the previous 24h, and so are elevated by excessive GH secretion, or in pregnancy or puberty.
- The definitive test is the oral glucose tolerance test (OGTT) with GH measurement. Method as described (p528) but insert IV cannula with three-way tap and citrate (see p558) 1h before test. Collect samples for GH, glucose, insulin at: 0, 30, 60, 90, 120, 150mins.
  Interpretation of OGTT: GH does not fall to <2mu/L in: acromegaly, anorexia nervosa, poorly controlled DM, hypothyroidism, Cushing's.
- MRI (or CT) scan of pituitary fossa.
- T4, basal serum PRL, testosterone (if male)—hypopituitarism?
- May need full triple stimulation test if hypopituitarism is suspected (p588). 558
- ECG. Visual fields and acuity. Skin thickness.
- Obtain old photos. New photo of full face, torso, hands on chest.

Treatment *Trans-sphenoidal surgery* on younger patients or if pressure symptoms. In 60% this reduces GH secretion to <5μg/mL.[1] 6 weeks after surgery readmit for OGTT with GH measurement, T4, PRL, testosterone, triple stimulation test. If GH fails to suppress below 2.0mu/L irradiation or bromocriptine will be required. Steroids should be stopped before these tests and triple stimulation test done on day 4 only if no signs of steroid deficiency (postural hypotension, fever, nausea, anorexia). *Post-op follow-up* every year (OGTT with GH measurement, T4, PRL, ECG, visual fields, x-rays—see above, photos).

External irradiation: For older patients. Follow-up as for surgery.

Medical management: Bromocriptine is used as an adjunct or if the patient is not a good operative risk. Start with 2.5mg PO at night. Increase by 2.5mg every 3 days up to 5mg/6h. On its own, it only provides adequate control in mild disease. Follow-up 2 weeks after maximum dose as for surgery. SE: nausea, postural hypotension.

Somatostatin analogues such as *octreotide* eg 0.1–0.2mg/8h SC have displaced dopamine agonists as the first line in somatotroph adenomas[1] (SE: gallstones).

1 A Levy 1994 *BMJ* i 1087

Diabetes insipidus (DI)

This is due to impaired water resorption by the kidney because of reduced ADH secretion from the posterior pituitary (cranial DI), or impaired response of the kidney to ADH (nephrogenic DI).

Symptoms Polyuria; dilute urine; polydipsia; water deficit if not drinking.

Causes of cranial DI Head injury, hypophysectomy, histiocytosis, metastases, pituitary tumour, sarcoidosis, vascular lesion, meningitis, inherited (autosomal dominant). Idiopathic DI (50%) is often self-limiting, and MRI may reveal an infundibuloneurohypophysitis (known to be lymphocytic, and possibly autoimmune[1]).

Causes of nephrogenic DI Low potassium, high calcium, drugs (lithium, demeclocycline), pyelonephritis, hydronephrosis, pregnancy (rare as a primary cause; due to placental production of vasopressinase; can exacerbate underlying DI from any cause).

Investigations U&E, Ca^{2+}, plasma and urine osmolalities.
Plasma osmolality should be high, and urine low. Serum sodium may be high. In psychogenic polydipsia plasma osmolality is often low.
The water deprivation test will confirm the diagnosis.

The water deprivation test (If first morning urine has osmolality >800mosmol/kg, DI is excluded.) Stop drugs (chlorpropamide, clofibrate, carbamazepine) before the test.
- Light breakfast, no tea, no coffee, no smoking.
- Weigh at 0, 4, 6, 7, 8h. Stop if >3% body weight lost.
- Supervise carefully to stop patient drinking.
- Empty bladder, then no drinks and only dry food for 8h. Collect urine hourly, measure volume. Measure osmolality at 1, 4, 7, 8h. Stop test if osmolality >800mosmol/kg (DI is excluded).
- Venous sample for osmolality at: 0.5, 3.5, 6.5, 7.5h.
- If diuresis continues, desmopressin 20µg intranasally (or 1µg IM) at 8h.
- Water can be drunk after 8h. Measure urine osmolality at 8, 9, 10, 11, 12h.

Interpreting the water deprivation test: Check plasma osmolality is >290mosmol/kg to ensure that the test has provided adequate stimulus for ADH release. The *normal* response is for urine osmolality to be >800mosmol/kg with a small rise only in osmolality after desmopressin. In *psychogenic polydipsia* the urine is also concentrated (>400mosmol/kg) but rather less than in the normal response. In *diabetes insipidus* the urine is abnormally dilute (<400mosmol/kg). However, in *cranial DI* the urine osmolality increases by more than 50% following desmopressin; whereas in *nephrogenic DI* it increases by less than 45% following desmopressin.

Treatment *Cranial DI:* Find cause, do triple stimulation test (p558). Give desmopressin 10–20µg/12–24h intranasally (use the smallest dose which controls polyuria: higher doses ↑risk of hyponatraemia). *Nephrogenic:* Treat cause. No high-protein meals/excess salt may help polyuria. If it persists, try bendrofluazide (=bendroflumethiazide) 5mg PO/24h.

Emergency treatment The diagnosis must be made. This can be done if: suitable cause, large urine output, urine osmolality low (around 150mosmol/kg), despite dehydration.
- Plasma U&E.
- IV fluids—5% dextrose, 2 litres in first hour.
- Continue fluids to rehydrate and then to keep up with urine output.
- Desmopressin 1µg IM (lasts 12–24h).

1 H Imura 1993 *NEJM* **329** 683

13. Haematology

Relevant pages elsewhere: Transfusion (p102); normal values (p753).

Further reading: D Nathan 1995 *Genes, Blood, and Courage,* Harvard University Press, ISBN 0-674-34473-L. Dayem Saif, introduced when he is a 6-year old with a stature of a 2-year, old has an Hb of 1.5g/dL: as low as his chance of survival with thalassaemia. This story about laboratory medicine and its stormy application at the bedside is definitely worth reading when feeling hemmed in by difficult patients, for it demonstrates that there are no difficult patients, only difficult times. The book portrays the vital nature of the doctor–patient relationship, and warns us against labelling people, unless the label is a poem: Dayem is Arabic for *Immortal Sword.*

On the taking of blood and of holidays

This is not one of those passages about how you should be kind to the patient, explain in full what you are going to do, talk him or her through venepuncture, label the bottles carefully, and make a plan for communicating the results. Be all this virtue as it may, there is something else which needs communicating about the most menial of our tasks: the *act* of taking blood. It is partly to do with the fact that as blood is life, and, because, as Ruskin taught us, 'there is no wealth but life' we are led to the conclusion that what is special about taking blood is that for once we are being given something valuable by the patient. What is this wealth? The answer is time. For while the blood is flowing into our tube we cannot be disturbed. We are excused from answering our bleeps, and from making polite conversation (a few grunts in reply to patients' enquiries about the colour of their blood is quite sufficient)—and we can indulge in that almost unimaginable luxury, at least as far as life on the wards is concerned, of being *alone with our own thoughts*. Thinking of this sacred time as a sort of hypnotic holiday is excellent. For however many nights we have been awoken, this little holiday will be worth an hour's sleep—if our mind is furnished and ready to empty itself of all objectivity. The best sight in haematological practice is, during venepuncture, to watch for those occasions when, owing to some chance characteristic of flow, the blood streaming into our tube breaks up into countless globules, and before coalescing again, these globules jostle together like the overcrowded chain of events which led us to this bedside. During this time, allow your own thoughts to coalesce into a more peaceful order if you can, and let William Blake help you in the task of furnishing your mind to banish objectivity, for he knew some truths about haematology unknown to strictly rational practitioners of this art:

> The Microscope knows not of this nor the Telescope: they alter
> The ratio of the Spectators Organs but leave Objects untouch'd
> For every space larger than a red globule of Mans blood
> Is visionary, and it is created by the Hammer of Los:*
> And every space smaller than a Globule of Mans blood opens
> Into eternity of which this vegetable Earth is but a shadow.
> The red Globule is the unwearied Sun by Los* created
> To measure Time and Space to mortal Men . . .

*Los, the *globe of fire,* is a symbol used by Blake to encompass the exultant energy of creation, the poet-imagination, and the burning brightness where all his noble images were pounded out of eternity and compounded into the most compressed verse and that we have (*se?* Ackroyd 1996 *Blake,* Minerva). These lines are from his poem *Milton,* section 29, lines 17–24, p516 in our *Blake: Complete Writings* edited (1925–1969) by Geoffrey Keynes—the surgeon, who, incidentally, led the way to lumpectomy for breast cancer, in preference to the much-hated radical mastectomy.

Anaemia is a low haemoglobin due to a low red cell mass. If the low Hb is due to dilution from an increased plasma volume (eg in pregnancy), the 'anaemia' is called physiological. A low Hb (at sea level) is <13.5g/dL for men and <11.5g/dL for women. It may be due to reduced production or increased loss of RBC and has many causes. These will often be distinguishable by history, examination, and inspection of the blood film.

Symptoms These may be due to the underlying cause or to the anaemia itself and include fatigue, dyspnoea, palpitations, headache, tinnitus, anorexia, bowel disturbance—and angina if there is pre-existing coronary artery disease.

Signs Pallor (look for pale conjunctivae), retinal haemorrhages. In severe anaemia (Hb <8g/dL) there may be signs of a hyperdynamic circulation eg tachycardia, murmurs and cardiac enlargement. Later heart failure may occur and in this state rapid blood transfusion may be fatal.

Anaemia due to excessive red cell destruction is called haemolytic anaemia. Suspect haemolysis if there is a reticulocytosis, mild macrocytosis, haptoglobin↓ (p584), bilirubin↑ and urobilinogen↑.

The next step in determining the cause of anaemia is to look at the MCV (normal mean cell volume is 76–96 femtolitres, 10^{15} fl = 1 litre).

Low MCV (microcytic) The common cause is:
- Iron-deficiency anaemia (IDA) (with a microcytic, hypochromic blood film showing anisocytosis and poikilocytosis (p576). It may be confirmed by showing serum iron↓ and ferritin↓ (more representative of total body iron) with total iron binding capacity (TIBC) ↑.
- Thalassaemia (suspect if the MCV is too low for the level of anaemia and the red cell count is raised).
- Congenital sideroblastic anaemia (very rare).

These last two are iron-loading conditions and will show serum iron ↑; ferritin ↑; but TIBC ↑.

Normal MCV (normocytic) Causes:
- Anaemia of chronic disease (ACD)
- Bone marrow failure
- Haemolysis
- Hypothyroidism
- Renal failure
- Pregnancy

If there is a reduced white cell or platelet count suspect bone marrow failure and perform a bone marrow biopsy.

High MCV (macrocytic) Causes:
- B12 or folate deficiency
- Alcohol
- Marrow infiltration
- Hypothyroidism
- Reticulocytosis (eg haemolysis)
- Myelodysplastic syndromes
- Liver disease
- Antifolate drugs (eg phenytoin)

Blood transfusion Avoid unless Hb dangerously low. The decision will depend on severity and cause. If risk of haemorrhage (eg active peptic ulcer) transfuse up to 8g/dL. In severe anaemia with heart failure, transfusion is vital to restore Hb to safe level, eg 6–8g/dL, but must be done with great care. Give packed cells slowly with 10–40mg frusemide (=furosemide) iv/po with alternate units (dose depends on previous exposure to diuretics; do not mix with blood). Check for rising JVP and basal crepitations and consider CVP line. If CCF gets worse, and immediate transfusion is essential, try a 2–3 unit exchange transfusion, removing blood at same rate as transfused.

Iron-deficiency anaemia (IDA)

This is common (seen in up to 14% of menstruating women). The main cause is <u>blood loss</u>, particularly <u>menorrhagia</u> or GI bleeding (from oesophagitis, peptic ulcer, carcinoma, colitis, diverticulitis, or piles).

In the Tropics, <u>hookworm</u> (causing GI blood loss) is the most common cause of IDA.

<u>Poor diet</u> may cause IDA in <u>babies</u> (but rarely in adults), those on special diets, or wherever there is poverty.

<u>Malabsorption</u> (eg in coeliac disease) is a rare cause of IDA.

Signs of chronic IDA: <u>koilonychia</u> (p25), <u>atrophic glossit</u>is, and, rarely, post-cricoid webs. ▶*Iron deficiency without an obvious source of bleeding mandates a careful GI workup.*

Tests: Faecal <u>occult blood</u>, <u>sigmoidoscopy, barium</u> studies, microscope <u>stool for ova.</u>

Treatment: If MCV↓, and good history of menorrhagia, <u>oral iron</u> may be started without further tests; otherwise, <u>treat the cause</u>. Give oral iron, eg as <u>ferrous sulfate</u> 200mg/12–8h PO. SE: constipation; black stools. Hb should rise by 1g/dL/week (with a reticulocytosis). Continue until Hb is normal and for 3 months to replenish stores. IM iron is almost never needed. If it is (because the oral route is impossible), use iron sorbitol and consult the *Data Sheet*.

Refractory anaemia

The usual reason for iron deficiency anaemia to fail to respond to iron replacement is that the patient has rejected the pills. Negotiate on concordance issues (p3). Is the reason for the problem GI disturbance (altering the dose of elemental iron may help). There may be continued blood loss, malabsorption or misdiagnosis (eg thalassaemia). Occasionally there is myelodysplasia with abnormal marrow maturation. This is refractory to most treatments and may be pre-leukaemic.

The anaemia of chronic disease

This is associated with many of diseases: eg <u>infection</u>, <u>collagen vascular disease</u>, <u>rheumatoid arthritis</u>, <u>malignancy</u>, <u>renal failure</u>. There is mild normocytic anaemia (eg Hb >8g/dL), sometimes confused with iron-deficiency anaemia but TIBC↓ and serum ferritin normal or ↑. *Treatment* is of the underlying disease. <u>Erythropoietin lack</u> is a cause of the anaemia of <u>renal failure</u>—genetically engineered erythropoietin is effective in raising the haemoglobin level (dose example: 75–450 units/kg/week; SE: flu-like symptoms, hypertension, mild rise in the platelet count).

Sideroblastic anaemia

<u>Hypochromic</u> RBCs are seen on the blood film with <u>sideroblasts</u> in the marrow (<u>erythroid precursors with iron deposited in mitochondria</u> in a ring around the nucleus). It may be <u>congenital</u> (rare, x-linked) or <u>acquired, and</u> is usually <u>idiopathic</u>, but may follow <u>alcohol</u> or <u>lead</u> excess, <u>myeloproliferative</u> disease, <u>malignancy</u>, <u>malabsorption</u>, <u>anti-TB</u> drugs. *Treatment* is <u>supportive; pyridoxine</u> may help (eg 10mg/24h PO; higher doses may cause neuropathy). <u>Iron loading</u> (haemosiderosis, ie <u>endocrine, liver, and cardiac damage) can be a problem</u> as GI iron absorption is increased.

The peripheral blood film

▶Many haematological (and other) diagnoses can be made by careful examination of the peripheral blood film. It is also necessary for interpretation of the FBC indices.

576

Acanthocytes: RBCs show many spicules (in abetalipoproteinaemia).

Anisocytosis: Variation in size, eg in megaloblastic anaemia, thalassaemia as well as iron-deficiency anaemia (IDA).

Basophilic stippling of RBCs is seen in lead poisoning, thalassaemia and other dyserythropoietic anaemias.

Blasts: Nucleated precursor cells (eg in myelofibrosis or leukaemia). They are not normally seen in peripheral blood.

Burr cells: Irregularly shaped cells occurring in uraemia.

Dimorphic picture: A mixture of RBC sizes, eg partially treated iron deficiency, mixed deficiency (Fe with B_{12} or folate deficiency), post-transfusion, sideroblastic anaemia.

Howell–Jolly bodies: Nuclear remnants seen in RBCs post-splenectomy; rarely leukaemia, megaloblastic anaemia, IDA, hyposplenism (eg coeliac disease, neonates, thalassaemia, SLE, lymphoma, leukaemia, amyloid).

Hypochromia: Less dense staining of RBCs seen in IDA, thalassaemia and sideroblastic anaemia (iron stores unusable).

Left shift: Immature white cells seen in circulating blood in any marrow outpouring, eg infection.

Leucoerythroblastic anaemia: Immature cells (myelocytes and normoblasts) seen in film. Due to marrow infiltration (eg by malignancy), hypoxia or severe anaemia.

Leukaemoid reaction: A marked reactive leucocytosis. Usually granulocytic eg in severe infection, burns, acute haemolysis, metastatic cancer.

Myelocytes, promyelocytes, metamyelocytes, normoblasts: Immature cells seen in the blood in leukoerythroblastic anaemia.

Normoblasts: Immature red cells, with a nucleus. Seen in leukoerythroblastic anaemia, marrow infiltration, haemolysis, hypoxia.

Pappenheimer bodies: Granules of siderocytes, eg lead poisoning, carcinomatosis, post-splenectomy.

Poikilocytes: Variably shaped cells, eg seen in IDA.

Polychromasia: RBCs of different ages stain unevenly (the young are bluer). This is a response to bleeding, haematinics (eg ferrous sulfate, B_{12}), haemolysis or dyserythropoiesis.

Reticulocytes: (NR: 0.8–2% of RBCs) Young, larger RBCs signifying active erythropoiesis. Increased in haemolysis, haemorrhage, and if B_{12}, iron or folate is given to marrow which lack these.

Right shift: Hypersegmented polymorphs (>5 lobes to nucleus) seen in megaloblastic anaemia, uraemia, and liver disease.

Rouleaux formation: Red cells stack on each other (the visual 'analogue' of a high ESR—see p618).

Schistocytes: Fragmented RBCs sliced by fibrin bands. Seen in intravascular haemolysis.

Spherocytes: Spherical cells; seen in haemolysis, hereditary spherocytosis, and burns.

Target cells: (Also called Mexican hat cells) These are RBCs with central staining, a ring of pallor, and an outer rim of staining seen in liver disease, thalassaemia, or sickle-cell disease—and, in small numbers, in iron-deficiency anaemia.

The neutrophils 2–7.5 × 10⁹/L (40–75% of white blood cells: but absolute values are more meaningful than percentages).

Increased in: Bacterial infections; trauma; surgery; burns; haemorrhage; inflammation; infarction; polymyalgia; PAN; myeloproliferative disorders and drugs (eg steroids). Marked increase in leukaemias; disseminated malignancy; severe childhood infection.

Decreased in: Viral infections; brucellosis; typhoid; kala-azar; TB. Also drugs, eg carbimazole; sulfonamides. They may be used up during septicaemia or destroyed by hypersplenism or neutrophil antibodies (seen in SLE and rheumatoid arthritis). There is reduced manufacture in B₁₂ or folate deficiency and in bone marrow failure (p610).

The lymphocytes 1.3–3.5 × 10⁹/L (20–45%).

Increased in: Viral infections—EBV, CMV, rubella; toxoplasmosis; whooping cough; brucellosis; chronic lymphatic leukaemia. Large numbers of abnormal ('atypical') lymphocytes are characteristically seen with EBV infection: these are T-cells reacting against EBV-infected B-cells. They have a large amount of clearish cytoplasm with a blue rim that flows around neighbouring RBCs. Other causes of 'atypical' lymphocytes: see p204.

Decreased in: Steroid therapy; SLE; uraemia; legionnaire's disease; AIDS; marrow infiltration; post chemotherapy or radiotherapy.

T-lymphocyte subset reference values: CD4 count: 537–1571/mm³ (low in HIV infection). CD8 count: 235–753/mm³; CD4/CD8 ratio: 1.2–3.8.

The eosinophils 0.04–0.44 × 10⁹/L (1–6%).

Increased in: Asthma and allergic disorders; parasitic infections (especially invasive helminths); PAN; skin disease especially pemphigus; urticaria; eczema; malignant disease (including eosinophilic leukaemia); irradiation; Löffler's syndrome (p702); during the convalescent phase of any infection.

The hypereosinophilic syndrome is seen when there is development of end-organ damage (restrictive cardiomyopathy; neuropathy; hepatosplenomegaly) in association with a raised eosinophil count (>1.5 × 10⁹/L) for more than 6 weeks. Steroids or cytotoxic drugs may give temporary relief.

The monocytes 0.2–0.8 × 10⁹/L (2–10%).

Increased in: Acute and chronic infections (eg TB; brucellosis; protozoa); malignant disease (including M4 and M5 acute myeloid leukaemia—p602, and Hodgkin's disease); myelodysplasia.

The basophils 0–0.1 × 10⁹/L (0–1%).

Increased in: Viral infections; urticaria; myxoedema; post-splenectomy; CML; UC; malignancy; systemic mastocytosis (urticaria pigmentosa); haemolysis; polycythaemia rubra vera.

Macrocytic anaemia

Macrocytosis (MCV >96 femtolitres) is a common finding in routine blood counts, often without anaemia. Only ~5% of these will be from B_{12} deficiency, so it is wise to approach a diagnosis in an organized manner.

Causes of macrocytosis *MCV >110fL:* •Vitamin B_{12} or folate deficiency.

MCV 100–110 fL:	•Alcohol	•Liver disease	•*Drugs:* eg azathioprine
•Haemolysis	•Pregnancy	•Hypothyroidism	•Zidovudine (p218)
•Marrow infiltrated	•Myelodysplasia		•Hydroxyurea (=hydroxycarbamide)

Consider the conditions above in the history and examination. The diagnosis may be obvious at this stage. Alcohol is the most likely cause of macrocytosis without anaemia.

Tests The blood film may show hypersegmented polymorphs ($B_{12}\downarrow$) or target cells (liver disease). *Other tests:* ESR (malignancy), LFTs (include GGT), T_4, serum B_{12} (note: falsely low result if on antibiotics—microbiological assay), red cell folate (more reliable than serum folate—use an FBC bottle).

Bone marrow biopsy is indicated if the cause is not revealed by the above tests. It is likely to show one of these 4 states:

Megaloblastic—B_{12} or folate deficiency (or cytotoxic drugs). (A megaloblast is a cell in which cytoplasmic and nuclear maturation are out of phase—as nuclear maturation is slow.)

Normoblastic marrow—liver damage, myxoedema.

Increased erythropoiesis—eg bleeding or haemolysis.

Abnormal erythropoiesis—sideroblastic anaemia, leukaemia, aplastic anaemia.

If results indicate B_{12} deficiency, consider a Schilling test to help to identify the cause. This determines whether a low B_{12} is due to malabsorption (B_{12} is absorbed from the terminal ileum) or to lack of intrinsic factor—by comparing the proportion of an oral dose (1μg) of radioactive B_{12} excreted in urine with and without the concurrent administration of intrinsic factor. (The blood must be saturated by giving an IM dose of 1000μg of B_{12}.) If intrinsic factor enhances absorption, lack of it (eg pernicious anaemia) is likely to be the cause (if not, look for blind loops, diverticula, and terminal ileal disease as the cause of the low B_{12}).

Causes of a low B_{12} Pernicious anaemia (p582); post-gastrectomy (no intrinsic factor to ↑absorption from terminal ileum); poor diet (eg vegans); more rarely, disease of terminal ileum (where B_{12} is absorbed)—eg: Crohn's; resection; blind loops; diverticula; worms (*Dyphyllobothrium*).

Causes of low folate Dietary deficiency (eg in alcoholics), increased need (pregnancy, haemolysis, dyserythropoiesis, malignancy, long-term haemodialysis), malabsorption especially coeliac disease, tropical sprue, drugs (phenytoin and trimethoprim).

Note In ill patients with megaloblastic anaemia (eg with CCF) it may be necessary to treat before the results of serum B_{12} and folate are to hand. Use large doses, eg hydroxocobalamin 1mg/24h IM, with folic acid 5mg/24h PO (►folate given alone may precipitate subacute combined degeneration of the spinal cord). Blood transfusions are very rarely needed, but see p572.

Pernicious anaemia

Essence This disease affects all cells of the body and is due to malabsorption of B_{12} resulting from lack of gastric intrinsic factor because of autoimmunity to parietal cells. Atrophic gastritis is usually present. In B_{12} deficiency synthesis of thymidine, and hence DNA, is impaired and in consequence red cell production is reduced. In addition the CNS, peripheral nerves, gut and tongue may be affected.

Common features
Tiredness and weakness (90%)
Dyspnoea (70%)
Paraesthesiae (38%)
Sore red tongue (25%)
Diarrhoea, dementia

Other features
Retinal haemorrhages
Lemon tinge to skin
Retrobulbar neuritis
Mild splenomegaly
Fever

Subacute combined degeneration of the spinal cord: This may be seen in any cause of a low B_{12}. Posterior and lateral columns are often affected, not always together. Onset is usually insidious—with peripheral neuropathy. Joint-position and vibration sense are typically affected first (dorsal columns) followed by distal paraesthesiae (neuropathy). If untreated, stiffness and weakness ensue. The classical triad is: ●Extensor plantars ●Brisk knee jerks ●Absent ankle jerks. Less common signs (depending on the balance of damage to peripheral nerves, spinal tracts, and other CNS damage): cognition↓, vision↓, absent knee jerks with brisk ankle jerks and flexor plantars, Lhermitte's sign (p454). Pain and temperature sensation may be intact even when joint position sense is severely affected. CNS signs can occur without anaemia.

Associations Thyroid disease (~25%), vitiligo, Addison's disease, carcinoma of stomach (possibly, so have a low threshold for endoscopy).

Tests ●Hb↓ (3–11g/dL) ●MCV >~110fl ●Hypersegmented polymorphs ●Serum B_{12} is always↓ ●WCC & platelets↓ ●Megaloblasts in the marrow

Megaloblasts are abnormal red cell precursors with delicate nuclear chromatin, and in which nuclear maturation is slower than cytoplasmic maturation. Antibodies to parietal cells are found in 90%; there may also be antibodies to intrinsic factor, either at B_{12} binding sites (50%) or at ileal binding sites (35%). A Schilling test (p580) may be appropriate occasionally (expect it to show that <7% of an orally administered dose of labelled B_{12} is excreted—unless concurrent intrinsic factor is given).[1]

Treatment Replenish stores with hydroxocobalamin (B_{12}) 1mg IM alternate days for 1–2 weeks (or, if CNS signs, until improvement stops). Then 250µg/week until Hb normal; maintenance dose: 1mg IM every 2–3 months for life (child's dose: as for adult). Initial improvement is heralded by a marked reticulocytosis (but serum iron falls first, if looked for).

Practical hints Beware of diagnosing pernicious anaemia in those under 40 years old: look for GI malabsorption (small bowel biopsy, p522).
1 Watch for hypokalaemia as treatment becomes established.
2 Pernicious anaemia with high output CCF may require exchange transfusion (p572) after blood for FBC, folate, B_{12} and marrow sampling.
3 As haemopoiesis accelerates on treatment, additional Fe may be needed.
4 WCC and platelet count should normalize in 1 week. Hb rises ~1g/dL per week of treatment.

Prognosis Complete neurological recovery is possible. Most see improvement in the first 3–6 months. Patients do best if treated as soon as possible after the onset of symptoms: don't delay!

1 M Mouallem 1997 *Lancet* 349 136

An approach to haemolytic anaemia

Haemolysis is the premature breakdown of RBCs. It may occur in the circulation (intravascular) or in the reticuloendothelial system (extravascular). Normal RBCs have a lifespan of ~120 days. In sickle-cell anaemia, for example, the life span may be as short as 5 days. If the bone marrow does not compensate sufficiently, a haemolytic anaemia will result.

Causes of haemolysis These are either genetic or acquired.

Genetic:
1 Membrane: hereditary spherocytosis or elliptocytosis.
2 Haemoglobin: sickling disorders (p588), thalassaemia.
3 Enzyme defects: G6PD and pyruvate kinase deficiency.

Acquired:
1 Immune: either isoimmune (haemolytic disease of newborn, blood transfusion reaction), autoimmune (warm or cold antibody mediated) or drug-induced.
2 Non-immune: trauma (cardiac haemolysis, microangiopathic anaemia, p586), infection (malaria, septicaemia), membrane disorders (paroxysmal nocturnal haemoglobinuria, liver disease).

In searching for evidence of significant haemolysis (and, if present, its cause) try to answer these 4 questions:
● *Is there increased red cell breakdown?* Bilirubin↑ (unconjugated), urinary urobilinogen↑, haptoglobin↓ (binds free Hb avidly, and is then removed by the liver, so it is quite a good marker of intravascular haemolysis).
● *Is there increased red cell production?* Eg a reticulocytosis, polychromasia, macrocytosis, marrow hyperplasia.
● *Is the haemolysis mainly extra- or intravascular?* Extravascular haemolysis may lead to splenic hypertrophy. The features of intravascular haemolysis are methaemalbuminaemia, free plasma haemoglobin, haemoglobinuria, low haptoglobin, and haemosiderinuria.
● *Why is there haemolysis?* See below, and p586.

History Ask about family history, race, jaundice, haematuria, drugs, previous anaemia.

Examination Look for jaundice, hepatosplenomegaly, leg ulcers (seen in sickle-cell disease).

Tests FBC, reticulocytes, bilirubin, LDH, haptoglobin, urinary urobilinogen. Films may show polychromasia, macrocytosis, spherocytes, elliptocytes, fragmented cells or sickle cells—and nucleated RBCs if severe.

Further investigations include the direct Coombs' test (DCT). This will identify red cells coated with antibody or complement and a positive result usually indicates an immune cause of the haemolysis. The RBC lifespan may be determined by chromium labelling and the major site of RBC breakdown may also be identified. Urinary haemosiderin (stains with Prussian Blue) indicates chronic intravascular haemolysis.

The cause of the haemolysis may now be obvious, but further tests may be needed. Membrane abnormalities are identified on the film, and Hb electrophoresis will detect Hb variants. Enzyme assays are reserved for when other causes have been excluded.

A Coombs' test will detect the immune acquired causes, and the non-immune group are usually identifiable by associated features. Osmotic fragility testing may be used to detect hereditary membrane disorders.

Causes of haemolytic anaemia

Sickle-cell disease See p588.

Hereditary spherocytosis Autosomal dominant (AD) causing fragile RBCs and variable haemolysis with spherocytes on the film. Clinical features: mild anaemia (Hb 8–12g/dL), splenomegaly, and risk of gallstones. RBCs show increased fragility. Diagnosis is by osmotic fragility tests. Treatment of spherocytosis: folate replacement; splenectomy if warranted (but there are risks with ensuing hyposplenism).

Hereditary elliptocytosis Usually inherited as autosomal dominant. The degree of haemolysis is variable. If needed, splenectomy may help.

Glucose-6-phosphate dehydrogenase deficiency is the commonest RBC enzyme defect. Inheritance is sex-linked with 100 million affected in Africa, the Mediterranean and the Middle and Far East. Neonatal jaundice occurs, but most are symptomless with normal Hb and blood film. They are susceptible to oxidative crises precipitated by drugs (eg primaquine, sulfonamides, ciprofloxacin), exposure to the broad bean *Vicia fava* (favism) or illness. Typically there is rapid anaemia and jaundice with RBC Heinz bodies (denatured Hb stained with methyl violet). Diagnosis: enzyme assay. Don't do these tests till some weeks *after* a crisis (wait for jaundice to go) as young RBCs may have sufficient enzyme to make the results appear normal. Treatment: avoid precipitants.

Pyruvate kinase deficiency Usually inherited as autosomal recessive; homozygotes often have neonatal jaundice; later, chronic haemolysis with splenomegaly and jaundice. Diagnose by enzyme assay. Often well-tolerated. There is no specific therapy but splenectomy may help.

Drug-induced immune haemolysis Due to formation of new RBC membrane antigens (eg penicillin in prolonged, high-dose), immune complex formation (many drugs, rare), or presence of autoantibodies to the RBC: α-methyldopa, mefenamic acid, L-dopa (rare, Coombs' +ve).

Autoimmune haemolytic anaemia (AHA) Causes: warm or cold antibodies. They may be primary (idiopathic) or secondary, usually to lymphoma or generalized autoimmune disease, eg SLE. Warm AHA presents as chronic or acute anaemia. Treat by steroids (± splenectomy). Cold AHA: chronic anaemia made worse by cold, often with Raynaud's or acrocyanosis. Treatment: keep warm. Chlorambucil may help. Mycoplasma and EBV may produce cold agglutinins, but haemolysis is rare.

Paroxysmal cold haemoglobinuria is caused by Donnath–Landsteiner antibody (seen in mumps, measles, chickenpox, syphilis) sticking to RBCs in cold, which causes complement-mediated lysis on rewarming.

Cardiac haemolysis is due to cell trauma in a prosthetic aortic valve. It may indicate valve malfunction.

Microangiopathic haemolytic anaemia (MAHA) Suspect if marked fragmentation±many microspherocytes on the film. Includes haemolytic–uraemic syndrome and ITP (see p397). Treat underlying disease; blood and fresh frozen plasma transfusions for support.

Paroxysmal nocturnal haemoglobinuria RBCs are unusually sensitive to complement due to loss of complement-inactivating enzymes on their surface, causing pancytopenia, abdominal pain, or thrombosis (eg Budd–Chiari syndrome, p696) ± haemolysis. Diagnosis: Ham's test (*in vitro* acid-induced lysis). Treatments: anticoagulation; blood product replacement; consider stem cell transplant.

Factors exacerbating haemolysis Infection often leads to increased haemolysis. Also parvoviruses (*OHCS* p214) cause cessation of marrow erythropoiesis (aplastic anaemia with no reticulocytes—p610).

♯ Sickle-cell anaemia

There is severe haemolysis from homozygous inheritance of a gene causing an amino acid substitution in haemoglobin (β6 Glu → Val), so making HbS (the adult AA-genotype codes HbA, p590). It is common in black Africans and their worldwide descendants. The homozygote (ss) has sickle-cell *anaemia* and heterozygotes (AS) have sickle-cell *trait*, which causes no disability (and may protect from *falciparum* malaria) except in hypoxia—eg in unpressurized aircraft or anaesthesia, when veno-occlusive events may occur—so all those of African descent need a sickling test pre-op. Symptomatic sickling occurs in heterozygotes with genes coding other analogous amino acid substitutions (eg haemoglobin sc and sd diseases). Homozygotes (cc; dd) have asymptomatic mild anaemia.

Pathogenesis In the deoxygenated state the HbS molecules polymerize and cause RBCs to sickle. Sickle cells are fragile, and haemolyse; they also block small vessels to cause infarction.

Tests Sickling tests detect Hbs. Electrophoresis distinguishes ss, AS states, and other Hb variants. Film: all have target cells. Aim for diagnosis *at birth* (cord blood) so that pneumococcal prophylaxis (23-valent vaccine, p332, or penicillin V 125mg/12h PO) may be given.

The Patient Typically has an Hb of 6–8g/dL; reticulocytes 10–20%: (haemolysis is variable) and jaundice *early on*, eg with painful swelling of hands and feet (hand and foot syndrome)—also splenomegaly (rare if >10yrs, as the spleen infarcts). Young sicklers alternate periods of good health with acute crises (below). *Later*, chronic ill-health supervenes from previous crises: ie renal failure; bone necrosis; osteomyelitis; leg ulcers; iron overload (and alloimmunization) from many transfusions. Long-term lung complications may be associated with hypoventilation, atelectasis, and lung infiltrates caused by rib infarction—and is partly preventable by incentive spirometry—10 maximal inspirations/2h while awake. ◁1▷

Sickle-cell crises These may be from thrombosis (the aptly-named 'painful crises'), haemolysis (rare), marrow aplasia or sequestration.

Thrombotic crises (precipitated by cold, dehydration, infection, ischaemia eg muscular exertion) are most common and can cause severe pain, often in the bones. They may mimic an acute abdomen or pneumonia. CNS signs: fits, focal signs. Priapism may occur—ie prolonged erections; if for >24h arrange prompt cavernosus-spongeosum shunting to prevent impotence (priapism also occurs in CML—p604).

Aplastic crises: These are due to parvoviruses; characterized by sudden lethargy and pallor and few reticulocytes. Urgent transfusion is needed.

Sequestration/hepatic crises (serious; may need exchange transfusion) Spleen and liver enlarge rapidly from trapped RBCs; signs: RUQ pain, INR/LFT↑, Hb↓↓.

Management of chronic disease
- Consider hydroxyurea (=hydroxycarbamide) if frequent crises.[2]
- Chronic blood tranfusion programmes can keep HbS level <30%, but there is a high incidence of development of antibodies to red cell antigens. Marrow transplant can be curative but remains controversial.[2][3]
- Febrile children risk septicaemia: repeated admission is avoided by out-patient ceftriaxone (eg 2 doses, 50mg/kg IV on day 0 and 1). Admission may still be needed, eg if Hb <5g/dL; WCC <5 or >30,000 × 10⁹/L; T° >40°C; severe pain; dehydration; lung infiltration.[2] Seek expert advice.

Prevention Genetic counselling; prenatal tests (*OHCS* p210–12). Parental education can help prevent 90% of deaths from sequestration crises.[3]

◁4▷ PS Bellett 1996 *E-BM* 1 76 2 *Lancet* Round 1995 346 1408 2 J Williams *NEJM* 1993 329 472+501 3 R Grundy 1993 *Arch Dis Chi* 69 256

Management of sickle-cell crisis ►Seek expert help.

- Give *prompt*, generous analgesia, eg with opiates (p90).
- Crossmatch blood. FBC, reticulocytes, blood cultures, MSU, CXR.
- Rehydrate with IVI. ●Give O_2 by mask if $P_aO_2\downarrow$. ●Keep warm.
- Blind antibiotics (p182) if feverish, after infection screen.
- Measure PCV, reticulocytes, liver and spleen size twice daily.
- Give blood transfusion if PCV or reticulocytes fall sharply, or if there are CNS or lung complications—when the proportion of sickled cells should be reduced to <30%. If Hb <6g/dL it is safe to transfuse; if >9g/dL do a partial exchange transfusion.

Patient-controlled analgesia (PCA) An example with paediatric doses. First try warmth, hydration, and oral analgesia: ibuprofen 5mg/kg/6h PO (codeine phosphate 1mg/kg/4–8h PO up to 3mg/kg/day may also be tried, but is relatively ineffective). If this fails, see on the ward and offer prompt morphine by IVI—eg 0.1mg/kg. Start PCA with morphine 1mg/kg in 50mL 5% dextrose, and try a rate of 1mL/h, allowing the patient to deliver extra boluses of 1mL when needed. Do respiration and sedation score every ¼h + pulse oximetry if chest/abdominal pain.[4] For further advice, liaise with your local pain clinic service.

✢ Thalassaemia

Haemoglobin (Hb) is a tetrameric compound having 2 different pairs of peptide chains (α and β) with a haem molecule attached to each peptide. Hb is heterogeneous: adults have 95% HbA ($\alpha_2\beta_2$) and a little HbA$_2$ ($\alpha_2\delta_2$). HbF ($\alpha_2\gamma_2$) predominates in fetal life; adults have small amounts; larger amounts occur in β thalassaemia. The thalassaemias are genetic diseases of unbalanced Hb synthesis, as there is underproduction (or no production) of one chain. Unmatched globins precipitate, damaging RBC membranes, causing their destruction while still in the marrow. They are common in a band going from the Mediterranean to the Far East.

The β thalassaemias (β^0/β^0, β^+/β^+, or β^+/β^0) are caused by mutations in β-globin genes on chromosome 11, leading to ↓β chain production (β^+) or its absence (β^0). There are various combinations of mutations (eg β^0/β^0, β^+/β^+, or β^+/β^0). Severity correlates with genetic defect. The picture is usually one of severe anaemia presenting in the first year, often as failure to thrive. Death may result in 1 year without transfusion. With adequate transfusion, development is reasonably normal but symptoms of iron overload appear after 10 years as endocrine failure, liver disease, and cardiac toxicity. Death is usually at 20–30yrs due to cardiac siderosis. Long-term infusion of desferrioxamine (=deferoxamine) prevents iron loading. If transfusion is inadequate, there is anaemia with reduced growth and skeletal deformity due to bone marrow hyperplasia, eg bossing of skull. Also splenomegaly, bleeding and intermittent fever. The film shows very hypochromic, microcytic cells with target cells and nucleated RBCs. HbF↑↑, HbA$_2$ variable, HbA absent. Prevalence of carriers: Cypriot 1:7; south Italy 1:10; Greek 1:12; Turkish 1:20; English 1:100.

β thalassaemia minor (eg β/β^+): This is the heterozygous state, recognized as MCV <75fl, HbA$_2$ >3.5% + mild, well-tolerated anaemia (Hb >9g/dL); it may worsen in pregnancy. Splenomegaly is rare.

The α thalassaemias The α globin genes are on chromosome 16. If all 4 α genes are deleted, death is *in utero*. If just one gene functions, anaemia is mild (+MCV↓). Some patients will have β^+/β^+ thalassaemia too, but less severely, as there are fewer unmatched α chains.

α chain deficiency leads to excess β chains and β_4 tetramers (=Hb H; the fetal equivalent, Hb Barts, is physiologically useless γ_4). α^0/α^+ causes haemoglobin H disease with Hb ~8g/dL ± hypersplenism. α/α^+ is 'silent'.

Thalassaemia intermedia and Hb variants These cause quite severe anaemias which are usually transfusion-independent, eg Hb C thalassaemia (one parent has the Hb C trait, and the other has β^+). Sickle-cell β^0 thalassaemia produces a picture similar to sickle-cell anaemia. HbE trait coupled with β^0 is common in India, and is similar to β^+/β^+ thalassaemia.

Diagnosis FBC, MCV, film, iron, HbA$_2$, HbF, Hb electrophoresis.

Treatment ●Transfusion to keep Hb >9g/dL. ●Iron-chelating agent, eg desferrioxamine (=deferoxamine) to protect against cardiac disease and diabetes mellitus. ●Large doses of ascorbic acid also increase iron output. ●Perform splenectomy if hypersplenism exists—give pneumococcal vaccination (p332) ± meningococcal vaccination. ●Give folate supplements. ●A histocompatible marrow transplant can offer the chance of a cure.[1] Adopt a holistic approach to guide the patient through a difficult life.[2]

Prevention Approaches are genetic counselling or antenatal diagnosis using fetal blood or DNA, then 'therapeutic' abortion.

1 D Weatherall 1993 *NEJM* 329 877 2 Thalassaemia Soc: 0181 348 0437; D Nathan 1995 *Genes, Blood & Courage* 0674-34471

Bleeding disorders

After trauma, 3 processes halt bleeding: constriction, gap-plugging by platelets, and the coagulation cascade. Disorders of haemostasis fall into these 3 groups. The pattern of bleeding is important—vascular and platelet disorders lead to prolonged bleeding from cuts, and to purpura and bleeding from mucous membranes. Coagulation disorders produce delayed bleeding after injury, into joints, muscle and the GI and GU tracts.

Vascular defects Causes may be congenital (Osler–Weber–Rendu syndrome, p706), acquired (eg senile purpura, steroid drugs, trauma, pressure, vasculitis, connective tissue disease, scurvy, and painful bruising syndrome). Scurvy produces perifollicular haemorrhage. The painful bruising syndrome is seen in women who develop tingling under the skin followed by bruising over limbs/trunk, resolving without treatment.

Causes of too few platelets *Production↓*: marrow failure; megaloblastosis. *Survival↓*: immune thrombocytopenic purpura (ITP); viruses; DIC; drugs; SLE; lymphoma; thrombotic thrombocytopenic purpura; hypersplenism; genetic disease.[1] *Platelet aggregation*: heparin causes this in 5% of patients.

ITP may be chronic ($♀:♂≈3:1$) or acute ($♀:♂≈1:1$, eg in children, OHCS p275, 2 weeks after infection, with sudden self-limiting purpura). *Cause:* Antiplatelet autoantibodies lead to phagocytic destruction. Chronic ITP runs an indefinite fluctuating course of bleeding, purpura (especially dependent pressure areas) and epistaxis, often in young women. There is no palpable splenomegaly. CNS, conjunctival and retinal haemorrhage is rare. Tests: antiplatelet IgG autoantibody +ve and many megakaryocytes in marrow. Also: ANA+ve in 44%; WCC↑ or ↔ ± eosinophilia. If symptomatic or platelets $<20 × 10^9$/L, consider prednisolone (start at 3mg/kg/day; aim to keep platelets $>30 × 10^9$/L—only takes a few days to work) ± splenectomy (cures ≤80%). In non-responders, try cyclophosphamide. Platelet transfusions are no use (except during splenectomy). IV immunoglobulin may raise the platelet count, but the effect is not sustained.

Causes of ↓platelet function Marrow diseases/dysplasia, NSAIDs, urea↑.

Coagulation disorders Congenital (eg haemophilia, von Willebrand's p710) or with: anticoagulation; liver disease; DIC; malabsorption (vit. K↓).
- •*Haemophilia A* This factor VIII deficiency is inherited as a sex-linked recessive in 1/10,000 ♂ births—often because of a 'flip tip' inversion in the tip of the X chromosome. There is a high rate of new mutations (30% of affected children have no family history). *Presentation* depends on severity and is often early in life or after surgery/trauma—with bleeds into joints and muscle, leading to crippling arthropathy and haematomas with nerve palsies due to pressure. *Diagnose* by ↑KCCT and factor VIII assay. *Management:* Seek expert advice. Avoid NSAIDs and IM injections. •Minor bleeding: pressure and elevation of the part. Desmopressin (0.4μg/kg/12–24h IVI in 50mL 0.9% saline over 20mins) raises factor VIII levels, and may be sufficient. •Major bleeds (eg haemarthrosis) require factor VIII levels to be ↑ to 50% of normal. Life-threatening bleeds (eg obstructing airway) need levels of 100%, eg with virally inactivated lyophilized factor VIII. Genetic counselling: OHCS p212.
- •*Haemophilia B* (Christmas disease) is due to factor IX deficiency and behaves clinically like haemophilia A.
- •Acquired haemophilia is due to antibodies to factor VIII.
- •Liver disease produces a complicated bleeding disorder with synthesis of clotting factors↓, absorption of vitamin K↓, and abnormalities of platelet function. Malabsorption leads to low uptake of vitamin K (needed for synthesis of factors II, VII, IX, and X). Treatment is parenteral vitamin K (10mg) or fresh frozen plasma for acute haemorrhage.

Anticoagulants See p596. DIC See p598.

The intrinsic and extrinsic pathways of blood coagulation

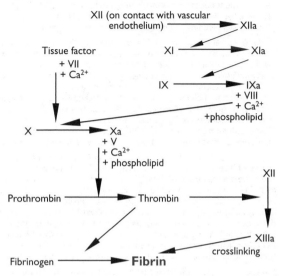

EXTRINSIC SYSTEM

INTRINSIC SYSTEM

XII (on contact with vascular endothelium) ⟶ XIIa

XI ⟶ XIa

Tissue factor
+ VII
+ Ca²⁺

IX ⟶ IXa
+ VIII
+ Ca²⁺
+phospholipid

X ⟶ Xa
+ V
+ Ca²⁺
+ phospholipid

Prothrombin ⟶ Thrombin ⟶ XII

XIIIa
crosslinking

Fibrinogen ⟶ **Fibrin**

The fibrinolytic system causes fibrin dissolution and acts via the generation of plasmin. The process starts by the release of tissue plasminogen activator (t-PA) from endothelial cells, a process stimulated by fibrin formation. t-PA converts inactive plasminogen to plasmin which can then cleave fibrin, as well as several other factors. t-PA and plasminogen both bind fibrin thus localizing fibrinolysis to the area of the clot.

Mechanism of fibrinolytic agents
1 *Alteplase* (=rt-PA=Actilyse®; from recombinant DNA) is a fibrinolytic enzyme imitating t-PA, as above. Plasma $t_{1/2} \approx 5$mins.
2 *Anistreplase* (=anisoylated plasminogen streptokinase activator complex =APSAC®) is a complex of human plasminogen and streptokinase (so anaphylaxis is possible). Plasma $t_{1/2} \approx 90$mins.
3 *Streptokinase* is a streptococcal exotoxin and forms a complex in plasma with plasminogen to form an activator complex which forms plasmin from unbound plasminogen. Initially there is rapid plasmin formation which can cause uncontrolled fibrinolysis. However, plasminogen is rapidly consumed in the complex and then plasmin is only produced as more plasminogen is synthesized. The activator complex binds to fibrin and so produces some localization of fibrinolysis.
4 *Urokinase* is produced by the kidney and is found in urine. It also cleaves plasminogen, but expense has limited its use.

1 One genetic cause of thrombocytopenia is autoimmune lymphoproliferative syndrome (ALPS) with splenomegaly, lymphadenopathy + other autoimmune features, mentioned here because of its interesting pathogenesis related to faulty apoptosis (programmed cell death of lymphocytes activated via routine infections) due to mutation of the gene known as 'Fas'. Apoptosis is essential immunological function, and is regulated by the Fas/Apo-1 receptor (*Blood* 1997 **89** 1341)

An approach to bleeding

There are 3 sets of questions to be answered:

1 *Is there an emergency?*—needing resuscitation or immediate referral?
- Is the patient about to exsanguinate (shock, coma, p762–767)?
- Is there hypovolaemia (postural hypotension, oliguria)?
- Is there CNS bleeding (meningism, CNS, and retinal signs)?

2 *Why is the patient bleeding?* Is bleeding normal, given the circumstances (eg trauma or parturition), or does the patient have a bleeding disorder?
- Is there unexplained bleeding, bruising, or purpura?
- Past or family history of bleeding—trauma, dentistry, surgery? Drugs (warfarin). Alcohol. Liver disease. Recent illness.
- Is the pattern of bleeding indicative of vascular, platelet, or coagulation problems (p592)? Are venepuncture sites bleeding (DIC)? Look for associated conditions (eg with DIC, p598).
- Is a clotting screen abnormal? Check FBC, platelets, INR, KCCT + thrombin time. Consider bleeding time, FDP (below), and factor VIII assay.

3 *If a bleeding disorder, what is the mechanism?* Management depends on degree of bleeding. If shocked, resuscitate (p766–7). If bleeding continues, and a clotting disorder is shown to exist, discuss need (and dose) for fresh frozen plasma (FFP) with a haematologist. If platelets↓, give platelets IVI (aim for >50 × 10⁹/L), except in ITP where steroids ± IV immunoglobulin may be used (especially in pregnancy, *OHCS* p142): consult an expert. Is there overdose with anticoagulants (p794)? In haemophiliac bleeds, *consult early* for coagulation factor replacement. *Never give IM injections.* Acutely, coagulation deficiencies may be treated by FFP + vitamin K (phytomenadione 2.5–10mg IV slowly, as castor oil free Konakion MM®).

Coagulation tests (Sodium citrate tube; false results if under-filled)

1 *Prothrombin time (PT):* Thromboplastin is added to test the extrinsic system. PT is expressed as a ratio compared to control [International Normalized Ratio, INR, normal range (NR) = 0.9–1.2]. Prolonged by: coumarins (eg warfarin); vitamin K deficiency; liver disease (as above).

2 *Thrombin time:* Thrombin is added to plasma to convert fibrinogen to fibrin. NR: 10–15sec, ↑ in heparin treatment, DIC or afibrinogenaemia.

3 *Kaolin cephalin clotting time (KCCT, or APTT, = PTT = partial thromboplastin time):* Kaolin activates the intrinsic system. Normal range 35–45sec, prolonged in heparin treatment or haemophilia.

Investigation of a bleeding disorder

Platelets: If low do FBC, film, bone marrow biopsy.
INR: If long, look for liver disease, or anticoagulant use.
KCCT: If long, consider factor VIII or IX deficiency, or heparin.
Bleeding time: If long, consider von Willebrand's disease (p710), or platelet disorders. Aspirin prolongs the bleeding time.

Disorder*	INR	KCCT	Thrombin time	Platelet count	Bleeding time	Notes
Heparin	↔	↑↑	↑↑	↔	↔	
DIC	↑↑	↑↑	↑↑	↓	↑	FDP↑, p598
Liver disease	↑	↑	↔↑	↔↓	↔↑	AST↑
Platelet defect	↔	↔	↔	↔	↑(↑)	
Vit K deficiency	↑↑	↑	↔	↔	↔	
Haemophilia	↔	↑↑	↔	↔	↔	see p592
von Willebrand's	↔	↑↑	↔	↔	↑(↑)	see p710

Special tests may be available (factor assays: ►consult a haematologist).
*After OTS, p215. FDP = fibrin degradation products

✠ Anticoagulants

▶Consider bleeding as a cause of any symptom in anyone on anticoagulants.

The main indications for anticoagulation ●DVT; pulmonary emboli.
●To prevent stroke in AF, or from prosthetic heart valves. Treat indefinitely.
●To prevent thrombosis/pulmonary emboli post-op in high-risk patients (p82).

Types of anticoagulant *Standard unfractionated* (~13,000 daltons) heparin
(IV or SC) acts fast, and is used as initial therapy, eg for 3 days to cover the
time before warfarin is effective, see below. Heparin (fractionated or
unfractionated) is the only anticoagulant used perioperatively. It inactivates
thrombin, and binds to plasma antithrombin III (so inactivating coagulation
enzyme Xa); monitor by *activated partial thromboplastin time* (APTT).

Low molecular weight heparin fragments (5000 daltons, eg dalteparin, enoxaparin, tinzaparin)[1] $T_{1/2}$ is 2–4-fold longer than standard heparin, and response
is more predictable, so it needs to be given once or twice daily SC. No
monitoring is needed. It can allow heparin to be started in out-patients. It
inactivates factor Xa (but not thrombin). *Dose example in prophylaxis:*
Dalteparin 2500iu SC 2h pre-op +12h post-op, then 5000iu daily for 5 days.
SE: Bleeding (at operative site, intracranial, retroperitoneal).
CI: Uncontrolled bleeding/risk of bleeding (eg peptic ulcer); endocarditis.

Warfarin is the most widely used coumarin (use phenindione if warfarin-
sensitive). It is used orally once daily as long-term anticoagulation. The
therapeutic range is narrow, varying with the condition being treated
(see opposite)—and is measured as a ratio compared with a standard
prothrombin time (the *international normalized ratio, INR*). Warfarin dis-
turbs vitamin K synthesis (hence active clotting factors↓). CI: Peptic
ulcer; bleeding disorders; severe hypertension; liver failure; endocarditis;
cerebral aneurysms. Use with caution in the elderly and those with past
GI bleeds. Use in pregnancy: OHCS p151. ▶Interactions: p752.
In the UK, warfarin tablets are 1mg (brown), 3mg (blue), or 5mg (pink).

Beginning anticoagulation ●Heparin 5000–10,000iu IV over 5min.
●Then add 25,000iu to 50mL 0.9% saline (=500iu/mL) in a syringe pump.
●Give 1000–2000iu/h IVI (2.8mL/h=1400iu/h). Check APTT (activated par-
tial thromboplastin time) at 6h. Institute the 5-day sliding scale below.

Measure APTT every 10h (every 4h if APTT >7, and stop the IVI).[2]

APTT	5–7	4–5	3–4	2½–3	1½–2½	1.2–1.4	<1.2
Change rate (iu/h) by	−500	−300	−100	−50	0	+200	+400

●Start warfarin 10mg PO at ~17.00 on day 1. Do INR 16h later (let lab know
he's on warfarin). If <1.8 (as is likely) the 2nd dose of warfarin is 10mg at
17.00h (24h after first dose). If >1.8, give warfarin 0.5mg PO at 17.00h.
●Use the sliding scale below to keep INR in the target range. Do INR daily
for 5 days, then alternate days until stable, then weekly or less often.[3]

INR	<2	2	2.5	2.9	3.3	3.6	4.1
Third dose	10mg	5mg	4mg	3mg	2mg	0.5mg	0mg
Maintenance	≥6mg	5.5mg	4.5mg	4mg	3.5mg	3mg	*

*Miss a dose; give 1-2mg the next day (if INR >4.5, miss 2 doses).

●Stop heparin when INR >2, and tell the lab he's no longer on heparin.

Antidotes Consult a haematologist. Stop anticoagulation; if further
steps needed, protamine sulfate can counteract heparin: 1mg IVI neutral-
izes 100u heparin given within 15min. Max dose: 50mg (if exceeded, may
itself have anticoagulant effect). Give oral vitamin K 10–20mg PO, and
do INR ~8h later. *If bleeding:* Give vitamin K *slowly* IV (Konakion MM®) for
warfarin poisoning: 5mg for serious bleeding, 0.5–2mg for simple
haematuria or epistaxis; consider 0.5mg if INR >7 without any bleeding.
This takes some hours to act and may last for weeks. If serious bleeding,
and INR↑, give a concentrate of factors II, IX and X (+ VII if available, or, if
unavailable, use fresh frozen plasma IVI).

Warfarin: guidelines for target levels for INR

The target level represents a balance between too little anticoagulation (and risk of thrombo-embolism) and too much anticoagulation (risk of bleeding). Since the risks of thrombo-embolism vary with the clinical situation, optimum INR varies. Recommendations are likely to change as further trials are done: check with a haematologist.

Choose a target INR within the range (not the range itself). This reduces the chance that the INR will stray outside the optimum range.[2]

The incidence of fatal bleeding due to warfarin is ~0.3/100 patient years. Severe bleeding is ~10-fold more common.

- Prosthetic heart valves. US guidelines are an INR of 2.5–3.5. A recent European trial suggests 3–4.9.[4] With higher risk valves (caged ball; tilting disc; mitral and aortic valves), aim perhaps for 4–4.9; with lower risk valves aim eg for ~3.
- Atrial fibrillation: US guidelines[5] are 2–3. A recent European trial suggests 2–3.9—but another trial has found that INR levels of >2 confer no added protection from stroke (but if the ratio was 1.7 the risk of stroke was 2-fold higher than if the ratio was 2).[6] So cautious doctors may favour a mid-Atlantic range of 2.5–3.5 (which offers a margin of error at both ends), particularly if the risk of stroke is low (no diabetes mellitus or past stroke or TIA, no hypertension; aged <65yrs).[7] An alternative (but a slightly less good one) for these low-risk patients is aspirin, particularly if the risk of bleeding is high (serious co-morbidity, or difficulty with monitoring INR).[8]
- Pulmonary embolism and above-knee DVT. Aim for INR of 2–3.

Duration of anticoagulation in DVT/PE (A rough guide)
6 weeks if the cause will go away (eg post-op immobility); 6 months if no cause found; indefinitely for identified, enduring causes.

1 A Schafer 1996 *NEJM* 334 724 2 S Fihn 1995 *NEJM* 333 54 3 Modified Fennerty regimen 1992 *Drug Ther Bul* 30 77 4 J Hirsh 1992 *Chest* 102 3125 5 S Cannegieter 1995 *NEJM* 333 11 & European Atrial Fibrillation Study Group 1995 *NEJM* 333 5 6 E Hylek 1996 *NEJM* 335 540 7 F Rosendaal 1996 335 587 8 J Mant 1997 *BMJ* i 1563

⚕ Leukaemia and the houseofficer

Leukaemic patients often fall ill suddenly. Aim to start safe treatment while awaiting advice. Major concerns are infection, bleeding, hyperviscosity (p618), and keeping IV lines open—and the line to your patient's hopes and fears. If you take time to explain and encourage, then accepting even the most difficult treatments may become possible.

In those with nonspecific confusion/drowsiness, do blood cultures and exclude hypoglycaemia, as well as the tests on p446.

Neutropenic regimen (for patients with a WCC ≤1.0 × 10^9/L)
►Close liaison with a microbiologist is essential.
● Full barrier nursing is often impossible, simple hand-washing is probably most important. Use a side room.
● Look for infection (mouth, perineum, axilla, IVI site). Do swabs.
● Avoid IM injections (the danger is an infected haematoma).
● Wash perineum after defecation. Swab moist skin with chlorhexidine. Avoid unnecessary rectal examinations. Give hydrogen peroxide mouth washes/2h and Candida prophylaxis (p195).
● TPR every 4h. High-calorie diet; no salads (Pseudomonas risk).

After taking cultures (blood, urine, sputum, Hickman line) and CXR, treat any known infection. If T° >38°C for >4–6h, or the patient is toxic, assume septicaemia, and start 'blind' broad-spectrum antibiotics, eg piperacillin and netilmicin ± vancomycin (p180). Check local preferences.

If there are chest signs consider treatment for *Pneumocystis* (co-trimoxazole ie trimethoprim 20mg/kg and sulfamethoxazole 100mg/kg per day PO/IV in 4 divided doses) but remember TB.

Continue antibiotics until afebrile for 5 days and neutrophils recover (>0.5 × 10^9/L). If fever persists despite antibiotics, consider CMV or fungal infection (eg Candida or Aspergillus, p244).

There may be a rôle for genetically engineered, recombinant human granulocyte-colony stimulating factor (rhG-CSF, or recombinant human granulocyte macrophage-colony stimulating factor (Gm-CSF). These stimulate neutrophil production (Gm-CSF stimulates production of all granulocytes and monocytes, and may allow intensive chemotherapy[1]—in theory!).

Other dangers *Cell lysis syndrome*: Prevent K^+↑ and urate↑ after massive destruction of cells by giving a high fluid intake ± allopurinol precytotoxics. *Hyperviscosity*: If WCC is >100 ×10^9/L WBC thrombi may form in brain, lung, and heart (leucostasis). Avoid transfusing before lowering WCC eg with hydroxyurea (=hydroxycarbamide) or leukopheresis as blood viscosity rises (risk of leucostasis↑). If transfusion vital, keep Hb <9g/dL.

Disseminated intravascular coagulation (DIC) A pathological activation of coagulation mechanisms may occur in any malignancy (also infection, trauma, or obstetric bleeding) Release of procoagulant agents leads to clotting factor and platelet consumption (consumption coagulopathy). Fibrin strands fill small vessels, slicing (haemolysing) passing RBCs. *Signs:* Extensive bruising, old venepuncture sites start bleeding, renal failure, gangrene, bleeding anywhere (eg uterus, lungs, CNS). *Tests:* Consult lab, as special bottles (kept in fridges) are used. Film: broken RBCs (schistocytes). Platelets↓; PT↑; APTT↑; fibrinogen↓ (correlates best with severity); fibrin degradation products↑. Blood may not clot in plain bottles.
Treat the cause where possible and give supportive treatment, eg accurate fluid balance, monitor urine volume hourly by catheter. Give 2 units fresh frozen plasma IV at once while expert advice is sought; platelets and blood may be needed. The rôle of heparin is controversial: prechemotherapy low-dose heparin may prevent DIC in acute promyelocytic leukaemia (a common cause of DIC).

1 *Drug Ther Bul* 1993 31 33

Acute lymphoblastic leukaemia (ALL)

Most leukaemias are caused by specific gene mutations, deletions or translocation. ALL manifests as a neoplastic proliferation of lymphoblasts.

Immunological classification *Common (c) ALL:* (~75%) Defined by reaction with specific antilymphoblast antibody. Phenotypically pre-B (ie the cells carry the same surface antigen as the pre-B lymphocyte). Any age may be affected, commonly 2–4yr-olds. ♂:♀ ≈1:1.

T-cell ALL: Any age but peak in adolescent males, eg presenting with a mediastinal mass and a high WCC.

B-cell ALL: Rare. Bad prognosis. Immunoglobulins present on blast cells.

Null-cell ALL: Undifferentiated, lacking any markers.

Morphological classification The FAB system (French, American, British) divides ALL into 3 types: (L1, L2, L3) by microscopic appearance.

The Patient Signs are due to marrow failure: anaemia, infection, and bleeding. Also: bone pain, arthritis, splenomegaly, lymphadenopathy, thymic enlargement, CNS involvement—eg cranial nerve palsies.

Common infections: (Eg relating to pancytopenia following chemotherapy): Zoster, CMV, measles, candidiasis, *Pneumocystis pneumonii* pneumonia, bacterial septicaemia. Consider use of immune serum for patients in contact with measles or zoster when on chemotherapy.

Diagnosis Characteristic cells in blood and bone marrow.

Treatment ●*Supportive care:* Blood and platelet transfusions, IV antibiotics (p598) at the first sign of infection.
- *Preventing infections:* The neutropenic regimen (p598); barrier nursing; prophylactic antibiotics (eg co-trimoxazole to prevent *Pneumocystis pneumonii* pneumonia—but beware: this may worsen neutropenia).
- *Chemotheraphy:* As in most leukaemias, patients are entered into national trials. A typical programme is in 3 steps:

1 *Remission induction:* This may be achieved with vincristine, prenisolone, L-asparaginase, and daunorubicin.

2 *CNS prophylaxis:* Intrathecal (or high-dose IV) methotrexate; CNS irradiation.

3 *Consolidation:* Courses of high-dose chemotherapy, eg—mercaptopurine (daily), methotrexate (weekly), and vincristine and prednisolone (monthly) for 2 years. Relapse is common in blood, CNS, or testis. Cure rate in children: ~70%. More details: *OHCS* p190.

Haematological remission means no evidence of leukaemia in the blood, a normal or recovering blood count, and less than 5% blasts in a normal regenerating bone marrow.

Marrow transplant (p602) Consider if poor prognosis. Often this is the only way to cure those showing t(9;22)—see below.[1]

Quality of life Think of ingenious ways of making life better (especially while barrier nursed). Wigs for alopecia after chemotherapy. Avoid repeated venepuncture by using a Hickman CVP line—a central line with a long, Dacron®-cuffed, subcutaneous portion (risk of infection↓).

Bad prognosis if:[2] Adult; male; Philadelphia translocation [t(9;22) (q34:q11)], *OHCS* p190; presentation with CNS signs or WCC >100 × 10⁹/L; B cell phenotype. Cure rates for children are 70–90%; for adults only 35% (0–20% if >60yrs old, where there is a second peak in incidence).

The future may lie in tailoring therapy to the exact gene defect. PCR can monitor elimination of affected cells by standard drugs, monoclonal antibodies, gene-targeted retinoids, cytokines, vaccines, or T-cell infusions.[3]

1 D Scheinberg 1995 *Lancet* 346 455   2 D Hoelzer 1993 *NEJM* 329 1343

Acute myeloid leukaemia (AML)

This neoplastic proliferation of blast cells is derived from marrow myeloid elements. It is a very rapidly progressive malignancy (death in ~2 months if untreated, with ~20% 3-year survival after chemotherapy).

Morphological classification (FAB—ie French, American, and British)

M1:	Undifferentiated blast cells	M5:	Monocytic
M2:	Myeloblastic	M6:	Erythroleukaemia
M3:	Promyelocytic	M7:	Megakaryoblastic leukaemia
M4:	Myelomonocytic		
M4eo:	Myelomonocytic with dysplastic eosinophils		

Incidence 1 in 10,000/yr. Increases with age. AML is getting more common as long-term complication of chemotherapy eg for lymphoma.

The Patient needs assessing in the following 3 areas:

Marrow failure	Leukaemic infiltration	Constitutional upset
Anaemia	Bone pain; tender sternum	Malaise
Infection:	CNS signs (cord compression,	Weakness
often Gram −ve	cranial nerve lesions)	Fever
Bleeding eg	Gum, testes, orbit (proptosis)	*Other features* poly-
petechiae	Hepatosplenomegaly	arthritis; skin/peri-
DIC	Lymphadenopathy	anal involvement

Diagnosis WCC variable. Blast cells may be few in the peripheral blood, so diagnosis depends on bone marrow biopsy. Differentiation from ALL depends on finding granules in the abnormal cells and Auer rods (may represent amalgamating granules). Cytogenetic analysis (eg type of mutation) may affect treatment recommendations, and helps guide prognosis.

Complications Infection is the major problem, related to both the disease and its treatment. Be alert to septicaemia (p598). Intra-oral infections are common. The place for prophylactic antibiotics is uncertain.

Chemotherapy causes ↑plasma urate levels (from tumour lysis)—so give allopurinol with chemotherapy, and keep well-hydrated with IV fluids.

Big nodes can cause 'mass effects', eg dyspnoea. Leucostasis (WBC thrombi, causing pulmonary or CNS infarcts) may occur if WCC↑↑: get help.

Treatment *Supportive care:* Blood and platelet transfusions. Barrier nursing, IV antibiotics. *Pitfalls in diagnosis of infection:* AML itself causes fever, common organisms present oddly, few antibodies are made, rare organisms—particularly fungi (especially candida or aspergillus).

Chemotherapy is very intensive, resulting in long periods of neutropenia + platelets↓. The main drugs used include daunorubicin, cytosine arabinoside and thioguanine (=tioguanine). Prognosis: ~20% long-term survival.

Bone marrow transplant (BMT)[1] Allogeneic transplants from histocompatible siblings or from unrelated donors (accessed via international computer-held databases) or syngeneic transplants from a twin may be indicated in first remissions. The idea is to destroy all leukaemic cells and the entire immune system by cyclophosphamide + total body irradiation, and then repopulate the marrow by transplantation from a matched donor infused IVI. BMT allows the most intensive chemotherapy regimens because marrow suppression is not an issue. Cyclosporin (=ciyclosporin) ± methotrexate may be used to reduce the effect of the new marrow attacking the patient's body (graft versus host disease). Complications: graft versus host disease; infections (CMV is common); veno-occlusive disease, relapse of leukaemia. Autologous transplantation is also effective. *Prognosis post bone marrow transplant:* Perhaps 60% long-term survivors. Gonadal function appears to return to normal after induction.

---

1 MRC-AML10 1998 *Lancet* 351 700—looked at relapse after 1st remission: adding autologous BMT to 4 courses of chemotherapy (starting eg with daunorubicin, cytarabine + thioguanine) ↓risk of relapse & improved survival.

Chronic lymphocytic leukaemia (CLL)

This is a monoclonal proliferation of well-differentiated lymphocytes—almost always (99%) B cells. The patient is usually over 40. Men are affected × 2 as often as women. CLL constitutes 25% of all leukaemias.

Staging (*Correlates with survival*) 0 Absolute lymphocytosis >15×10⁹/L. I Stage 0 + enlarged lymph nodes. II Stage I+enlarged liver or spleen. III Stage II+anaemia (Hb <11g/dL). IV Stage III + platelets <100 × 10⁹/L.

Symptoms (None in 25%.) Bleeding, weight↓, infection and anorexia.

Signs Enlarged, rubbery, non-tender nodes. Late hepatosplenomegaly.

Film Lymphocytosis may be marked. Often normochromic normocytic anaemia. Autoimmune haemolysis may contribute to this. Thrombocytopenia from marrow infiltration (rarely antiplatelet antibodies).

Complications 1 Autoimmune haemolysis. 2 Infection—bacterial (mostly of respiratory tract, as a result of hypogammaglobulinaemia)—or viral (altered cell-mediated immunity). 3 Bone marrow failure.

Natural history Some remain in *status quo* for years, or even regress. Usually nodes slowly enlarge (± lymphatic obstruction). Death is often via infection (zoster, pneumococcus, meningococcus, TB, candida, aspergillosis) or transformation to aggressive lymphoma (Richter's syn.).

Treatment *Chemotherapy* is often not needed, but may postpone marrow failure. Chlorambucil is used to ↓ lymphocyte count. Dose: eg 0.1–0.2mg/kg daily PO. Steroids are used, eg in autoimmune haemolysis.
Radiotherapy: Use for relief of lymphadenopathy or splenomegaly.
Supportive care: Transfusions, prophylactic antibiotics, occasionally IV human immunoglobulin.

Prognosis Often good: depends on stage.

Chronic myeloid leukaemia (CML)

CML is characterized by uncontrolled proliferation of myeloid cells. It accounts for 15% of leukaemias. It is a myeloproliferative disorder (p612) having features in common with these diseases: eg splenomegaly (often massive). It commonly presents with constitutional symptoms. It occurs most often in middle age. There is a slight male predominance.

Philadelphia chromosome (Ph¹) A hybrid chromosome comprising translocation between the long arm of chromosome 9 and the long arm of chromosome 22—t(9;22). The Philadelphia chromosome is present in granulocyte, RBC, and platelet precursors in >95% of those with CML. Those without Ph¹ have a worse prognosis. (Some patients have a masked translocation—cytogenetics do not show the Ph¹, but the bcr/abl gene rearrangement is detectable by molecular genetic techniques.)

Symptoms Mostly chronic and insidious, eg weight↓, tiredness, gout, fever, sweats, bleeding, or abdominal pain. 10% are detected by chance.

Signs Splenomegaly, variable hepatomegaly, anaemia, bruising.

Tests WBC↑↑ (often >100 × 10⁹/L), Hb↓ or normal, platelets variable. urate and alk phos↑; B₁₂↑. Leucocyte alk phos↓ (on stained film).

Natural history Variable; median survival 3–5yrs; 3 phases: *chronic*, lasting months or years of few, if any, symptoms→ *accelerated phase*, with increasing symptoms, spleen size, and difficulty in controlling counts→ *blast transformation*, with features of acute leukaemia ± death.

Treatment Hydroxyurea (=hydroxycarbamide) 0.5–2g/24h PO is the mainstay in the chronic phase. Busulfan is rarely used. Monitor FBC to avoid pancytopenia. Treatment of transformed CML is poor. Some types have lymphoblastic characteristics (treat as for ALL). Treatment of myeloblastic transformation rarely achieves lasting remission. Another option is autologous bone marrow transplant starting with chemotherapy and whole-body radiotherapy followed by autografting of patient's previously stored haemopoietic stem cells. Allogeneic transplantation, from an HLA-matched donor, should be considered if eg <55yrs, during chronic phase.[1] ~50–60% of transplanted patients will be cured. Trials show that α-interferon may have a rôle, with improved median survival compared with standard chemotherapy (eg 5.5yrs vs 4.7yrs).[2] It is toxic.

1 JA Hansen 1998 *NEJM* **338** 962   2 L Kumar 1995 *Lancet* **346** 984

Hodgkin's lymphoma [Thomas Hodgkin, Guy's,UK 1798–1866]

Lymphomas are malignant proliferations of lymphoid tissue. Histology divides into Hodgkin's and non-Hodgkin's types. In the former, characteristic cells with mirror-image nuclei occur (Reed–Sternberg cells)—often containing the Epstein–Barr genome, so suggesting one cause.

Classification (In order of incidence)	**Prognosis**
Nodular sclerosing	Good
Mixed cellularity*	Good
Lymphocyte predominant (probably non-Hodgkin's)	Good
Lymphocyte-depleted*	Poor

*Higher incidence and worse prognosis if HIV+ve.[1]

The Patient Often presents with enlarged, painless nodes, eg in neck or axillae. Rarely there may be alcohol-induced pain or features due to mass effects of nodes. 25% have constitutional upset, eg fever, weight loss, night sweats, pruritus, and lethargy. The term *Pel–Ebstein fever* implies fever alternating with long periods (15–28 days) of normal or low temperature: it is, at best, rare—and some have called it mythical.*

Signs: Lymphadenopathy (note position, consistency, mobility, size, tenderness). Look for weight loss, anaemia, hepatosplenomegaly.

Tests Node biopsy for diagnosis. FBC, film, ESR, LFTs, urate, Ca^{2+}, CXR, bone marrow biopsy, abdominal CT/MRI (p738), lymphangiography rarely. Staging laparotomy involves splenectomy with liver and lymph node biopsy but may not influence final outcome and is rarely done nowadays.

Staging (Influences treatment and prognosis.)
I Confined to single lymph node region.
II Involvement of 2 or more regions on same side of the diaphragm.
III Involvement of nodes on both sides of the diaphragm.
IV Spread beyond the lymph nodes.

Each stage is subdivided into A (no systemic symptoms other than pruritus) or B—presence of weight loss >10% in last 6 months, unexplained fever >38°C or night sweats. These indicate more extensive disease. Extranodal disease may be indicated by subscripted E, eg I-A$_E$.

Treatment Radiotherapy for stages IA and IIA. Chemotherapy for IIA through to IVB. Chemotherapy examples: 'ABVD'—**A**dreamycin, **B**leomycin, **V**inblastine, and **D**acarbazine and MOPP—**M**ustine (=chlormethine), **O**ncovin® (vincristine), **P**rocarbazine, and **P**rednisolone. More intensive regimens are used, eg for advanced disease. Autologous marrow transplants are useful in relapsed disease. *Peripheral stem-cell transplantation:* Autologous or allogeneic transplantation of blood progenitor cells help restore marrow function after myeloablative therapy—as do agents which stimulate progenitor cells, eg rhG-CSF (Filgrastim®, p598).[2]
Complications of treatment: Hypothyroidism; lung fibrosis and other radiation SE (p692). Chemotherapy—nausea, alopecia, infertility in men, infection and second malignancies, especially acute myeloid leukaemia and non-Hodgkin's lymphoma. Both may produce myelosuppression.

5-year survival Depends on stage and grade, from >90% in IA lymphocyte-predominant disease to <40% with IVB lymphocyte-depleted.

Emergency presentations Infection; marrow failure (rare in Hodgkin's); svc obstruction. This latter presents with JVP↑, a sensation of fullness in the head, dyspnoea, blackouts, and facial oedema; ►*Arrange same day radiotherapy*; high-dose corticosteroids may also be useful.

---

*Pel-Ebstein fever was dismissed by Richard Asher (*Talking Sense*, Pitman), as a fever existing only thanks to its having been exotically named (the 1885 patients of Dr PK Pel had no histology, and fevers in Hodgkin's are *usually* non-specific). Another unfair reason for consigning it to myth is the fact that the 1975 paper proving its existence (and its relation to cyclical changes in node size) does not come up in literature searches as Wilhelm *Ebstein* (1836-1912) is misspelled *Epstein* throughout (*Cancer* 1975 **36** 2026) 1 U Tirelli 1994 BMJ i 1148 2 L Kumar 1995 *Lancet Rev.* **346** s9

Non-Hodgkin's lymphoma

This group includes all lymphomas without the Reed–Sternberg cell and is a very diverse group. Most are B-cell proliferations. Not all are centred on lymph nodes. An example of extra-nodal tissues generating lymphoma is mucosa-associated lymphoid tissue—MALT (gastric MALT is associated with *H pylori*, and may only regress when this is eradicated[■]). Incidence has doubled since 1970 (to 1:10,000) perhaps from immunosuppression from sunlight exposure, HIV, HTLV-1, EBV, and petrochemicals.[1]

The Patient ●Typically an adult with lymphadenopathy. ●Extra-nodal spread occurs early, so presentation may be in skin, bone, gut, CNS, or lung. ●Often symptomless. ●Pancytopenia occurs (marrow dysplasia). ●Infection is common. ●Systemic signs as in Hodgkin's.

Examine all over. Note nodes (if any is >10cm across, staging is advanced[2]). Do ENT exam if GI lymphoma (GI and ENT lymphoma often co-exist).

Diagnosis & staging As for Hodgkin's (staging is less important as 70% have widespread disease at presentation). Always do node biopsy and CT/MRI (chest, abdomen, and pelvis), FBC, U&E, LFT. Consider Ba meal, lymphangiogram, cytology of pleural or peritoneal effusion; CSF cytology if CNS signs.

Histology This is something of a quagmire, as classificatory systems are complex and changing (none is satisfactory). It is the job of the histologist to tell the clinician whether the lymphoma is low- or high-grade.

Low-grade lymphomas are more indolent but are incurable; the high-grade types are more aggressive, but long-term cure is achievable.

The low grade group includes lymphocytic (comparable to CLL but mainly in lymphoid tissue), immunocytic, and centrocytic lymphomas. In the high grade are centroblastic, immunoblastic and lymphoblastic types. The Revised European-American classification of Lymphoid Hyperplasia (REAL) system is one classificatory system making use of genotypic analysis (immunoglobulin and T-cell receptor gene rearrangements) and it associates lymphoma types with specific chromosome breaks).

Survival This is worse if the patient is elderly or symptomatic, or there is bulky disease, or anaemia at presentation. Histology is also important, but is by no means straightforward. Typical 5-year survival figures for treated patients might be 30% for high-grade lymphomas, and over 50% for low-grade lymphomas, but the picture is very variable.

Treatment If symptomless and low grade, none may be needed (some may remit). Chlorambucil or cyclophosphamide can control symptoms. Splenectomy may help. Radiotherapy can be used for local bulky disease. Purine analogues (eg 2-chlorodeoxyadenosine, fluarabine) are under trial.

If high grade, a variant of CHOP: cyclophosphamide, doxorubicin hydrochloride, vincristine (Oncovin®) with prednisolone may be used; other regimens are under trial.[2] If the histology is lymphoblastic, treat as ALL. In advanced disease, uncertainty is much greater.[3][■]

Burkitt's lymphoma (A lymphoblastic lymphoma mainly in African children). It is associated with Epstein–Barr virus (EBV) infection and shows a 14q+/8q- chromosomal translocation (immunogenic loci and myc oncogene). Jaw tumours are common, usually with GI involvement. Histology: 'starry sky' appearance (isolated histiocytes on background of abnormal lymphoblasts). Spectacular remission may result from a single dose of a cytotoxic drug—eg cyclophosphamide 30mg/kg IV.

Causes of lymphadenopathy See p50. Also angioimmunoblastic lymphadenopathy (skin rashes, fever—seen in the elderly; histology is characteristic; >50% progress to lymphoma).

1 N O'Connon 1995 *Lancet* 345 1522 & N Harris 1994 *Blood* 84 1361–92 2 *Lancet* 1997 349 34 & 664 3 S O'Reilly 1992 *BMJ* i 1682 & *Cancer* 1982 49 2112–35[■]

Bone marrow, and bone marrow failure

The bone marrow is responsible for haemopoiesis and, in adults, is found in the vertebrae, sternum, ribs, skull and proximal long bones, although it may expand in some anaemias (eg thalassaemia). All cells are thought to arise from an early, pluripotent stem cell which divides in an asymmetric way to produce a committed progenitor and other stem cells. Committed progenitors then undergo further differentiation before their release as formed elements into the blood.

Bone marrow failure usually produces pancytopenia, often with sparing of lymphocyte counts. Bone marrow biopsy will help find the cause.

Causes of pancytopenia Bone marrow failure, below; hypersplenism; SLE, megaloblastic anaemia, paroxysmal nocturnal haemoglobinuria.

Causes of marrow failure
1 Stem cell failure: eg aplastic anaemia—this can be toxic (chloramphenicol, benzene), immunological, congenital, or viral (eg hepatitis B; parvoviruses infect marrow erythroblasts, see *OHCS* p214).
2 Infiltration: from malignancy, TB.
3 Fibrosis: eg myelofibrosis.
4 Abnormal differentiation of a genetically damaged clone of cells, eg myelodysplasia (a premalignant condition), HIV.

Aplastic anaemia *Presentation:* pancytopenia with a hypoplastic marrow (ie the marrow stops producing cells). *Causes:* as above.

Incidence: 10–20 per million per year. Presents as bleeding, anaemia or infection. In approximately 50% of there is response to androgens ± immunosuppressive therapy.

Treatment of aplastic anaemia: The principle is to support the blood count (see below) while undertaking definitive treatment, which, for the severely affected young patient, is marrow transplantation (if there is a histocompatible sibling donor). Otherwise cyclosporin (=ciclosporin) and anti-thymocyte globulin may be effective.

Bone marrow support The symptoms of bone marrow failure are due to the pancytopenia. Red cells survive for ~120 days, platelets for an average 8 days, and neutrophils for 1–2 days so early problems are mainly from neutropenia and thrombocytopenia.

Erythrocytes: A one-unit transfusion should raise the Hb by about 1g/dL. See p102. Transfusion may drop the platelet count so it may be necessary to give platelets before and after.

Platelets: Spontaneous bleeding is unlikely if platelets >20 × 10^9/L, but risk of traumatic bleeds is great if <40 × 10^9/L. Platelets are stored at 22°C, should not be put in the fridge, and may require irradiation prior to use (eg if marrow transplant, or severely immunosuppressed). Indications for transfusion: counts <10 × 10^9/L (not in ITP, p592), excessive bleeds, and DIC. Crossmatching is not needed but platelets should be ABO compatible (+Rh matched, if of child-bearing age). 4u of fresh platelets should raise the count to >40 × 10^9/L in an adult. Check the dose required with the lab.

Neutrophils: Use a 'neutropenic regimen' if the count <0.5 × 10^9/L. See p598. The place of neutrophil transfusions is unclear. They may be tried in proven, continued bacteraemia but are short-lived, expensive, and may transmit infection or cause pneumonitis without offering any benefit.

Bone marrow biopsy Ideally an aspirate *and* trephine should be taken, usually from the posterior iliac crest, although aspirates may also be taken from the anterior iliac crest or the sternum. Aspirates should be smeared promptly onto slides (≥8). Thrombocytopenia is rarely a contraindication. Severe coagulation disorders may need to be corrected. Apply pressure afterwards (lie on that side for 1–2h if platelets are low).

The myeloproliferative disorders

These form a group of disorders characterized by proliferation of precursors for myeloid elements—RBCs, WBCs, and platelets. While the cells proliferate they also retain the ability to differentiate. The 4 disorders share several features, including the fact that all may present with constitutional symptoms such as fever, weight loss, night sweats, itch and malaise.

Classification is by the cell type which is proliferating:*

RBC	→	Polycythaemia rubra vera (PRV).
WBC	→	Chronic myeloid leukaemia (CML, p604).
Platelets	→	Essential thrombocythaemia.
Fibroblasts	→	Primary myelofibrosis (reactive and not part of the malignant clone).

*Each may undergo transformation to acute leukaemia.

The blood count reflects 2 processes: the *proliferating cell line*—may involve other myeloid elements (eg in PRV, RBC↑; but there may be rises in WBC ± platelets too)—and *marrow infiltration* which may ↓normal cell numbers.

Polycythaemia may be relative (plasma volume↓) or absolute (RBC mass↑). The way to distinguish these is by red cell mass estimation using radioactive chromium. Relative polycythaemia is often due to dehydration (eg alcohol or diuretics). Absolute polycythaemia may be primary (polycythaemia rubra vera, PRV) or secondary, eg from smoking, chronic lung disease, tumours (fibroids, hepatoma, hypernephroma), or altitude.

Polycythaemia rubra vera *Cause:* Neoplasia of a clone from one multipotent cell whose erythroid progenitor offspring are unusual in being sensitive eg to insulin-like growth factor ± interlukin-3, and in not needing erythropoietin to avoid apoptosis (p593).[1] *Incidence:* 1.5/100,000/yr; peak age: 45–60yrs. *Signs:* ●↑PCV ●↑WBC ●↑Platelets or normal ●↓MCV ●↑Spleen (in 60%). *Presentation* is determined by hyperviscosity (CNS signs, p618; angina; Raynaud's, p706); itch—typically after a hot bath) and ↑RBC turnover (gout). It may also present with bruising, or after a routine FBC. *Diagnosis:* Raised red cell mass (>125% of predicted—⁵¹Cr studies) and splenomegaly in the presence of normal P_aO_2. Marrow shows erythroid hyperplasia. Leucocyte alk phos (LAP) usually↑ (LAP↓ in CML). B_{12}↑. *Treatment:* Refer. Aim to keep PCV <50%, eg by venesection or hydroxyurea (=hydroxycarbamide) if platelet count or WCC difficult to control. In older patients consider IV ³²P (it is leukaemogenic) or busulfan eg 4mg/day PO. *Prognosis:* Variable—many often remain well for many years but others will die from myelofibrosis, leukaemia, or thrombotic disorders from hyperviscosity and/or malfunctioning platelets. Do FBC every 3 months.

Essential thrombocythaemia is characterized by ↑↑ platelet counts, (500–1000 × 10⁹/L, + abnormal morphology and function). *Presentation:* Bleeding; thrombosis; mnoneuritis multiplex from microvascular occlusion. *Treatment:* Busulfan or hydroxyurea (=hydroxycarbamide) may be needed for symptoms or if the platelet count is >800 × 10⁹/L, however platelet count correlates poorly with the risk of thrombosis. Aspirin is useful, especially if there is any evidence of a thrombotic diathesis. *Causes of* ↑platelet count: Kawasaki disease (OHCS p750); myeloproliferative or inflammatory disease (eg rheumatoid); bleeding; post-splenectomy. ~50% of those with unexplained thrombocytosis will have malignancy.

Primary myelofibrosis (myelofibrosis) There is intense marrow fibrosis with resultant haemopoiesis in the spleen and liver (myeloid metaplasia) causing massive splenomegaly. *Presentation:* Variable—constitutional upset, splenomegaly, bone marrow failure. *Film:* Leuco-erythroblastic (p576); tear-drop RBCs. Hb↓. Marrow tap: dry. *Treatment:* Supportive (p610), iron and folate supplements. *Other causes of marrow fibrosis:* Any myeloproliferative disorder, lymphoma, secondary carcinoma, TB, leukaemia, irradiation.

1 R Schwartz 1998 *NEJM* 338 613

Myeloma

Myeloma is a plasma cell neoplasm which produces diffuse bone marrow infiltration and focal osteolytic deposits. An M band (M for mono-clonal—not IgM) is seen on serum and/or urine electrophoresis.

Incidence 5/100,000. Peak age: 70yrs. Sex ratio: equal.

Classification Based on the principal neoplastic cell product:

IgG	55%
IgA	25%
Light chain disease	20%

60% of IgG and IgA myelomas also produce free immunoglobulin (Ig) light chains which are filtered by the kidney and may be detectable as Bence Jones protein (these precipitate on heating and redissolve on boiling). They may cause renal damage or, rarely, amyloidosis.

The Patient ●Bone pain/tenderness is common, and often postural, eg back, ribs, long bones, and shoulder—not extremities. (25% have no clinical or x-ray signs of bone disease at presentation.) ●Pathological fracture (eg rib). ●Lassitude (from anaemia, renal failure, or dehydration via proximal tubule dysfunction, from light chain precipitation). ●Pyo-genic infection. ●Amyloid. ●Neuropathy. ●Signs of hyperviscosity (p618): ●Visual acuity↓ ± haemorrhages/exudates on fundoscopy. ●Bleeding.

Diagnosis Many plasma cells in marrow; an M band or urine light chains on serum/urine electrophoresis (Bence Jones proteins, p650) is sup-portive evidence. Other tests: FBC, ESR↑, marrow. Alk phos usually nor-mal (unless healing fracture). Non-myeloma immunoglobulins↓; urea, creatinine, urate and Ca²⁺↑ in ~40%; bone x-ray: punched-out lesions (pepper-pot skull), osteoporosis. Bone scintigrams may be normal.

Treatment[1] *Supportive:* Bone pain, anaemia, and renal failure are the main problems so give analgesia and transfusions as needed. Advise high fluid intake. Solitary lesions may have *radiotherapy*, and may heal.

Chemotherapy: None is curative. 1st-line is usually melphalan, either as a 4-day course each month, or combined (eg with the ABCM regimen—Adriamycin, Bleomycin, Cyclophosphamide, Melphalan). ~60% respond so that the paraprotein level falls before reaching a plateau phase. Treatment is usually stopped at this point, and restarted when the pro-tein level begins to rise (escape phase). High-dose chemotherapy and autologous marrow transplantation improve results. Allogeneic trans-plantation may be curative in young patients. If hypercalcaemia is a prob-lem, use bisphosphonates (see below and p644). Monitor FBC and paraprotein.

Death is commonly due to renal failure, infection or haemorrhage.

Survival Worse if urea >10mmol/L or Hb <7.5g/dL. 50% alive at 2yrs.

Dangers

1 Ca²⁺↑: p644. Use IV saline 0.9% 4–6 litres/day with careful fluid bal-ance. Consider steroids, eg hydrocortisone 100mg/8h IV. Bisphos-phonates or mithramycin may be needed in refractory disease.

2 Hyperviscosity (p618), causing cognition↓, disturbed vision, and bleed-ing. Plasmapheresis can remove light chains (so helping renal function).

3 Acute renal failure may be precipitated by IVU. See p382.

1 IC MacLennan 1994 *BMJ* i 1033

Ⓡ Paraproteinaemia

Paraproteinaemia denotes presence in the <u>circulation of immunoglobulin produced by a single clone</u> of plasma cells or their precursors. The paraprotein is recognized as a sharp M band (M for Monoclonal, not IgM) on serum electrophoresis*. There are 6 major categories:

1 *Multiple myeloma:* See p614.

2 *Waldenström's macroglobulinaemia:* This is a lymphoplasmacytoid malignancy <u>producing an IgM paraprotein,</u> lymphadenopathy and splenomegaly. CNS and ocular symptoms of hyperviscosity may occur (p618). <u>Chlorambucil and plasmapheresis* (p618) may help.</u>

3 *Primary amyloidosis:* See below.

4 *Monoclonal gammopathy* (benign paraproteinaemia) is common (3% >70yrs) and may be misdiagnosed as myeloma (but paraprotein level is stable, immunosuppression and urine light chains are absent and there is little plasma cell marrow infiltrate.

5 *Paraproteinaemia <u>in lymphoma or leukaemia:</u>* Eg 5% of CLL.

6 *Heavy chain disease:* Production of free heavy chains. α chain disease is the most important, causing <u>malabsorption</u> from <u>infiltration of small bowel wall. It may terminate in lymphoma.</u>

Amyloidosis

This is a disorder characterized by extracellular deposits of an abnormal, degradation-resistant protein called amyloid. Various proteins, under a range of stimuli, may polymerize to form amyloid fibrils—which are detected by +ve staining with Congo Red and by showing apple-green birefringence in polarized light.

Classification

1 *Systemic:*
- Immunocyte dyscrasia (fibrils of immunoglobulin light chain fragments, known as 'AL' amyloid).
- Reactive amyloid ('AA' amyloid—a non-glycosylated protein).
- Hereditary amyloid (eg type 1 familial amyloid polyneuropathy).

2 *Localized:* ●Cutaneous. ●Cerebral. ●Cardiac. ●Endocrine.

AL amyloid (primary amyloidosis): This is associated with monoclonal proliferation of plasma cells—eg in myeloma. Clinical features include carpal tunnel syndrome, peripheral neuropathy, purpura, cardiomyopathy and macroglossia (a large tongue).

AA amyloid (secondary amyloidosis): This can occur in association with chronic infections (eg TB, bronchiectasis), inflammation (especially rheumatoid arthritis) and neoplasia. It tends to affect kidneys, liver and spleen and commonly presents as proteinuria, nephrotic syndrome[1] and hepatosplenomegaly.

The diagnosis of amyloidosis is made after Congo Red staining of affected tissue. The rectum is a favourite site for biopsy.

Treatment rarely helps. AA amyloid may improve if the primary disease is treated. Immunosuppression may cause deposits to regress.

An interesting, but rare, complication of amyloid is the intravascular absorption of factor X, causing a long prothrombin time and KCCT, and a serious coagulopathy.

1 BMJ 1996 i 1087 *Electro*phoresis and plasma*pheresis* look as though they should share endings, but they do not: Greek *phoros=bearing* (*esis=process*), but *aphairesis* is Greek for *removal.*

617

The erythrocyte sedimentation rate (ESR)

The ESR is a nonspecific indicator of the presence of disease. It measures the rate of sedimentation of RBCs in anticoagulated blood over 1 hour. If certain proteins cover red cells these will stick to each other in columns (the same phenomenon as rouleaux on the blood film, p576)—and so they will fall faster. The ESR rises with age and anaemia. A simple, reliable[1] way to allow for this is to calculate the upper limit of normal, using the Westergren method, to be (for men) age in years ÷ 2. For women the formula is (years + 10) ÷ 2. In those with a slightly abnormal ESR the best plan is probably to wait a month and repeat the test. The same advice does not hold true for patients with a markedly raised ESR (>100mm/h). In practice, most will have signs pointing to the cause—usually paraproteinaemias, other malignancy (almost always disseminated), connective tissue diseases (eg giant cell arteritis), rheumatoid arthritis, renal disease, sarcoidosis, or infection. There is a group of patients whose vague symptoms would have prompted nothing more than reassurance—were it not for a markedly raised ESR—and in whom there are no pointers to specific disease. The underlying disease (in one survey) turned out to include myeloma, giant cell arteritis, abdominal aneurysm, metastatic prostatic carcinoma, leukaemia, and lymphoma. Therefore it would be wise (after history and examination) to consider these tests: FBC, plasma electrophoresis, U&E and creatinine, PSA, chest and abdominal x-rays, and biopsy of bone marrow or temporal artery.

Some conditions *lower* the ESR, eg polycythaemia, sickle-cell anaemia, and cryoglobulinaemia. Even a slightly raised ESR in these patients should prompt one to ask: *What else is the matter?*

If ready-prepared vacuum ESR tubes (Seditainer) are used, then lower values are recorded compared with the reference method, as follows:

Seditainer:	Reference:	Seditainer:	Reference:	Seditainer:	Reference:
10	11	30	40	50	75
15	18	35	47	55	87
20	25	40	56	60	100
25	32	45	65	65	118

For CRP (an alternative to the ESR), see p650.

Hyperviscosity syndromes

These occur if the plasma viscosity rises to such a point that the microcirculation is impaired.

Causes: Myeloma (p614), Waldenström's macroglobulinaemia (p616, IgM ↑viscosity more than the same amount of IgG), polycythaemia. High leucocyte counts in leukaemia may also produce the syndrome (leucostasis).

Presentation: Visual disturbance, retinal haemorrhages, headaches, coma, and GU or GI bleeding.

The visual symptoms ('slow-flow retinopathy') may be described as 'looking through a watery car windscreen'. Other causes of slow-flow retinopathy are carotid occlusive disease and Takayasu's disease (p708).

Treatment: Removal of as little as 1 litre of blood may relieve symptoms. Plasmapheresis may help: in this process blood is withdrawn and allowed to settle in a container. The supernatant plasma is discarded, and the RBCs returned to the patient after being resuspended in a suitable medium.

The spleen and splenectomy

The spleen was a mysterious organ for many years; we now know it plays a vital immunological rôle by acting as a reservoir for lymphocytes, and in dealing with bacteraemias. Splenomegaly is a commonish problem and its causes can be divided into massive (into the RIF) and moderate.

Causes of massive splenomegaly CML, myelofibrosis, malaria (hyperreactive malarial splenomegaly), schistosomiasis, leishmaniasis, 'tropical splenomegaly' (idiopathic—Africa, SE Asia) and Gaucher's syndrome. *Moderate splenomegaly:* Infection (eg malaria, EBV, endo-carditis, TB), portal hypertension, haematological (haemolysis, leukaemia, lymphoma), connective tissue disease (RA, SLE), sarcoidosis, primary antibody deficiency (OHCS p201), CML, idiopathic. *Others:* p152.

Splenomegaly can be uncomfortable, and may lead to *hypersplenism* (ie pancytopenia as cells become trapped in the spleen's reticuloen-dothelial system, with symptoms of anaemia, infection, or bleeding). When faced with a mass in the left upper quadrant it is vital to recog-nize the spleen: ●It moves with respiration. ●It enlarges towards the RIF. ●You may feel a notch. ●'You can't get above it' (ie the top margin dis-appears under the ribs). Abdominal x-ray may help. When hunting the cause for enlargement look for lymphadenopathy and liver disease. Appropriate tests: FBC, ESR, LFTs and liver, marrow, or lymph node biopsy.

Splenectomy[1] This may be indicated for severe splenic trauma, splenic cysts, splenic (and adjacent organ) tumours, and as part of the treatment of ITP (p592), autoimmune haemolysis, and, occasion-ally, for the staging of Hodgkin's disease. Post-splenectomy, mobilize early (transient ↑platelets predisposes to thrombi). ►*The main prob-lem post-splenectomy is lifelong increased risk from infection.* Consider those with partial splenectomy also at risk. Reduce this risk by giving:
●Patient-held cards alerting health professionals to the infection risk.
●Pneumococcal vaccine (p332), >2 weeks pre-op to ensure good response. Avoid in pregnancy. Re-immunize every 5–10 years.
●*Haemophilus influenzae* type b vaccine (p192) ± meningococcal vaccine.
●Prophylactic oral antibiotics (phenoxymethylpenicillin) continuously until aged 16yrs, or for 2yrs post-splenectomy, whichever is longer.
●'Stand-by' amoxicillin, to start *at once* if any symptoms of infection.
●Warnings of risk of severe malaria, and other tropical infections.
●Urgent hospital admission if infection develops despite the above.

1 Working Party of British Committee for Standards in Haematology 1996 *BMJ* i 430

Thrombophilia[1,2]

Thrombophilia (inherited or acquired) is a primary coagulopathy resulting in a propensity to thrombosis. Note: thrombocytosis (platelets↑) and polycythaemia also cause thrombosis. It is *not* rare, and it *is* treatable—and needs special precautions in *surgery*, *pregnancy*, and *enforced inactivity*. Be alert to it in non-haemorrhagic stroke, eg if <60 years old, thrombosis at <45 years (or family history). Risk is increased by obesity, immobility, trauma (accidents or surgery), pregnancy, and malignancy.

Inherited—*Activated protein C (APC) resistance:* The commonest cause of inherited thrombophilia and, in many populations, the commonest cause of thrombo-embolism. The molecular defect is a single point mutation in factor V (V Leiden). Thrombotic risk is increased in pregnancy and those on oestrogen-containing oral contraceptives (risk ↑ by 30–35-fold in FV:Q heterozygous carriage, and by several hundred-fold in homozygous carriage—and screening *might* be appropriate with the newly available modified test for APC resistance[3]). There is ↑ risk of MI.
Antithrombin III deficiency: This affects 1:2000. Heterozygotes' thrombotic risk is 4-fold greater than with protein C or S deficiency. Homozygosity is lethal. *Protein C and protein S deficiency:* These vitamin K dependent factors act together to neutralize factors V and VIII. Heterozygotes deficient for either protein risk thrombosis, and skin necrosis (especially if using oral anticoagulants). Homozygous deficiency for either protein causes neonatal purpura fulminans—fatal if untreated.

Acquired Common causes are new progesterones in the Pill (*OHCS* p66) and the *antiphospholipid syndrome* when serum antiphospholipid antibodies are found (lupus anticoagulant and/or anticardiolipin antibody)—predisposing to venous and arterial thrombosis, thrombocytopenia, and recurrent fetal loss in pregnant women. Most do not have SLE.

Investigation *Consider special tests if recurrent or unusual thrombosis:*
Venous thrombo-embolism <40yrs   Thrombo-embolism in the family
Arterial thrombosis <30 yrs   Recurrent fetal loss
Skin necrosis (especially if on warfarin)   Neonatal thrombosis

Liaise with a haematologist. Do FBC with platelets; prothrombin time; thrombin time; activated partial thromboplastin time; and fibrinogen concentration. Further tests: activated protein C resistance (ratio), lupus anticoagulant and anticardiolipin antibodies, and looking for antithrombin III and proteins C and S deficiency (this phenotype is associated with heterozygosity or homozygosity for the factor V Leiden mutation in ≥95% of individuals). Haematologists may recommend looking directly for the V Leiden mutation, eg if already on warfarin, and other results are confusing.
    Ideally investigate while well, not pregnant, and not anticoagulated.

Treatment Treat acute thromboses with heparin, then warfarin. In antithrombin III deficiency unusually high doses of heparin may be needed (dose is difficult to determine in those with lupus anticoagulant). Ensure full heparinization. Liaise with a haematologist about introducing warfarin, and treatment duration. *Prevention:* Avoid the Pill. Advise elastic stockings. Risk of recurrent thrombosis following DVT, PE, stroke, or TIA if antiphospholipid antibody +ve is ~30%/year.[3] Aspirin or warfarin (INR <3) ↓risk to ~20%. If INR >3 on warfarin excess risk is ~nil. Pregnancy is a problem: warfarin is teratogenic. Get expert help, eg aspirin + heparin (≤10,000u/12h sc for those with ≥2 fetal losses).[4] For those with <2 fetal losses, either giving no treatment or aspirin alone might be appropriate).
    Before medium-to-major (especially orthopaedic) surgery, liaise with a haematologist. Antithrombin III cryoprecipitate may be indicated, as well as more thorough prophylaxis against post-op thromboses.

ng Ther Bul 1995 33 6 & 35 2 Brit. Soc. Haematol Guidelines 1992 *J Clin Path* 46 97-103
Khamashta *NEJM* 1995 332(15) 993 4 F Cowchock *Am J Obstet Gynecol* 1992 166 1318
AT Hattersley 1996 *Lancet* 348 343 and B Dahlback 1996 *Lancet* 347 1346e

Immunosuppressive drugs

As well as being used in leukaemias and cancers, these are used in organ and marrow transplants, rheumatoid arthritis, psoriasis, chronic hepatitis, asthma, giant cell arteritis, polymyalgia, SLE, PAN, and inflammatory bowel and other disease (so this page could figure in almost any chapter).

Prednisolone When you start long-term steroids, explain about:
- Not stopping steroids suddenly. Collapse may result, as endogenous production takes time to restart.
- Increasing the dose at times of illness/stress (eg 'flu or pre-op).
- Carrying a steroid card saying what dose is taken, and the reason.
- The importance of monitoring, eg ESR in polymyalgia. In *any* drug intervention ask ►"How will I monitor therapy?" Better still ask "Can the patient monitor himself?" eg peak flow in asthma. It is no good teaching self-monitoring if you do not also teach in detail, with written advice, about what action to take if things go wrong, eg "start prednisolone 5mg tablets, 6 a day if your morning peak flow is less than 25% of usual. Less than 25% means. . . Telephone (eg the ward or GP) if. . ." It is hard to find the right balance in teaching self-monitoring. Is it better to have a perfectly controlled disease and a patient made neurotic by a peak flow machine (for instance) or a happy-go-lucky person stumbling from one crisis to the next? The answer will depend in part on the nature and severity of the disease, and the personality of the patient. If one of the crises includes death, neurosis may seem a price worth paying. Discussing these issues with the patient in a truthful but humorous way may be the right approach. We know that ~½ of adolescents with leukaemia do not follow their doctor's directions when off the ward. Facing this issue in advance is likely to be helpful.
- Avoid concurrent drugs bought over the counter, eg aspirin, ibuprofen; the danger is steroid-associated GI bleeds: if NSAIDs are essential ask the patient to come to you for advice. You might consider an NSAID combined with misoprostol, a prostaglandin analogue (Arthrotec®, p664).
- Interactions: [Prednisolone]↓ by antiepileptics (below) and rifampicin.
- SE: TB reactivation; oedema, osteoporosis, cataract, euphoria, BP↑, glucose↑, pneumocystis, UTI, toxoplasmosis, aspergillus, serious chickenpox/zoster, so try to avoid contacts (and the need for varicella-zoster immunoglobulin). ●Avoid pregnancy. ►Neutropenic regimen: p598.

Azathioprine ●SE: peptic ulcer, marrow suppression, WCC↓. Do FBCs.
- Interactions: [Azathioprine]↑ by mercaptopurine.

Cyclosporin (=ciclosporin) In transplant patients 6mg/kg/day may be needed; in rheumatoid arthritis, keep the dose <4mg/kg/day.
- Monitor U&E and creatinine every 2 weeks for the first 3 months, then monthly if dose >2.5mg/kg/day (every 2 months if less than this). ►Reduce the dose if creatinine rises by >30% on 2 measurements *even if the creatinine is still in normal range*. Stop if the abnormality persists.
- Monitor blood levels in transplant patients.
- SE: nephrotoxicity, hepatotoxicity, oedema, gum hyperplasia, tremor, paraesthesiae, BP↑, confusion, seizures, lymphoma, skin cancer.
- Interactions are legion. Always check. Examples: [Ciclosporin]↑ by ketoconazole, diltiazem, nicardipine, verapamil, the Pill, erythromycin. [Ciclosporin]↓ by barbiturates, carbamazepine, phenytoin, rifampicin. Avoid concurrent nephrotoxics: gentamicin, amphotericin. Concurrent NSAIDs augment hepatotoxicity: monitor LFTs.

Methotrexate ●SE: hepatitis, lung fibrosis, CNS signs, teratogenicity.
- [Methotrexate]↑ by NSAIDs, aspirin, penicillin, probenecid.

Cyclophosphamide ●SE: carcino- and terato-genic, haemorrhagic cystitis, marrow suppression (especially if using allopurinol concurrently).

14. Biochemistry

Relevant pages in other chapters: Reference intervals (p754); IV fluids on the surgical wards (p100); acute renal failure (p384 and p386).

On being normal in the society of numbers

Biochemistry reduces our patients to a few easy-to-handle numbers: this is the discipline's great attraction—and its greatest danger. The normal range (reference interval) is usually that which includes, say, 95% of patients. If variation is randomly distributed, 2.5% of our results will be 'too high', and 2.5% 'too low' on an average day, when dealing with apparently normal people. This statistical definition of normality is the simplest. Other definitions may be *normative*—ie stating what an upper or lower limit *should* be. For example, the upper end of the reference interval for plasma cholesterol may be given as 6mmol/L because this is what biochemists state to be the *desired* maximum. 40% of people in some populations will have a plasma cholesterol greater than this. The WHO definition of anaemia in pregnancy is an Hb of <11g/dL, which makes 20% of mothers anaemic. This 'lax' criterion has the presumed benefit of triggering actions which result in fewer deaths by haemorrhage. So do not just ask "What is the normal range?"—also enquire about who set the range, for what population, and for what reason.

The top end of the range of normal blood pressure has been defined as being a blood pressure which, if it were treated with hypotensives, would do more harm than good. ►Normal values can have hidden historical, social and political desiderata—just like the normal values novelists ascribe to their characters: ' . . . *Conventions and traditions, I suppose, work blindly but surely for the preservation of the normal type; for the extinction of proud, resolute and unusual individuals. . . Society must go on, I suppose, and society can only exist if the normal, if the virtuous, and the slightly deceitful flourish, and if the passionate, the headstrong, and the too-truthful are condemned to suicide and to madness. Yes, society must go on; it must breed, like rabbits. That is what we are here for . . . But, at any rate, there is always Leonora to cheer you up; I don't want to sadden you. Her husband is quite an economical person of so normal a figure that he can get quite a large proportion of his clothes ready-made. That is the great desideratum of life. . .*'[1]

1 Ford Madox Ford 1915 *The Good Soldier*, Penguin, pages 214 and 228

The essence of biochemistry

Only do a test if the result will influence management. Make sure you look at the result! Explain to the patient where this test fits in to his or her overall plan of management. ►Do not interpret biochemical results except in the light of clinical assessment (unless forced by examiners). ►If there is disparity, trust clinical judgment and repeat biochemistry.

The reference intervals (normal range) are usually defined as the interval, symmetrical about the mean, containing 95% of results on the population studied. The more tests you run, the greater the probability of an 'abnormal' result of no clinical significance: see p624.

Artefacts Correct calcium for albumin (p642).

Anion gap reflects unmeasured anions (p630).

Biochemistry results: major disease patterns (↑ = raised, ↓ = lowered)
Dehydration: Urea↑, albumin↑ (useful to plot change in a patient's condition). Haematocrit (PCV)↑, creatinine ↑.
Renal failure: Creatinine↑, urea↑, anion gap↑, K⁺↑ (p640), HCO₃⁻↓.
Thiazide and loop diuretics: Sodium↓, bicarbonate↑, potassium↓, urea↑.

Bone disease:	Ca^{2+}	PO_4^{3-}	Alk phos
Osteoporosis	normal	normal	normal
Osteomalacia	↓	↓	↑
Paget's	normal	normal	↑↑
Myeloma	↑	↑,normal	normal
Bone metastases	↑	↑,normal	↑
Primary hyperparathyroidism	↑	↓,normal	normal,↑
Hypoparathyroidism	↓	↑	normal
Renal failure (low GFR)	↓	↑	normal,↑

Hepatocellular disease: Bilirubin↑, AST↑, (alk phos, mildly ↑, albumin↓).

Cholestasis: Bilirubin↑, GGT↑↑, alk phos↑↑, usually extrahepatic cholestasis if >350iu/L (AST↑).

Myocardial infarct: AST ↑ (also LDH ↑, CK↑, p280).

Diabetes mellitus: Glucose↑, bicarbonate↓.

Addison's disease: Potassium↑, sodium↓.

Cushing's syndrome: May show potassium↓, bicarbonate↑, Na⁺↑.

Conn's syndrome: May present with potassium↓, bicarbonate↑ (and high blood pressure). Sodium↑ or normal.

Diabetes insipidus: Sodium↑ (both hypercalcaemia and hypokalaemia may cause nephrogenic diabetes insipidus).

Inappropriate ADH secretion: Na⁺↓ with normal or low urea and creatinine.

Excess alcohol intake: Evidence of hepatocellular disease. Early evidence in GGT ↑, MCV↑, ethanol in blood before lunch.

Some immunodeficiency states: Normal serum albumin but *low* total protein (low as immunoglobulins are missing—also making crossmatching difficult because expected haemagglutinins are absent; OHCS p201).

What biochemical derangements might be rapidly fatal? See p627.

The laboratory and ward tests

►Laboratory staff like to have contact with you.

A laboratory decalogue
1. Interest someone from the laboratory in your patient's problem.
2. Fill in the request form fully.
3. Give clinical details, not your preferred diagnosis.
4. Ensure that the lab knows whom to contact.
5. Label specimens as well as the request form.
6. Follow the hospital labelling routine for crossmatching.
7. Find out when analysers run, especially batched assays.
8. Talk with the lab before requesting an unusual test.
9. Be thoughtful: at 4.30pm the routine results are being sorted.
10. Plot results graphically: abnormalities show sooner.

Artefacts and pitfalls in laboratory tests
- Do not take blood sample from an arm which has IV fluid running into it.
- Repeat any unexpected result before acting on it.
- For clotting time do not use sample from heparinized IV catheter.
- Serum K^+ is overestimated if sample old or haemolysed (this occurs if venepuncture is difficult).
- If using Vacutainers, fill *plain* tubes first—otherwise anticoagulant contamination from previous tubes can cause errors.[1]
- Calcium analysis is affected by albumin (p642).
- INR may be underestimated if citrate bottle underfilled.
- Drugs may cause *analytic* errors (eg prednisolone cross-reacts with cortisol). Be suspicious if results unexpected.
- Food may affect result (eg bananas raise urinary HMAA—p554).

The use of dipsticks Store dipsticks with container lid on in a cool, dry place, not refrigerated. If improperly stored, or past expiry date, do not use. For urine dipstick dip briefly in urine, run edge of strip along container and hold strip horizontally. Read at specified time—check instructions for the stick you are using.

Urine specific gravity (SG) can be measured by dipstick. It is not a good measure of osmolality. Causes of low SG (<1.003) are: diabetes insipidus, renal failure. Causes of high SG (>1.025) are: diabetes mellitus, adrenal insufficiency, liver disease, heart failure, acute water loss. Hydrometers underestimate SG by 0.001 per 3°C above 16°C.

Sources of error in interpreting dipsticks results
Bilirubin: False +ve: phenothiazines. False –ve: urine not fresh, rifampicin.
Urobilinogen: False –ve: urine not fresh.
Ketones: L-dopa affects colour (can give false +ve).
Blood: False +ve: myoglobin, profuse bacterial growth. False –ve: ascorbic acid.
Urine glucose: Depends on test. Pads with glucose oxidase are not affected by other reducing sugars (unlike Clinitest®) but can give false +ve to peroxide, chlorine; and false –ve with ascorbic acid, salicylate, L-dopa.
Protein: Highly alkaline urine can give false +ve.
Blood glucose: Sticks use enzymatic method and are glucose specific. Major source of error is applying too little blood (large drop to cover pad is necessary), and poor timing. Reflectance meters increase precision but introduce new sources of error.

1 WA Bartlett 1993 BMJ ii 868

Laboratory results: when to take action NOW

- On receiving a dangerous result first check its name and date.
- Go to the bedside. If the patient is conscious, turning off any IVI (until fluid is checked: a mistake may have been made) and ask the patient how he or she is. *Any fits, faints, collapses, or unexpected symptoms?*
- Be sceptical of an unexpectedly wildly abnormal result with a well patient. Could the specimens have got muddled up? Is there an artefact? Was the sample taken from the 'drip' arm? A low calcium, for example, may be due to a low albumin (p642).
- When in doubt, repeat the test.

The values chosen below are somewhat arbitrary, and must be taken as a guide only. Many results less extreme than those below will be just as dangerous if the patient is old, immunosuppressed, or has some other pathology such as pneumonia.

Plasma biochemistry (beware electrocardiological ± CNS events, eg fits)

Calcium (uncuffed and corrected for albumin) >3.5mmol/L *If shortening Q–T interval on ECG (p264) then dangerous hypercalcaemia: see p644.*

Calcium (uncuffed and corrected for albumin) <2mmol/L+symptoms such as tetany or long Q–T = *Dangerous hypocalcaemia. See p642.*

Glucose <2mmol/L = *Hypoglycaemia. IVI; glucose 50mL 50% IVI if coma.*

Glucose >20mmol/L = *Dangerous hyperglycaemia. Is parenteral insulin needed? See p784.*

Potassium <2.5mmol/L = *Dangerous hypokalaemia, esp. if on digoxin (p640).*

Potassium >6.5mmol/L = *Dangerous hyperkalaemia. See p386*

Sodium <120mmol/L = *Dangerous hyponatraemia. See p638*

Sodium >155mmol/L = *Dangerous hypernatraemia. See p638*

Blood gases

PaO₂ <8kPa = *Respiratory failure. Give O₂. Go to p352.*

pH <7.1 = *Dangerous acidaemia. Go to p630 to determine the cause.*

Haematology results

Hb <7g/dL with low mean cell volume (<75fL) or history of bleeding *This patient may need urgent transfusion (no spare capacity). See p102.*

Platelets <40 × 10⁹/L. *He may need a platelet transfusion; call a haematologist.*

Plasmodium falciparum seen on the film *Start antimalarials now. See p196.*

ESR >30mm/h + headache *Could the patient have giant cell arteritis? Go to p674.*

CSF results

>1 neutrophil seen *Is there meningitis (usually >1000 neutrophils)? See p442.*

Organisms on Gram stain *Talk to a microbiologist. Urgent blind treatment: p442.*

▶If results are conflicting, equivocal, or inexplicable, get prompt help.

Intravenous fluid therapy

(See also p100 and p636.)

If fluids cannot be given orally they are normally given intravenously. Alternatives are via a central venous line or subcutaneously.

Three principles of fluid therapy

1 **Maintain normal daily requirements.** About 2500mL fluid containing roughly 100mmol sodium and 70mmol potassium per 24h are required. A good regimen is 2 litres 5% dextrose and 1 litre of 0.9% saline every 30h with 20–30mmol of potassium per litre of fluid. Postoperative patients may need more fluid and more saline depending on operative losses. If the serum sodium is rising then more dextrose and less saline is required.

2 **Replace additional losses.** The amount and type of fluid lost is a guide (check fluid charts, drainage bottles etc). Remember that febrile patients have increased losses too. In practice the problem is usually whether to give saline or dextrose. Most body fluids (eg vomit) contain salt, but less than plasma, and thus replacement will require a mixture of saline and dextrose. Shocked patients require resuscitation with a colloidal plasma expander eg Dextran® or Haemaccel®, or saline, but not dextrose (caution in liver failure, see below). Note that Dextran® interferes with platelet function and may prolong bleeding. Patients with acute blood loss require transfusion with packed cells or whole blood. As a holding measure, colloid or saline may be used while blood is being crossmatched. If more than 1L is required then O-negative or group-specific blood should be used (see p766).

3 **Special cases.** Patients with *heart failure* are at greater risk of pulmonary oedema if given too much fluid. They also tolerate saline less well since Na^+ retention accompanies heart failure. If fluids iv must be given use with care. Patients with *liver failure*, despite being oedematous and often hyponatraemic, have increased total body sodium, and saline should not be used in resuscitation; salt-poor albumin solution or blood should be given.

A note on fluids. *0.9% saline ('normal saline')* has about the same sodium content as plasma (150mmol/L) and is isotonic with plasma. *5% dextrose* is isotonic but only contains 278mmol/L glucose ie 50g/L (dextrose is glucose), and is a way of giving water, since the liver rapidly metabolizes all the glucose leaving only water. It provides little energy.

More concentrated glucose solutions exist, and may be used in the treatment of hypoglycaemia. They are hypertonic, and irritant to veins. Therefore, care in their use is needed, and infusion sites should be inspected regularly, and flushed with saline after use. *Dextrose-saline (one-fifth normal saline)* is also isotonic, containing 30mmol/L of sodium and 4% glucose (222mmol/L). It has roughly the concentration of saline required for normal fluid maintenance, when given 10 hourly.

▶Hypertonic and hypotonic saline solutions are available, but are for specialist use only.

▶Examine patients regularly to assess fluid balance, and look for signs of heart failure (p296) which can result if excess fluid is given. Excessive dextrose infusion may lead to water overload (p638).

▶Daily weighing helps to monitor overall fluid balance, as will the fluid balance charts.

Acid–base balance

Arterial blood pH is closely regulated in health to 7.40 ±0.05 by various mechanisms including bicarbonate, other buffers, and the kidney. Acid-base disorders needlessly confuse many people, but if a few simple rules are applied then interpretation, and diagnosis are easy.

- pH< 7.35 is an acidosis; pH> 7.45 is an alkalosis.
- CO_2 is an acidic gas (normal concentration 4.7–6.0 kPa).
- HCO_3^- is alkaline (normal concentration 22–28mmol/L).
- 1° changes in HCO_3^- are termed metabolic, and of CO_2 respiratory.

1 Look at the pH: is there an acidosis or alkalosis?
2 Is the CO_2 abormal? If so, is change in keeping with change in pH (ie if there is an acidosis, is CO_2 raised)? if so it is a *respiratory* problem. If there's no change, or an opposite one, then the change is compensatory.
3 Is the HCO_3^- abnormal, and if so, is the change in keeping with the change in pH? If so the problem is a *metabolic* one.

An example
pH 7.05, CO_2 2.0kPa, HCO_3^- 8.0mmol/L.
There is an acidosis, and the CO_2 is low, and so is a compensatory change. The HCO_3^- is low, and is thus the cause; ie a metabolic acidosis.

Metabolic acidosis pH↓, HCO_3^-↓
To help diagnosis work out *anion gap* (AG):

$$AG = [K^+] + [Na^+] - [Cl^-] - [HCO_3^-] \text{ (plasma concentrations).}$$

Normal range: 8–16mmol/L. It is a measure of the difference between cation, and unestimated anions—'fixed' or organic acids—eg phosphate, ketones, lactate.

Causes of metabolic acidosis and increased anion gap:
Due to increased production of fixed/organic acids.
- Lactic acid (shock, infection, hypoxia)
- Urate (renal failure)
- Ketones (diabetes mellitus, alcohol)
- Drugs/toxins (salicylates, biguanides, ethylene glycol, methanol)

Causes of metabolic acidosis and normal anion gap:
Due to loss of bicarbonate, or ingestion of H^+ ions.
- Renal tubular acidosis
- Diarrhoea
- Drugs (acetazolamide)
- Addison's disease
- Pancreatic fistulae
- Ammonium chloride ingestion

Metabolic alkalosis pH↑, HCO_3^-↑
- Vomiting
- K^+ depletion (diuretics)
- Burns
- Ingestion of base

Respiratory acidosis pH↓ CO_2↑
- Any lung, neuromuscular or physical cause of respiratory failure (p352).
► Look at the P_aO_2. It will probably be low. Is oxygen therapy required?
► If so use care if COPD is the underlying cause, as too much oxygen may make matters worse (p348).

Respiratory alkalosis pH↑, CO_2↓
A result of hyperventilation.
CNS causes: Stroke, subarachnoid haemorrhage, meningitis.
Other causes: Anxiety, altitude, fever, pregnancy, drugs eg salicylates.

A note on terminology: to aid understanding we have used the terms acidosis and alkalosis; where a purist would use acid-, alkalaemia.

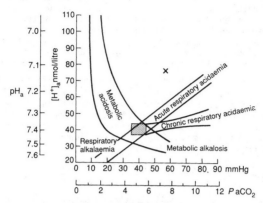

The shaded area represents normality. This method is very powerful. The result represented by point X, for example, indicates that the acidaemia is in part respiratory and in part metabolic. Seek a cause for each.

The biochemistry of kidney function[1]

The kidney controls the elimination of many substances. It also makes erythropoietin, renin, and 1,25-dihydroxycholecalciferol. Filtered sodium is exchanged with potassium and hydrogen ions by a pump in the distal tubule. Glucose spills over into urine when plasma concentration is above renal threshold for reabsorption ($\approx$10mmol/L, but varies from person to person, and is lower in pregnancy).

Creatinine clearance is a measure of glomerular filtration rate (GFR)—the volume of fluid filtered by glomeruli per minute. About 99% of this fluid is reabsorbed. Creatinine once filtered is only slightly reabsorbed. Thus:

[Creatinine]^{plasma} × creatinine clearance = [creatinine]^{urine} × urine flow rate

To measure creatinine clearance (normal value is >100mL/min). Collect urine over 24h. At start void and discard urine; from then on, and at end of 24h, void into bottle. Take sample for plasma creatinine once during 24h. Use formula above. Take care with units. Major sources of error are calculation (eg units) and failure to collect all urine. If urine collection is unreliable use formula:[2]

$$\text{creatinine clearance (mL/min)} = \frac{(140 - \text{age in years}) \times (\text{wt in kg})}{72 \times \text{serum creatinine in mg/dL}}$$

For women multiply above by 0.85. Unreliable if: unstable renal function; very obese; oedematous. (The protein : creatinine ratio in a spot morning urine is an alternative way to monitor chronic renal decline: see p370.) The conversion factor from µmol/L to mg/dL is 88.4; mg/dL=µmol ÷ 88.4.

Abnormal kidney function

There are three major biochemical pictures.

●*Low GFR* (classic acute renal failure)

Plasma biochemistry: The following are raised: urea, creatinine, potassium, hydrogen ions, urate, phosphate, anion gap.
The following are lowered: calcium, bicarbonate.

Other findings: Oliguria.

Diagnosis: Low GFR (creatinine clearance).

Causes: Early acute oliguric renal failure (p384), long-standing chronic renal failure (p388).

●*Tubular dysfunction* (damage to tubules)
Plasma biochemistry: The following are lowered: potassium, phosphate, urate, bicarbonate. There is acidosis. Urea and creatinine are normal.

Other findings (highly variable): Polyuria with glucose, amino acids, proteins (lysozyme, β2-microglobulin), and phosphate in urine.

Diagnosis: Test renal concentrating ability (p566).

Cause: Recovery from acute renal failure. Also: hypercalcaemia, hyperuricaemia, myeloma, pyelonephritis, hypokalaemia, Wilson's disease, galactosaemia, metal poisoning.

●*Chronic renal failure:* As GFR reduces; creatinine, urea, phosphate and urate all increase. Bicarbonate (and Hb) decrease. Eventually potassium increases and pH decreases. There may also be osteomalacia.

Assessment of renal failure may need to be combined with other investigations to reach diagnosis, eg urine microscopy (p370), radiology (p372), or renal biopsy (in glomerulonephritis), or ultrasound.

1 R Gabriel *Postgraduate Nephrology* 3 ed, Butterworths   2 D Cockcroft 1976 *Nephron* 16 31

Creatinine clearance: worked example

Suppose:
urine creatinine concentration = **u** mmol/L;
plasma creatinine concentration = **p** µmol/L;
24h urine volume = **v** /mL.

There are 1440 minutes per 24h (used below to convert urine rate from volume per 24h into volume per minute). **p**/1000 is used to convert micromoles to millimoles.

Creatinine clearance = u × v/1440 ÷ p/1000mL/min.

$$u \times v/p \times 0.7$$

Thus, if: **u** = 5mmol/L; **p** = 120 µmol/L; **v** = 2500mL;
creatinine clearance = 5 × (2500/120) × 0.7
= 73mL/min

Urate and the kidney

Causes of hyperuricaemia High levels of urate in the blood (hyper-uricaemia) may result from increased turnover or reduced excretion of urate. Either may be drug-induced.

- *Drugs:* Cytotoxics; thiazides; ethambutol.
- *Increased cell turnover:* Lymphoma; leukaemia; psoriasis; haemolysis; muscle necrosis (p394).
- *Reduced excretion:* Primary gout (p666); chronic renal failure; lead nephropathy; hyperparathyroidism.
- In addition: Hyperuricaemia may be associated with hypertension and hyperlipidaemia. Urate may be raised in disorders of purine synthesis such as the Lesch–Nyhan syndrome (*OHCS* p752).

Hyperuricaemia and renal failure Severe renal failure from any cause may be associated with hyperuricaemia, and very rarely this may give rise to gout. Sometimes the relationship of cause and effect is reversed so that it is the hyperuricaemia which causes the renal failure. This can occur following cytotoxic treatment (*tumour lysis syndrome*) eg in leukaemia; and in muscle necrosis.

How urate causes renal failure In some instances ureteric obstruction from urate crystals occurs. This responds to retrograde ureteric catheterization and lavage. More commonly, urate precipitates in the renal tubules. This may occur at plasma levels $\geq$1.19mmol/L.

Prevention of renal failure Before starting chemotherapy, ensure good hydration; consider alkalinization of the urine; and initiate allopurinol (a xanthine oxidase inhibitor) which prevents a sharp rise in urate following chemotherapy. The dose is: 200–800mg/24h. It increases the toxicity of azathioprine. There is a remote risk of inducing xanthine nephropathy.

Treatment of hyperuricaemic acute renal failure Prompt rehydration and alkalinization of the urine after excluding bilateral ureteric obstruction. Once oliguria is established, haemodialysis is required and should be used in preference to peritoneal dialysis.

Gout See p666.

Electrolyte physiology

Most sodium is extracellular, and is pumped out of the cell by the sodium pump, in exchange for K+, which requires energy from ATP.

Osmolarity is the number of osmoles per *litre* of solution.

Osmolality is the number of osmoles per *kg* of solvent (norm 280–300).

A mole is the molecular weight expressed in grams.

To estimate plasma osmolality: $2[Na^+ + K^+] + Urea + Glucose$. If the measured osmolality is greater than this (ie an osmolar gap of >10mmol/L), consider: diabetes mellitus, high blood ethanol, methanol, or ethylene glycol.

Fluid compartments For 70kg man: *total fluid* = 42 litres (60% body weight). *Intracellular fluid* = 28 litres (67% body fluid), *extracellular fluid* = 14 litres (33% body fluid). *Intravascular component* = 3 litres plasma (5 litres of blood).

Distribution between intra- and extravascular compartments is determined by osmotic equilibrium, and the 'oncotic pressure' exerted by non-diffusible proteins.

Fluid balance over 24h is roughly:

Input (/mL water)	Output (/mL water)
drink: 1500	urine: 1500
in food: 800	insensible loss: 800
metabolism of food: 200	stool: 200
total: **2500**	total: **2500**

Control of sodium *Renin* is produced by the juxtaglomerular apparatus in response to decreased renal blood flow, and catalyses the formation of angiotensin I from angiotensinogen. This is then converted by angiotensin-converting enzyme (ACE) to angiotensin II. The latter has several important actions including efferent renal arteriolar constriction (so increasing perfusion pressure); peripheral vasoconstriction; and stimulation of the adrenal cortex to produce aldosterone, which activates the sodium pump in the distal renal tubule leading to reabsorption of sodium and water from the urine, in exchange for potassium and hydrogen ions.

High GFR (p632) results in high sodium loss.

High renal tubular blood flow and haemodilution decrease sodium reabsorption in the proximal tubule.

Control of water Controlled mainly by sodium concentration. An increased plasma osmolality causes thirst, and the release of antidiuretic hormone (ADH) from the posterior pituitary which increases the passive water reabsorption from the renal collecting duct, by opening water channels to allow water to flow from the hypotonic luminal fluid into the hypertonic renal interstitium.

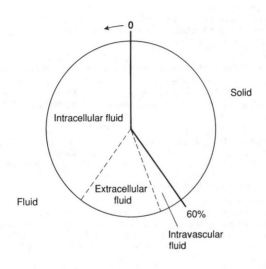

✂ Sodium: hyponatraemia

►Do not base treatment on plasma sodium concentration alone.

Patients with a low plasma Na⁺ may exhibit signs of water excess—such as confusion, fits, hypertension, cardiac failure, oedema, anorexia, nausea, muscle weakness, haemodilution, ie PCV <40% (<35% if ♀).

Diagnosis See tree opposite. The key question is: is the patient dehydrated? History and urine analysis are your guides.

Causes of hyponatraemia
●Diuretics, especially thiazides.
●Water excess, either orally, or as excess 5% dextrose IV.
●Others—see tree opposite.

Management
Treat specific cause. Assess renal function: if poor, dialysis may be needed.

If not dehydrated, renal function good, and if Na >125mmol/L, treatment rarely needed. If Na <125mmol/L, restrict water to 0.5–1 litre/day if tolerated. Consider frusemide (=furosemide) 40–80mg/24h IV slowly/PO for a few days only. SIADH (below) is occasionally treated by producing nephrogenic diabetes insipidus with demeclocycline.

If dehydrated and kidney function good, 0.9% saline can be given. In *emergency* (seizures, coma) consider rapid IVI of 0.9% saline or hypertonic saline (eg 1.8% saline) at 70mmol Na⁺/h. Aim for a gradual increase in plasma sodium to above 125mmol/L. Watch out for heart failure, and central pontine myelinosis. ►Seek expert advice.

Syndrome of inappropriate ADH secretion (SIADH)
This is an important cause of hyponatraemia, but is over-diagnosed. The diagnosis is made by finding a concentrated urine (sodium >20mmol/L) in presence of hyponatraemia (<125mmol/L) or low plasma osmolality (<260mmol/kg), and absence of hypovolaemia, oedema, or diuretics.

Causes:
●*Malignancy* (lung small-cell; pancreas; prostate; lymphoma; others).
●*CNS disorders* (meningoencephalitis; abscess; stroke; subarachnoid, subdural haemorrhage; head injury; Guillain–Barré; vasculitis, eg SLE).
●*Chest disease* (TB; pneumonia; abscess; aspergillosis).
●*Metabolic* disease (porphyria; trauma).
●*Drugs* (opiates; chlorpropamide; psychotropics; cytotoxics).

Hypernatraemia

The Patient Look for thirst, confusion, coma, and fits—with signs of dehydration: dry skin, ↓skin turgor, postural hypotension, and oliguria if water deficient. Laboratory features: ↑PCV, ↑albumin, ↑urate.

Causes Usually due to water loss in excess of sodium loss.
●Fluid loss without water replacement (eg diarrhoea, vomit, burns).
●Incorrect IV fluid replacement.
●Diabetes insipidus (p566). Suspect if large urine volume. This may follow head injury, or CNS surgery, especially pituitary.
●Osmotic diuresis. (for diabetic coma, see p784).
●Primary aldosteronism: suspect if BP↑, K⁺↓, alkalosis (HCO₃↑).

Management: Give water orally if possible. Otherwise dextrose 5% IV slowly (~4L/24h) guided by urine output and plasma sodium. Some authorities recommend giving 0.9% saline since this causes less marked fluid shifts and is hypotonic in a hypernatraemic patient. Avoid hypotonic solutions.

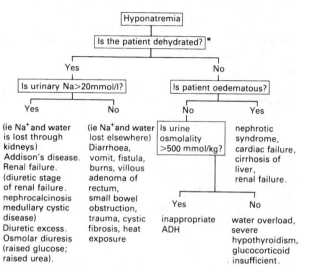

Hyponatremia

Is the patient dehydrated? *

Yes

Is urinary Na>20mmol/l?

Yes

(ie Na⁺ and water is lost through kidneys) Addison's disease. Renal failure. (diuretic stage of renal failure. nephrocalcinosis medullary cystic disease) Diuretic excess. Osmolar diuresis (raised glucose; raised urea).

No

(ie Na⁺ and water lost elsewhere) Diarrhoea, vomit, fistula, burns, villous adenoma of rectum, small bowel obstruction, trauma, cystic fibrosis, heat exposure

No

Is patient oedematous?

No

Is urine osmolality >500 mmol/kg?

Yes

inappropriate ADH

No

water overload, severe hypothyroidism, glucocorticoid insufficient.

Yes

nephrotic syndrome, cardiac failure, cirrhosis of liver, renal failure.

NB: in cirrhosis, hyponatremia may precede oedema

⚡ Potassium

General points Most potassium is intracellular, and thus serum potassium levels are a poor reflection of total body potassium. The concentrations of potassium and hydrogen ions in extracellular fluid tend to vary together. This is because these ions compete with each other in the exchange with sodium which occurs across most cell membranes (sodium is pumped out of the cell) and in the distal tubule of the kidney (sodium is reabsorbed from the urine). Thus if hydrogen ion concentration is high, fewer potassium ions will be excreted into the urine. Similarly K^+ will compete with H^+ for exchange across cell membranes and extracellular K^+ will accumulate.

Hyperkalaemia

▶A plasma potassium >6.5mmol/L needs urgent treatment (p386) but first ensure that this is not an artefact (eg due to haemolysis inside the bottle).

Signs and symptoms Cardiac arrhythmias. Sudden death. *ECG:* Tall tented T-waves; small P-wave; wide QRS complex becoming sinusoidal, VF.

Causes
Oliguric renal failure
- K^+ sparing diuretics
- Rhabdomyolysis (p394), burns
- Metabolic acidosis (DM)
- Excess K^+ therapy
- Addison's disease (see p552)
- Massive blood transfusion
- Drugs, eg ACEi, suxamethonium
- Artefact. Haemolysis of sample; delay in analysis—K^+ leaks out of RBCs; thrombocythaemia—platelet leak K^+ as sample clots in tube.

Treatment Treat underlying cause. ▶In emergency see p386.

Hypokalaemia

If <2.5mmol/L needs urgent treatment. Note that hypokalaemia exacerbates digoxin toxicity.

Signs and symptoms Muscle weakness, hypotonia, cardiac arrhythmias, cramps and tetany. *ECG:* Small or inverted T-waves; prominent U-wave (after T-wave); prolonged P-R interval; depressed ST segment.

Causes
- Diuretics
- Vomiting, and diarrhoea
- Pyloric stenosis
- Villous adenoma rectum
- Intestinal fistulae
- Cushing's syndrome/steroids/ACTH
- Conn's syndrome
- Alkalosis
- Purgative and liquorice abuse
- Renal tubular failure (p632)

If on diuretics, then a raised bicarbonate is the best indication that the hypokalaemia is likely to have been long-standing. Magnesium may be low, and hypokalaemia is often difficult to correct until magnesium levels are restored to normal. In hypokalaemic periodic paralysis, intermittent weakness lasting up to 72h appears to be caused by K^+ shifting from the extracellular to the intracellular fluid. See *OHCS* p756. Suspect Conn's syndrome if hypertensive, hypokalaemic alkalosis in someone not taking diuretics (p554).

Treatment *If mild:* (>2.5mmol/L, no symptoms) give oral potassium supplement (at least 80mmol/24h eg Sando-K® 2 tabs bd). If patient taking thiazide diuretic, hypokalaemia >3.0mmol/L rarely needs treating. *If severe:* (<2.5mmol/L, dangerous symptoms) give IV potassium cautiously, not more than 20mmol/h, not more than 40mmol/L. Do not give potassium if oliguric. ▶Never give potassium as a fast 'stat' bolus dose.

Calcium physiology and hypocalcaemia

General points About 40% of plasma calcium is bound to albumin. Usually it is total plasma calcium which is measured although it is the unbound, ionized portion which is important. Therefore, *adjust calcium level for albumin as follows*: Add 0.1mmol/L to calcium concentration for every 4g/L that albumin is below 40g/L, and a similar subtraction for raised albumin. However, many factors affect binding (eg other proteins in myeloma, cirrhosis, individual variation) so be cautious in your interpretation. If doubt over a high Ca^{2+} take blood specimens uncuffed (remove tourniquet after needle in vein, but before taking blood sample), and with the patient fasted.

The control of calcium metabolism

- *Parathyroid hormone (PTH):* A rise in PTH causes a rise in plasma Ca^{2+} and a decrease in plasma PO_4^{3-}. This is due to $\uparrow Ca^{2+}$ and $\uparrow PO_4^{3-}$ reabsorption from bone; and $\uparrow Ca^{2+}$ but $\downarrow PO_4^{3-}$ reabsorption from the kidney. PTH secretion enhances active vitamin D formation. PTH secretion is itself controlled by ionized plasma calcium levels.
- *Vitamin D:* Calciferol (Vit D_3), and ergocalciferol (Vit D_2) are biologically identical in their actions. Serum Vit D is converted in the liver to 25-hydroxy Vit D (25OH VitD). In the kidney a second hydroxyl group is added to form the biologically active 1,25-dihydroxy Vit D (1,25(OH)$_2$VitD), also called calcitriol, or the much less active 24,25(OH)$_2$Vit D. Calcitriol production is stimulated by $\downarrow Ca^{2+}$ $\downarrow PO_4^{3-}$, and PTH. Its actions include $\uparrow Ca^{2+}$ and $\uparrow PO_4$ absorption from the gut; $\uparrow Ca^{2+}$ and $\uparrow PO_4^{3-}$ reabsorption in the kidney; enhanced bone turnover; and inhibition of PTH release. Disordered regulation of 1,25(OH)$_2$VitD underlies familial normocalcaemic hypercalciuria which is a major cause of calcium oxalate renal stone formation (p376).
- *Calcitonin:* Made in C cells of the thyroid, this causes a decrease in plasma calcium and phosphate, but its physiological rôle is unclear. It is a marker for medullary carcinoma of the thyroid.
- Thyroxine (=levothyroxine) may $\uparrow$ plasma calcium although this is rare.
- Hypomagnesaemia prevents PTH release, and may cause hypocalcaemia.

Hypocalcaemia

▶ Apparent hypocalcaemia may be artefact of hypoalbuminaemia (above).

The Patient Tetany, depression, perioral paraesthesiae, carpo-pedal spasm (wrist flexion and fingers drawn together) especially if brachial artery occluded with blood pressure cuff (*Trousseau's sign*), neuromuscular excitability eg tapping over parotid (facial nerve) causes facial muscles to twitch (*Chvostek's sign*). Cataract if chronic $Ca^{2+}\downarrow$. ECG: Q-T interval $\uparrow$.

Causes It may be a consequence of thyroid or parathyroid surgery. *If phosphate raised* then either chronic renal failure (p388), hypoparathyroidism or pseudohypoparathyroidism (p546). If phosphate $\leftrightarrow$ or $\downarrow$ then either osteomalacia (high alkaline phosphatase), overhydration or pancreatitis.

Treatment If *symptoms mild give* calcium 5mmol/6h PO. Do daily plasma calcium levels. ▶In chronic renal failure see p388. If necessary add alfacalcidol; start at 0.5–1µg/24h PO. If *symptoms are severe*, give 10mL (2.32mmol) calcium gluconate 10% IVI over 30mins (bolus injections are only needed very rarely). Repeat as necessary.

⚜ Hypercalcaemia

Signs and symptoms ('Bones, stones, groans and psychic moans') Abdominal pain; vomiting; constipation; polyuria; polydipsia; depression; anorexia; weight loss; tiredness; weakness; BP↑; confusion; pyrexia; renal stones; renal failure; corneal calcification; cardiac arrest. ECG Q–T interval↓.

Causes and diagnosis Most commonly malignancy (myeloma, bone metastases, PTHrP↑, p546) and 1° hyperparathyroidism. Pointers to malignancy are: low plasma albumin, lowish chloride, hypokalaemia, alkalosis, raised phosphate and raised alkaline phosphatase. Other investigations (eg isotope bone scan, CXR, FBC) may also be of diagnostic value.

Treat the underlying cause. If Ca^{2+} >3.5mmol/L, or BP↓, severe abdominal pain, vomiting, pyrexia, confusion, aim to reduce calcium as follows:
- **Bloods:** Measure U&E's, Mg^{2+}, creatinine, Ca^{2+}, PO_4^{3-}, Alk phos.
- **Fluids:** Rehydrate with IVI 0.9% saline eg 4–6 litres in 24h as needed. Correct hypokalaemia and hypomagnesaemia (mild metabolic acidosis does not need treatment). This will reduce symptoms, and ↑renal Ca^{2+} loss. Monitor U&E during treatment.
- **Diuretics:** Frusemide 40mg/12h IV, once rehydrated. ▶Avoid thiazides.
- **Bisphosphonates:** A single dose of pamidronate (30mg IVI over 4h in 0.9% saline, p686) will lower Ca^{2+} over 2 to 3 days. Maximum effect is at 1 week. They inhibit osteoclast activity, and so bone reabsorption.
- **Steroids:** Occasionally used, eg in sarcoidosis.
- **Salmon calcitonin:** Now rarely used (8u/kg/8h IM). More side-effects than bisphosphonates, but quicker onset. Again inhibits osteoclasts.
- **Other:** Chemotherapy may ↓ Ca^{2+} in malignant disease eg myeloma.

Magnesium

Magnesium is distributed 65% in bone and 35% in cells. Its level tends to follow those of Ca^{2+} and K^+. Magnesium excess is usually caused by renal failure, but rarely requires treatment in its own right.

Magnesium deficiency causes paresthesiae, fits, tetany, arrhythmias. Digitalis toxicity may be exacerbated. *Causes:* Severe diarrhoea; ketoacidosis; alcohol; total parenteral nutrition (monitor weekly); accompanying hypocalaemia; accompanying hypokalaemia (especially with diuretics). *Treatment:* If needed, give magnesium salts, PO or IV (dose example: 10mmol $MgSO_4$ IVI over 3min–2h, depending on severity; monitor Mg^{2+} often).

Hypermagnesaemia As levels rise these effects occur: neuromuscular depression, then ↓BP; then CNS depression, then coma.

Zinc

Zinc deficiency This may occur in parenteral nutrition or inadequate diet. Rarely it is due to a genetic defect. *Signs and symptoms:* Look for red, crusted skin lesions especially round nostrils and corners of mouth. *Diagnosis:* Therapeutic trial of zinc (plasma levels are unreliable as they may be low, eg in infection or trauma, without deficiency).

Selenium

An essential element present in cereals, nuts, and meat. Low soil levels in some parts of Europe, and China cause deficiency states. Required for the antioxidant glutathione peroxidase, which ↓harmful free radicals. It is also antithrombogenic, and is required for sperm motility proteins. Deficiency may increase the frequency of neoplasia and atheroma; and may lead to a cardiomyopathy or arthritis. Serum levels are a poor guide. Toxic symptoms may also be found with over-energetic replacement.

1 GN Hortobagyi 1996 *NEJM* 335 1785-9 & *E-BM* 1997 2 73   2 MP Rayman 1997 *BMJ* i 387

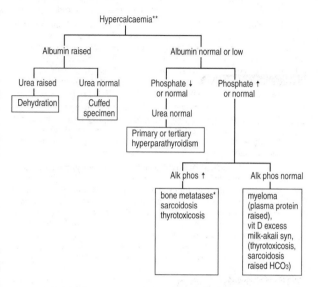

*Most common primary: breast, kidney, lung, thyroid,
prostate, ovary, colon.

NB: the best discriminating features between bone metastases and
hyperparathyroidism (the commonest two causes of hypercalaemia) are
low albumin, low chloride, alkalosis (all suggesting metastases).
Raised plasma PTH strongly supports hyperparathyroidism.

**This biochemical flow diagram must be taken in conjunction with
clinical picture and is a guide only.

Metabolic bone disease: 1. Osteoporosis

Osteoporosis implies <u>reduced bone density</u>. If trabecular bone is mostly affected, <u>crush fractures of vertebrae</u> are common (accounting for the littleness of little old ladies—and their dowager's hump); if cortical bone is mostly affected, <u>fracture of a long bone</u> is more likely, eg femoral neck: *the big cause of death and orthopaedic expense, especially in older women.*

Prevalence: 5%. $\female:\male \approx 4:1$ *Risk of future osteoporotic fracture* is increased if:
- Slender or anorectic
- Smoker or <u>alcoholic</u>
- Prolonged rest; old age
- Hyperparathyroidism
- >5mg/day prednisolone
- Vertebral deformity
- Early menopause
- Cushing's disease
- <u>Malabsorption</u>
- <u>Thyrotoxicosis</u>
- Myeloma
- Amenorrhoea
- Osteoporosis in family
- <u>Primary biliary cirrhosis</u>
- <u>Rheumatoid arthritis</u>
- Hypogonadism
- Past low-trauma fracture
- Mastocytosis (*OHCS* p602)

Diagnosis: <u>X-ray</u> (easier with hindsight afforded by bone fracture). <u>Serum Ca^{2+}, PO_4^{3-}, and alk phos normal</u>. <u>Bone densitometry</u> may be used, but its rôle is unclear: screening is probably not effective, and it is less effective than taking into account risk factors in the prediction of hip fracture.[□] Biopsy specimens may be unrepresentative.

Prevention: <u>Exercise: good, Ca^{2+}-rich diet; avoid smoking and excess alcohol</u>. HRT almost halves the risk of fractures <u>if given for 5–10 yrs post menopause</u> (only while treatment continues), and should be considered for those at ↑risk. It also ↑ bone density in established osteoporosis, and ↓ further fractures. <u>Unopposed oestrogens risk endometrial cancer—so give combined HRT</u>, eg *conjugated oestrogens* 0.625mg/24h PO continuously, with *norgestrel* 0.15mg daily from days 17–28 (eg <u>Prempak C 0.625®</u>). Not *all* women will be candidates for HRT, eg if past DVT or PE, or breast cancer, or ↑risk of breast cancer—see *OHCS* p19.

Treatment: •Strongly consider HRT—see above.
- <u>Bisphosphonates</u>: Didronel PMO® (14 days of etidronate 400mg/day and 76 days of Ca^{2+} in <u>90-day cycles</u>). It is licenced in vertebral osteoporosis, and ↓fracture rate[1,2]. Alendronate[3] is licenced for osteoporosis treatment at any site. SE: abdo pain, nausea, and oesophaegeal ulceration. ▶Read manufacturer's instructions to patients before prescribing.
- Others: <u>Vitamin D is effective</u>[2] (watch serum Ca^{2+}). Calcitonin is rarely used due to SE and cost. <u>Ca^{2+} tablets</u> are only of use if Ca^{2+} intake is low.

2. Paget's disease of bone

There is <u>increased bone turnover</u> associated with <u>increased numbers of osteoblasts and osteoclasts</u> with <u>resultant remodelling, bone enlargement, deformity, and weakness</u>. Rare in the under-40s. Incidence rises with age (3% over 55 years old). Commoner in temperate climes, and Anglo-Saxons. It may be asymptomatic or cause <u>pain</u> and enlargement of skull, femur, clavicle—and bowed (<u>sabre</u>) tibia—also <u>pathological fractures</u>, <u>nerve deafness</u> (bone overgrowth), and <u>high-output CCF</u>. *X-rays:* Localized enlargement of bone. <u>Patchy cortical thickening with sclerosis</u>, <u>osteolysis, and deformity</u> (*osteoporosis circumscripta* of the skull). Affinity for axial skeleton, long bones, and skull.

Blood biochemistry: Ca^{2+} and PO_4^{3-} normal; <u>alk phos markedly raised</u>.

Complications: Bone sarcoma (1% of those affected for >10yrs). Symptoms of nerve compression eg deafness. *Treatment:* If analgesia fails, *alendronate* (a <u>bisphosphonate</u>—inhibits osteoclasts) may be tried (40mg/24h PO before food for 6 months) to reduce pain and/or deformity. It is more effective than etidronate or calcitonin, and as effective as IV pamidronate.

1 N Watts 1990 *NEJM* 323 73 2 *Drug Ther Bul* 1992 34 45 3 D Black 1996 *Lancet* 348 1535

Understanding <u>Dexa bone scan results</u>: WHO osteoporosis criteria

Typical sites examined are the <u>lumbar spine</u> (preferably 3 vertebra) and <u>hip</u>. Bone mineral density (BMD, in grams/cm²) is compared with that of young healthy women (if it is a woman being tested). The 'T-score' relates to the number of standard deviations the BMD is from the average. If the T score is:

>0	BMD is better than the reference
0 to −1	BMD is in the top 84%: no evidence of osteoporosis
−1 to −2.5	Osteopenia, with risk of later osteoporotic complication, so consider preventive measures (see opposite).
−2.5 or worse	BMD is in the bottom 2.5% of the population: osteoporosis is present—severe if there is one or more fragility fracture.

An example of a <u>suitable indication for densitometry is before embarking on prednisolone treatment</u> (>6 months, at >7.5mg/day; steroids contribute to osteoporosis by promoting <u>osteoclast bone resorption</u>, and <u>decreasing muscle mass</u> and ↓GI Ca^{2+} absorption).

Metabolic bone disease: 3. Osteomalacia

In osteomalacia there is a normal amount of bony tissue but a reduced quantity of mineral content. Thus there is an excess of uncalcified osteoid and cartilage. Rickets is the result if this process occurs during the period of bone growth; osteomalacia is the result if it occurs after fusion of the epiphyses.

Forms

Vitamin D deficiency: Due to malabsorption (p522), poor diet, or lack of sunlight.

Renal osteomalacia: Renal failure leads to 1,25-dihydroxycholecalciferol (1,25(OH)$_2$ vitamin D—p642) deficiency.

Drug-induced: Anticonvulsants may induce liver enzymes, leading to a breakdown of 25-hydroxycholecalciferol.

Vitamin D resistance: A number of mainly inherited conditions in which the osteomalacia responds to high doses of vitamin D, see below.

Liver disease: Reduced production of 25-hydroxy vitamin D (25(OH)-vitamin D), and malabsorption of vitamin D, eg cirrhosis (p506).

Tests *Plasma:* Mildly ↓Ca^{2+}; PO$_4^{3-}$↓; alk phos↑; 25(OH) vitamin D↓, except in resistant cases; 1,25(OH)$_2$ vitamin D↓ in renal failure; PTH (p642) high.

Biopsy: Shows incomplete mineralization.

X-ray: Cupped, ragged metaphyseal surfaces (in rickets). In osteomalacia there is a loss of cortical bone; also, apparent partial fractures without displacement may be seen especially on the lateral border of the scapula, inferior femoral neck and medial femoral shaft (Looser's zones).

Signs and symptoms *Rickets:* Knock-kneed; bow-legged. Features of hypocalcaemia (p642). Children with rickets are ill.

Osteomalacia: Bone pain; fractures (neck of femur); proximal myopathy (waddling gait).

Treatment Calcium-with-vitamin D (400 units) tablets: 1–2 tablets/day.
- If due to malabsorption give parenteral calciferol 7.5mg monthly.
- If vitamin-D-resistant give calciferol 10,000 units/24h PO.
- If due to renal disease give alfacalcidol (1α-hydroxy vitamin D) 1µg/24h PO and adjust dose according to plasma calcium.
- Monitor plasma calcium.

➤ Vitamin D therapy (esp. alfacalcidol) can cause dangerous hypercalcaemia.

Vitamin D-resistant rickets exists in two forms. Type I with low renal 1α-hydroxylase activity, and type II with end organ resistance to 1,25(OH)$_2$ vitamin D. Both are treated with large doses of 1,25(OH)$_2$ vitamin D.

X-linked hypophosphataemic rickets Dominantly inherited—due to a defect in renal phosphate handling (probably Na$^+$/PO$_4^{3-}$ transporter). Rickets develops in early childhood, and is associated with poor growth. Plasma phosphate is low, alkaline phosphatase high, and there is phosphaturia. Treatment is with high doses of oral phosphate, and 1,25(OH)$_2$ vitamin D. Hypophosphataemic osteomalacia may develop in patients consuming phosphate binders eg aluminium hydroxide, or some rare tumour, and is accompanied by severe muscle weakness.

See also renal osteodystrophy, p388.

Proteins: in plasma

Electrophoresis distinguishes a number of bands (see figure).

Albumin is synthesized in the liver; $t_{1/2} \approx 20$ days. It binds *bilirubin, free fatty acids, calcium* and some *drugs. Low albumin* results in oedema. *Causes:* Liver disease, nephrotic syndrome, burns, protein-losing enteropathy, malabsorption, malnutrition, late pregnancy, artefact (eg from arm with IVI), posture (5g/L higher if upright), genetic variations, malignancy. *High albumin—Causes:* Dehydration; artefact (eg haemostasis).

α_1 **zone** Absence (or $\downarrow\downarrow$) suggests α_1-antitrypsin deficiency, an autosomal recessive disease causing cirrhosis and emphysema: unopposed phagocyte proteases increase the nomal age-related decline in FEV$_1$ from ~35mL/yr to 80mL/yr, exacerbated by smoking (eg $\downarrow$ by 300mL/yr). Signs: dyspnoea; weight$\downarrow$; cor pulmonale; PCV$\uparrow$; LFT$\uparrow$ (hepatocytes cannot secrete the protein).

α_2 **zone** is mainly α_2 macroglobulin and haptoglobin (p584). May be increased in nephrosis with an associated decrease in other bands.

β **zone** is *low* in active nephritis, glomerulonephritis, and SLE.

γ **zone** is *diffusely raised* in: chronic infections, liver cirrhosis (with a low albumin and α-globulin), sarcoidosis, SLE, RA, Crohn's, TB, bronchiectasis, PBC, hepatitis and parasitaemia. It is *low* in: nephrotic syndrome, malabsorption, malnutrition, immune deficiency (severe illness, diabetes mellitus, renal failure, malignancy or congenital).

Paraproteinaemia See p616.

Acute phase response The body responds to a variety of insults with, amongst other things, the synthesis, by the liver, of a number of proteins (normally present in serum in small quantities)—eg α_1-antitrypsin, fibrinogen, complement, haptoglobin and C-reactive protein. An increased density of the α_1- and α_2-fractions, often with a reduced albumin level, is thus seen with conditions such as infection, malignancy (especially α_2-fraction), trauma, surgery and inflammatory disease.

C-reactive protein (CRP) helps monitoring of inflammation. The best test is quantitative, normal <0.80mg/L. Like the ESR, it is raised in many inflammatory conditions, but changes more rapidly; increases in hours and falling within 2–3 days of recovery. Therefore, it can be used to follow the response to therapy (eg antibiotics) or activity of disease (eg Crohn's disease). If the CRP has fallen 3 days after the onset of treatment for infection then consider that your choice of antibiotics was appropriate. CRP is raised by active rheumatic disease (rheumatoid arthritis, rheumatic fever, seronegative arthritides, vasculitides), tissue injury or necrosis (acute MI, transplanted kidney or bone marrow rejection, malignancies—especially breast, lung, GI), burns, infection—bacterial much more than viral infection. It is very useful for diagnosis of post-operative or intercurrent infections when the ESR may still be elevated. If the CRP has not started to fall 3 days after surgery then complications must be considered (eg infection, PE). CRP is *not* raised by SLE, leukaemia (fever, blast crisis, or cytotoxins), ulcerative colitis, pregnancy, osteoarthritis, anaemia, polycythaemia, or heart failure. Its highest levels are seen in bacterial infections (>10mg/L). Absence of an elevated CRP significantly reduces the pre-test probability of other investigations for bacterial infection, eg bone or gallium scan, and so may be a cheaper, more comfortable alternative.

IN URINE (If protein >0.15g/24h then pathological. See p370.)

Albuminuria Usually caused by renal disease.

Bence Jones protein consists of light chains excreted in excess by some patients with myeloma (p614). They are not detected by dipsticks and may occur with normal serum electrophoresis.

Haemoglobinuria p586 Myoglobinuria p394 Microalbuminuria p396, 532.

C-reactive protein	
Marked elevation	*Normal-to-slight elevation*
Bacterial infection	Viral infection
Abscess	Steroids/oestrogens
Crohn's disease	Ulcerative colitis
Connective tissue diseases	SLE
(except SLE)	
Neoplasia	
Trauma	
Necrosis (eg MI)	

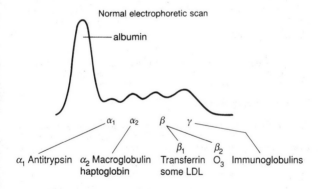

Normal electrophoretic scan

albumin

α_1 α_2 β γ

α_1 Antitrypsin α_2 Macroglobulin   Transferrin O_3 Immunoglobulins
haptoglobin   some LDL

β_1 β_2

Plasma enzymes

▶Reference intervals vary from laboratory to laboratory.

Raised plasma levels of specific enzymes can be very useful indications of specific disease. But remember that, for example, 'cardiac enzymes' may be raised for reasons other than cardiac pathology. The major causes of *raised enzymes* are given below. ●Reference intervals: p754.

Alkaline phosphatase Liver disease (suggests cholestasis). Bone disease (isoenzyme distinguishable, reflects laying down of osteoid, ie osteoblast activity) especially Paget's, growing children, healing fractures, osteomalacia, metastases, hyperparathyroidism and renal failure. The placenta makes its own isoenzyme, accounting for the raised alk phos of pregnancy.

Alanine-amino transferase (ALT; SGPT). Liver disease (suggests hepatocyte damage). Also raised in shock.

Aldolase Skeletal muscle. Also heart and liver disease.

α-Amylase Acute pancreatitis. Also severe uraemia, diabetic ketoacidosis. Not raised in chronic pancreatitis (little tissue remaining).

Aspartate-amino transferase (AST; SGOT). Liver disease (suggesting hepatocyte damage). Following myocardial infarct (p280). Also skeletal muscle damage, and haemolysis.

Creatine kinase Levels are raised in *myocardial infarction* (p280; isoenzyme can be distinguished, 'CK-MB', normally <5% total); *muscle damage* (rhabdomyolysis, p394; prolonged running; haematoma; seizures; IM injection; defibrillation; bowel ischaemia; dermatomyositis, p670)—and *drugs* (eg statins, p277). ▶A raised CK doesn't necessarily mean an MI.

Gamma-glutamyl transpeptidase (GGT, γGT) Levels raised in liver disease (particularly alcohol-induced damage).

Lactate dehydrogenase (LDH) Following myocardial infarct (p280). Liver disease (suggests hepatocyte damage). May also be raised in haemolysis, pulmonary embolism, and tumour necrosis.

Tumour markers

Tumour markers are rarely sufficiently specific to be of diagnostic value. Their main value is in monitoring the course of an illness and the effectiveness of treatment. Reference ranges vary between laboratories.

Alpha-fetoprotein ↑In hepatocellular ca (p510), germ-cell tumours (not pure seminoma) hepatitis; cirrhosis; pregnancy; open neural tube defects.

CA 125 Raised in carcinoma of the ovary, breast, and hepatocellular carcinoma. Also raised in pregnancy, cirrhosis and peritonitis.

CA 153 Raised in carcinoma of the breast and benign breast disease.

CA 19-9 Raised in colorectal and pancreatic carcinoma, and cholestasis.

Carcino-embryonic antigen (CEA) Useful in monitoring gastrointestinal neoplasms, especially colorectal carcinoma. Also raised in cirrhosis, pancreatitis, and smoking.

Human chorionic gonadotrophin Raised in pregnancy and germ-cell tumours. For hydatidiform moles and choriocarcinoma, see OHCS p26.

Neurone specific enolase (NSE) Raised in small cell carcinoma of lung.

Placental alkaline phosphatase (PLAP) Raised in pregnancy, carcinoma of ovary, seminoma, and smoking.

Prostate specific antigen See opposite.

Prostate specific antigen (PSA)

As well as being a marker of prostate cancer, PSA is (unfortunately) raised in benign prostatic hypertrophy. See prostate cancer (p392) and p393 for advising men who ask for a PSA test. PSA cannot predict if a cancer will cause ill health—also 25% of large benign prostates give PSA up to 10; levels may be higher if no recent ejaculation. Some labs give plasma reference intervals (nmol/L) as follows:

Healthy males <40 years old:	PSA <4 in 100%	
Healthy males >40 years old:	PSA <4 in 96%	
	PSA 4–10 in 4%	PSA will be ~50%
Benign prostatic hypertrophy:	PSA <4 in 91%	lower after 6 months
	PSA 4–10 in 8%	on 5α reductase
	PSA >10 in 1%	inhibitors (to ↓ pros-
Prostatic cancer:	PSA <4 in 15%	tate size: see p134)[1]
	PSA 4–10 in 20%	
	PSA >10 in 65%	

The above is a rough guide only (different labs have different reference ranges, and populations vary; more specific assays are also becoming available, which may partly solve these problems). It is shown to illustrate the common problem of interpreting a PSA of ~8—and as a warning against casual requests for PSAs in the (vain) hope of simple answers.

1 S Taneja 1997 *BMJ* i 371

Hyperlipidaemia MND

High serum cholesterol, and to a lesser extent triglicerides, are major risk factors for coronary heart disease (CHD). Half the UK have a serum cholesterol putting them at significant risk of CHD. But treatment must be in consideration with other risk factors: smoking, BP↑, DM, family history—see risk equation, p740. Benefits of treatment must be set against cost, and imposition of diets and tablet-taking (with expensive follow-up plans). Screen people wisely: for some it may be better not to know.[1]

Trial evidence that treating hypercholesterolaemia is worthwhile
- '4S' study.[2] Secondary prevention trial (patients all had ischaemic heart disease) using simvastatin 20mg in 4444 men aged 35–70, (cholesterols of 5.5–8.0mmol/L). Number needed to treat (NNT, p748) to prevent one fatal MI was 25 (over 6yrs), and 14 for non-fatal events.
- WOSCOPS.[3] Primary prevention trial in Scotland with over 6,500 men (cholesterol >6.5mmol/L) taking pravastatin 40mg. NNT to prevent one fatal MI was 142 (over 5 years), and for all cardiac events was 55.
- CARE[4] study. Secondary prevention trial with 40mg of pravastatin in >4,000 people post-MI with 'normal' cholesterol (<6.2mmol/L). NNT for fatalities was 91 over 5yrs, and for non-fatal MI was 38.

Do plasma lipids in those < 70yrs old if: (Evidence is scant if >70.)
- Family history of hyperlipidaemia.
- Family or personal history of CHD before 65 or risk↑, eg DM, BP↑.
- Xanthomata or xanthelasmata. • Corneal arcus before 50yrs old.

Management[5,6] (Cholesterol >5.2mmol/L and aged <60–70yrs)
- Exclude 1° or 2° hyperlipidaemias. Treat as appropriate.
- Lifestyle advice. Aim for BMI of 20 to 25. Diet with <10% of calories from saturated fats and plenty of gel-forming fibre (p482). Exercise.
- HRT if appropriate (if no DVT/PE, or breast cancer or ↑risk of breast cancer).
- Give a statin (below) to all who have had a past myocardial infarct if cholesterol >4.8mmol/L (5.5mmol/L if just angina)—and to those with known CHD who fail to respond to the measures above.
- If no overt heart disease, risk factor tables (p740) give cut-off points for R₂.[5]
- 'Statins' are first choice (see p277); they ↓cholesterol synthesis in the liver (eg simvastatin 10–40mg PO at night). CI: porphyria, LFT↑. SE: myositis (stop if CK ≥↑700u/L; if muscle aches, check CK; risk is 1/100,000 treatment years[5]); abdo pain; LFT↑ (stop if AST ≥100u/L).
- Second-line therapy. Fibrates eg bezafibrate (useful in familial mixed hyperlipidaemias); anion exchange resins eg cholestyramine; and nicotinic acid (HDL↑; LDL↓; SE: severe flushing; reduced by giving aspirin 300mg ½h pre-dose).
- Hypertriglyceridaemia responds best to fibrates, nicotinic acid, or fish oil.

Primary hyperlipidaemias Risk of CHD↑↑. Lipids travel in blood packaged with proteins as lipoproteins. There are 4 classes: chylomicrons (mainly triglyceride); low-density lipoprotein (LDL, mainly cholesterol, the lipid correlating most strongly with CHD); very low density lipoprotein (VLDL, mainly triglyceride); high density lipoprotein (HDL, mainly phospholipid, correlating inversely with CHD—it's 'good'). See opposite.

Secondary hyperlipidaemias These are caused by diabetes mellitus; alcohol abuse; T₄↓; renal failure, nephrosis, cholestasis.

Xanthomata These yellowish lipid deposits may be: eruptive (itchy nodules in crops in hypertriglyceridaemia); tuberous (yellow plaques on elbows and knees); planar—also called palmar (orange-coloured streaks in palmar creases), virtually diagnostic of remnant hyperlipidaemia; or deposits in tendons, eyelids (xanthelasmata), or cornea (arcus).

1 BMJ 1993 i 1355 2 Lancet 1994 344 1388 3 NEJM 1995 333 1301 4 N Eng J Med 1996 335 1001 5 Drug Ther Bul 1996 34 89 using corrected Sheffield tables 5 Brit. Hyperlipidaemia Soc. 1997 Guidelines i 53

Primary hyperlipidaemias[1]

chol=plasma cholesterol mmol/L
Trig=plasma triglyceride (mmol/L); blue numerals=**WHO** phenotype

Lipoprotein lipase deficiency[I]	Chol <6.5 chylomicrons↑ <u>Trig</u> 10–30	Eruptive xanthomata; lipaemia retinalis; hepatosplenomegaly (HSM)
Familial hypercholesterolaemia[IIa]	Chol 7.5–16 LDL↑ Trig <2.3	<u>Tendon xanthoma;</u> arcus; xanthelasma
Familial defective apoprotein B-100[IIa]	Chol 7.5–16 LDL↑ Trig <2.3	Tendon xanthoma; arcus; xanthelasma
<u>Polygenic hypercholesterolaemia</u>[IIa]	Chol 6.5–9 LDL↑ Trig <2.3	*The commonest 1° lipidaemia* <u>xanthelasma; corneal arcus</u>
Familial combined hyperlipidaemia[IIa,IIb,IV or V]	Chol 6.5–10 LDL↑ VLDL↑ Trig 2.3–12 HDL↓	*Next commonest 1° lipidaemia* xanthelasma; arcus;
Remnant particle disease[III]	Chol 9–14 LDL↑ Trig 9–14	Palmar striae; tubero-eruptive xanthoma
Familial hypertriglyceridaemia[IV or V]	Chol 6.5–12 VLDL↑ Trig 10–30 Chylomicrons	Eruptive xanthoma; lipaemia retinalis; HSM

PRIMARY HDL ABNORMALITIES
hyperalphalipoproteinaemia HDL chol >2 HDL↑   –
hypoalphalipoproteinaemia HDL ""<0.92 HDL↓   –

►**What are the priorities in treating diet-resistant hyperlipidaemia?**[1]*

Top priority: *Treat those with ischaemic heart disease if cholesterol >5.2.*
2nd priority: *Treat those with many risk factors, eg BP↑ ± DM if chol >6.5.*
3rd priority: *Treat asymptomatic adult males if cholesterol >7.8.*
4th priority: *Treat post-menopausal women if cholesterol >7.8mmol/L.*

*LDL may also trigger these actions: if >3.4, or >5, or >6 or >6mmol/L for each of the priorities above, respectively. Aim for a level of <3.4mmol/L.

Xanthelasma: IIa, IIb, IV, V } Same.
Corneal arcus: IIa, IIb, IV, V
Lipaemia Retinalis: I, IV, V.
Eruptive Xanthoma: I, III, IV, V
Hepatosplenomegaly: I

The porphyrias

The acute porphyrias are rare genetic diseases caused by errors in the pathway of haem biosynthesis resulting in the toxic accumulation of porphobilinogen and δ-aminolaevulinic acid (porphyrin precursors). Characterized by acute neurovisceral crises, due to the increased production of porphyrin precursors, and their appearance in the urine. Some forms have cutaneous manifestations. Prevalence: 1–2 per 100,000.

Acute intermittent porphyria is a low-penetrant autosomal dominant condition; 28% have no family history (eg as the culprit porphobilinogen deaminase gene has undergone one of its 50 mutations *de novo*). ~10% of those with the gene have neurovisceral symptoms. Attacks are intermittent, more common in women, and may be precipitated by many drugs (see below). Urine porphobilinogens are raised during attacks and often (50%) between them (the urine may go deep red on standing). Faecal porphyrin levels are normal. There are no skin manifestations.

Variegate porphyria and *hereditary coproporphyria* are autosomal dominants. Signs: photosensitive blistering skin lesions and/or acute attacks. The former is prevalent in Afrikaners in South Africa. Porphobilinogen is high only in an attack, and other metabolites may be detected in faeces.

Features of an acute attack Colic ± vomiting ± fever ± wcc↑—so mimicking an acute abdomen (anaesthesia can be disastrous here)—also:
- Hypotension
- Hyponatraemia
- Hypokalaemia
- Hypotonia
- Proteinuria
- Psychosis/odd behaviour*
- Peripheral neuritis
- Paralysis
- Seizures
- Sensory impairment
- Sight may be affected
- Shock (± collapse)

Drugs to avoid in acute intermittent porphyria are legion (they may precipitate above symptoms ± quadriplegia, see *BNF/OTM*), they include: *alcohol*; several *anaesthetic agents* (barbiturates, halothane); *antibiotics* (chloramphenicol, sulfonamides, tetracyclines); *painkillers* (pentazocine); *oral hypoglycaemics*; *contraceptive pill*. (S Whatley 1995 *Lancet* **346** 1007)

Treatment of an acute attack Remove precipitants, then:
- Give IV fluids to correct electrolyte imbalance.
- High carbohydrate intake (eg Hycal®) by NG tube if necessary.
- IV haematin is probably the treatment of choice in most centres now.
- Nausea controlled with prochlorperazine 12.5mg IM.
- Sedation if necessary with chlorpromazine 50–100mg PO/IM.
- Pain control with: aspirin, dihydrocodeine or morphine.
- Seizures can be controlled with diazepam.
- Treat tachycardia and hypertension with propranolol.

Non-acute porphyrias
Porphyria cutanea tarda, *erythropoietic protoporphyria* and *congenitial porphyria*, are characterized by cutaneous photosensitivity alone, since there is no overproduction of porphyrin precursors, only porphyrins.

EtOH, lead, and Fe deficiency can cause abnormal porphyrin metabolism.
▶Offer genetic counselling (*OHCS* p212) to all patients and their families.

---

*__B__e sure I looked up at her eyes
Happy and proud; at last I knew
Porphyria worshipped me; surprise
Made my heart swell, and still it grew
While I debated what to do.
That moment she was mine, mine fair,

Perfectly pure and good: I found
A thing to do, and all her hair
In one long yellow string I wound
Three times her little throat around,
And strangled her . . .
[From *Porphyria's Lover*, Robert Browning]

Pulse oximetry[1]

▶ *Don't rely on vision to assess hypoxia. Early cyanosis is hard to detect.* Given optimal daylight one may detect an oxyhaemoglobin saturation of ≤80–75%. This corresponds to ≥5g/100mL of reduced ('blue') Hb, and is really quite hypoxic. Pulse oximetry allows non-invasive assessment of peripheral haemoglobin saturation with oxygen, transcutaneously on the finger or ear-lobe, and provides a useful tool with which to monitor patients.

Principles of oximetry In trying to measure the ratio of oxygenated to total Hb by looking through the skin there are many artefacts due to the tissues. These can be obviated by comparing colours at different stages during the cardiac pulse. Any difference is due to arterial blood alone (providing there are no confusing venous pulses—eg if the patient has tricuspid incompetence).

There are 2 light-emitting diodes (red and infrared), and a detector, which faces them through tissue ≤10mm thick. Diodes beam in sequence, and after correction for ambient light (don't have it too high) the oxyhaemoglobin saturation is given from an empirically determined table. Diodes flash up to 600 times per second, so read-outs appear continuous.

Errors Poor perfusion of the finger (or ear-lobe—better as it's nearer the heart, worse because devices tend to fall off). To get round this rub the digit, or put on some glyceryl trinitrate cream. Others include:
- Motion
- Excess ambient light
- Venous pulsation
- Dyshaemoglobinaemias
- Nail varnish
- Some skin pigmentation

Reference intervals An oxyhaemoglobin saturation of 90% is an interesting figure, because this is the knee of the sigmoid (f)-shaped oxyhaemoglobin dissociation curve (just above the horizontal line in the figure). Small changes in oxyhaemoglobin saturation *above* this level hardly make any difference to the arterial O_2 tension. *Below* this level, small changes really *do* matter. ≤80% is clearly abnormal and action is required (unless this is the patient's best, for example in chronic bronchitis and respiratory failure). For each 1% fall in oxyhaemoglobin saturation there is a sizeable drop in arterial O_2 tension. This is why on most pulse oximeters the alarm is set to 90%, and why this is a good target to aim for when you are reoxygenating someone. Nevertheless, individual circumstances may require you to set a lower goal.

Cautions Do not rely on pulse oximetry in carbon monoxide poisoning (see p794); also, in chronic obstructive pulmonary disease you need to know the P_aCO_2: if this is rising the P_aO_2 may give false reassurance. As with any bedside test, be sceptical, and seek occasional formal lab confirmation of blood gas results, whenever indicated (p353).

Indications Use pulse oximetry to monitor patients who are physically ill or at risk of biological compromise—eg during endoscopy, anaesthesia, or on the open ward, eg with pneumonia, myocardial infarction or pulmonary embolism—in fact whenever a life might be slipping through you fingers. Don't worry too much about not knowing the P_aCO_2, but enquire about symptoms of its excess (eg headache) and look for its signs (bounding pulse, and papilloedema, if it is chronic). Often P_aCO_2 matters less than the P_aO_2, and the time taken to do a blood gas might be better spent.

1 CD Hanning 1995 *BMJ* ii 367

15. Rheumatological & related illnesses

Relevant pages in other chapters: Charcot's joints (p476).
Eponymous syndromes: Behçet's disease (p694); Sjögren's syndrome
(p708); Wegener's granulomatosis (p710).

Points of note in the rheumatological history

Age, occupation, ethnic origin.

Presenting symptoms		**Past history**
Joints	Pain	Infection; trauma
	Morning stiffness	Diarrhoea; inflammatory
	Swelling	bowel disease
	Loss of function	Venereal disease
	Joints affected over	Gout
	course of disease	Previous operations
General	Nodules or lumps	
	Red eyes, dry eyes or mouth	*Treatments*
	Fever, rashes, ulcers	Current and previous
	Raynaud's phenomenon	Adverse reactions to
		medications

Social and family history
What can the patient do or not do?
Domestic situation
Family history of rheumatoid arthritis, osteoarthritis, gout, back disease.

Back pain

This is very common, and often self-limiting; *but be alert to sinister causes.*
Key points in the history: 1 Onset: sudden (related to trauma?) or gradual? 2 Are there motor or sensory symptoms? 3 Are bladder or bowel affected? Pain worse on movement and relieved by rest is often mechanical. If it is worse after rest, an inflammatory cause is likely.

Examination: 1 Movements of the spine: mark skin points 10cm above and 5cm below L5 in midline with patient erect. Ask patient to bend forward as far as possible. Measure distance between points. If <20cm, movement is restricted; 2 Neurological deficits: perianal sensation; UMN and LMN signs in legs; 3 Signs of generalized disease suggest malignancy.
Dorsal root irritation causes lancinating pain in the relevant dermatome, made worse by coughing and bending forward. *Lasègue's sign* is positive if straight leg raising on supine patient is painful and restricted to <45°. It suggests lumbar disc prolapse irritating nerve roots (although interobserver reproducibility is poor for this test, do not assume that there is some gold-standard which will reveal all: 20–30% of 'normals' with *no* back pain have *some* disc protrusion on MRI,■ but in finding out if this is significant, you have to rely on features and signs such as Lasègue's sign).

Neurosurgical emergencies ●*Acute cauda equina compression:* Alternating or bilateral root pain in legs, saddle anaesthesia (ie bilaterally around anus), and disturbance of bladder or bowel function.
●*Acute cord compression:* Bilateral pain, LMN signs at level of compression, UMN and sensory signs below, sphincter disturbance. Causes (same for both types of compression): bony metastasis (look for missing pedicle on x-ray), myeloma, cord or paraspinal tumour, TB (p198), abscess.
►Urgent treatment prevents irreversible loss: laminectomy for disc protrusions; decompression for abscess; radiotherapy for tumours.

Tests MRI (p738) is the best way to illustrate cord compression, myelopathy, intraspinal neoplasms, cysts, haemorrhages and abscesses (myelography, plain x-rays and CT are problematic). FBC, ESR (↑ in myeloma, infections, tumours), U&E, PSA, and *technetium* scan 'hot spot' may support diagnosis of neoplastic or inflammatory lesion.

Causes Age determines the most likely causes.
● 15–30yrs: Prolapsed disc, trauma, fractures, ankylosing spondylitis (p668), spondylolisthesis (eg L5 shifts forward on S1), pregnancy.
● 30–50yrs: Degenerative joint disease, prolapsed disc, malignancy (lung, breast, prostate, thyroid, kidney).
● >50yrs: Degenerative, osteoporosis, Paget's, malignancy, myeloma. Lumbar artery atheroma (which may itself cause disc degeneration[1]).
Rarer causes: Spinal stenosis (bony encroachment), cauda equina tumours, spinal infection (usually staphylococcal, also *Proteus, E coli, S typhi*, TB). Often no systemic signs of infection.

Treatment Specific causes need specific treatment. Usually no cause is found, so treat empirically: avoid precipitants; teach safe lifting skills with back straight. Analgesia, and carrying on with life is better than bed rest (>3 days is rarely justifiable) or physiotherapy.[2] There are rôles for rehabilitation exercises, manipulation, corsets, and, sometimes, laminectomy.[3]

Features which may indicate sinister back pain
● Young (<20y) or old (>55)
● Violent trauma
● Alternating sciatica
● Bilateral sciatica
● Weak legs
● Weight loss
● PUO; ESR↑ (>25mm/h, p618)
● Taking systemic steroids
● Progressive, continuous, nonmechanical pain
● Systemically unwell; drug abuse; HIV +ve
● Spine movement in *all* directions painful
● Localized bony tenderness
● CNS deficit at more than one root level
● Pain or tenderness of thoracic spine
● Bilateral signs of nerve root tension
● Past history of neoplasia

1 L Kauppila 1993 *BMJ* i 1267 2 DoH 1994 *Back Pain* HMSO■ ◁3▷ A Malmivaara 1995 *NEJM* 332 351

✚ Arthritis

The Patient with arthritis will suffer pain, stiffness (especially early morning), loss of function, and signs of inflammation at one or more joints.

Diagnosis ▶Assume there is septic arthritis if a joint is red and tender (acute onset). Aspirate the joint and look for blood, crystals and pus (culture and Gram stain). Sepsis may completely destroy a joint within 24 hours of onset. On microscopy, finding WBCs in the aspirate fluid suggests sepsis, but does not prove it—for example, the diagnosis may be pseudogout (are there needle-shaped crystals phagocytosed within WBCs?). If in doubt, treat for sepsis as described below.

Causes—*Monoarthritis:*
Sepsis (eg *Staphs, streps, pseudomonas brucella, gonococci,* TB, *salmonella*)
Trauma
Gout
Pseudogout
Spondyloarthritides
Osteoarthritis
Rheumatoid arthritis (rarely)
Haemarthrosis
Local malignant deposit

Polyarthritis:
Viruses (eg mumps, rubella, EBV hepatitis B, enteroviruses, HIV)
Rheumatoid or osteoarthritis
Spondyloarthritides
SLE
Henoch–Schönlein purpura
TB
Drug allergies
Acute rheumatic fever
Gonorrhoea
Crystal-induced arthritides

Assess Extent of joint involvement (include spine), symmetry, disruption of joint anatomy, limitation of movement (by pain or contracture), effusions and periarticular involvement. See p35 for a full assessment. Associated features: dysuria or genital ulcers, skin or eye involvement, lungs, kidneys, heart, GI (eg mouth ulcers, bloody diarrhoea) and CNS.

Radiology: Affected joints looking for erosions, calcification, widening or loss of joint space, changes in underlying bone (eg sclerotic areas, osteophytes), sacroiliac joints if a spondyloarthritis is possible; CXR in RA, SLE, and TB. In septic arthritis, x-rays are likely to be normal, as may be ESR and CRP (if CRP↑, expect it to fall once treatment gets under way).

Joint aspiration: OHCS 656. Microscopy (+culture): any blood, crystals or pus?

Blood: Culture if sepsis is possible. Do FBC and ESR. Urate, urea and creatinine if systemic disease. Rheumatoid factor, antinuclear antibody, and other autoantibodies. In trauma, arthroscopy may help. Consider HIV serology.

Treatment is determined by the cause. If **septic arthritis** is suspected, give flucloxacillin (for staphs—adult: ½–1g/6h slowly IV) *plus* benzylpenicillin 1.2g/4h IV until sensitivities are known. In infants, *Haemophilus* is common so give cefotaxime too (50mg/kg/12h IV slowly). Look for atypical mycobacteria and fungi if HIV +ve. Ask a microbiologist how long to continue treatment (eg 2 weeks IV then 4 weeks of oral therapy).[1] The rôle of repeated aspiration, lavage, and surgery is uncertain.[1,2] Ask an orthopaedic surgeon's advice. Beware inviting in new pathogens. Splints may be helpful in immobilizing the joint in the early days of treatment. If a joint prosthesis is present, surgery with removal of all foreign material may be required. Vigorous physiotherapy follows antibiotics.

---

1 RA Hughes 1996 *Reports on Rheumatic Diseases* 7 1–4   2 1992 Report of the Working Group Of Brit Soc for Rheumatology and the Royal College of Physicians Research Unit *J R Col Phys Lond* 26 83–5

Synovial fluid in health and disease*

Aspiration of synovial fluid is used primarily to look for infectious or crystal (gout and pseudogout—p666) arthropathies.

	Appearance	Viscosity	wbc/mL	Neutrophils
Normal	Clear, colourless	High	<200	<25%
Non-inflammatory[1]	Clear, straw	High	<5000	<25%
Haemorrhagic[2]	Bloody, xantho-chromic	Variable	<10,000	<50%
Acute inflammatory[3]	Turbid, yellow	Decreased		
•Acute gout			~14,000	~80%
•Rheumatic fever			~18,000	~50%
•Rheumatoid arthritis			~16,000	~65%
Septic	Turbid, yellow	Decreased		
•TB			~24,000	~70%
•Gonorrhoeal			~14,000	~60%
•Septic (non-gonococcal)[4]			~65,000	~95%

[1] Eg, degenerative joint disease, trauma.
[2] Eg, tumour, haemophilia, trauma.
[3] Includes eg Reiter's, pseudogout, SLE etc.
[4] Includes *Staphs*, *Streps*, Lyme, and *Pseudomonas* (eg post-op).

For inflammatory causes of arthritis: Synovial fluid wbc >2000/mL is 84% sensitive and 84% specific; synovial fluid neutrophil count >75% is 75% sensitive and 92% specific.

* Wallach, *Interpretation of Diagnostic Tests: A synopsis of Laboratory Medicine*, 5e, Little, Brown and Company, Boston, 1992. There is much individual variation in wbc/mL values.

Rheumatoid arthritis (RA)

Typically a persistent, symmetrical, deforming, peripheral arthropathy. Peak onset: 4th decade. ♀:♂>3:1. Prevalence: 3%. Genetics: HLA DR4 linked. Immunogenesis is said to be via presentation of the culprit (unknown) antigen to T-helper cells, with subsequent cytokine-mediated synovial neutrophil exudate, which releases cartilage-degrading enzymes.▣

Presentation See PLATE 5. Typically with swollen, painful, and stiff hands and feet, especially in the morning. This gradually gets worse and larger joints become involved. Less common presentations are: 1 Relapsing/remitting monoarthritis of different large joints (palindromic). 2 Persistent monoarthritis (often of knee). 3 Systemic illness (pericarditis, pleurisy, weight↓) with minimal joint problems at first. (Commoner in men.) 4 Vague limb girdle aches. 5 Sudden-onset widespread arthritis.

Signs At first, sausage-shaped fingers and MCP joint swelling. Later, ulnar deviation and volar subluxation (partial dislocation) at MCP joints, Boutonnière and swan-neck deformities of fingers (OHCS p670), or Z-deformity of thumbs. The wrist subluxes and the radial head becomes prominent (piano-key). Extensor tendons in the hand may rupture and adjacent muscles waste. Similar changes occur in the feet. Larger joints may be involved. Atlanto-axial joint subluxation may threaten the cord.

Extra-articular Anaemia. Nodules. Lymphadenopathy. Vasculitis. Carpal tunnel syndrome. Multifocal neuropathies. Splenomegaly (5%; but only 1% have Felty's syndrome: leucopenia, lymphadenopathy, weight loss, p698). Eyes: episcleritis, scleritis, keratoconjunctivitis sicca. Pleurisy. Pericarditis. Pulmonary fibrosis. Osteoporosis. Amyloidosis.

Tests X-ray of RA joints show excess soft tissue, juxta-articular osteoporosis, loss of joint space, then bony erosions ± subluxation. Complete carpal destruction may be seen. Rheumatoid factor +ve in 75% (Sjögren's 100%, SLE 30%, MCTD 30%, PSS 30%, p670), ANA +ve in 30%.

Treatment ●Regular exercise. ●Physiotherapy. ●Occupational therapy. ●Household aids and personal aids (orthoses), eg wrist splints. ●Intralesional steroids (for joint injection technique, see OHCS p656–8). ●Surgery—to improve function, not for cosmetic effect. ●Oral drugs: if no contraindication (asthma, active peptic ulcer) start an NSAID eg ibuprofen 400–800mg/8h pc (ie after food)—cheapest and least likely to cause GI bleeds or naproxen 250–500mg/12h (good as twice daily dose, and is more anti-inflammatory than ibuprofen, and may cause less GI bleeding than other NSAIDs). Diclofenac 25–50mg/8h pc is similar to naproxen and is available combined with misoprostol (Arthrotec®, an ulcer-protecting agent, p490): consider this if there is a history of dyspepsia and NSAIDs vital. One cannot predict which NSAID a patient will respond to. If 1–2 week trials of 3 NSAIDs do not control pain, or if synovitis for >6 months, try disease-modifying drugs (DMDs). DMD side-effects are many and serious. ►Regular monitoring is essential. If DMDs fail, consider cytotoxics (eg azathioprine, methotrexate). ●DMD side-effects: *Gold:* Marrow↓, proteinuria, LFTs↑. *Penicillamine:* Marrow↓, proteinuria, taste↓, oral ulcers, myasthenia, Goodpasture's. *Sulfasalazine:* (the best tolerated DMD, and most often used) Marrow↓, sperm count↓, hepatitis, oral ulcers. *Chloroquine:* Permanent retinopathy, tinnitus, headache. Rash with any of them. See OHCS p672 for dosages. ●The rôle of steroids: we know these can reduce erosions when given in early disease—eg prednisolone 7.5mg/day PO.▣ It is *not* known if all such patients should have this. One problem is ↓bone density over long periods. Another problem is that it would be difficult to keep patients to <7.5mg/day, as, for the first months, there may be great symptomatic improvement, which then tails off, leaving patients wanting higher doses, and risking cataract, fluid retention, and peptic ulcers.

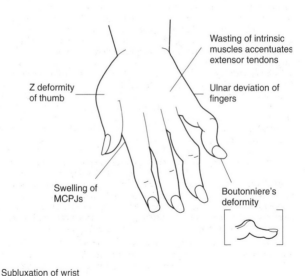

Wasting of intrinsic muscles accentuates extensor tendons

Ulnar deviation of fingers

Z deformity of thumb

Swelling of MCPJs

Boutonniere's deformity

Subluxation of wrist

Prominent radial head

Swan neck deformity

Osteoarthritis (OA)

OA, the commonest joint condition, is symptomatic three times more often in women, and the mean age of onset is 50yrs. It is usually primary, but may develop secondary to any joint disease or joint injury.

The Patient He or she may complain of pain on movement, worse at end of day; background pain at rest; stiffness; joint instability. Most commonly affected are DIP joints, first metacarpophalangeal, first metatarsophalangeal, cervical and lumbar spine, next the hip, then knee. There may be joint tenderness, derangement, ± bony swelling (eg Heberden's nodes, ie bony lumps at DIP joints), poor range of movement, effusions.

Radiology Loss of joint space, subchondral sclerosis and cysts, marginal osteophytes. **Other investigations** are normal.

Treatment Simple analgesics (eg paracetamol). If the pain is very bad, give NSAIDs (see p664). Reduce weight. Consider joint replacement. Do exercises (eg regular quadriceps exercises in knee OA) and keep active.

Crystal arthropathy

Gout In the acute stage there is severe pain, redness and swelling in the affected joint—often the metatarsophalangeal joint of the big toe (podagra). Attacks are due to hyperuricaemia (p634) and the deposition of sodium monourate crystals in joints, and may be precipitated by trauma, surgery, starvation, infection and diuretics. After repeated attacks, urate deposits (tophi) are found in avascular areas, eg pinna, tendons, joints, eye—and chronic tophaceous gout is said to exist. 'Secondary' causes of gout: polycythaemia, leukaemia, cytotoxics, renal failure.

Diagnosis depends on finding urate crystals in tissues and synovial fluid (serum uricate not always↑). Synovial fluid microscopy: negatively birefringent crystals; neutrophils (+ ingested crystals). X-rays may show only soft-tissue swelling in the early stages. Later well-defined 'punched out' lesions are seen in juxta-articular bone. There is no sclerotic reaction, and joint spaces are preserved until late. *Prevalence:* ~½–1%. ♂:♀ ≈ 5:1.

Treatment of acute gout is with an NSAID such as prompt ibuprofen or naproxen 750mg stat, then 250mg/8h PO pc. If contraindicated (eg peptic ulcer), give colchicine 1mg PO initially, then 0.5mg/2h PO until the pain goes or D&V occurs, or 10mg has been given. Do not repeat within 3 days. Note: in renal failure, NSAIDs and colchicine are problematic: steroids may be very effective, but have their own SE (get expert help).

Prevention of attacks: Avoid purine-rich foods (offal, oily fish), obesity and alcohol excess. No aspirin (it ↑ serum urate). Consider reducing serum urate with long-term allopurinol, but not until 3 weeks after an attack. Allopurinol: 100–300mg/24h PO pc, adjusted in the light of serum urate levels (typically 200mg/24h; max 300mg/8h). SE: rash, fever, WCC↓; if troublesome, substitute a uricosuric, eg probenecid 0.5g/12h PO.

Pseudogout (Calcium pyrophosphate arthropathy) Risk factors:–Old age –Dehydration –Intercurrent illness –Hyperparathyroidism –Myxoedema/DM –PO_4^{3-}↓ Mg^{2+}↓ –Any arthritis (RA,OA) –Haemochromatosis –Acromegaly

The Patient: Two typical presentations: 1 *Acute pseudogout:* Less severe and longer-lasting than gout; affects different joints (mainly knee).
2 *Chronic calcinosis:* Destructive changes like OA, but more severe; affecting eg knees, also wrists, shoulders, hips. *Tests:* Calcium deposition on x-ray (eg triangular ligament in wrist). Joint crystals are weakly positively birefringent in plane polarized light.

Treatment of pseudogout: This is symptomatic, eg with NSAIDs (p672).

X-ray findings in OA

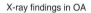

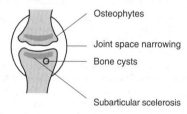

X-ray findings in gout

Spondyloarthritides

Ankylosing spondylitis (AS) *Prevalence:* 1 in 2000. Men present earlier: ♂:♀ ≈6:1 at 16yrs old, and ≈2 at 30yrs old. >95% HLA B27 +ve.

Symptoms: The typical patient is a young man presenting with morning stiffness, backache, sacroiliac pain, progressive loss of spinal movement (spinal ankylosis) who later develops kyphosis, neck hyperextension (question mark posture), and spino-cranial ankylosis. Other features:

Thoracic excursion↓	Periosteitis of calcaneum or	Amyloidosis
Chest pain	ischial tuberosities	Carditis; iritis
Hip/knee involvement	Plantar fasciitis	Lung fibrosis (apex)

Tests: Radiology may show: a 'bamboo spine', squaring of the vertebra, erosions of the apophyseal joints, obliteration of the sacroiliac joints (sacroiliitis also occurs in Reiter's disease, Crohn's disease and chronic polyarthritis). Other tests: FBC (normochromic anaemia); ESR↑.

Treatment: Exercise, not rest, for backache. If able to co-operate with an intensive exercise regimen to maintain posture and mobility, he may keep happy and employed, despite chronic progressive illness. NSAIDs may relieve pain and stiffness. Rarely, spinal osteotomy is useful.

Mortality: 1.5-fold higher than expected (eg from secondary amyloid or cardiovascular causes), but most never need hospital treatment.[1]

Enteropathic arthropathies Inflammatory bowel disease and GI bypass surgery (and possibly Whipple's disease, p712) are associated with spondyloarthritis and large joint mono- or oligo-arthropathy.

Psoriatic arthritis See *OHCS* p586.

Reiter's syndrome *Presentation:* A triad of *urethritis, conjunctivitis* and *seronegative arthritis.* A typical patient is a young man with recent NSU—which may be asymptomatic; it may also follow dysentery (and epidemics have occurred eg in war). Often large joint mono- or oligo-arthritis; it may be chronic or relapsing. *Other features:* Iritis, keratoderma blenorrhagica (brown, aseptic abscesses on soles and palms); mouth ulcers; circinate balanitis (painless serpiginous penile rash); enthesopathy (plantar fasciitis, Achilles tendonitis) and aortic incompetence (rare). *Tests:* First of 2-glass urine test shows debris in urethritis. (In prostatitis there is more matter in the last sample.) Also look for neutrophils, and macrophages containing neutrophils (Peking cells) in synovial fluid. X-rays: periosteitis at ligamentous insertions; rheumatoid-like changes if chronic. *Management:* Rest; splint affected joints; NSAIDs. Recovery may take months.

Universal truths and some comments about spondyloarthritides

These conditions are seronegative arthritides (rheumatoid factor is –ve), but exclude seronegative RA. These features are held in common:
- Involvement of spine (spondylo-) and sacroiliac (SI) joints—also called 'axial arthritis'.
- Asymmetrical large-joint oligo- (ie few joints) or monoarthritis.
- Inflammation then calcification of tendon insertions sites (enthesopathy), eg plantar fasciitis, Achilles tendinitis, costochondritis.
- Extra-articular manifestations: uveitis, aortic regurgitation, upper zone pulmonary fibrosis, amyloidosis.
- HLA B27 association (88–96% of those with ankylosing spondylitis).

The spondyloarthritides show considerable overlap with one another. They are treated with physical and occupational therapy, advice about posture, and NSAIDs (if necessary for symptom control).

Other diseases associated with arthritis (seronegative)

Lyme disease (p232), psoriasis, Behçet's (p694), leukaemia (p600), pulmonary osteoarthropathy (p342), endocarditis, acne, acromegaly (p564), Wilson's disease (p712), familial Mediterranean fever (p186), sarcoid, sickle-cell (p588), haemochromatosis (p509)—and **reactive arthritis** eg from:

Yersinia (p225)	Chlamydia trachomatis	Campylobacter
Salmonella/Shigella	& Chl pneumoniae (p334)	Ureaplasma; HIV
Vibrio parahaemolyticus	Borrelia burgdorferi (p232)	Clostridium difficile

Lipopolysaccharide antigen stimulation (IgA antibodies) may be important in reactive arthritis. Reactive arthritis is treated with NSAIDs, physiotherapy, and steroid joint injections. Antibiotics only help after yersinia or chlamydial infection.[1]

Chronic arthritis in children may take several forms:
- Juvenile ankylosing spondylitis (mainly boys over 9 years)
- Juvenile rheumatoid arthritis (mainly post-pubertal girls)
- Juvenile psoriatic arthritis
- Juvenile chronic arthritis, or Still's disease, is most common. It may be a systemic illness, polyarticular, or pauciarticular (associated with ANA and chronic uveitis). See OHCS p758.

1 K Lehtinen 1993 *Annals of Rheumatic Diseases* 52 174-6

Connective tissue diseases—1

Essence The connective tissue diseases (CTDs or collagen vascular diseases) form an unholy alliance, like Yorkist pretenders to a Lancastrian throne. And they often seem as sinister to the student. Unholy, because the rightful heirs to the title (like the true diseases of collagen, eg Ehlers–Danlos syndrome, OHCS p746) are excluded. Alliance, because clinically they have much in common. They overlap with each other, affect many organ systems, are associated with systemic fever and malaise, tend to run a chronic course, often respond to steroids, and are often associated with anaemia of chronic disease and a raised ESR. But their pathologies vary.

670

Included in this group are: systemic lupus erythematosus (p672), RA (p664), progressive systemic sclerosis, polymyositis, dermatomyositis, mixed connective tissue disease, Sjögren's syndrome (p708), relapsing polychondritis, polyarteritis nodosa (p674), polymyalgia rheumatica (p674), giant cell arteritis (p674), Wegener's granulomatosis (p710), Behçet's syndrome (p694), Takayasu's arteritis (p708).

Systemic lupus erythematosus The group 'prototype' (p672).

Progressive systemic sclerosis (PSS) There are 3 forms: •*CREST syndrome:* calcinosis (subcutaneous tissues), Raynaud's phenomenon, disordered oesophageal motility, sclerodactyly, and telangiectasia. •*Generalized progressive systemic sclerosis* with kidney involvement; BP↑↑; polyarthritis; myopathy; lung and GI fibrosis. No treatment works; give symptomatic support. Prognosis varies from weeks (malignant hypertension) to years, and is shorter than in CREST. •*Scleroderma:* This is tightening and fibrosis of the skin. ♀:♂≈4. It typically presents in years after childbirth (it has been thought of as a graft-vs-host phenomenon, in which the 'graft' is residual circulating fetal cells, ie a microchimera).[1]• *Diagnostic criteria:* Proximal skin scleroderma, or any 2 of: sclerodactyly, digital pitting scars, pulp loss, bibasilar lung fibrosis. NB: morphoea (localized skin sclerosis) rarely, if ever, progresses to PSS. Characteristic autoantibodies *may* occur (in any of the 3 forms)—to topoisomerase (Scl-70), RNA polymerases, and centromeres.

Mixed connective tissue disease (MCTD) combines features of SLE, PSS, and polymyositis. Renal or CNS involvement is rare. Anti-RNP (ribonuclear protein) antibody is present (without other types of ANA; there is a speckled pattern of staining). Prognosis is probably the same as SLE.

Relapsing polychondritis attacks the pinna, nasal septum and larynx, the last causing stridor. It is associated with aortic valve disease, arthritis and vasculitis. Treat with steroids.

Polymyositis and dermatomyositis

Insidious, symmetrical, proximal muscle weakness results from muscle inflammation. Dysphagia, dysphonia (problems with the mechanics, not the idea, of speech production/phonation), facial oedema, or respiratory weakness may develop. 25% have a purple (heliotrope) rash on cheeks, eyelids and light-exposed areas, ± nail-fold erythema. Raynaud's, lung involvement, polyarthritis, retinitis (like cotton-wool patches), and myocardial involvement occur, with associated malignancy in >10% of patients >40yrs, but this figure is controversial. Diagnosis is by muscle enzyme (CK) levels, electromyography (EMG—shows fibrillation potentials), and muscle biopsy. Rest and prednisolone help (start with 60mg/24h PO). Immunosuppressives (p622) and cytotoxics are also used, but often the patient remains disabled. One good, small randomized trial (N=15) has shown great benefit from immune globulin 2g/kg once monthly—so much so that wheelchairs have given way to the climbing of stairs and to running.

A more aggressive form with prominent vasculitis occurs in children.

1 J Nelson 1998 *Lancet* **351** 559 (fetal cells are 33-fold commoner in scleroderma patients than in controls)

Systemic lupus erythematosus

SLE is a non-organ-specific, autoimmune vasculitis in which antinuclear antibodies (ANA) occur. ♀:♂ ≈9:1. *Prevalence:* ~0.2%. *Commoner in:* pregnancy; Afro-Caribbeans; Asians—and if HLA B8, DR2 or DR3 +ve. ~10% of relatives of SLE patients are affected. It's a remitting and relapsing illness, with peak age at diagnosis being 30–40yrs (in the UK).

The Patient ●*Musculoskeletal symptoms* (95%): Joint/muscle pain, myositis, proximal myopathy. Non-erosive polyarthritis with periarticular and tendon involvement. Deforming arthropathy rarely may occur due to capsular laxity (Jaccoud's arthropathy). Aseptic bone necrosis.
●*Skin* (81%): Photosensitive malar butterfly rash (hyperkeratosis, follicular plugging over nasal bridge, spreading to cheeks); scarring alopecia; livedo reticularis (net-like rash); Raynaud's; purpura; oral ulcers; urticaria; conjunctivitis; bullae. Discoid lupus (ears, cheeks, scalp, forehead, chest) is a 3-stage rash: erythema → pigmented hyperkeratotic oedematous papules → atrophic depressed lesions.
●*Renal* (≤75%): Proteinuria; casts; oedema; uraemia; glomerulonephritis, eg necrotizing-proliferative combined with membranous nephropathy.
●*CNS* (≤18%): Depression; psychosis; fits; hemi- or paraplegia; cranial nerve lesions; cerebellar ataxia; chorea; meningitis. *Eye:* Retinal exudates.
●*Pulmonary* (48%): Pleurisy (± pleural effusion); pneumonia; fibrosing alveolitis; obliterative bronchiolitis; pulmonary oedema (rare).
●*CVS* (38%): ▶BP↑; pericarditis (± effusion); Libman–Sacks endocarditis.
●*Blood:* Normocytic anaemia (75%); Coombs' +ve haemolysis; WCC↓; lymphopenia; INR↑; platelets↓ (lymphocyte; clotting factor and platelet antibodies); ESR↑; CRP ↔ (unless intercurrent infection); B-cell lymphoma.
●*Other:* Fever (77%); splenomegaly; lymphadenopathy; recurrent abortion.[1]

Immunology 80% are ANA +ve. High titre of ANA directed against double-stranded DNA is almost exclusive to SLE. Its absence doesn't exclude it. 40% are Rh factor +ve. 11% have false +ve syphilis serology from IgG anticardiolipin antibodies. Antibodies to Ro (SS-A), La (SS-B), and UI ribonuclear protein help define overlap syndromes (see Sjögren's, p708).

Monitoring activity BP, urinalysis, FBC, U&E ± complement: C3d↑, C3↓, C4↓ (better than ESR), double-stranded (anti-ds) DNA antibody titres.

Treatment Refer to an expert. ●Sun-block creams (OHCS p599) ●NSAIDs.
●*Hydroxychloroquine* if joint or skin symptoms are not controlled by NSAID, eg 6mg/kg/24h PO for 4 weeks, then 200mg/24h. (SE: irreversible retinopathy—check vision at least annually).
●*Prednisolone* for exacerbations (0.75–1mg/kg/24h PO for 6–10 weeks, then reduce) with hydroxychloroquine (≤ 6mg/kg/24h). Relapses may be preventable by additional prednisolone as soon as anti-dsDNA rises.[2]
●*Low-dose steroids* may be of value in chronic disease.
●*Cyclophosphamide* helps renal function more than steroids.[3] Dose example: 0.5–3mg/kg/day PO; intermittent pulses of 20mg/kg/month IV—give fewer SE. Its rôle in CNS disease is unclear. *Azathioprine* 1–2.5mg/kg/day PO is used as a steroid-sparing drug (SE: lymphoma).
●*Cyclosporin (=ciclosporin)* or *methotrexate* may be advised by experts.

Drug lupus Can be caused by isoniazid, hydralazine (if >50mg/24h in slow acetylators), procainamide, chlorpromazine, anticonvulsants. Lung and skin signs prevail over renal and CNS. It remits if drug is stopped. Sulfonamides and the Pill may exacerbate idiopathic SLE.

Antiphospholipid syndrome SLE may be seen with arterial or venous thromboses, stroke, migraine, miscarriages, myelitis, myocardial infarct, multi-infarct dementia—and ↑*cardiolipin* (a phospholipid) antibody (IgG and IgM). Aspirin or anticoagulation (INR ≈ 3) may be needed: see p624.[4]

1 *Lupus* 1996 66 659 2 H Bootsma 1995 *Lancet* 345 1595 3 P Venables 1993 BMJ ii 663 4 BMJ 1993 ii 883

Connective tissue diseases—vasculitis

Essence Vasculitis occurs in non-organ specific autoimmune diseases (eg RA, SLE), but may be less important than the glomerulonephritis or synovitis. It is the principal feature in certain other connective tissue diseases (CTDs) which may or may not be autoimmune (eg PAN, Wegener's). There is a third group of CTDs in which the importance of vasculitis is unknown (eg progressive systemic sclerosis). Vasculitis also occurs in conditions that are not usually included in the CTDs (eg drug reactions).

Polyarteritis nodosa (PAN) Commoner in males by 4:1. Some cases are associated with HBsAg. It is a necrotizing vasculitis which causes aneurysms of medium-sized arteries.

The Patient: General features: fever, malaise, weight↓, arthralgia.
- Renal: (75%) Main cause of death. Hypertension, haematuria, proteinuria, renal failure, intrarenal aneurysms, vasculitis.
- Cardiac: (80%) Second biggest cause of death. Coronary arteritis and consequent infarction. ↑BP and heart failure. Pericarditis. In Kawasaki's disease (childhood PAN variant, OHCS p750) coronary aneurysms occur.
- Pulmonary: Pulmonary infiltrates and asthma occur in vasculitis (some say that lung involvement is incompatible with PAN, calling it then Churg–Strauss syndrome).
- CNS: (70%) Mononeuritis multiplex, sensorimotor polyneuropathy, seizures, hemiplegia, psychoses.
- GI: (70%) Abdominal pain (any viscus may infarct), malabsorption because of chronic ischaemia.
- Skin: Urticaria, purpura, infarcts, livedo (p672), nodules.
- Blood: WCC↑, eosinophilia (in 30%), anaemia, ESR and CRP raised.

Diagnosis is most often made from clinical features in combination with renal or mesenteric angiography. ANCA may be +ve (p675).

Treatment: Treat hypertension meticulously. Refer to experts. Use high-dose prednisolone, and then cyclophosphamide.

Other vasculitides Wegener's granulomatosis (p710). Behçet's disease (p694). Takayasu's arteritis (p708).

Polymyalgia rheumatica (PMR)

Common in old ladies who have aching and morning stiffness in proximal limb muscles for >1 month ± mild polyarthritis, depression, fatigue, fever, and anorexia. It overlaps with giant cell arteritis. Both may cause CNS signs, claudication, angina, pulmonary infarcts, and hypopituitarism.[1] *Tests* ESR usually >40mm/h; CK usually ↔; alk phos↑ (portal inflammation). If ESR <40, but the story is good, do not rule out PMR. *Treat* with prednisolone 15mg/24h PO (↓to 7.5–10mg/24h over 2–3 months; then reduce dose slowly). Some will require steroids for 2–3 years. Monitor with ESR.

Giant cell (cranial/temporal) arteritis (GCA)

Cranial arteritis is associated with polymyalgia in 25% of people. Common in the elderly, it is rare under 55yrs. *Symptoms:* Headache, scalp and temporal artery tenderness (eg on combing hair), jaw claudication, amaurosis fugax, or sudden blindness in one eye. *Tests:* ESR↑, CRP↑, platelets↑, alk phos↑, Hb↓. ►If you suspect GCA, do an ESR, start prednisolone 1mg/kg/24h PO *immediately*. Some advocate higher doses (?IV) if visual symptoms[2] (ask an ophthalmologist). Skip lesions occur, so don't be put off by –ve biopsy. Consider temporal artery biopsy in the next few days. Note: the immediate risk is blindness but longer term, the main cause of death and morbidity in GCA is steroid treatment!. Reduce prednisolone after 5–7 days in the light of symptoms and ESR; ↑dose if symptoms recur. Typical course: 2yrs, then complete remission.

1 M Radhamanohar 1992 *Care of the Elderly* 4 162   2 R Lamb 1995 *BMJ* ii 455

Plasma autoantibodies: disease associations

Antinuclear antibody	+ve in	*Smooth muscle antibody*	+ve in
Systemic lupus erythematosus	99%	Chronic active hepatitis	40–90%
Rheumatoid arthritis	32%	Primary biliary cirrhosis	30–70%
Juvenile rheumatoid arthritis	76%	Idiopathic cirrhosis	25–30%
Chronic active hepatitis	75%	Viral infections	80%
Sjögren's syndrome	68%	(low titres)	
Progressive systemic sclerosis	64%	'Normal' controls	3–12%
'Normal' controls	0–2%	(↑ with age: 20% at 70yrs)	

Gastric parietal cell antibody		*Antibody to mitochondria*	
Pernicious anaemia (adults)	>90%	Primary biliary cirrhosis	60–94%
Atrophic gastritis: females	60%	Chronic active hepatitis	25–60%
males	15–20%	Idiopathic cirrhosis	25–30%
Autoimmune thyroid disease	33%	'Normal' controls	0.8%
'Normal' controls	2–16%		

Antibody to reticulin	
Coeliac disease	37%
Crohn's disease	24%
Dermatitis herpetiformis	17–22%
'Normal' controls	0–5%

Thyroid antibodies	Microsomal	Thyroglobulin
Hashimoto's thyroiditis	70–91%	75–95%
Graves' disease	50–80%	33–75%
Myxoedema	40–65%	50–81%
Thyrotoxicosis	37–54%	40–75%
Juvenile lymphocytic thyroiditis	91%	72%
Pernicious anaemia	55%	?
'Normal' controls	10–13%	6–10%
	(50% in older women)	

Rheumatoid factor	+ve in		
Rheumatoid arthritis	70–80%	Still's disease	rarely +ve
Sjögren's syndrome	≤100%	Infective endocarditis	≤50%
Felty's syndrome	≤100%	SLE	≤40%
Progressive systemic sclerosis	30%	'Normal' controls	5–10%

It is also associated with viral hepatitis, infectious mononucleosis, TB and leprosy.

Cytoplasmic anti-neutrophil cytoplasmic antibody cANCA (Target: proteinase B):
Wegener's disease   ≥90% (also α_1-antitrypsin deficiency)

Perinuclear anti-neutrophil cytoplasmic antibody pANCA Target: myeloperoxidase[et al]
Microscopic polyangiitis   ~75%[1] (It's a vasculitis in kidney & lung)

1 G Cambridge 1998 *Reports on Rheumatic Diseases* (Nº 13) pANCA may also be +ve in: PAN; Churg-Strauss syndrome (p674); vasculitic rheumatoid arthritis; biliary cirrhosis; UC/Crohn's; sclerosing cholangitis; crescentic GN (p380); chronic active hepatitis. There is confusing cross-reaction with thyroid microsomal antigen (and ANA). ANCA levels may correlate better with vasculitis activity than ESR/CRP (*OTM* 3010-12).

The eye in systemic disease

The eye plays host to many diseases: the more you look, the more you'll see, and the more you'll enjoy medicine, for the eye is beautiful, and its signs are legion.

Vascular retinopathy (See also p300.) This may be *arteriopathic* (arteriovenous nipping: arteries nip veins where they cross) or *hypertensive*—with arteriolar vasoconstriction and leakage (hard exudates, macular oedema, haemorrhages, and, rarely, papilloedema). Thickened arterial walls are shiny ('silver wiring'). Narrowed arterioles lead to localized infarction of the superficial retina, seen as cotton-wool spots and flame haemorrhages. Leaks from these appear as hard exudates ± macular oedema/papilloedema (rare). The grading of hypertensive retinopathy I–IV is considered obsolescent by some, partly because changes due to arteriopathy and those due to hypertension are confused, and also because some grades exist in normotensive, non-diabetic people.

Emboli passing through the retina produce *amaurosis fugax* (p436; any carotid bruits?—p40). *Retinal haemorrhages* are common in leukaemia; comma-shaped conjunctival haemorrhages and retinal new vessel formation may occur in sickle-cell disease; optic atrophy in pernicious anaemia. Note also Roth spots (retinal infarcts) in endocarditis (p312).

Retinal vein occlusion is caused by BP↑, age, or hyperviscosity (p618). Suspect in any acute fall in acuity. If it's the central vein, the fundus is like a stormy sunset (those angry red clouds are haemorrhages). In branch vein occlusion, changes are confined to a wedge of retina. Get expert help.

Metabolic disease Diabetes: p532. Hyperthyroid exophthalmos: p543. Lens opacities: hypoparathyroidism. Conjunctival and corneal calcification may occur in hypercalcaemia, including hyperparathyroidism. In gout, conjunctival deposits of monosodium urate may give sore eyes.

Granulomatous disorders Syphilis, TB, sarcoid, leprosy, brucellosis, and toxoplasmosis all inflame the eye; either front chamber (anterior uveitis/iritis) or back chamber (posterior uveitis/ choroiditis). Refer to an ophthalmologist. In sarcoid there may be cranial nerve palsies.

Collagen diseases cause inflammation of the eye coat (episcleritis/ scleritis). Conjunctivitis is found in Reiter's; episcleritis in PAN and SLE; uveitis in ankylosing spondylitis and Reiter's (p668). Scleritis in rheumatoid arthritis and Wegener's is potentially damaging to the eye. Refer patients with eye pain immediately. In dermatomyositis there is orbital oedema with retinopathy showing cotton-wool spots (microinfarcts).

Keratoconjunctivitis sicca (Sjögren's syndrome, p708.) There is reduced tear formation (<10mm in 5min on Schirmer filter paper test), producing a gritty feeling in the eyes. Decreased salivation also gives a dry mouth (xerostomia). It is associated with collagen diseases. Treatment is with artificial tears (tears naturale, or hypromellose drops).

Systemic infections Septicaemia may seed to the internal eye causing infection in the vitreous (endophthalmitis). Syphilis can cause chorioretinitis or iritis; congenital syphilis causes a pigmented retinopathy.

AIDS and HIV (►See p214.) Those who are HIV+ve may develop CMV retinitis, characterized by cotton-wool retinal spots with flame haemorrhages ('pizza pie' fundus, signifying superficial retinal infarction). This may be asymptomatic but can cause sudden visual loss. If it is present it implies full-blown AIDS, and a CD4 count <100. Cotton-wool spots on their own indicate HIV retinopathy and may occur before the full HIV picture.

Candidiasis of the vitreous is found mostly in IV drug abusers and is hard to treat. Kaposi's sarcoma may affect the lids or conjunctiva.

Differential diagnosis of 'red-eye'

	Conjunctiva	Iris	Pupil	Cornea	Anterior chamber	Intraocular pressure	Appearance
Acute glaucoma	Both ciliary and conjunctival vessels injected. Entire eye is red	Injected	Dilated, fixed, oval	Steamy, hazy	Very shallow	Very high	
Iritis	Redness most marked around cornea. Colour does not blanch on pressure	Injected	Small, fixed	Normal	Turgid	Normal	
Conjunctivitis	Conjunctival vessels injected, greatest toward fornices. Blanch on pressure. Mobile over sclera	Normal	Normal	Normal	Normal	Normal	
Subconjunctival hemorrhage	Bright red sclera with white rim around limbus	Normal	Normal	Normal	Normal	Normal	

After RD Judge, GD Zuidema, FT Fitzgerlad 1989 *Clinical Diagnosis* 5 ed, Little Brown, Boston/Toronto.

Skin manifestations of systemic diseases

Erythema nodosum Painful, red nodular lesions on anterior shins (± thighs/forearms). Associated with: sarcoid; drugs (sulfonamides, oral contraceptive, dapsone); bacterial infections (streptococcus, mycobacterium—TB, leprosy). Less common associations: Crohn's; UC; BCG vaccination; leptospirosis; yersinia; various viral and fungal infections.

Erythema multiforme 'Target' lesions (symmetrical ± central blister, on palms/soles, limbs and elsewhere). Often with mouth, genital and eye ulcers and fever (= Stevens–Johnson syndrome). Associated with: drugs (barbiturates; sulfonamides); infections (herpes; mycoplasma; orf, p174); collagen disorders. 50% are idiopathic. Get expert help in severe disease.

Erythema chronicum migrans Starts as a small papule, then enlarges to a red ring (eg 50mm across) with raised border and central fading. It lasts from 48h–3 months. May be multiple. Cause: Lyme disease (p232).

Erythema marginatum Pink coalescent rings on trunk which come and go. It is seen in rheumatic fever (or rarely other causes eg drugs).

Pyoderma gangrenosum Recurring nodulo-pustular ulcers, ~10cm wide, with tender red/blue overhanging necrotic edge, healing with cribriform scars. *Site:* eg leg; abdomen; face. *Associations:* UC; Crohn's; autoimmune hepatitis; neoplasia; Wegener's; myeloma. ♀:♂ >1:1. *Differential:* Behçet's, warfarin necrosis, rheumatoid vasculitis, 3°syphilis, blastomycosis, skin amoebiasis. *Treatment:* Get help. Saline cleansing, high-dose oral or intralesional steroids ± ciclosporin ± topical antibiotic. *Lancet* 1997 350 1720

Vitiligo *Vitellus* is Latin for *spotted calf:* typically white patches ± hyper-pigmented borders. Sunlight makes them itch. *Associations:* Autoimmunity: Graves', Addison's, and Hashimoto's diseases, diabetes mellitus, alopecia areata, hypoparathyroidism, premature ovarian failure. Treat by camouflage cosmetics, sunscreens, ± steroid creams ± dermabrasion.[1]

Specific diseases & their skin manifestations

Diabetes mellitus Recurrent infections; ulcers; *necrobiosis lipoidica* (shiny area on shin with yellowish skin and telangiectasia); *granuloma annulare* (OHCS p578); fat necrosis at insulin injection site.

Gluten-sensitive enteropathy (coeliac disease) *Dermatitis herpetiformis* (itchy blisters eg in groups on knees, elbows and scalp). It is postulated that gluten induces circulating immune complexes, which react with elements in the dermis. The itch (which can drive patients to suicide) responds to dapsone 100–200mg/24h PO within 48h—and this may be used as a diagnostic test. The maintenance dose may be as little as 50mg/week. In 30% this will need to be continued, in spite of having a gluten-free diet. SE (dose related): haemolysis, hepatitis, agranulocytosis. Contraindications: G6PD-deficiency. Risk of lymphoma↑ (with coeliac disease *and* dermatitis herpetiformis)—so surveillence is needed.[2]

Malabsorption Dry pigmented skin, easy bruising, hair loss, leuconychia.

Hyperthyroidism *Pretibial myxoedema* (red oedematous swellings above lateral malleoli, progressing to thickened oedema of legs and feet), *thyroid acropachy* (clubbing + subperiosteal new bone in phalanges).

Neoplasia *Acanthosis nigricans:* pigmented rough thickening of skin in axillae or groin with warty lesions, associated especially with carcinoma of the stomach; *dermatomyositis* (p670); *skin metastases;* *acquired icthyosis:* dry scaly skin associated with lymphoma; *thrombophlebitis migrans:* successive crops of tender nodules affecting blood vessels throughout the body, associated with carcinoma of the pancreas (especially body and tail tumours).

Crohn's Perianal/vulval ulcers; erythema nodosum; pyoderma gangrenosum.

Liver disease Reddened palms; spider naevi; gynaecomastia; decrease in secondary sexual hair; jaundice; bruising; scratch marks.

1 G Agarwal 1997 *BMJ* ii 889 & UK Vitiligo Society, tel 0171 388 8905 2 B Bardur 1994 *BMJ* i 13

Skin diagnoses not to be missed

Malignant melanoma ♀:♂ ≈1.5:1. UK incidence: 3500/year, 800 deaths (up 80% in last 15yrs). Sunlight is a major cause, partricularly in the early years. They can be tricky to diagnose, but most have ≥1 major component on the Glasgow check-list:[1] They may occur in pre-existing moles.

Major	Minor	Less helpful features:
●Change in size	●Inflammation	●Asymmetry/irregular border
●Change in shape	●Crusting/bleeding	●Irregular colour
●Change in colour	●Sensory change	●Elevation
	●Diameter >7mm	●Irregular border

Neighbouring 'satellite' lesions may occur. If smooth, well-demarcated, and regular it is unlikely to be a melanoma. *Treatment:* OHCS p584.

Squamous cell carcinoma This usually presents as an ulcerated lesion, with hard, raised edges. They may begin in solar keratoses (below), or be found on the lips of smokers or in long-standing gravitational leg ulcers. Metastases are rare, but local destruction may be extensive. *Treatment:* Total excision. Note: the condition may be confused with a keratoacanthoma—a fast-growing, benign, self-limiting papule plugged with keratin.

Basal cell carcinoma (Rodent ulcer) This epithelioma has malignant potential—in an indolent fashion. If left untreated, extensive local destruction may occur. Caucasians who have enjoyed decades in the sun are particularly at risk. The lesion is an ulcerated nodule with raised, pearly margins—usually on the face above a line joining the chin to the ear lobe. Early removal eg by curettage is usually curative. Cryotherapy is an alternative. Radiotherapy is valuable in the elderly, but should be avoided in the young because of scarring and telangiectasia.

Senile or actinic keratoses These occur on sun-exposed areas, appearing as crumbly, yellow-white crusts. Malignant change may occur. Treatment: cautery; cryotherapy; 5% 5-fluorouracil cream which is used twice daily (with this sequence of events: erythema → vesiculation → erosion → ulceration → necrosis → healing epithelialization). Healthy skin is unharmed. Treatment is usually for 4 weeks, but may be prolonged. There is no significant systemic absorption if the area treated is <500cm². Avoid in pregnancy. The hands should be washed after applying the cream.

Secondary carcinoma The most common metastases to skin are from breast, kidney, and lung. The lesion is usually a firm nodule, most often on the scalp. See acanthosis nigricans (p678).

Mycosis fungoides is a lymphoma (cutaneous T-cell lymphoma, as in Sézary syndrome) which is usually confined to skin. It causes itchy, red plaques.

Leukoplakia This appears as white patches (which may fissure) on oral or genital mucosa. Frank carcinomatous change may occur.

Leprosy Suspect in any anaesthetic hypopigmented lesion.

Syphilis Any genital ulcer is syphilis until proved otherwise. Secondary syphilis: papular rash—including palms (p233).

Others Kaposi's sarcoma (p702); Paget's disease of the breast (p706).

Bowen's disease (*Intra-epidermal carcinoma-in-situ*) starts as a lazy, non-invasive, scaly, red plaque, but it can change into a squamous cell epithelioma. Confirm by biopsy. *Treatment:* Excision, cautery, cryosurgery, radiotherapy—or topical 5-FU. Penile Bowen's disease is called Queyrat's erythroplasia (it's velvety).

1 MF Healsmith 1994 *Br J Derm* **130** 48

16. Oncology

Relevant pages in other chapters:
Leukaemias and lymphomas (p598–603)
Immunosuppressive drugs (p622)
Pain (p90)
Dying at home (*OHCS* p442)
Facing death (p7)

For specific cancers, see the relevant chapter.

Looking after people with cancer

There are no simple or complex rules which guarantee success. However, there is no doubt that getting to know your patient, making an agreed management plan, and seeking out the right expert for each stage of treatment *all* need to be central activities in oncology. These issues centre around communication, and the personal attributes of the doctor as physician. There is nothing unique about oncology in this regard—it is simply that in oncology these issues are often highly focused.

Psychological support Examples include: allowing the patient to express anger, fear—or any negative feeling (anger can anaesthetize pain).
- Counselling, eg with a breast cancer nurse, to prepare for mastectomy.
- Alternative therapy. This is one way for the patient to stay in charge, and maintain autonomy. Beware of leading patients to have unrealistic hopes, but equally, it is not our place to dilute hope with cynicism.
- Biofeedback and relaxation therapy can ↓side-effects of chemotherapy.[1]
- Cognitive and behavioural therapy reduces psychological morbidity associated with cancer treatments. See *OHCS* p638–96.
- Group therapy (*OHCS* p472) is known to reduce pain and mood disturbance, and reduce the frequency of maladaptive coping strategies.
- Meta-analyses have suggested that psychological support can have at least some effect on improving outcome measures such as survival.[2]

Hints on breaking bad news[3]

1 Choose a quiet place where you will not be disturbed. This may be impossible—but at least give the matter some thought.
2 Find out what the patient already knows or surmises (often a great deal). The picture is often confusing as surmises are not static and change rapidly, so that when you try to verify what your patient is telling you by going over the same ground again, you may get quite a different impression—both may be valid and relevant.
3 Find out how much the person wants to know. You can be surprisingly direct about this. "Are you the sort of person who, if anything were amiss, would want to know all the details?"
4 Share information about diagnosis, treatments, prognosis, and specifically listing supporting people (eg nurses) and institutions (eg hospices). Try asking "Is there anything else you want me to explain?" Do not hesitate to go over the same ground repeatedly.
5 'Cancer' has very negative connotations for many people. Address this, and explain that ~50% of cancers are cured in the developed world.[4,5]
6 Follow-through. The most important thing here is to leave the patient with the strong impression that, come what may, you are with him or her whatever, and that this unwritten contract will not be broken.

At the start, treatment may be aimed at curing the patient, or interrupting disease progression. If and when the disease does progress, emphasis will shift further toward palliative treatment. But it is never too early to think about palliation. It is an important component of treatment right from the start.

1 L Fallowfield 1995 *BMJ* ii 1316 2 TJ Meyer 1995 *Health Psych* 14 101 3 R Buckman 1992 *How to Break Bad News*, PaperMac 0-333 54564-7 4 S Hellman 1997 *Lancet* 349 *suppl* 1 5 S Sontag *Illness as Metaphor*

Oncology and genetics

Inherited cancer syndromes	Gene	Chromosome location	
Familial polyposis (colorectum)	APC	5q	
von Hippel–Lindau (kidney, CNS)	VHL	3p	(page 710)
Multiple endocrine neoplasia type I (pituitary, pancreas, thyroid)	??	11q	(page 546)
Multiple endocrine neoplasia type 2	RET	10q	(page 546)
Basal cell naevus synd. (CNS, skin)	PTCH	9q	
Retinoblastoma (eye, bone)	Rb	13q	(OHCS page 506)
Li Fraumeni syndrome (multiple)	TP53	17p	(OHCS page 752)
Neurofibromatosis type I (CNS; rare)	NF1	17q	(page 474)
Neurofibromatosis type 2 (common) (meningiomas, auditory neuromas)	NF2	22	(page 474)

Examples of commoner cancers having a familial subset[1]

Breast and ovarian cancers	BRCA1	17q
	BRCA2	13q
Hereditary non-polyposis colon ca	MSH2	2p
	MLH1	3p
	PMS2	7p
Familial melanoma	INK4A	9p

BRCA gene mutations Predisposing mutations are present in 1 in 500 persons. They will account for most of the cancers in families where many individuals are involved—but if the family only has 2–3 affected individuals, mutations here are much less likely to be to blame, even if the diagnosis is before 60yrs old. BRCA mutations confer a lifetime incidence for breast or ovary cancer of ~80%. The sister or daughter of a lady with such a mutation has a 50% chance of having the mutation, and hence a 40% lifetime risk of breast or ovary cancer. Options for such a person include regular mammography, ovarian ultrasound screening, quantification of serum markers, or even prophylactic tamoxifen. None of these interventions has been shown to be effective, which is why some women choose prophylactic mastectomy/oophorectomy.

Women with families with fewer affected members should not routinely be offered these options, but they may request entry into trials of surveillance. If no mutation is found, no risk quantification can be given. Even if a mutation *is* found, quantification may be wrong as research on which the calculation is based was done on families with *large numbers of affected individuals*. So looking for mutations may help by providing (uncertain) reassurance if they are not found. But we must set against this the disadvantage of raising the spectre of genetic predisposition to cancer, and imperfections in risk quantification. Screening is expensive.

Other cancers Most cancers show *some* familial clustering. If you have a first-degree relative <45yrs old with *colorectal cancer*, your lifetime risk is 1-in10 (1-in-6 if 2 such relatives have it). Screening colonoscopy is sometimes offered to these patients, eg every 3 years. A genetic locus for predisposition to *prostate cancer* has been found. Men with at least 1 first-degree relative with prostate cancer have a >3-fold ↑risk of prostate cancer[2]—and the cancers behave more aggressively (5-year relapse-free survival is 29% with familial cancers vs 52% in non-familial disease).[3]

Analysis of tumour DNA may show a 'replication error repair' (RER) phenotype. This reflects mutations in genes contributing to DNA repair. Genetic testing in family members where there are many affected individuals is not controversial. Some authorities may consider it worthwhile to do genetic testing when only a few individuals in the family are involved, and possibly when just one member is involved, if that individual is much younger than expected—but concrete evidence of benefit is lacking.[1]

1 C Caldas 1997 *Lancet* 349 suppl 16　2 *Internat J Cancer* 1997 70 679–81　3 *J Clin Onc* 1997 15 1478–80

✝ Oncological emergencies

►A patient with cancer who becomes acutely ill may be made more comfortable using simple measures. Pain control is important (p90 and *OHCS* p778), but treat specific problems with specific treatment.

Hypercalcaemia Often seen in carcinoma of breast, bronchus, prostate; also myeloma. It is due to bone metastases or ectopic PTH secretion.

Signs: Malaise; nausea/vomiting; polydipsia; polyuria; dehydration; weight↓; constipation; fits; psychosis; confusion; drowsy; coma.

Management: **1** Treat malignancy, stop thiazide diuretics, and consider loop diuretic. Mobilize patient if possible. **2** Hydrate: 3–4 litres of 0.9% saline IV over 24h. If mild, give phosphate tablets 500mg/12h PO. If no improvement in 24h, **3** Give bisphosphonate, eg disodium pamidronate (opposite)—up to 90mg/course. *Infuse slowly,* eg 30mg in 300mL 0.9% saline over 3h. Expect response in 3–5 days.[1]

Superior vena caval obstruction Typically with lung carcinoma (80%) or lymphoma (17%). If tests do not clinch diagnosis of underlying cancer, treat on basis of most likely cause (eg elderly smoker likely to have lung cancer; but lymphoma more likely in fit young men).

The Patient: May have distended thoracic/neck veins ± dyspnoea, oedema, feeling of fullness in head, headache—and may not be able to do up the top button of his shirt. *Signs:* JVP↑; plethoric face; tachypnoea.

Investigations: Sputum cytology (eg might detect cells from small cell carcinoma); CXR; CT thorax. Note that bronchoscopy might be hazardous.

Management: Dexamethasone 4mg/6h PO. Chemotherapy (small cell carcinoma and lymphoma). Urgent (same day) radiotherapy (squamous cell carcinoma).

Cord compression Thoracic 70%; lumbosacral 20%; cervical 10%.

The Patient: Back pain; weakness; upper motor neurone and sensory signs (cord level can often be found). Urine retention (treat urgently).

Tests: Plain x-ray of spine; myelogram; CT scan; MRI.

Management: Discuss with neurosurgeon and radiotherapist. Dexamethasone (4–8mg/6h PO). Radiotherapy. Surgery indicated if: no previous histology; progression of condition while on radiotherapy; previous radiotherapy to maximum dose; spine mechanically unstable.

Raised intracranial pressure (p780) In setting of cancer consider dexamethasone; radiotherapy; occasionally surgery to remove solitary metastasis. Surgery also indicated for some primary CNS tumours.

Tumour lysis syndrome Lysis of rapidly growing tumour (especially lymphomas, leukaemias, and myeloma) due to effective treatment can cause rise in urate, potassium, and phosphate leading to renal failure. Prevention is with adequate hydration before starting therapy and allopurinol 300mg/24h PO started the day before therapy. Treat hyperkalaemia; haemodialysis if renal failure.

Inappropriate ADH secretion p638; **febrile/neutropenic regimen** p598.

---

1 GN Hortobagyi 1996 *NEJM* 335 1785–9 & *E-BM* 1997 2 73

Treatment of hypercalcaemia with disodium pamidronate	
Calcium (mmol/L)	**Pamidronate (mg)**
up to 3	15–30
3–3.5	30–60
3.5–4	60–90
>4	90

Infuse slowly, eg 30mg in 300mL 0.9% saline over 3h. Expect response in 3–5 days.

✠ Symptom control in severe cancer

Pain ▶Do not be miserly with analgesia: aim to *eliminate* pain.

Types of pain: Don't assume the cancer is the cause (eg abdominal pain may be from constipation). Seek the mechanism. Nerve destruction pain, for example, may respond to amitriptyline (eg10–75mg at night) rather than opiates. Bone pain may respond to NSAIDs. Back pain may respond to radiotherapy, or a nerve block. Identify each symptom and type of pain.
Management 1. Pain is affected by mood, morale, and meaning. Explain its origin to both the patient and relatives. 2. Modify the pathological process where possible, for example with: radiotherapy; hormones; chemotherapy; surgery. 3. Plan rehabilitation goals. 4. Give analgesics, by mouth if possible. Do not use the patient's pain to prompt the drug round—aim to prevent pain with regular prophylactic doses (eg 4-hourly). Work up the ladder until pain is relieved (see table). Monitor response carefully. Laxatives (eg co-danthrusate 10mL PO at night) and anti-emetics (below) are often needed with analgesic.

Giving oral morphine: Start with aqueous morphine 10mg/4h PO (or 30mg rectal suppository). Double the dose at night (the aim is to promote 8 hours' sleep). Most patients need no more than 30mg/4h PO. A few need much more. Aim to change to slow-release morphine (MST) given every 12h, when daily morphine needs are known. If the disease process modifies morphine's metabolism to its more active 6-glucuronide form it may become ineffective (morphine-resistant pain, also confusingly termed 'paradoxical pain')—and methadone, which has a different pathway, may be effective.[1] NSAIDs and ketamine are alternatives.[2]

Vomiting Be meticulous in preventing vomiting *from before the first dose* of chemotherapy, to avoid anticipatory vomiting before the next dose. Give orally if possible. If severe vomiting prevents this, give the drug rectally or subcutaneously by syringe driver.

Cause:	Anti-emetic to try:
Drugs, radio- or chemotherapy	Ondansetron 4–8mg/8–12h PO/IV
Uraemia, hypercalcaemia	Haloperidol 0.5–2mg/24h (max 20mg) PO
Intracranial pressure ↑	Cyclizine 50–100mg/24h PO
Intestinal obstruction	Cyclizine 50–100mg/24h PO
Oesophageal reflux	Metoclopramide 10mg/8h PO (≤0.5mg/kg/day)
Delayed gastric emptying	Metoclopramide 10mg/8h PO (≤0.5mg/kg per day); cisapride 10mg/8h PO; see p491
Gastric irritation	Stop drugs (eg NSAIDs)

Breathlessness Consider supplementary O_2 or morphine. Is there a malignant pericardial effusion? If so, only start treatments such as pericardiocentesis, pericardiectomy, pleuropericardial windows, external beam radiotherapy, percutaneous balloon pericardiotomy, or pericardial instillation of immunomodulators or sclerosing bleomycin if there is a good prospect for improving quality of life.

Pruritus (itching) p48.

Venepuncture problems Repeated venepuncture with the attendant risk of painful extravasation and phlebitis is avoided by a *Hickman line*—a double-lumen line which tunnels under the skin to access the heart via a large vein. It is inserted with strict aseptic technique. Patients can look after their own lines (and give their own drugs, so that they can stay at home or at work). Problems: ●Infection.
●Blockage (flush with 0.9% saline or dilute heparin eg every week).
●Axillary, subclavian, or superior vena cava thrombosis/obstruction.
●Line slippage (allow up to ~4cm over a 2-month period: measure the distance from its tip to the skin).
Even more convenient portable delivery devices are available, allowing drugs to be given at a preset time, without the patient's intervention.

The analgesic ladder (See p90 for NNT.)

Rung one	*non-opioid*	aspirin; paracetamol; NSAID
Rung two	*weak opioid*	codeine; dihydrocodeine; dextropropoxyphene
Rung three	*strong opioid*	morphine; diamorphine; buprenorphine (sublingual)

If one drug fails to relieve pain, move up ladder; do not try other drugs at the same level. In new, severe pain, jump on in at rung three.

Syringe drivers (eg for drugs marked ⌐═─) or **suppositories** are used when *dysphagia* or *vomiting* make oral drugs useless. For *pain* try oxycodone 30mg suppositories (eg 30mg/8h, ≈30mg morphine). *Agitation:* try diazepam 10mg suppositories (eg 10mg/8h).

Other agents to know about

- Bisacodyl tablets (5mg), 1–2 at night help *opiate-constipation*.
- Cholestyramine 4g/6h PO (1h after other drugs): *itch* in jaundice.
- Enemas, eg Arachis oil, may help *resistant constipation*.
- H_2 antagonists (eg cimetidine 400mg/12h PO) help *gastric irritation*— eg associated with gastric carcinoma.
- Haloperidol 0.5–10mg PO helps *agitation, nightmares, hallucinations* and *vomiting*. ⌐═─
- Hydrogen peroxide 6% cleans an unpleasant-feeling *coated tongue*.
- Hyoscine hydrobromide 0.4–0.8mg sc/8h or 0.3mg sublingual: *vomiting* from upper GI obstruction or noisy *bronchial rattles*. ⌐═─
- Nerve blocks may lastingly relieve *pleural* or other *resistant pains*.
- Low residue diets may be needed for *post-radiotherapy diarrhoea*.
- Metronidazole 400mg/8h PO mitigates anaerobic *odours* from tumours; so do charcoal dressings (Actisorb®). Aerosol masking attempts often make equally unpleasant compound smells.
- Naproxen 250mg/8h with food: *fevers* caused by malignancy or bone pain from metastases (consider splinting joints if this fails).
- Pineapple chunks release proteolytic enzymes when chewed, eg for a *coated tongue*. (Sucking ice or butter also helps the latter.)
- Spironolactone 100mg/12h PO + bumetanide 1mg/24h PO may help distressing symptoms of *distension* which accompanies *ascites*.
- Steroids: most useful is dexamethasone: give 8mg IV stat to relieve symptoms of *superior vena cava* or *bronchial obstruction*—or *lymphangitis carcinomatosa*. Tabs are 2mg (≈15mg prednisolone). 4mg/12–24h PO may *stimulate appetite*, or reduce ICP↑ *headache*, or induce (in some patients) a satisfactory sense of euphoria.
- Table fans ± supplemental humidified oxygen helps hypoxic *dyspnoea*.
- Chlorpromazine helps air hunger (eg 12.5mg IV, 25mg suppository).
- Thoracocentesis (± bleomycin pleurodesis) in pleural effusion.

1 D Bowsher 1993 BMJ i 473 2 R Twycross 1993 BMJ i 793 See C Regnard 1992 *A Guide to Symptom Control in Advanced Cancer*, 2e, Haigh & Hochland; R Twycross 1990 *Symptom Control in Terminal Cancer*, Sobell Publications, Oxford and R Twycross, S Lack 1990 *Therapeutics in Terminal Care*, Churchill Livingstone

Cancer treatments

Invasive cancer affects 30% of the population; 20% die from cancer. Management involves close liaison between the patient, surgeons, physicians, oncologists, haematologists and the general practitioner. See p683.

Surgery Usually, a biopsy is offered to establish diagnosis. Surgery may be the most common, and sometimes the only, treatment—as is the case for some tumours in the GI tract, soft tissue sarcomas and gynaecological tumours and for advanced cancers of the head and neck.

Radiotherapy Uses ionizing radiation to kill tumour cells. Radiation is by naturally occurring isotopes, or by artificially produced x-rays. The quantity of radiation is the *absorbed dose*; its SI unit is the gray (Gy). 3-D treatment plans using CT/MRI allow high-dose radiation to be delived accurately.

Sometimes germ-cell tumours (seminoma, teratoma) and lymphomas appear to be particularly sensitive to irradiation which is therefore a major part of management particularly for local disease. Many head-and-neck tumours, gynaecological cancers, and localized prostate and bladder cancers are curable with radiotherapy. Radiotherapy may also be used in symptom control, eg bone metastases and SVC obstruction.

Side-effects of radiation: See p692.

Chemotherapy The choice of agent, its administration and dosage require expert guidance. Over twenty substances are in common use. Some major classes are: alkylating agents (eg cyclophosphamide, clorambucil, busulfan); antimetabolites (eg methotrexate); vinca alkaloids (eg vincristine, vinblastine); antitumour antibiotics, eg actinomycin D). Chemotherapy is an important treatment in: germ-cell tumours and some leukaemias and lymphomas; ovarian cancer (following surgery, although only 20% will be cured); and small cell lung cancer (although most patients will still die within 18 months). Chemotherapy has a part to play in the treatment of: some breast cancers; advanced myeloma; sarcomas; and some childhood cancers (such as Wilms' tumour).

Common side-effects: Vomiting; alopecia; marrow suppression—consider pretreatment pneumococcal vaccination, (p332). Each drug has its own spectrum of unwanted effects. *Extravasation of chemotherapeutic agent* (IVI leaks subcutaneously): maintain a high index of suspicion. Signs: pain; burning; swelling; infusion slows. Management: Stop infusion. Withdraw 5mL of blood. Remove needle. Elevate limb and apply cold pack over area for about 15mins. Do not use same site for infusion until all signs have disappeared. If ulceration, seek advice from plastic surgeon.

Communication ▶ *Include the patient in the decision-making process.* It is known that younger, female patients particularly want this—and giving of information and the sharing of decisions is known to reduce treatment morbidity. So although this is exhausting (sometimes the same ground needs to be covered many times) it is definitely worth spending time in this area. One widely-liked aid in this regard is for the specialist to videotape her consultation, to give to the patient for repeated viewing. A huge amount is forgotten or fails to register the first time.

Side-effects of radiotherapy[1]

Radical radiotherapy (aiming to cure) typically gives 40–60Gy of radiation (1Gy =,1 Gray = 100 rads) in daily doses of 1.8–2.75Gy over 3–7 weeks. Palliative radiotherapy, to prevent, relieve, or delay symptoms gives between 6–8Gy as a single fraction and 30Gy in up to 10 fractions.

Early reactions include nausea, diarrhoea, and skin erythema and usually resolve in a few weeks. Acute bone marrow depression may also occur but tends to be transient.

Late reactions usually take months or years to develop and are more common after radical radiotherapy and with higher radiation doses. Brain, bowel, and spinal cord are particularly susceptible to late reactions as these tissues have limited ability to self-repair. Concurrent use of actinomycin D, doxorubicin, and bleomycin increase risk of late reactions.

Skin Erythema; dry desquamation with itch; moist desquamation. Patients should keep treated areas dry and clean and avoid soap. Radiotherapy markings should not be removed during treatment.

Mouth and GI tract Prior dental assessment if treatment to oral cavity; antiseptic mouth washes and avoidance of smoking and spicy food. Aspirin mouth wash for pain, and treat oral thrush (p500). Treat dysphagia with Mucaine® mixture 15mins before meals.

Pelvic area Low residue diet helpful if change in bowel habit. Treat diarrhoea with codeine phosphate or loperamide. Culture MSU if urinary frequency or dysuria, and give potassium citrate mixture.

Central nervous system irradiation can lead to demyelination, and neurone necrosis. Brain irradiation of children of 18–24Gy can lead to cognitive dysfunction after 1 year, especially if <6 years old at onset of treatment. Spinal cord irradiation may lead to myelopathy; inner ear irradiation (eg for nasopharyngeal carcinoma) may damage the cochlea causing hearing loss. About 1% of women receiving supraclavicular or axillary radiotherapy for breast cancer develop brachial plexus damage with paraesthesia, finger numbness, shoulder pain, and arm weakness on the irradiated side (exclude axillary tumour recurrence); subcutaneous axillary fibrosis may contribute to frozen shoulder (arrange physiotherapy during radiotherapy to prevent this) and lymphoedema.

Genitourinary irradiation may induce renal failure and hypertension if bilateral (avoid kidney irradiation if possible). Periureteric fibrosis causes urinary obstruction requiring drainage in 25% after pelvic irradiation (so investigate, do not presume tumour recurrence). Bladder shrinkage and chronic cystitis after radical bladder or prostate radiotherapy may require surgery. Gonad irradiation affects reproductive function so store eggs or sperm pre-radiotherapy if children may be wanted later. Vaginal stenosis and dyspareunia are reduced after pelvic irradiation by early (at 2 weeks) resumption of intercourse or use of dilators. Pelvic irradiation can cause large bowel strictures, fistulae, and abscesses. If present, do not presume recurrence.

Other effects Cataracts; hypothyroidism may develop after neck treatment, and jaws may necrose (beware mandibular tooth extraction after radiotherapy). Pneumonitis occurs in 6% after lung radiotherapy (fever, cough, dyspnoea within 3–6 months of starting treatment) and chronic lung fibrosis can also occur.

1 *Drug Ther Bul* 1997 35 13

17. Eponymous syndromes

► *Common things happen commonly, but many people have rare diseases.*
Note: for paediatric and orthopaedic syndromes, see OHCS p742–58.

Alice in Wonderland syndrome Disturbance of one's view of oneself (intrapsychic time passes too fast) seen in epilepsy, migraine, or on falling asleep.

Arnold–Chiari malformation The cerebellar tonsils and medulla are malformed and herniate through the foramen magnum. This may cause progressive hydrocephalus with mental retardation, optic atrophy and ocular palsies, and spastic paresis of the limbs. It may also cause syringomyelia (p476) or focal cerebellar and brainstem signs such as ataxia, dysphagia, oscillopsia, and nystagmus. There may be an association with bony abnormalities of the base of the skull (basilar impression). MRI is better than CT in aiding diagnosis.

Baker's cyst Posterior herniation of capsule of the knee joint leads to escape of synovial fluid into one of the posterior bursae, stiffness and knee swelling (transilluminable in the popliteal space). *Tests:* Ultrasound. *Differential:* DVT (may co-exist). *Treatment:* Aspiration is possible, but recurrence is common.

Barrett's oesophagus In chronic reflux oesophagitis (p491), squamous mucosa undergoes metaplastic change and the squamocolumnar junction (*ora serrata*) appears to migrate caudally. The length affected may be a few cm only or all the oesophagus. It carries a 40-fold ↑ risk of adenocarcinoma. Loss of the tumour-suppressor gene 'p53' may be important.☐ *Presentation:* ●Retrosternal pain, radiating to back, worsened by hot or cold foods ●Dysphagia ●Vomiting ●Haematemesis ●Melaena. Once diagnosed, surveillance programmes vary depending on age and general health.☐ If pre-malignant changes are found, some advocate oesophageal resection especially in younger, fit patients; others favour laser ablation with frequent endoscopic ultrasound monitoring.
Management: Regular endoscopy and intensive anti-reflux measures, including long-term proton pump inhibitors ± epithelial laser ablation or photodynamic therapy (PDT) aiming for resolution of metaplasia. PDT involves light-induced activation of an orally administered photosensitizer such as 5-aminolaevulinic acid which causes the accumulation of protoporphyrin IX in GI mucosal cells. Local laser light at 630nm then causes necrosis—which is confirmed by finding squamous re-epithelialization. This can prevent the need for surgery.

Bazin's disease Skin TB (localized areas of fat necrosis with ulceration and an indurated rash, characteristically on adolescent girls' legs=*erythema induratum*).

Behçet's disease (♂:♀≈2:1; HLA-B5/51 associated) multi-organ disease of unknown (?viral) cause *Joints:* Arthritis. *Eyes:* Pain, vision↓, floaters, iritis, hypopyon, retinal vein occlusion *via* retinal vasculitis and retinal infiltrates. *Mouth, scrotum, labia:* Painful ulcers (heal by scarring). *Gut:* Colitis. *CNS:* Meningoencephalitis, ICP↑, brainstem signs, dementia, myelopathy, encephalopathy, cerebral vein thrombosis. *Treatment:* Prednisolone (start at 20–60mg/24h PO) or colchicine; steroid cream for ulcers. In non-responsive uveitis consider chlorambucil 0.2mg/kg/day PO, ciclosporin or IFN-α [*Lancet* 1997 **350** l818]. [*Hulusi Behçet, 1919*]

Berger's disease (IgA nephropathy) The commonest glomerulonephritis (p380) in the West—causing episodic haematuria with viral infections. IgA is deposited in glomeruli; microscopy shows mesangial proliferation. Heavy proteinuria and hypertension indicate a poor prognosis. 15–20% go on to end-stage renal failure. Secondary IgA nephropathy may be associated with ankylosing spondylitis, coeliac disease, and HIV. *Treatment:* Alternate-day prednisolone may help, as may phenytoin (IgA levels↓), as may tonsillectomy.☐

Bickerstaff's brainstem encephalitis Acute, progressive cranial nerve dysfunction, ataxia, coma and apnoea may lead to a (reversible) brain death picture (not true brain death: no structural brain damage has been proven).

Bornholm disease (Devil's grip) This is caused by coxsackie B virus. It usually presents in young children or adults with sudden severe pain in the chest and abdomen, on one side. There may be no pain in other muscles. Rhinitis is usually present. *Differential diagnosis:* MI, acute abdomen. *Treatment:* Analgesics. *Prognosis:* Recovery in 2 weeks. [*Bornholm Island, Denmark*]

Brown-Séquard syndrome This results from a lesion in one (lateral) half of the spinal cord (eg hemisection). There is ipsilateral paralysis and joint position sense loss below the lesion. There is ipsilateral analgesia and thermoanaesthesia at the level of the lesion, but there is contralateral loss of these modalities a few segments below the lesion (because of the pattern of decussation of these fibres in the cord). The reflexes are brisk and the tone is increased ipsilaterally. There are also sphincter disturbances. Causes: trauma, infection, neoplasia, MS, degenerative disease. *[Charles Brown-Séquard, 1811–94]*

Budd–Chiari syndrome Hepatic vein obstruction (usually by thrombosis or tumour) presents with sudden epigastric pain and shock, or more insidiously with signs of portal hypertension, jaundice, and cirrhosis. It may follow the use of oral contraceptives. *Treatment:* Surgery may be indicated.

Buerger's disease (Thromboangiitis obliterans; endarteritis obliterans) This is inflammation of arteries, veins and nerves with thrombosis in the middle sized arteries found *only* in male cigarette smokers. It may lead to gangrene.

Caplan's syndrome This is rheumatoid arthritis coupled with necrotic lung granulomata in coal miners. These cause cough, dyspnoea, and haemoptysis. CXR: bilateral nodules (0.5–5cm). *Treatment:* Steroids (carefully exclude TB first).

Charcot–Marie–Tooth syndrome (Peroneal muscular atrophy) This presents at puberty or in early adult life and begins with foot drop and weak legs. The peroneal muscles are the first to atrophy. The disease spreads to the hands and then the arms. Sensation is usually diminished, as are the reflexes. The cause is unknown. It seldom becomes totally incapacitating.

Creutzfeldt–Jakob disease See Jakob–Creutzfeldt disease (p702)

Curtis-Fitz-Hugh syndrome Chlamydial perihepatitis in sexually active women. It may simulate biliary pain and cause chronic peritonitis with ascites.

Devic's syndrome (Neuromyelitis optica) This condition is increasingly being considered as a variant of multiple sclerosis. There is massive demyelination of the optic nerves and chiasm and also of the spinal cord. The prognosis is variable, and complete remission may occur.

Dressler's syndrome (Post-myocardial infarction syndrome) This develops 2–10 weeks after an MI or heart surgery. It is thought that myocardial necrosis stimulates the formation of autoantibodies against heart muscle. *The Patient:* He or she may suffer recurrent fever and chest pain, ± pleural and pericardial rub (from serositis). Cardiac tamponade may occur, so avoid anticoagulants. *Treatment:* Steroids and anti-inflammatory agents are used.

Dubin–Johnson syndrome A familial metabolic disorder which leads to failure of excretion of conjugated bilirubin. There is intermittent jaundice with pain in the right hypochondrium. It does not cause hepatomegaly. *Tests:* Alk phos ↔; bile in the urine. Liver biopsy shows diagnostic pigment granules.

Dupuytren's contracture Palmar fascia contracts so that the fingers (typically the right 5th finger) cannot extend. There is a nodular thickening of the connective tissue over the 4th and 5th fingers. *Prevalence:* ~10% of males over 65yrs (>if +ve family history). *Associations:* Smoking, alcohol use, heavy manual labour, trauma, diabetes mellitus, phenytoin treatment, Peyronie's disease, AIDS. It may be thought of as being a marker of disturbed metabolism of free radicals derived from O_2: ischaemia (the primary event) → increased xanthine oxidase activity → reduced oxygen → superoxide free radicals → fibroblast proliferation → type III collagen → palmar fibrosis. Allopurinol (binds xanthine oxidase) has been observed to reduce symptoms—but surgery may be needed (M Frey 1997 *Lancet* **350** 164). *[Baron Guillaume Dupuytren, 1831]*

Ekbom's syndrome (Restless legs syndrome) The patient (who is usually in bed) is seized by an irresistible desire to move his legs in a repetitive way accompanied by an unpleasant sensation deep in the legs. The pathogenesis is unknown, but a defect in the basal ganglia has been suggested. *Treatment:* Many drugs have been tried; carbamazepine (p450) and clonazepam (1–4mg PO nocte) have shown benefit.

Fabry's disease An X-linked disorder of glycolipid metabolism due to deficiency of galactosidase-A. Ceramide trihexoside is deposited in the skin (angiokeratoma corporis diffusum), kidneys, and vasculature. Most die in the 5th decade. Cardiac manifestations include infarction, angina, short PR interval, rhythm disturbances, LVH, CCF, mitral valve lesions, congestive and hypertrophic obstruction cardiomyopathies.

Fanconi anaemia (*OHCS* p748) Aplastic anaemia with congenital deafness and absence of radii. It may terminate in acute myeloid/monomyelocytic leukaemia.

Felty's syndrome This is rheumatoid arthritis, splenomegaly and leucopenia. Usually in long-standing disease. Recurrent infections are common. Hypersplenism also produces anaemia and thrombocytopenia. Lymphadenopathy, pigmentation and persistent skin ulcers occur. Rheumatoid factor ↑↑. Splenectomy may improve the neutropenia.   [*Augustus Felty, 1934*]

Foster Kennedy syndrome This is optic atrophy of one eye with papilloedema of the other, caused by a tumour on the inferior surface of the frontal lobe—on the side of the optic atrophy.   [*Foster Kennedy, 1884–1952*]

Friedreich's ataxia (autosomal recessive or, rarely, sex-linked) Idiopathic cord degeneration. The spinocerebellar tracts degenerate causing cerebellar ataxia and dysarthria, nystagmus and dysdiadochokinesis. Loss of corticospinal tracts occurs (∴ weakness and extensor plantars) and peripheral nerve damage, so the tendon reflexes are paradoxically depressed (differential diagnosis p426). There is dorsal column degeneration resulting in loss of postural sense. Pes cavus is characteristic and there is often a scoliosis. Cardiomyopathy may cause cardiac failure. Typical age at death: ~50yrs.   [*Nikolaus Friedreich, 1863*]

Froin's syndrome CSF protein↑ and xanthochromia but normal cell count—seen in CSF below a block in spinal cord compression. [*Georges Froin, born 1874*]

Gardner's syndrome A dominantly inherited disorder with multiple premalignant colonic polyps, bone tumours (benign exostoses), and soft-tissue tumours such as epidermal cysts, dermoid tumours, fibromas and neurofibromas. Fundoscopy reveals black spots (congenital hypertrophy of retinal pigment epithelium) and is valuable in detecting carriers of the gene (on the long arm of chromosome 5) before symptoms develop. Median age at onset: 20yrs. Symptoms: bloody diarrhoea. Careful follow-up is needed. Subtotal colectomy with fulguration of rectal polyps aims to prevent malignancy.

Gélineau's syndrome (narcolepsy) The patient, usually a young man, succumbs to irresistible attacks of inappropriate sleep ± vivid, psychic hallucinations, cataplexy (p428), and sleep paralysis (on waking, while fully alert, there is paralyisis of speech and willed movement). Associations: encephalitis; head injury; MS; HLA DR2. *Treatment:* Methylphenidate (*OHCS* p206) 10mg PO after breakfast and lunch. It is an amphetamine, and may cause dependence and psychosis. Modafinil (eg 200mg PO mané) is said to be better. SE: anxiety, aggression, dry mouth, euphoria, insomnia, BP↑, dyskinesia, alk phos↑. (*Neurology* 1998 **50** s43).

Gerstmann's syndrome Finger agnosia, left/right disorientation, dysgraphia and acalculia. Although these features do not occur together more often than predicted by chance, when they do, they suggest a dominant parietal lobe lesion.

Gilbert's syndrome This inherited metabolic disorder is quite a common cause of *unconjugated* hyperbilirubinaemia. Prevalence is estimated at 1–2%. The onset is shortly after birth, but it may be unnoticed for many years. Liver biopsy is normal, but should rarely be required clinically. Jaundice occurs during intercurrent illness. A rise in bilirubin on fasting or after IV nicotinic acid can confirm the diagnosis. Prognosis is excellent.   [*Nicolas Gilbert, 1901*]

Gilles de la Tourette syndrome *Presentation:* Motor tics (p428), blinking, nodding, stuttering ± irrepressible, explosive, occasionally obscene verbal ejaculations and gestures, usually beginning in childhood. There may be remissions. There may be a witty, innovatory, phantasmogoric picture, 'with mimicry, antics, playfulness, extravagance, impudence, audacity, dramatizations, . . . surreal associations, uninhibited affect, speed, 'go', vivid imagery and memory, and

hunger for stimuli'—also grunting, sniffing, throat-clearing, twirling round in circles, nipping people, making obscene gestures (copropraxia), repeating self and others (palilalia, echolalia), repeating others' movements (echopraxia). *Diagnosis:* Motor or vocal tics for >1yr (may not be concurrent). *Association:* Obsessive-compulsive disorder. *Prevalence:* 1:2000. A dominant gene with variable expression may be responsible. *Treatment:* Haloperidol (eg 3mg/4h PO) or clonidine (50µg/12h PO) may help the severely affected. Tics may be brought under control through the medium of dance. [Georges Gilles de la Tourette].

Goodpasture's syndrome Proliferative glomerulonephritis+lung symptoms (haemoptysis) caused by antibasement membrane antibodies (binding kidney's basement membrane and the alveolar membrane). *Tests:* CXR: infiltrates, often in the lower zones. Kidney biopsy: crescentic nephritis. Many die in the first 6 months. *Treatment:* Vigorous immunosuppressive treatment and plasmapheresis (p618) may help (*NEJM* 1992 **326** 373 & 1380). [Ernest Goodpasture, 1919]

Guillain–Barré polyneuritis *Incidence:* 1–2/100,000/year. *Signs:* A few weeks after surgery, 'flu vaccination, or infection (eg URTI, mycoplasma, zoster, HIV, CMV, EBV, Campylobacter jejuni) an ascending neuropathy occurs (?from cell-mediated hypersensitivity to myelin ± antibody-mediated demyelination). In 40%, no cause is found. It may advance fast, affecting all limbs at once. Unlike other neuropathies, proximal muscles are more affected, and trunk, respiratory, and cranial nerves (especially VII) may be affected. Sensory symptoms are common (eg backache) but signs are usually hard to detect. It is the progressive respiratory involvement that is the chief danger. *Rarer features:* Papilloedema (? from ↓CSF resorption), pandysautonomia, Miller Fisher syndrome (ataxia, ophthalmoplegia, areflexia). *Tests:* Nerve conduction studies; vital capacity 4 hourly. CSF: protein↑ (eg by 10g/L) ± lymphocyte count↑. Treat on ITU. ▶Ventilate sooner rather than later, eg if FVC <1.5 litres; P_aO_2 <10kPa; P_aCO_2 >6kPa. Immunoglobulin 0.4g/kg/24h IV for 5 days is as good as plasma exchange, and more convenient (*E-BM* 1997 **2** 151). *Prognosis:* Good; ~85% make a complete or nearly complete recovery. 10% are unable to walk alone at 1 year. Complete paralysis is compatible with complete recovery. *Mortality:* 10%. [Georges Guillain & Jean Barré, 1916]

Henoch–Schönlein purpura (HSP) This presents with purpura (ie purple spots/nodules which do not disappear on pressure—signifying intradermal bleeding) often over buttocks and extensor surfaces. There may be associated urticaria. The typical patient is a young boy. There may be a nephritis (with crescents, in ⅓ of patients—an IgA nephropathy—we could think of HSP as being a systemic version of Berger's p694), joint involvement, abdominal pain (± intussusception), which may mimic an 'acute abdomen'. The fault lies in the vasculature; the platelets are normal. It often follows respiratory infection, and it usually follows a benign course over months. Complications (worse in adults): massive GI bleeding, ileus, haemoptysis (rare) and renal failure (rare).

Horner's syndrome Pupil constriction (miosis), sunken eye (enophthalmos), ptosis and ipsilateral loss of sweating (anhydrosis) due to interruption of the sympathetic supply to the face. This may occur in the brainstem (demyelination; vascular disease), the cord (syringomyelia), the thoracic outlet (Pancoast's tumour, p706), or on the sympathetic nerves' trip on the internal carotid artery into the skull (carotid aneurysm), and thence to the orbit. [Johann Horner, 1869]

Huntington's chorea is an autosomal dominant condition (gene on chromosome 4) with full penetrance. Onset is usually in middle age. Thus the child of an affected parent lives under a Damocles' sword, having a 50% chance of becoming affected. Onset is insidious, and the course is relentlessly progressive with: chorea; personality change (eg more irritable) preceding dementia and death. Epilepsy is common. *Pathology:* Marked reduction in GABA-nergic and cholinergic neurones in the corpus striatum. *Treatment:* No treatment prevents progression. Counselling and support of the patient and the family are of the most value. For the treatment of chorea, see p40. [George Huntington, 1872]

Jakob–Creutzfeldt disease (JCD, CJD) is a human spongiform encephalopathy (scrapie is a form of the disease found in sheep, and bovine spongiform encephalopathy, BSE, is a related encephalopathy found in cows). The cause is thought to be a 'prion', ie a protein (PrPSc) which is an altered form of a normal protein (PrPc) having the unusual property of causing the normal protein to transform into the abnormal prion protein (thus accounting for the infectious nature of the disease). The abnormal protein accumulates leading to neuronal damage and tiny cavities. In the genetically determined form of the disease (Gerstmann–Sträussler syndrome), it is thought that the 'normal' protein is abnormally unstable and readily transforms to the abnormal type.

Prion infectivity is uncertain as BSE has now been transmitted through several generations of mice without the appearance of abnormal prion protein.▫

Molecular strain typing and and mouse experiments (*BMJ* 1997 ii 831) indicate that spread to humans can occur *via* infected offal (scrapie-infected protein was fed to UK cows in the 1980s before offal was 'banned' from the food chain; note that not all abattoirs will have been scrupulous in removing offal from carcasses). This 'new-variant' type (nvCJD) has its own epidemiology (opposite).▫ Other routes of infection: corneal transplants; hormones made from human pituitaries. Signs: (after a long incubation), dementia, focal CNS signs, myoclonus, vision↓. Tests: CSF gel electrophoresis. See http://www.bse.org.uk [*Hans Creutzfeldt, 1920, Alfons Jakob, 1921*]

Kaposi's sarcoma (KS) This indolent sarcoma is either derived from capillary endothelial cells or from fibrous tissue associated with a new serologically identifiable human γ-herpesvirus (KSHV=HHV-8▫). It presents as purple papules or plaques on skin and mucosa (any organ). It metastasizes to lymph nodes. There are 2 types: **1** Endemic (Central Africa), featuring peripheral, slow-growing lesions in older men with rare visceral involvement and a good response to chemotherapy. **2** KS in HIV +ve patients (particularly in homosexual men), where it is diagnostic of AIDS (p212). Pulmonary Kaposi's sarcoma may present as breathlessness. Lymphatic obstruction predisposes to cellulitis. Other groups affected: Jews and transplant patients. Diagnosis is by biopsy. *Treatments* (eg if extensive disease or for cosmetic reasons): Local radiotherapy, interferon α (10–18mu/day), and chemotherapy with doxorubicin, bleomycin, vinblastine (intralesional) and dacarbazine—have all been used with success in open trials.▫ Get expert help. [*Moricz Kaposi, 1887*]

Korsakoff's syndrome This is a ↓ability to acquire new memories. It may follow Wernicke's encephalopathy. It is due to thiamine deficiency (eg in alcoholics). The patient may have to relive his grief each time he hears of the death of a friend. He will confabulate to fill in the gaps in his memory. *Treatment*: See *Wernicke's*, p712. [*Sergei Korsakoff (more accurately transliterated Korsakov), 1887*]

Leriche's syndrome Absent femoral pulses, intermittent claudication of buttock muscles, pale cold legs, and impotence. It is due to aortic occlusive disease (eg a saddle embolism at its bifurcation). [*René Leriche, 1940*]

Löffler's eosinophilic endocarditis A restrictive cardiomyopathy + eosinophilia (eg 120 × 10⁹/L). These infiltrate many organs. It may be an early stage of tropical endomyocardial fibrosis and overlaps with the idiopathic hypereosinophilic syndrome (HES), but is probably distinct from eosinophilic leukaemia. It presents with increasingly severe heart failure (75%), and mitral regurgitation (49%). *Treatment*: Digoxin + diuretics often only help if combined with suppression of the eosinophilia, eg with prednisolone or hydroxyurea (=hydroxycarbamide).

Löffler's syndrome (pulmonary eosinophilia) Allergic eosinophil infiltration of the lungs. Allergens include: *Ascaris lumbricoides, Tricinella spiralis, Fasciola hepatica, Strongyloides stercoralis, Ancylostoma duodenale, Toxocara canis*, sulfonamides, hydralazine, nitrofurantoin, and chlorpropamide. Often symptomless, and the diagnosis is suggested by an incidental CXR (diffuse fan-shaped shadows)—or there may be cough, fever, and an eosinophilia (eg 20%). *Treatment*: Eradicate allergens. If idiopathic, steroids are tried. [*Wilhelm Löffler, born 1887*]

Lown–Ganong–Levine syndrome Acceleration of conduction of cardiac impulses with a normal QRS complex. Atrial impulses may bypass the AV node using a fast-conducting accessory pathway, but rejoin the bundle of His—so producing a short P-R interval and atrial arrhythmias (*but* no delta wave).

Signs which may distinguish new-variant JCD from 'old' JCD include:
- An early age at presentation (median 29 years; range 16–48 years).
- Prolonged duration of illness (median 14 months; range 11–21 months).
- Emotional features are an early sign (anxiety, withdrawal, apathy, depression, personality change—also insomnia).
- Sensory disturbance (eg cold legs, foot pain hyperaesthesia, dysaesthesia).
- Involuntary movements (myoclonus, chorea) ± dysarthria may occur early.
- Normal EEG (standard JCD has a characteristic spike and wave pattern).
- MRI *may* show a characteristic signal in the posterior thalamic area.
  CT is normal in both forms of the illness, and CSF tests detecting 14-3-3 protein cannot be relied upon (and are +ve in new and standard variant).
- Homozygosity for methionine at codon 129 of the PrP gene.

M Pocchiariai 1998 *BMJ* i 563 & M Zeidler 1997 *Lancet* 350 903 (*N*=22, so conclusions are provisional)

McArdle's glycogen storage disease (Type V) The cause is myophospho-rylase deficiency (as shown on muscle biopsy). Inheritance: autosomal recessive. Stiffness follows exercise. Venous blood from exercised muscle shows low levels of lactate and pyruvate. There may be myoglobinuria. *Treatment:* Avoid extreme exercise. Oral glucose and fructose may help.

Mallory–Weiss tear Vomiting *causes* haematemesis via an oesophageal tear.

Marchiafava–Bignami syndrome Wine induces degeneration of the corpus callosum, leading to seizures, ataxia, tremor, excitement and apathy.

Marchiafava–Micheli syndrome (Paroxysmal nocturnal haemoglobinuria) An intracorpuscular defect causes haemolysis (hence haemoglobinaemia and haemoglobinuria) during the night, in young adults.

Marfan's syndrome This is an autosomal dominant connective tissue disease, caused by mutations of the fibrillin-1 gene (15q21.1) causing abnormalities in the synthesis, secretion, or matrix incorporation of fibrillin (a glycoprotein in elastic fibres)[1]—and arachnodactyly (long spidery fingers), high-arched palate, armspan > height, lens dislocation ± unstable iris, and aortic dilatation (β-blockers appear to slow this). Aortic incompetence may occur, eg if pregnant. Echocardiogram screening may be helpful. Homocystinuria may give a similar picture.

Marfan's	vs	Homocystinuria
●Autosomal dominant		●Autosomal recessive
●Upwards lens dislocation		●Downwards lens dislocation
●Aortic incompetence		●Heart rarely affected
●Normal mentality		●Mental retardation
●Scoliosis, flat feet, herniae		●Recurrent thromboses; osteoporosis
Life expectancy is ~halved		●+ve urine cyanide-nitroprusside test
from cardiovascular risks		●Response to pyridoxine

Meigs' syndrome The association of a pleural effusion with a benign ovarian fibroma or thecoma. It is a transudate. Ascites may also be present. The mechanism of the effusion is unknown. *[Joseph Meigs, 1937]*

Ménétrier's disease There is hyposecretion of gastric acid, gross mucosal hypertrophy into folds up to 4cm high, epigastric pain, GI bleeding, protein loss from the stomach, ↓gastric mobility, oedema, weight↓, D&V. It may be due to a trophic effect of a hormone, or it may be a response to regurgitation of the small bowel contents through the incompetent pylorus. Total gastrectomy may be indicated. Gastric carcinoma may follow. Less severe forms of the disease are known as Schindler's disease. *[Pierre Ménétrier 1859–1935]*

Meyer–Betz syndrome (Paroxysmal myoglobinuria) A necrotizing disease of exercising muscles, causing muscle tenderness (± weakness, swelling, bruising), chills, pallor, abdominal pain, fever, WCC↑, LFT↑, DIC, P_aO_2↓, and shock. First urine turns pink, and then as more myoglobin is excreted it becomes deep red/brown. Oliguria or anuria may follow. ♂:♀ >1:1. *Diagnosis:* Muscle biopsy, CPK↑, serum myoglobin↑. *[Hans Meyer, 1824–1895 & Vladimir Betz 1834–1894]*

Mikulicz's syndrome A variant of Sjögren's syndrome, with epithelial salivary gland hyperplasia, blocking of ducts and symmetrical enlargement. Lacrimal glands may also enlarge. The patient complains of a dry mouth. *[Johann von Mikulicz-Radecki, 1892]*

Milroy's syndrome (Lymphoedema praecox) An inherited malfunction of the lymphatics causing asymmetric swelling of young girls' legs. *Management:* ●Reassure that it is benign; only 10% progress to the other leg over 10–20yrs. ●Treat any infection proactively (eg insect bites). ●Good foot hygiene. ●If support stockings (OHCS p598) do not help, try a Lymphapress® device for active compression at night. Surgery with skin grafts is very rarely needed for 'elephantiasis leg'.

Münchausen's syndrome The patient gains many hospital admissions through deception, feigning illness, hoping for a laparotomy (*laparotimophilia migrans*), or bleeding alarmingly (*haemorrhagica histrionica*) or presenting with curious fits (*neurologica diabolica*) or false heart attacks (*cardiopathia fantastica*).

Myalgic encephalomyelitis (=*Chronic fatigue syndrome*) see OHCS p471.

Nelson's syndrome If bilateral adrenalectomy is performed, feedback inhibition of ACTH is removed. Browning of the skin due to this excess ACTH production is known as Nelson's syndrome.

Ogilvie's syndrome There is functional ('pseudo') GI obstruction caused by malignant retroperitoneal infiltration. (Other causes include lumbar spine fracture, U&E imbalance.) A water-soluble contrast enema or colonoscopy allows decompression, and excludes mechanical obstruction. Management is conservative. Correct U&E. Caecal exteriorization is rarely needed.

Ortner's syndrome This is recurrent laryngeal nerve palsy caused by a large left atrium associated with mitral stenosis.

Osler–Weber–Rendu syndrome This is hereditary haemorrhagic telangiectasia. There are punctiform lesions on mucous membranes. It presents with epistaxis or GI bleeding. The natural history is variable.

Paget's disease of breast is an intra-epidermal, intraductal cancer. Any red, scaly lesion around the nipple should bring to mind Paget's disease, and a biopsy is indicated. ►Never diagnose eczema of the nipple without a biopsy. *Treatment:* Mastectomy is usual to excise underlying ductal tumour. [*Sir James Paget, 1874*]

Pancoast's syndrome Apical lung cancer + ipsilateral Horner's syndrome, caused by invasion of the cervical sympathetic plexus. Also shoulder and arm pain (brachial plexus invasion C8–T2) ± hoarse voice/bovine cough (unilateral recurrent laryngeal nerve palsy and vocal cord paralysis). [*Henry Pancoast, 1932*]

Peutz–Jeghers' syndrome Benign intestinal (usually jejunal) hamartomatous polyps occurring with dark freckles on lips, oral mucosa, lips, face, palm, and soles. There may be GI obstruction, or massive GI haemorrhage. Autosomal dominant. Malignant change occurs in ≤3%, typically with duodenal polyps. *Treatment:* Usually conservative. Local excisions may be needed. Hamartomas are an excessive focal overgrowth of normal, mature cells in an organ composed of identical cellular elements. (See OTS.)

Peyronie's disease Fibrosis in the penis leads to angulation which makes coitus most inconvenient. Associations: Dupuytren's contracture, premature atherosclerosis. Surgery and prostheses aid penetration. External penile splints ('supercondoms') also help. [*François de la Peyronie, 1743*]

Pott's syndrome This is spinal TB. Rare in the West, this tends to affect young adults, giving pain, and stiffness of all back movements. ESR↑. Abscess formation and spinal cord compression may occur. Disc spaces may be affected in isolation or with vertebral involvement either side (usually anterior margins early). X-rays: narrow disc spaces and vertebral osteoporosis early, with bone destruction leading to wedging of vertebrae later. Whereas in the thoracic spine paraspinal abscesses may be seen on x-ray and kyphosis on examination, with lower thoracic or lumbar involvement, abscess formation may be by psoas muscle in the flank, or in the iliac fossa. The bacillus reaches the spine via the blood. T10–L1 are the most commonly affected vertebrae. *Treatment* is with antitubercular therapy (p200). [*Sir Percival Pott, 1779*]

Prinzmetal (variant) angina Angina occurring at rest, due to coronary artery spasm, causes ECG shows ST elevation. *Treatment:* As for ordinary angina (p278); nifedipine is said to be particularly useful. *Association:* Circle of Willis occlusion from intimal thickening (moyamoya disease; *Lancet* 1998 **351** 183).

Raynaud's syndrome This is episodic digital ischaemia, precipitated by cold or emotion. Fingers ache and change colour: pale → blue → red. It may be idiopathic (Raynaud's disease—prevalence: 3–20%; ♀:♂>1:1, abating at menopause) or have an underlying cause (Raynaud's phenomenon):

Scleroderma and SLE	Rheumatoid arthritis	Thorax outlet obstruction
Trauma	Arteriosclerosis	Use of vibrating tools
Leukaemia	Thrombocytosis	Mixed cryoglobulinaemia
Cold agglutinins	Drugs; PRV (p612)	Monoclonal gammopathies

Treatment: Keep warm; stop smoking. Nifedipine 10–20mg/8h PO helps some.

Electrically heated mittens are available (Raynaud's Association, 40 Blagden Crescent, Alsager, Cheshire, UK, ST2 2BG). Sympathectomy may help severe disease (lower limb). Iloprost eg 0.5 nanograms/kg/min IVI (available from Schering for named patients) may salvage digits with ulceration and near-gangrene; effects last up to 16 weeks. Relapse is common.

Refsum's syndrome This is the association of polyneuritis, nerve deafness, night blindness (pigment retinopathy), cerebellar ataxia, ichthyosis, cardiomyopathy, deafness, and anosmia with a high CSF protein (but no cells). Lipid metabolism is abnormal, leading to excessive phytanic acid in fat, the liver, kidneys, and nerves. Plasmalogens (a kind of phospholipid)↓, plasma phytanic acid and pipecolic acid↑. Autosomal recessive. *Treatment:* Diet; plasmapheresis.

Rotor syndrome Defective excretion of conjugated bilirubin, producing cholestatic jaundice (autosomal dominant with impaired penetrance).

Sjögren's syndrome This is the association of a connective tissue disease (rheumatoid arthritis in 50%) with keratoconjunctivitis sicca (↓lacrimation causing dry eyes) or xerostomia (↓salivation causing dry mouth). Lymphocytes and plasma cells infiltrate secretory glands (also lungs and liver) causing fibrosis. The connective tissue disease is usually severe and rheumatoid factor is always present. Anti-Ro (SSA) and anti-La (SSB) antibodies are variably present. Gland biopsy shows sialadenitis. Involvement of other secretory glands is common causing dyspareunia, dry skin, dysphagia, otitis media, and pulmonary infection. Other features: peripheral neuropathy, renal involvement, hepatosplenomegaly. There is an association with other connective tissue diseases, renal tubular acidosis, adverse drug reactions and lymphoma. *Tests:* Conjunctival dryness may be quantified by putting a strip of filter paper under the lower lid and measuring the distance along the paper that tears are carried (Schirmer's test). Less than 10mm in 5mins is positive. *Treatment:* Hypromellose (artificial tears) ± occlusion of the punctum which drains tears. Xerostomia may respond to frequent cool drinks, or artificial saliva sprays (Luborant®).   [Henrik Sjögren, 1933]

Stevens–Johnson syndrome Drugs (sulfonamides, penicillin, sedatives), viruses or other infection (eg orf, *Herpes simplex*), neoplasia or other systemic disease induce a systemic illness with fever, arthralgia, myalgia ± pneumonitis and conjunctivitis. Vesicles develop in mucosa of mouth, GU tract, and/or the conjunctivae. The skin develops the typical target lesions of erythema multiforme, often on the palms. They may blister in the centre. The signs may also include polyarthritis and diarrhoea. *Treatment:* Calamine lotion for the skin, steroids (systemic and as eye-drops) were once used, but ask a dermatologist and ophthalmologist. Prognosis is good, but the illness may be severe for the first 10 days before resolving over 30 days. Damage to the eyes may persist and at worst, blindness may result.   [Albert Stevens and Frank Johnson, 1922]

Sturge–Weber syndrome The association of a facial port wine stain (haemangioma) with contralateral focal fits. There may also be glaucoma, exophthalmos (p543), strabismus, optic atrophy, and spasticity with a low IQ. The fits are caused by a corresponding capillary haemangioma in the brain. Skull x-ray shows cortical calcification, but angiography is usually normal.

Takayasu's arteritis (Aortic arch syndrome) An idiopathic arteritis causes narrowing of the first centimetres of the innominate, carotid, and subclavian arteries with the adjacent aorta, as well as renal arteries. *The Patient* is typically a woman 20–40yrs old. Eyes—amblyopia, blindness, cataracts, atrophy of the iris, optic nerve and retina. CNS—hemiplegia, headache, vertigo, syncope, convulsions. CVS—pulselessness; systolic murmurs above and below the clavicle; aortic regurgitation; aortic aneurysm. Renal—BP↑ *Diagnosis:* ESR >40mm/h (if disease is active); aortography. *Treatment:* Prednisolone (starting example: 40mg/24h PO); angioplasty, reconstructive surgery and endarterectomies may be tried. *Prognosis:* 10yr survival: ~90%.   [Mikito Takayasu, 1908]

Tietze's syndrome An idiopathic costochondritis. There is pain in the costal cartilage, often localized. It is enhanced by motion, coughing, or sneezing. The second rib is most commonly affected. The diagnostic key is *localized* tenderness which is marked (flinches on prodding). *Treatment:* Simple analgesia, eg aspirin. Its importance is that it is a benign cause of what at first seems to be alarming, eg cardiac, pain. In lengthy illness local steroid injections may be used.

Todd's palsy Focal CNS signs (eg hemiplegia) following a seizure. The patient seems to have had a stroke, but recovers in <24 hours.   [Robert Todd, 1856]

Vincent's angina Pharyngeal infection with an ulcerative gingivitis caused by *Borrelia vincentii* (a spirochaete) + fusiform bacilli (Gram −ve, non-sporing variously called *Bacteroides, Fusobacterium,* or *Fusiforms*). Try penicillin V 250mg/6h PO combined with metronidazole 400mg/8h PO.   *[Jean-Hyacinthe Vincent, 1898]*

Von Hippel–Lindau syndrome This predisposition to renal cysts/carcinomas, phaeochromocytoma, and haemangioblastoma (in lateral lobes of the cerebellum) ± aneurysms and tortuosities of the retinal vessels, leading to subretinal haemorrhages presents in young adults with headache, dizziness, unilateral ataxia, or blindness. The culprit gene acts by binding elongin A. *Lancet* 1997 350 1756.

Von Willebrand's disease This is an autosomal dominant deficiency of factor VIII which behaves like a platelet abnormality (platelet adherence to connective tissue ↓)—so there is post-operative, traumatic or mucosal bleeding (nose bleeds, menorrhagia). Haemarthroses and muscle haematomas are rare. *Tests:* Prolonged bleeding time, but normal platelet count and whole blood clotting time. Von Willebrand factor (vWF) is low (its action helps platelet adhesion and prolongs factor VIII t½: synonym: factor VIII-related antigen—VIIIR:Ag). Factor VIII clotting activity (VIII:C) may be low. *Treatment:* (p592) factor VIII cryoprecipitate; vasopressin.

Waterhouse–Friedrichsen's syndrome and meningococcaemia (Haemorrhage into the adrenal cortex with a fulminant necrotizing meningococcaemia, causing purpura, rash, fever, meningitis, coma, and DIC). There is shock as normal vascular tone requires cortisol to set activity of alpha and beta adrenergic receptors—and aldosterone is needed to maintain extracellular fluid volume. Sepsis is only one cause of adrenal haemorrhage; others are coagulopathic states, pregnancy diseases, shock, and other stresses. It is best to think of meningococcal endotoxin as a potent initiator of inflammatory and coagulatory cascades. *Treatment:* ▶▶Benzylpenicillin 1.2g/4h IV, hydrocortisone 200mg/4h IV, and expert help for renal failure and DIC—difficult and controversial; antithrombin III (AT-III) may help; heparin is ineffective if AT-III↓.

New approaches (offered here more as examples of how to think about meningococcaemia, than as properly validated or recommended options):
●*Extracorporeal membrane oxygenation:* This may help cardiorespiratory failure.
●*Terminal fragment of human bactericidal/permeability-increasing protein (rBPI₂₁):* This endotoxin-binding part of neutrophil azure granules can ↓cytokines.
●*Heparin with protein C concentrate.* Protein C is a naturally-occuring anticoagulant, and deficiency (as in meningococcaemia) leads to intravascular thrombosis. It can reverse coagulopathy, and could help prevent limb gangrene.
●*Plasmapheresis* (± fresh fresh-frozen plasma/ cryoprecipitate) may remove cytokines, and may help by correcting acidosis.
●*Thrombolysis* (rTPA) may help limb re-perfusion (*Lancet* 1997 350 1566).

Weber's syndrome Ipsilateral third-nerve palsy with contralateral hemiplegia, due to midbrain infarction after occlusion of the paramedian branches of the basilar artery (which supplies the cerebral peduncles).

Wegener's granulomatosis A potentially fatal granulomatous vasculitis. *Diagnostic criteria:* ●Necrotizing granulomas in respiratory tract ●Generalized necrotizing arteritis ●Glomerulonephritis. Any organ *may* be involved—eg nasal ulceration with epistaxis, rhinitis, sinus involvement, otitis media, multiple cranial nerve lesions, oral ulcers, gum hypertrophy ± bleeding and microabscesses, lung symptoms and variable shadows on CXR (eg multiple nodules), hypertension and glomerulitis. The patient is also systemically ill. *Eye signs* (seen in 50%): proptosis ± ptosis (orbital granuloma), conjunctivitis, corneal ulcers, episcleritis, scleritis, uveitis, retinitis. *Tests:* ANCA (p675) may help diagnostically and in disease monitoring. *Treatment:* High-dose steroids may be backed up by cyclophosphamide which has revolutionized prognosis in these patients. Dose example: 3–4 pulses of 500mg cyclophosphamide IV separated by 7–10 days with mesna to reduce cyclophosphamide-induced chemical cystitis.

Wernicke's encephalopathy Thiamine deficiency (often in alcoholics) with a triad of nystagmus, ophthalmoplegia (external recti commonly) and ataxia. Other eye signs such as ptosis, abnormal pupillary reactions, and altered consciousness may occur. Consider this diagnosis in all those with any of the above signs: it may present with headache, anorexia, vomiting, and confusion. *Tests:* Red cell transketolase↓ or plasma pyruvate↑. *Treatment:* Urgent thiamine to prevent irreversible Korsakoff's syndrome (p702). Dose examples: thiamine 200–300mg/24h PO; maintenance: 25mg/24h PO. If the oral route is quite impossible, consider Pabrinex®, 2–3 pairs of high-potency ampoules/8h IV over 10mins for ≤2 days, then daily for 5–7 days. An IM (gluteal) preparation is available (dose example: 1 pair/12h IM for up to 7 days). Have resuscitation facilities to hand as anaphylaxis can occur.   [Karl Wernicke, 1875]

Whipple's disease A cause of GI malabsorption which usually occurs in men >50yrs old. Other features: arthralgia, pigmentation, weight↓, lymphadenopathy, ± cerebellar or cardiac signs. Jejunal biopsy shows intact villi, but the cells of the lamina propria are replaced by macrophages which contain PAS +ve glycoprotein granules. Similar cells are found in nodes, spleen, and liver. *Cause:* Tropheryma whippelii. *Tests:* PCR may help diagnosis. *Treatment:* Co-trimoxazole or prolonged tetracycline may bring a remission.   [George Whipple, 1907]

Wilson's disease (Hepatolenticular degeneration) A disorder of copper metabolism due to an autosomal recessive gene on chromosome 13 which leads to copper deposition in liver and brain, causing cirrhosis and basal ganglia destruction. *Prevalence:* 29/million. *Presentation:* The patient may be a child or young adult with tremor, chorea, dysarthria, dysphagia, drooling, weakness, fits, and mental deterioration—or just cirrhosis. Examination may reveal wasting. Diagnosis is by clinical evidence and demonstration of copper in tissues (eg liver, or cornea—seen by expert using slit lamp). Kayser–Fleischer rings may be seen (brown pigmentation in the periphery of the cornea (not iris) from copper deposit). Serum caeruloplasmin and *total* serum copper both usually ↓. Urine: copper >100µg/24h. Contact your local lab. *Treatment* with penicillamine (aids copper elimination) is effective if given early. 500mg/ 6–8h PO ac for first year then 250mg/6–8h. Monitor FBC and platelets, and test urine for blood and protein frequently.   [Samuel Wilson, 1912].

Zollinger–Ellison syndrome This is the association of peptic ulcer with a gastrin-secreting pancreatic adenoma (or simple islet cell hyperplasia). Gastrin excites excessive acid production which can produce many ulcers in the duodenum and stomach. Rarely, adenomas are located in the stomach or duodenum. 50–60% are malignant, 10% are multiple and 30% of cases are associated with multiple endocrine adenomatosis (type 1). Incidence: 0.1% of patients with duodenal ulcer disease.

Suspect in those with multiple peptic ulcers resistant to drugs, particularly if there is associated diarrhoea and steatorrhoea or a family history of peptic ulcers (or of islet cell, pituitary, or parathyroid adenomas). *Tests:* Raised fasting serum gastrin level (>1000pg/mL) with a raised basal gastric acid output of >15mmol/h (the latter test is of less importance). *Treatment:* Proton pump inhibitors (PPIs) such as lanzoprazole and omeprazole (p492) are more effective than H_2 blockers. These PPIs bind irreversibly with parietal cell potassium hydrogen ATP-ase. SE: headaches, rash, diarrhoea. Dose: of omeprazole: 20mg/24h–60mg/12h PO (start with 60mg/day and adjust according to response). Measuring intragastric pH helps determine the best dose (aim to keep pH at 2–7; a daily dose of 60mg typically achieves this). The hazards of long-term use are unknown. Ask an expert about the possibility of excising the tumour after location by ultrasound, CT scans, or angiography, provided there is not already disseminated malignancy (usually in the liver). Some say that surgery should be reserved for when medical treatment fails. Streptozotocin may also have a rôle here. *Prognosis:* 5-year survival with metastases: ~20% (M Langman 1991 BMJ ii 482 & OTM 3e 1996).

18. Radiology

Relevant pages in other chapters:
The chest x-ray (p326); IVU (p372); ultrasound in obstetrics (OHCS p118); sedation (OHCS p773).

We thank Dr S Vinjamuri for his help with this chapter

Delegation, audit, and changing rôles in the radiology department

Once upon a time, people could say with confidence that the radiographer was the person who produced diagnostic images using x-rays, ultrasound, nuclear medicine, and magnetic resonance—while the radiologist was the doctor who *interpreted* those images. Pressure of work is radically changing rôles, as illustrated in this (controversial) flow diagram.[1]

Radiologists join with physicists and others to create a new image
↓
Techniques are refined and radiologists are trained in the new work
↓
Medicolegal and clinical demands increase requests for the new image
↓
Radiologists have to delegate to keep on top of their workload
↓
Radiographers take on extra supervised work
↓
Radiologists become so busy they can no longer fully supervise the work
↓
Radiographers start giving out 'provisional' reports
↓
Provisional reports turn out to be comparable with definitive reports
↓
Radiographers provide definitive reports
↓
Radiographers become increasingly busy, and expensive to train and retain
↓
Others may take on jobs once done by radiographers (taking x-rays)

What determines the feasability of changing rôles is *audit*, and the establishment of *protocols* agreed among the professionals concerned. Training and audit help ensure that no one practises beyond their capabilities, and patients must be informed whenever someone dealing with them steps outside traditional rôles. Audit entails showing that there is no increase in radiation dose to the patient (eg in radiographer-performed barium enemas), no film wastage, no increased referral to other services, and unchanged disease detection rates, all for less money.

So if nurses are requesting x-rays (as they do in some casualty departments) and radiographers are reporting them, who needs doctors? The answer is 3-fold. Doctors are needed to mend the bones if they are broken; doctors are required for training and development within their department—and doctors are *fast*.[1,2] Radiologists can report films accurately 2–3 times faster than anyone else. On this view, they are a bargain.

1 AH Chapman 1997 *Lancet* **350** 581   2 DC Haiart 1991 *BJCP* **45** 43–5

Radiology and imaging

CT (computerized tomography) and MRI (magnetic resonance imaging) have revolutionized the practice of neurology and neurosurgery. For other areas of the body, the decision whether to use conventional radiology, nuclear medicine, ultrasound, or CT is not always clear-cut and may depend on local availability. Generally, do plain films before contrast, and do ultrasound where possible (cheap and non-invasive). The more expensive CT and MRI are to be held in reserve for when the preliminary investigations are indecisive or inadequate. However, because a hospital bed is such an expensive resource, if an expensive test can make a quick diagnosis, money may be saved. An example of using expensive tests in cost-containment is using early CT in the investigation of abdominal masses, rather than leaving CT to be the last in a long line of often inconclusive tests. This philosophy is all the more telling in some emergencies—eg severe head injury with Glasgow coma scale <8 (p764), which requires CT as the first test.

Every physician should be able to read the plain chest and plain abdominal film, and recognize common medical disorders presenting on hand and skull radiographs. There is no substitute for examining the x-rays of your patient yourself to gain experience in the appearances of normal and abnormal films.

There are 4 basic steps in interpreting any radiograph:

1. **Check the film is technically correct** Is the film named, dated, right/left orientated, and marked as to whether AP (anteroposterior), PA (posteroanterior), erect, or supin?. Penetration is important (vertebral bodies just visible through heart on a CXR) when commenting on diffuse shadowing. Check for rotation (eg asymmetry of clavicles on a CXR) as this may affect the appearances of normal structures (eg the hila).

2. **Describe the abnormalities seen** This may be a change in the appearance of normally visualized structures, or an area of increased opacity or translucency. There are 4 main radiographic densities: bone, air, fat, water (ie soft tissue, which is mostly water). A border is only seen at an interface of 2 densities, eg heart (water) and lung (air); this 'silhouette' is lost if air in the lung is replaced by consolidation (water). This is the silhouette sign and can be used to localize pathology (eg right middle lobe pneumonia or collapse causing loss of distinction of the right heart border).

3. **Translate these into pathology** (For example: pleural fluid, consolidation, collapse).

4. **Suggest a differential diagnosis.**

The order of scrutiny is unimportant, but it is advisable to have a structured approach so as not to miss any major abnormality.

▶Remember. . . *Treat the patient not the film.*

Check that the film is technically correct, only then:
- Comment on any obvious abnormality.
- Systematically consider: heart, mediastinum, lung fields, the diaphragm, soft tissues (remember both breasts) and bones.
- Re-study the 'review areas': the apices, the hila, behind the heart, and the costo-phrenic angles (for small effusions).
- Consider if you need a lateral film.

The diaphragm Check expansion (normally 6 ± 1 anterior ribs or 9 ± 1 posterior ribs). Overinflation may suggest COPD or asthma. Right hemidiaphragm is higher than the left by up to 3cm in 95% of cases. The lateral costo-phrenic angles should be sharp and acute—ill-defined in hyperinflation or with effusion. On a lateral view, the right hemi-diaphragm is the one that passes through the heart shadow to the anterior chest wall while the left ends at the posterior heart border.

The root of the neck and trachea The trachea is central, but slight deviation to the right may be seen inferiorly. A paratracheal line is commonly seen—loss of this suggests paratracheal lymphadenopathy.

Mediastinum and heart. Look for the landmarks. The cardio-thoracic ratio is the ratio of the heart width to the chest width. It should be <50%—(essential to have a PA film as the heart is magnified on AP or supine films). Observe patterns of cardiac enlargement (see figure). Mediastinal widening may be due to aortic dissection, lymph nodes, thymus, thyroid, or tumour.

The hila Composed of pulmonary arteries and veins with nodes and airways. Left usually higher than right (~1cm) but of equal density. Look for change in density—tumour, lymph nodes, or just rotated film?

The lung fields Increased translucency may be:
1 Pneumothorax—absent vascular markings and lung edge visible.
2 Bullous change—eg in emphysema.
3 Hyperinflation in COPD.
4 Pulmonary hypertension—p366.
5 Pulmonary embolus—localized oligaemic lung fields.

Abnormal opacities may be classifed as:

1 *Consolidation:* Diffuse margins, or opacity+air bronchogram within it (silhouette sign) but little volume change (unlike collapse).

2 *Collapse:* Characteristic patterns are seen (see p327), and loss of volume causes shift of the normal landmarks (hila, fissures, etc.).

3 *'Coin' lesions:* (ie a solitary pulmonary nodule) have an enormous differential diagnosis. Treat as tumour until proved otherwise. See p343.

4 *'Ring' shadows:* Either airways (pulmonary oedema, bronchiectasis), or cavitating lesions, eg pulmonary infarct (triangular with a pleural base), abscess (bacterial, fungal, amoebic, hydatid) or tumour.

5 *Linear opacities:* Septal lines (Kerley B lines—interlobular lymphatics seen with fluid, tumour, dusts, etc.). Atelectasis.

6 Diffuse lung shadowing: See p326.

- **Check** the name, the date and orientation (right/left).

- **Is it erect or supine?** The gas pattern is best seen on supine films, but many surgeons prefer erect films to demonstrate fluid levels. Free intraperitoneal air is best seen on an erect CXR when it is subdiaphragmatic. Causes include a perforated viscus (eg peptic ulcer, colon), or after surgery (eg laparoscopy) or prolonged vaginal intercourse. Beware of misdiagnosing gas in bowel adjacent to the diaphragm.

- **Is any contrast evident?** Always ask for the control film. Calcification is otherwise easy to miss.

- **Observe the gas pattern and position** Small bowel is recognized by its central position and valvulae conniventes, which reach from one wall to the other. Large bowel is more peripheral and the haustrae go only part of the way across the lumen. Abnormal position may point to pathology, eg gas is central in ascites; it is displaced to the left lower quadrant by splenomegaly. If the transverse colon is >5.5cm wide, consider toxic dilatation (eg from UC). Confirm by finding numerous broad-based pseudopolyps projecting into the lumen, and loss of normal haustral pattern.

- **Look for extraluminal gas**

  Air in the liver or biliary system: After passing a stone, after ERCP (p498), or with gas-forming infection.

  Air in GU system: Entero-vesical fistula.

  Air in the peritoneum: Perforated ulcer/diverticulum, prolonged vaginal intercourse.

  Air in the colonic wall (Pneumatosis coli): Infective colitis.

  Air elsewhere: There may also be air in a subphrenic abscess.

- **Look for calcification in the abdomen or pelvis** Calcification in arteries (atherosclerosis, the egg-shell calcification in an aneurysm), lymph nodes, phleboliths (smooth, round), renal calcification or ureteric stones (usually jagged; look along the line of the ureter), adrenal (TB), pancreatic (chronic pancreatitis), liver or spleen, gallstones (only 10% opaque), bladder (stone, tumour, TB, schistosomiasis), uterus, dermoid cyst, which may contain teeth.

- **Bones of spine and pelvis** Look for metastases (osteolytic or osteoblastic), Paget's disease, Looser's zones (osteomalacia), collapse, osteoarthritis (p666); the 'rugger-jersey' spine of osteomalacia.

- **Soft tissues** The psoas lines are obliterated in retroperitoneal inflammation, haemorrhage, or peritonitis. Note kidney size and shape (normally 2–3 vertebral bodies length and parallel to the psoas line).

- **Meteorism** Localized peritoneal inflammation can cause a localized ileus. This may be seen on the plain film as a 'sentinel loop' of intraluminal gas and can provide a clue to the site of pathology.

Cholecystitis	Pancreatitis
Appendicitis	Diverticulitis

(In young patients, even localized inflammation can produce a generalized ileus).

...in skull views (SXR)

...ne chief reason for requesting a skull x-ray is trauma (in some centres, and in some circumstances, CT or MRI will be done in preference).

▶If the Glasgow coma scale score is ≤8/15 after acute head injury, the patient needs an urgent CT scan: *do not delay this for skull x-rays.*

The chief things to look for are: ●Presence of a linear skull fracture (increases likelihood of intracranial haematoma from 1:1000 to 1:30 if alert, and from 1:100 to 1:4 if consciousness impaired). ●Presence of a depressed skull fracture (needs elevating if depressed by an amount which is greater than the width of vault). ●Presence of a calcified pineal, shifted >3mm from the midline—but not all the population has a conveniently calcified gland. ●The status of the cranio-cervical junction.

Skull radiographs may be useful in other clinical situations:
●**Bone density and thickness** *Diffuse increase in vault density* is seen in Paget's disease and fluorosis (excessive fluoride ingestion, eg from insecticides, causing mottled enamel, and osteofluorosis, which is a combination of osteosclerosis and osteomalacia).
Diffuse increase in thickness is seen in acromegaly, thalassaemia and meningiomas (especially parasagittal or sphenoidal ridge) and Paget's.
Localized increase in bone density is seen in Paget's disease, osteomyelitis, malignancy (eg leukaemia and histiocytosis).
Lucent areas: trauma, malignancy (myeloma), Paget's, hyperparathyroidism.
●**Intracranial calcification** May be normal (pineal) or may reflect a tumour (7% of gliomas, 10% of meningiomas, >70% of craniopharyngiomas are calcified), vascular malformation (sinuous tram-line occipital calcification seen in Sturge–Weber syndrome; ring calcification of cerebral aneurysms) or old infection (TB, toxoplasmosis).
●**The sella turcica** Normally, widest AP diameter of the pituitary fossa is 11–16mm and depth 8–12mm in adults. Enlargement occurs with pituitary adenoma; erosion of the posterior clinoids with raised intracranial pressure; erosion of the lamina dura of the dorsum sellae with tumour or aneurysm.
●**Air sinus** Thick mucosa (chronic sinusitis); enlarged in acromegaly; fluid level after trauma (eg in maxillary sinus with infraorbital fracture; sphenoid sinus with basal skull fracture—you'll miss this if you do not turn lateral SXR on its side, ie the position in which the film was taken).

The hand x-ray

Cast your eye over the entire film looking for:
●**Deformities** Ulnar deviation/subluxation (rheumatoid arthritis), syndactyly/polydactyly, short metacarpals (pseudohyperparathyroidism).
●**Joints** Erosions and bone destruction of the arthritides, effusions (seen as joint space widening and pericapsular soft tissue). Check the joints involved and symmetry (DIP, PIP, wrists).
●**Loss of bone density**—diffuse: osteoporosis; localized: cysts (osteoarthritis—Heberden's nodes at DIP joints, Bouchard's nodes at PIP joints; simple cyst; sarcoid), avascular necrosis, erosions (below).
●**Erosions eg of terminal phalangeal tufts** seen in sarcoid, hyperparathyroidism, and scleroderma (the latter allowing the nail to curve—'pseudoclubbing') and subperiosteal erosions along the radial border of the middle phalanges (an early sign of hyperparathyroidism). Coarse trabeculations are seen in chronic haemolytic anaemia, Paget's disease, and the lipidoses (eg Gaucher's syndrome, *OHCS* p748).
●**Soft tissues**—generalized increase in thickness seen in acromegaly (spade-like hands), localized thickness, eg gouty tophi, arterial, pericap-
'ar or soft-tissue calcification (eg CREST, p670).

The spine

Cervical spine

In major trauma the first x-ray to be performed after resuscitation is a cross-table lateral of the cervical spine. All seven cervical vertebrae

must be seen, along with C7–T1 junction: do not accept an incomplete x-ray—try traction on the arms, or a swimmer's view. Occasionally subluxations do not show up without flexion and extension views (perform only on the advice of a senior colleague).

▶ If a cervical spine injury is suspected you must immobilize the neck until it is excluded.

▶ A cross-table portable cervical spine x-ray in the best hands will miss up to 15% of injuries.

When examining the film, follow 4 simple steps:

●Alignment: Of anterior and posterior vertebral body, posterior spinal canal and spinous processes. A step of <25% of a vertebral body implies unifacet dislocation; if >50% it is bifacetal. 40% of those <7yrs old have anterior displacement of C2 on C3 (pseudosubluxation); still present in 20% up to 16yrs. 15% show this with C3 on C4. In this physiological subluxation, the posterior spinal line is maintained. Angulation between vertebrae >10% is abnormal.

●*Bone contour:* Trace around each vertebra individually. Look for avulsion fractures of the body or spinous process. A wedge fracture is present if the anterior height differs from posterior by >3mm. Check odontoid (open mouth view but can be seen on lateral view); don't mistake vertical cleft between incisors for a peg fracture!—epiphyses in children can be mistaken for fractures; the distance between the odontoid and anterior arch of C1 should be <3mm (may be increased in children). Type 1 fractures are of the odontoid peg, type 2 of its base, and type 3 fractures extend into the body of C2.

●*Cartilages:* Check that intervertebral disc space margins are parallel.

●*Soft tissues:* If the space between the lower anterior border of C3 and the pharyngeal shadow is >5mm suspect retropharyngeal swelling (haemorrhage; abscess)—this is often useful indirect evidence of a C2 fracture. Space between lower cervical vertebrae and trachea should be <1 vertebral body.

Thoracic and lumbar spine

Wedge fractures are common, particularly in the osteoporotic. Suspect metastatic secondaries (often seen in the vascular pedicles), especially if adjacent vertebrae are involved. A spondylolysis (usually at L5/S1) is seen as a defect in the pars interarticularis on the lateral, or more easily the oblique film (look for 'Scottie dog'—the 'collar' is the defect); it may be congenital or acquired, the latter being a fatigue fracture, acute trauma or pathological fracture (tumour; TB; Paget's). If L5 slips forward on S1 this is a spondylolisthesis. Prolapsed intervertebral disc cannot be diagnosed from a plain film; MRI gives better definition than CT, and both have largely replaced radiculograms.

Specific conditions: Ankylosing spondylitis, p668 (sacroiliitis; syndesmophytes; bamboo spine); osteomalacia ('rugger-jersey' spine); Scheuermann's disease (apophysitis resulting in fixed smooth kyphosis in adolescents); spina bifida occulta (present in up to 20% of population: may be minor abnormal neurology in legs).

Principal source: American College of Surgeons (1988), Advanced Trauma Life Support (ATLS) course manual, and PA Driscoll 1993 *BMJ* ii 855

Contrast studies

These are performed either with an IV contrast agent or with an oral contrast such as barium or Gastrograffin.

Contrast reactions to IV reagents occur in ~1/1000 patients and death by anaphylaxis in 1/40,000. Reactions include hives, bronchospasm and/or pulmonary oedema. Ask about a history of atopy (p28) or allergy to iodine or seafood. Take advice from your radiologists—premedication with corticosteroids (eg: prednisolone 40mg PO 12h prior and 2h prior) is effective in reducing the incidence of reactions. The newer non-ionic contrast agents available should be used in this situation. When renal function is impaired, ensure good hydration (IV fluids) pre- and post-study (diuresis confers no additional benefit).[1]

Angiography Used to image aorta, big arteries and branches (atheromatous stenosis and thrombosis, embolism, aneurysms, A-V fistulas, and angiomatous malformations), and for the investigation of tumours. It may be combined with interventions, eg balloon dilatation, embolization, marking for identification intra-operatively, etc. Digital subtraction angiography (DSA) provides reverse negative views and requires less contrast.

- *Cardiac and coronary angiography:* (See p272.)
- *Angiography in peripheral vascular disease:* (See p128).
- *Pulmonary angiography:* Used for visualization of emboli and vascular abnormalities and assessment of right heart pressures. It is the most accurate procedure for diagnosis of PE but is often reserved for those who on clinical grounds have a massive PE and intervention (such as thrombolysis) is being considered (p774).
- *Cerebral angiography:* For intracranial and extracranial vascular disease, atherosclerosis, aneurysms and arterio–venous malformations.
- *Selective visceral angiography:* Used to locate the source of GI bleeding (acute or chronic) when this has not been found by endoscopy. It may be used to selectively infuse drugs or embolic material into the bleeding territory. Coeliac axis angiography is used for intrahepatic pathology (haemangiomas, site and blood supply of hepatic tumours pre-operatively) and is used for selective embolization (especially for carcinoid secondaries in the liver). Late films give good views of the portal vein. Splenic phlebography, performed by percutaneous puncture of the spleen and injection of contrast, may be a useful test in portal hypertension for imaging and pressure measurements.
- *Renal angiography:* Originally used to distinguish tumour from cyst (now superseded by ultrasound and CT). Widely used for the embolization of vascular tumours and for the investigation of renal hypertension (secondary to atheroma or fibromuscular hyperplasia).

1 R Solomon 1994 *NEJM* **331** 1416

GI studies with contrast

Barium swallow This is a method for investigating dysphagia, if endoscopy is not available, or if motility needs to be observed.

Barium meal This is a method of outlining oesophageal, gastric, and duodenal pathology. Endoscopy is often the preferred method of investigating upper GI phenomena as it allows biopsy and, in some instances, therapeutic intervention (p498).

Barium follow-through (=small bowel meal, or small bowel series) The small volume of dense barium used for a barium meal is not suitable for this test, in which barium via a transpyloric tube is followed to the ileocaecal valve—so do not request this test as an add-on to a barium meal request.[1] If *both* are needed, do each separately. *Indications:*
- When trying to diagnose Crohn's disease, or in GI bleeding when endoscopy and barium enemas are normal.
- If there is difficulty in diagnosing malabsorption—eg if complications such as lymphoma are suspected.
- Intermittent GI obstruction.

Small bowel barium enema The indications are the same as for the barium follow-through—but the route is reversed. It may be more sensitive in Crohn's disease, and in outlining tiny small-bowel tumours—but it is more uncomfortable, and the dose of radiation is higher.

Barium enema Use the 'double contrast' technique of air and barium which gives improved demonstration of surface mucosal pattern. Distending the gut wall allows pathology to be more readily seen. Used for demonstration of structural lesions (eg tumour, diverticula, polyps, ulcers, fistulae) as well as abnormal peristalsis, reflux etc. If GI perforation or fistula is suspected, often Gastrograffin is the contrast of choice to prevent contaminating the operative field with barium.

Cleansing the colon is the most important determinant of quality of barium enemas—regimens vary; contact your radiology department. Note that colonoscopy (p498) allows biopsy, and is the most accurate way to assess the colon—but it is more likely to cause perforation, and it is hard to reach the caecum. It is not so widely available as barium enema. In white men, sigmoidoscopy may be the best way to rule out colorectal carcinomas—whereas in black women, who have more proximal cancers, barium enema may be the investigation of choice.[2]

Cholangiography may be performed in a variety of ways.
- *Endoscopic retrograde cholangiopancreatography (ERCP):* (See p498.)
- *Oral cholecystography:* Was the first investigation to be used to visualize the gall bladder. Patient is given oral contrast 12–24h prior to the study. Failure of gall bladder opacification is considered abnormal and indicative of gallstone disease, but may also be due to acute pancreatitis, peritonitis or cholecystitis. Unlikely to work if serum bilirubin >34µmol/L.
- *Intravenous cholecystography:* Is seldom indicated but may be useful in suspected choledocholithiasis and now rarely performed. In order to carry out the investigation, serum bilirubin should be <50µmol/L. Contraindicated in patients with severe hepato-renal disease, allergy to contrast and IgM paraproteinaemia (precipitates out with contrast).
- *Percutaneous transhepatic cholangiography:* May be used to demonstrate dilated ducts in obstructive jaundice and may be combined with external drainage or internal drainage (using an endoprosthesis across the stricture). Contraindications: bleeding tendency, cholangitis, ascites, allergy.

1 D Martin 1994 *Medicine in Practice* 1 7 2 Cancer 1997 **80** 193 http://www.giradiology.com

Ultrasound

▶*Ultrasound is easy to do—and easy to misinterpret.* Its rôle overlaps with CT, but it is much cheaper and involves no radiation. In one 3-hour session an ultrasonographer can do 18 or so scans—all for the price of a single CT scan, but definition is less precise.[1] Ultrasound machines are portable, and need little maintenance.

Because imaging by ultrasound entails no ionizing radiation, it has completely taken over conventional radiology in obstetrics (except for pelvimetry, see *OHCS* p118). Also, it is often the first line of investigation of abdominal organs and cardiac lesions. It is also used to guide needle aspiration, or biopsy of masses and collections. However, it is quite operator-dependent and reliability of results may vary. The use of Doppler allows one to assess, qualitatively, patency and direction of flow through vessels, but does not give an accurate quantitative measurement.

Abdominal scan This is often the initial investigation for abdominal masses. It may be used to assess: 1 Liver size and texture (eg fatty liver, shrunken cirrhotic liver), masses within it (cysts *vs* tumour). 2 The biliary system (dilation in obstructive jaundice, p484; the cause, ie stone *vs* tumour, is less reliably seen). 3 Doppler of the portal and splanchnic veins is used to rule out thrombosis and assess direction of flow in the portal veins in cirrhosis. 4 The gall bladder (thickening and gallstones within it). 5 The pancreas (pseudocysts, abscesses and sometimes tumour). 6 The aorta and major vessels for aneurysm. 7 The kidneys (size, texture, hydronephrosis in obstruction, polycystic disease, tumour). Often ultrasound is the initial investigation for haematuria and is better than IVU for bladder pathology (but see p374). It is good for showing fluid and lymphoceles around transplanted kidneys. The adrenals are less reliably imaged and only fairly large are masses identified.

Pelvic scan ●Ultrasound is the best imaging technique for monitoring normal and abnormal pregnancy, fetal growth and development, localization of the placenta, ectopic pregnancy. ●Testicular masses—hydrocele *vs* tumour. ●Ovarian and uterine masses (tumours, cysts and fibroids). For further details, see obstetric ultrasound: *OHCS* p118–9.

Cardiovascular ultrasound (p274) M-mode echocardiography allows measurements of chamber size and accurate assessment of valve and wall motion. 2D echocardiography provides real-time images of the anatomy and spatial relationships. Duplex Doppler scanners include colour coding of flow directions and allow direct visualization of shunts and regurgitant flow. Doppler is also used in the assessment of carotid stenosis (p433).

Miscellaneous *Thyroid scan:* To distinguish cysts from tumours. Cannot distinguish benign from malignant nodule.

Orbit and eye: Assessment of retinal and choroidal detachment, localization of foreign bodies, and assessment of retro-orbital masses.

Large veins (eg femoral and popliteal veins): These may be assessed by Doppler ultrasound as an easy, non-invasive initial investigation when thrombosis is suspected (p92).

Other places where adventurous probes have entered: Oesophagus (trans-oesophageal echo, TOE, in mitral valve analysis, thoracic aortic aneurysm); *vagina* (ovarian cancer screening; fertility investigations, looking for mature follicles); *rectum* (TRUSS=transrectal ultrasound scan, for prostatic disease detection); *coronary arteries* (tiny device to delineate pathoanatomy).

1 S Mindel 1997 *Lancet* 350 426

Radioisotope scanning: 1

Bone scanning ^{99}Tcm-MDP (methylene diphosphonate) is the most commonly used radiotracer; it is retained in areas with increased osteoblastic activity. Imaging is done 3h post-injection (pi). Common indications: •Assessment of metastatic disease from a known primary •Assessment of extent of Paget's disease •Diagnosis of scaphoid fractures •Diagnosis of stress fractures •Identification of osteoid osteoma •Assessment of extent of arthritis •Characterization of metabolic bone disease.

Brain scanning ^{99}Tcm-HMPAO (hexamethyl propylene amine oxime) is the most commonly used radiotracer. Imaging is performed using single photon emission computed tomography (SPECT) within 30 minutes pi Tracer distribution reflects the distribution of the regional cerebral blood flow (rCBF). rCBF SPECT can be used to support a clinical diagnosis of dementia; localization of ictal focus in epilepsy prior to surgery; assessment of the vascular deficit/reserve in acute stroke; and other pathologies where cortical perfusion needs assessment.

Cardiac scanning *Myocardial perfusion imaging (MPI):* MPI is used mainly to evaluate atypical chest pain; to assess the extent of ischaemic heart disease; and to assess viable myocardium prior to revascularization. Exercise-induced coronary arterial spasm is detected by comparing imaging at rest and under stress. Any areas underperfused on exercise but better perfused at rest are reported as ischaemic. Dipyridamole, adenosine or dobutamine are used as stressors if arthritis, abnormal ECG (left bundle branch block, or on digoxin with changes to the ECG) preclude exercise, or those in whom the exercise test is inconclusive. SPECT imaging is performed after injection of ^{201}Tl (Thallium-201), ^{99}Tc^m-MIBI (methoxy isobutyl isonitrile) or ^{99}Tcm-Tetrofosmin.

Radionuclide ventriculography (RNV): Planar imaging performed after radiolabelling the red blood cells, and data acquisition by multi-gated acquisition (MUGA) where the data collection is synchronized to the ECG, provides objective and reproducible data on ventricular ejection fractions, regional wall motion abnormalities, and information on ventricular aneurysms.

Infarct avid imaging: Imaging with ^{99}Tcm-PYP (pyrophosphate) or with ^{111}In-Fab' (microsomal antibody fragment) may be used to identify sites of infarction 24–72 hours after the event, in patients with equivocal ECG and equivocal 'cardiac' enzyme (creatine kinase—CPK, CK-MB) levels.

Lung scanning ^{99}Tcm-MAA (macroaggregates of albumin) is commonly used to assess perfusion (Q̇) and ^{99}Tcm Technegas, ^{81}Krm, or ^{133}Xe may be used to assess ventilation (V̇). V̇/Q̇ scanning relies on the physiological principle of reduction in segmental perfusion and normal ventilation in pulmonary embolism. Matched reduction in perfusion and ventilation can be seen in parenchymal lung disorders. Scans are always interpreted with a current CXR and reports are in the form of probabilities (see opposite).

Testicular scans: ^{99}Tcm-pertechnetate may be used to differentiate orchitis (increased uptake) from testicular torsion (reduced uptake).

We thank Dr Sobhan Vinjamuri for help with this page (& p789-90)

Basic principles

Radioisotope scanning involves administrating a small amount of radioactive tracer and plotting its distribution throughout the body in general and in the organ that is to be studied in particular.

The radioactive tracer consists of a ligand (non-radioactive) which is complexed to a radionuclide. Technetium-99m (^{99}Tcm) is the commonest one used in all nuclear medicine imaging centres, others include Indium-111 (^{111}In), Iodine-123 (^{123}I), Gallium-67 (^{67}Ga) (all gamma ray emitters). The gamma rays emitted by the radioisotope are transformed into analogue and/or digital information by a gamma camera. Imaging performed by a rotating gamma camera is termed 'single photon emission computed tomography' or SPECT.

Since anatomic modalities (CT/MRI) image anatomy but rarely allow comment on functional significance of anatomical abnormalities, and since radioisotope studies provide physiological/functional information, correlative imaging provides complementary information of greater clinical relevance than either type of test individually.

Probabilistic diagnosis of pulmonary embolism with V̇/Q̇ scans

Radiology (V̇/Q̇ scan) is more accurate than clinical judgement, but a high clinical probability increases the likelihood of a PE whatever the V̇/Q̇ result. To give the best chance of an accurate diagnosis clinical judgement should be combined with the V̇/Q̇ result. Most patients with a PE do not have a high-probability scan, and the big difficulty arises with a moderate or low clinical suspicion and an intermediate or low probability scan: here the chances of a PE are from 4–88%. What is required is something to refine diagnosis. In good hands angiography is safe, reliable, and definitive; but if unavailable, looking for the presence of DVTs (ultrasound, p92, or venography) *may* help to provide further evidence in support of a PE; although PEs may occur without a DVT[2,3]. Spiral CT or MRI may help, and are being developed. So the situation is complex: seek advice!

Previous PE makes scans hard to interpret (a significant proportion are abnormal for some time after the first PE: be sure to tell the radiologist).

A high probability V̇/Q̇ scan (>90%) exists if: ≥ 2 big (>75% of a segment) segmental perfusion deficits or ≥ 4 involving >26% of a segment (ie a moderate deficit)—or one big + ≥3 moderate deficits.

A low probability (<15%) exists if: There are any number of *matched* ventilation–perfusion defects, whatever their size—or small perfusion defects (<25% of a segment)—or non-segmental defects. (No treatment required.)

An intermediate probability (~50%) lies between high and low probability.[1] A 'normal' scan means a <5% likelihood of PE. >40% of scans are non-diagnostic, alas, and angiography may be needed.

1 T Fennerty 1997 *BMJ* i 425 & PIOPED 1990 *JAMA* 263 2762 2 *E-BM* 1997 2 187 3 F Turkstra 1997 *Ann Int Med* 126 775–81

Radioisotope scanning: 2

Liver scans ^{99}Tcm-tin or sulfur colloid scans are taken up by macrophages (Kupffer cells in liver) and may be used to assess diffuse liver disease.

Hepatobiliary scans ^{99}Tcm-HIDA (hepatic iminodiacetic acid) is taken up by the hepatocytes, cleared into the gall bladder through intrahepatic channels, and then excreted into the gut via the cystic duct. This test is used mainly to diagnose acute cholecystitis (where the gall bladder is not visualized till 4 hours); for diagnosing biliary leaks post-surgery and for quantitative information on gall bladder kinetics.

Thyroid scans ^{99}Tcm-pertechnetate or ^{123}I-Iodide may be used for assessment of solitary thyroid nodules (up to 25% of cold nodules are malignant, warm or hot nodules are benign); assessment of congenital hypothyroidism and localization of ectopic thyroid tissue; diagnosis of autonomous functioning thyroid adenomas (AFTA) and differentiation of Graves' from Plummer's toxicosis (diffuse vs nodular). ^{131}I scans are useful in the assessment and follow-up of patients with well differentiated thyroid cancer.

Parathyroid scans Imaging is primarily indicated to localize a parathyroid adenoma once a biochemical diagnosis of primary hyperparathyroidism is made. Owing to the close proximity of the parathyroids to the thyroid gland, images are acquired in 2 phases, the first depicting the thyroid phase and the second depicting the thyroid + parathyroid phase. Subtracting the first set of images from the second set is said to be indicative of the parathyroid phase. A normal parathyroid gland is not visualised on subtraction. ^{99}Tcm-pertechnetate, ^{99}Tcm-MIBI (p733) at 5 min post-infusion (pi) or ^{123}I is used for the thyroid phase; ^{201}Tl or ^{99}Tcm-MIBI imaging at 2–3h pi used for the second phase.

Adrenal scans Phaeochromocytomas and other tumours of neuroectodermal origin can be localized using ^{123}I-MIBG (metaiodobenzylguanidine).

Renal scans Radioisotope scanning and computer-assisted analysis of the images of the kidneys (renography) provides vital functional information. Standard renography with ^{99}Tcm-DTPA or ^{99}Tcm-MAG3 provides data on split renal function; and uptake and excretory patterns of each kidney. Diuretic renography performed by injecting 0.5mg/kg of frusemide (=furosemide) at the end of a standard renogram helps to distinguish physiological dilatation of the renal pelvis from obstructive nephropathy. Captopril renography performed by repeating the standard renogram after administration of oral captopril (25–50mg) helps to confirm renovascular disorders (unilateral better than bilateral). ^{99}Tcm-DMSA (dimethyl succinic acid) is a renal cortical imaging agent and is useful in chronic pyelonephritis, renal scarring, and renal cortical cysts.

Inflammation/infection imaging ^{67}Ga-citrate is useful in the evaluation of PUO; localization of abscesses (5–10 days old); evaluation of chronic inflammation, eg in sarcoid; assessment of mediastinal lymphomas; and to assess prognosis and monitor therapy in pneumocystis carinii pneumonia.

^{111}In or ^{99}Tcm-labelled white blood cells are useful in the evaluation of abdominal and pelvic abscesses; evaluation of osteomyelitis; evaluation of prosthetic infection (especially hip); assessment of the activity and progression of disease; and to monitor response to treatment in patients with colitis (especially Crohn's disease).

Other scans Lymphangiography is useful to differentiate venous oedema from lymphatic oedema and to diagnose lymphatic obstruction. Oesophageal transit and gastric emptying studies help to assess upper GI motility. Radiolabelled red blood cell scans are useful in the localization of active upper GI bleeding. Meckel's scans help to localize abnormally functioning ectopic gastric mucosa (as in Meckel's diverticulum).

Computerized tomography (CT) scans

Computerized tomography can be performed with or without IV contrast. A dilute oral contrast agent prior to abdominal or pelvic scanning helps delineate the bowel. Density measurements (expressed as Hounsfield units) can be used to differentiate between masses (eg cysts, lipomas, or haematomas). In Hounsfield units, bone is +1000, water is 0, fat is −1000, and the remaining tissues fall between depending on consistency. Vascular lesions 'enhance' with IV contrast while non-vascular lesions do not.

The brain

Most suspected intracerebral lesions are now investigated by CT as a primary diagnostic procedure. CT is used for the diagnosis of hydrocephalus where the ventricles are dilated and sulci flattened against the inner skull. Unilateral mass lesions cause midline shift, compressing the lateral ventricles, and may have considerable surrounding oedema, seen as a low-density area. CT is also considered to establish whether the cause of a stroke is intracranial bleeding (haemorrhage is seen as a high density lesion). As the clot absorbs, the lesion becomes isodense, and, later, of low attenuation. Similarly, extradural and subdural haematomas are seen in the acute phase as high-density peripheral lesions—but they may be isodense, and a real problem arises if they are bilateral and isodense, because there is no tell-tale midline shift.[1] Chronic subdural haematomas appear hypodense. Cerebral infarction is seen as an area of low attenuation, often enhancing, with no mass effect. Cerebral atrophy is seen as deepening of the sulci and narrowing of the gyri.

When to consider a CT scan in a patient with headaches:
- Progressive worsening of symptoms, or change in their pattern.
- If associated with the onset of epilepsy (especially focal epilepsy).
- Any change in personality.
- CNS signs such as falling acuity, papilloedema, diplopia, deafness, dysphasia, ataxia, or focal weakness.
- Recent head injury, or falls (is there a subdural haemorrhage?).

The abdomen Most liver pathology can be imaged by ultrasound but CT can improve accuracy and reveal smaller lesions. The pancreas is well shown (small lesions can be missed). Acute pancreatitis causes general swelling and oedema of the gland. CT is particularly useful in delineating renal and adrenal masses. It has largely replaced lymphangiography in evaluation of para-aortic and retroperitoneal lymphadenopathy and is used in staging abdominal and haematological malignancy.

The chest CT is of great value in picking up small lesions such as pleural deposits, which may be missed on plain x-ray: it is able to find 40% more nodules than whole lung tomograms which demonstrate 20% more nodules than plain x-ray. CT is also useful for assessing mediastinal masses and aneurysms. Modern fast body scanners can even show intracardiac lesions (eg myxomas, p317) although transoesophageal ultrasound and ECG-gated MRI remain superior.

Spiral CT is being developed for diagnosing pulmonary emboli, and has attractions because 90% are diagnostic (compared with ~50% for V̇/Q̇ scans, p733) but availability is limited, and it entails significant radiation. But it may have a rôle when the chance of a non-diagnostic V̇/Q̇ scan is high (eg abnormal CXR). Sensitivity (in good hands) 90%; specificity: 92%.[2]

One can store a digital CT study more easily than a chest x-ray (1MB *vs* 4MB).

RJ Davenport 1994 *BMJ* ii 792   2 D Hansell 1998 *BMJ* i 490

Magnetic resonance imaging (MRI)

MRI uses measurements of magnetic movements of atomic nuclei to delineate tissues. Refer to a specialized text for the physics involved. Two types of images are produced:

- *T1 weighted images:* Provide good anatomical planes and better separation of cystic and solid structures due to the wide variance of T1 values among normal tissues. Fat appears as brightest (high signal intensity), the remaining tissues appearing as varying degrees of lower signal intensity (black). Flowing blood appears black.
- *T2 weighted images:* These provide the best detection of pathology and a decreased visualization of normal anatomy. Tumour surrounded by fat may be lost on T2 imaging. Fat and fluid appear brightest.

Advantages of MRI:
- Non-ionizing radiation
- Shows vasculature without contrast
- Images can easily be produced in any plane, eg sagittal and coronal (good for spinal cord, aorta, vena cava)
- Visualization of posterior fossa and other areas prone to bony artefact on CT, eg cranio-cervical junction
- High inherent soft tissue contrast
- Precise staging of malignancy, eg extending to within bone marrow and other areas occult to CT and other methods

Disadvantages of MRI:
- High cost of equipment
- Claustrophobia (in magnet tunnel for 30–120mins—hypnosis, music, or sedation may be needed)
- Long imaging time causes increased motion artefact
- Unable to scan very ill patients requiring monitoring equipment
- Unsuitable for those with metal foreign bodies (eg pacemakers, CNS vascular clips, cochlear implants, valves, shrapnel)
- Unable to image calcium

MRI machines are noisy brutes, and some people will become disorientated, suffering claustrophobia and terror (don't underestimate this). Good explanation, and someone to talk to during the procedure may help.

Positron emission tomography (PET)

Molecules labelled with positron-emitting radionuclides are injected, and post-anihilation event photon paths are analysed by crystal detectors to produce 3D images of function—eg of blood flow (labelled ammonia) or glucose metabolism (fluordeoxyglucose, FDG).

In cardiology it may help answer questions such as "Is this piece of non-functioning myocardium dead or just hibernating?" If hibernating (low blood flow but glucose metabolism is present), then angioplasty to its supply vessel could improve function.

PET in tumours PET can help if CT/MRI fails to distinguish cell death after radiotherapy from tumour recurrence. This helps plan stereotactic radiotherapy. Whole-body PET can disclose asymptomatic resectable tumours (glycolysis is ↑ in cancer cells, making them visible to PET).[1]

PET can prevent invasive tests eg by imaging epileptogenic foci, where no anatomic lesion is found on MRI. PET can also diagnose dementia (even before symptoms start), and distinguish Alzheimer's from other types (symmetrical hypometabolism in parietal and temporal lobes—not the frontal lobes, which are affected in Pick's dementia).

PET in research PET may help answer questions such as "Does schizophrenia have a physical basis in the brain?"—and it is interesting to note that it has already shown subtle changes affecting the hippocampus and temporal lobes. Here PET is leading to new models of schizophrenia involving a defect in self-monitoring arising from a white-matter neurodevelopmental encephalopathy affecting the interconnections of the associative areas of the brain—see *OHCS* p357 for further details.

Cost ≥£350/scan. Cost-effectiveness issues have yet to be resolved.

1 S Yasuda 1997 *Lancet* 350 1819 (N=1872; 14 treatable cancers were found, but PET missed 11; thyroiditis, sarcoid, and colonic adenomas cause 'false' +ves—but may need clinical attention).

An example of epidemiology at work

Some decades ago epidemiologists tested the hypothesis that smoking and hypertension were associated with cardiovascular disease. Painstaking cohort studies confirmed that these were indeed *risk markers* (a term that does not imply causality). Over the years, as evidence accumulates, the term risk marker may give way to *risk factor*—which implies causation, and the separate idea that risk-factor modification will cause a reduction in disease. Demonstrating a dose-response relationship (with the correct time sequence) is good evidence of a causal relationship—eg showing that the greater the number of cigarettes smoked, the greater the risk, or the lower the blood pressure achieved (up to a point!) by antihypertensives, the less the mortality from cardiovascular events. It is still possible that blood pressure is a risk marker of some other phenomenon, but this gets less likely if the relationship between BP and cardiovascular mortality is found to correlate *while keeping other known risk factors constant*. The work of the epidemiologist does not stop here. He or she can use actuarial statistics to weigh the relative merits and interactions of a number of risk factors, to give an overall estimate of risk for an individual. It is then possible to say things like: "If the 5-yr risk of a serious cardiac event in people with no overt cardiac disease is >15%, then drug treatment of hyperlipidaemia may begin to be cost-effective—and a 10% 5-yr risk may be a sufficient point to trigger antihypertensive treatment in someone with, say, a BP of 150/90." These figures are a guide only: only ~60% of those in the top 10% of the risk distribution will have an adverse coronary event in the 5-year period. Nevertheless this is more accurate than taking into account risk factors singly—and so we are led to our first important conclusion:

epidemiology improves and informs our dialogue with our patients
We can give patients good evidence on which to base their choices.

Risk equations (ideally as part of computerized medical records) may be given as follows (a, m, μ, and σ are variables relating risk-factors):[1]

> If $a = 11.1122 - (0.9119 \times \ln(\text{BP})) - (0.2767 \times \text{SMO}) - (0.7181 \times \ln(\text{FAT})) - (0.5865 \times \text{LVH})$
> and for males $m = a - (1.4762 \times \ln(\text{AGE})) = 0.1759 \times \text{DIAB}$
> and for females $m = a - 5.8549 + (1.8515 \times \ln(\text{AGE}/74)^2) - (0.3758 \times \text{DIAB})$
> and $\mu = 4.4181 + m$
> and $\sigma = e^{-(0.3155 - 0.278m)}$ and $v = (\ln(5) - \mu/\sigma$
> then **5 year risk** $\approx 1 - (e^{-(e^v)})$ if AGE is 30 to 74yr, BP is the mean systolic, eg 3 readings—and SMO, DIAB, and LVH are each 1 if the patient is a smoker, has diabetes or left ventricular hypertrophy, eg on ECG; if not present, each is 0. FAT is the ratio of total cholesterol to HDL. This is the EMIS formulation of the 'Dundee equations'; see also J Robson 1997 *BMJ* **ii** 277 & the corrected Sheffield tables for primary prevention of heart disease, *Lancet* 1996 **348** 1251

The essence of epidemiology

Epidemiology is the study of the distribution of clinical phenomena in populations. Its chief measures are prevalence and incidence.

The *period prevalence* of a disease is the number of cases, at any time during the study period, divided by the population at risk. If the population at risk is unclear, then the population must be specified—for example, the prevalence of uterine cancer varies widely, depending on whether you specify the general population (men, women, boys, and girls) or only women, or women who have not already had a hysterectomy.

The *incidence* of a disease is the number of new cases within the study period which must be specified, eg annual incidence. *Point prevalence* is the prevalence at a point in time. The *lifetime* prevalence of hiccups is ~100%; the (UK) incidence is millions/year—but the point prevalence may be 0 at 3am today if no one is actually having hiccups.

Association Epidemiological research is often concerned with comparing the rates of disease in different populations. For example, the rate of bronchial carcinoma in a population of men who smoke, compared with men who do not smoke. A difference in rates points to an association (or dissociation) between the disease and factors which distinguish the populations (in this case, smoking or not). If the rates are equal, association is still possible—with a confounding variable (eg both groups share the same very smoky environment).

Ways of accounting for associations: A causes B; B causes A; a third agent, P, causes A and B; it may be a chance finding.

There are 2 types of study which explore causal connections:

1 *Case–control (retrospective) studies:* The study group consists of those with the disease (eg lung cancer); the control group consists of those without the disease. The previous occurrence of the putative cause (eg smoking) is compared between each group. Case–control studies are retrospective in that they start after the onset of the disease (although cases may be collected prospectively).

2 *Cohort (prospective) studies:* The study group consists of subjects exposed to the putative causal factor (eg smoking); and the control group consists of subjects not so exposed. The incidence of the disease is compared between the groups. ▶A cohort study generates incidence data, whereas a case–control study does not.

Matching An association between A and B may be due to another factor P. To eliminate this possibility matching for P is often used in case-control studies. One powerful but unreliable (if numbers are small) way to do this in clinical trials is for the subjects to be allocated to groups randomly; check important 'P's have been distributed evenly between groups.

Overmatching Suppose that unemployment causes low income, and low income causes depression. If you matched study and control groups for income, then you would miss the genuine causal link between unemployment and depression. In general, avoid matching factors which may intervene in the causal chain linking A and B.

Masking If the subject does not know which of two trial treatments she is having, the trial is single blind. To further reduce risk of bias, the experimenter should also not know (double blind).
▶In a good treatment trial, the blind lead the blind.

Further reading: D Sackett 1991 *Clinical Epidemiology*, 2e, Little Bro
D Sackett 1997 Evidence-based Medicine: how to practice and t

Evidence-based medicine[1]

This is the conscientious and judicious use of current best evidence from clinical care research in the management of individual patients.

The problem 2,000,000 papers are published each year. Patients may benefit directly from a tiny fraction of these papers. How do we find them?

A partial solution 50 journals are scanned not by experts in neonatal nephrology or the left nostril, but by searchers trained to spot papers which have a direct message for practice, and meet pre-defined criteria of rigour (below). Summaries are then published in *Evidence-based Medicine*.[2] *Questions used to evaluate papers:* **1** Are the results *valid*? (Randomized? Blinded? Were all patients accounted for who entered the trial? Was follow-up complete? Were the groups similar at the start? Were the groups treated equally, apart from the experimental intervention?) **2** What *are* the results? (How large was the treatment effect? How precise was the treatment effect?) **3** Will the results help *my* patients (cost–benefit sum).[1]

Problems with the solution ●*The concept of scientific rigour is opaque.* What do we want? The science, the rigour, the truth, or what will be most useful to our patients? These may overlap, but they are not the same.
●Will the best be the enemy of the good? Are useful papers rejected due to of some blemish? Answer: *all* evidence needs appraising (often impossible!).
●By reformulating patients in terms of answerable questions, EBM risks missing the point of the patient's consultation. He might simply want to express his fears, rather than be used as a substrate for an intellectual exercise.
●Is the standard the same for the evidence for *all* changes to our practice? For example, we might want to avoid prescribing drug X for constipation if there is the slimmest chance that it might cause colon cancer. There are many other drugs to choose from. We might require far more robust evidence than a remote chance to persuade us to do something rather counter-intuitive, such as giving heparin in DIC. How robust does the data need to be? There is no science to tell us the answer to this: we decide off the top of our head (albeit a wise head, we hope).
●What about the correspondence columns of the journals from which the winning papers are extracted? It takes years for unforeseen but fatal flaws to surface, and be reported in correspondence columns.
●There is a danger that by always asking 'What is the evidence. . .' we will divert resources from hard-to-prove activities (which may be very valuable) to easy-to-prove services. An example might be physiotherapy for cerebral palsy. The unique personal attributes of the therapist may be as important as the objective regimen: she is impossible to quantify. It is a much easier management decision to transfer resources to some easy-to-quantify activity, eg neonatal screening for cystic fibrosis.
●Evidence-based medicine can never be always up to date. Reworking meta-analyses in the light of new trials takes time—if it is ever done at all.

Advantage~ **~nce-based medicine** ●It improves our reading habits.
●It lea~ ~stions, and then to be sceptical of the answers.
●~ ~ld like it (wasteful practices can be abandoned).
~ ~ presupposes that we keep up to date, and makes
~ ~ around the perimeter of our knowledge.
~ ~pens decision-making processes to patients.

~ ~doubt that, *where available*, evidence-based
~ ~what it is superseding. It may not have as
~ ~taining unimpeachable evidence is time-
~ ~rhaps impossible. Despite these caveats,
~ ~he most exciting medical development
~ ~scribing to its ideals and its journal.

WJ i 1122 & ii 259 **2** *Evidence-based Medicine* BMA, ~tel. 0171 383 6270. See L Ridsdale *Evidence-based* ~ *Effective Clinical Practice*, Blackwell

⊹ Six to five against

Your surgical consultant asks whether Gobble's disease is more common in men or women. You have no idea, and make a guess. What is the chance of getting it right? Common sense decrees that it is even chances; 'Sod's Law' predicts that whatever you guess, your answer will always be wrong. A less pessimistic view is that the balance is only slightly tipped against you: according to Damon Runyon, "all life is six to five against".[1] This might be called *Runyon's Law*.

Doctors as gamblers Given a set of information, different diagnoses have different odds. Any new information simply changes these odds.

Does a new symptom suggest a new disease, or is it due to the disease which is already known? Here the gambler scores over the intuitive clinician, as the answer is often counter-intuitive. Suppose that S is quite a rare symptom of Gobble's disease (occurring, say, in only 5% of patients). But suppose that S is a very common symptom of disease A (occurring in 90%). If we have a patient whom we already know has Gobble's disease and who goes on to develop symptom S, isn't S more likely to be due to disease A, rather than Gobble's disease? The answer is usually no: *it is generally the case that S is due to a disease which is already known, and does not imply a new disease.*[2]

The reason for this can be seen by considering the 'odds ratio', ie the ratio of [the probability of the symptom, given the known disease] to [the probability of the symptom given the new disease × the probability of developing the new disease].

This ratio is, usually, vastly in favour of the symptom being due to the old disease because of the prior odds of the two diseases. For example, a 50-year-old man with known carcinoma of the lung has some transient neurological symptoms and a normal CT scan. Are these symptoms due to secondaries in the brain or to transient ischaemic attacks (TIAs)? The chance of secondaries in the brain which cause transient neurological symptoms is 0.045 given carcinoma of the lung.[2] The chance of such secondaries not showing up on a CT scan is 0.1. Therefore the chance of this cluster of clinical symptoms is 0.0045 (ie 0.045 × 0.1). The chance of a normal CT scan and transient neurological symptoms given a TIA is 0.9. However, the chance of a 50-year-old man developing TIA is 0.0001. Therefore the odds ratio is 0.0045/(0.9 × 0.0001). That is, the odds ratio is ~50 to 1 in favour of secondaries in the brain.

Note: it is only very occasionally that the prior odds of a new disease are so high that the new disease is more likely. For example, someone presenting with anaemia already known to have breast cancer, who lives in an African community where 50% of people have hookworm-induced anaemia, is likely to have hookworm as well as breast carcinoma.

1 D Runyon 'A Nice Price', in *Runyon on Broadway*, 1950, Constable 2 J Bella 1985 *Lancet* i 326

Investigations change the odds

Diagnostic medicine is for gamblers (see p744). We treat investigations as though they tell us the diagnosis. But the logic of investigations is rather different. As you are taking a history and examining the patient, you make various wagers with yourself (often barely consciously) as to how likely various diagnoses are. The results of subsequent tests simply affect these odds. A test is, generally, only worthwhile if it alters the diagnostic odds in a way which is clinically important.

The effect of the test on the diagnostic odds *See CAD*

To work this out you need to know the *sensitivity* and *specificity* of the investigation. All investigations have false positive and false negative rates, as summarized below:

		Patients with the condition	Patients without the condition
TEST	Subjects appear to have the condition	True +ve (a)	False +ve (b)
RESULT	Subjects appear not to have the condition	False –ve (c)	True –ve (d)

Sensitivity: how reliably is the test +ve in the disease? a/a+c
Specificity: how reliably is the test –ve in health? d/d+b

Suppose we have a test of sensitivity 0.8 and specificity 0.9. The *likelihood ratio* of the disease given a +ve result (LR+) is the ratio of the chance of having a positive test if the disease is present to the chance of having a positive test if the disease is absent $[0.8/(1-0.9)]$; ie 8:1 in the above example. More generally:

LR+ = sensitivity/(1–specificity)

LR– (likelihood ratio of the disease given a negative result) = (1–sensitivity)/specificity. (1–0.8/0.9, ie 2:9 in the above example.)

Is there any point to this test? Work out the 'posterior odds' assuming first a positive and then a negative result to the test. This is done from the equation: *posterior odds = (prior odds) × (likelihood ratio)*.

For example, if your clinical assessment of a man with exercise-induced chest pain is that the odds of this being due to coronary artery disease (CAD) is 4:1 (80%), is it worth his doing an exercise tolerance test (sensitivity 0.72; specificity 0.8)?[1] If the test were positive the odds in favour of CAD would be $4 \times (0.72)/(1-0.8) = 14:1$ (93%). If negative, they would be $4 \times (1 - 0.72)/0.8 = 1.4:1$ (58%)

An experienced clinician is likely to have higher prior odds for the most likely diagnosis. The above example shows that with high prior odds, the test has to have a high sensitivity and specificity for a negative result to bring the odds below 50%.

Here is another example of likelihood ratios at work in showing by how much a given test result will raise or lower the pre-test probability of the target disease:[1] Joe is a 40-year-old man (not on NSAIDs) referred for endoscopy because of dyspepsia. Before the results of a bedside test for *Helicobacter pylori* are known, he has a 50% chance of harbouring this organism, which, if present, is the probable cause of an ulcer, for which endoscopy is needed for proper evaluation. The likelihood ratio for a –ve test result is 0.13 (sensitivity 88%, specificity 91%).[2] So if the test is –ve, the chance of Joe having *H pylori* is <1%—and it may be appropriate to send him home without endoscopy (eg if symptoms are of short duration and no weight loss/dysphagia). If the test is +ve the probability of *H pylori* infection is >90%, strongly suggesting the need for endoscopy.

1 C Hawke 1997 *BMJ* i 1690   2 P Moayeddi 1997 *BMJ* i 119

Numbers needed to treat (NNT)[1]

If the risk of dying from a myocardial infarction once a patient is in hospital is 10%, and a new treatment reduces this to 8%, this statistic may be made to look more impressive by saying that the new drug reduced mortality by 20%. When we hear this we think that 20% of people taking the drug would benefit—a price we might be prepared to pay, even if there were some bad side-effects. But if you gave the drug to 100 people with MIs only ~2 would be expected to derive any benefit. In terms of numbers needed to treat we might say that 50 patients would need treating for there to be one person saved. Worthwhile, but hard work—and expensive.

In some preventive studies in mild hypertension, 800 people may need treating according to a certain regimen to save one stroke. When expressed like this, the treatment seems less wonderful.

One of the strengths of the concept of *Number Needed to Treat* (NNT) is that it is context dependent. If a new antihypertension regimen is being considered, it could be compared with the old where the NNT was 800. If the new regimen is only marginally better, the NNT to prevent one death or stroke *by adopting the new regimen in place of the old* may run into thousands, as will your drugs bill if the new regimen is more expensive.

One problem with NNT-concepts occurs with trials where there is a large placebo effect, eg in pain relief. Say the placebo response rate is 40% and that of a new analgesic is 60%. NNT is 5. Perhaps it's better to say to patients about to start the new drug that 60% respond (p90).

Screening See Card.

Modified Wilson criteria for screening (1–10 spells iatrogenic—to remind us that in treating healthy populations we have an especial duty to do no harm.)

1 The condition screened for should be an **i**mportant one.
2 There should be an **a**cceptable treatment for the disease.
3 Diagnostic and **t**reatment facilities should be available.
4 A **r**ecognizable latent or early symptomatic stage is required.
5 **O**pinions on who to treat as patients must be agreed.
6 The test must be of *high discriminatory power* (see below), *valid* (measuring what it purports to measure, not surrogate markers which might not correlate with reality) and be *reproducible*—with safety **g**uaranteed.
7 The **e**xamination must be acceptable to the patient.
8 The untreated **n**atural history of the disease must be known.
9 A simple **i**nexpensive test should be all that is required.
10 Screening must be **c**ontinuous (ie not a 'one-off' affair).
Summary: screening tests must be cost-effective.

Informed consent: Rees' rule Before offering screening, there is a duty to quantify for patients their chance of being disadvantaged by it—from anxiety (may be devastating, eg while waiting for a false +ve result to be sorted out) and the effects of subsequent tests (eg bleeding after biopsy following an abnormal cervical smear), as well as the chances of benefit.

Problems These have all affected UK screening programmes.
1 Those most at risk do not present for screening, thus increasing the gap between the healthy and the unhealthy—the *inverse care law*.
2 The 'worried well' overload services by seeking repeat screening.
3 Services for investigating those testing positive are inadequate.
4 Those who are false positives suffer stress while awaiting investigation, and remain anxious about their health despite reassurance.
5 A negative result may be regarded as a licence to take risks.

1 J A Muir Gray 1995 *Bandolier* **11** 1

Examples of effective screening	*Unproven/ineffective screening*
Cervical smears for cancer	Mental test score (dementia)
Mammography for breast cancer	Urine tests (diabetes; kidney disease)
Finding smokers (+quitting advice)	Antenatal procedures (*ohcs* p95)
Looking for malignant hypertension	PSA screening (prostate cancer, p653)

750 Nomogram for calculating doses of gentamicin

1 Join with a straight line the serum creatinine concentration appropriate to the sex on scale A and the age on scale B. Mark the point at which this line cuts line C.[1]

2 Join with a line the mark on line C and the body weight on line D. Mark the points at which this line cuts lines L and M. These will give the loading and maintenance doses respectively.

3 Confirm the appropriateness of this regimen at an early stage by measuring serum levels, especially in severe illness and renal impairment.

4 Adjust dose if peak concentrations (1h after im dose; 30 mins after iv dose) outside the range 5–10mg/L. Trough concentrations (just before dose) above 2mg/L indicate the need for a longer dosage interval.

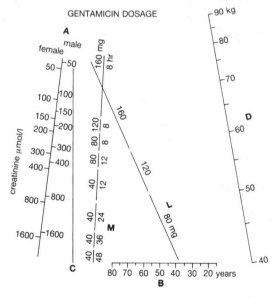

GENTAMICIN DOSAGE

The above allows for **thrice-daily** doses. Many now favour **once-daily doses** (eg 5mg/kg/day for a smallish person) because of fewer adverse effects and possibly better bactericidal activity. There is quite good evidence from meta-analyses backing up such assertions—provided there is no increase in cardiac output (eg in anaemia or Paget's disease), and the context is not one of ascites, burns, children or pregnancy.[2,3] The big problem is that we do not have good information on how to calculate (and monitor) once-a-day regimens.[4] The *Cooke & Grace* regimen:[5] one source provisionally recommends, for feverish neutropenic adults with serum creatinine <300μmol/L, a starting dose of gentamicin 5mg/kg iv over 30mins, with a serum trough value measured ~24h later. If this proves satisfactory (level <1mg/L) then perform twice-weekly monitoring. If the trough level is 1-2mg/L, halve the dose, and monitor the next trough (ie at 24h). These authors generally stopped gentamicin if this level was >2mg/L, and instituted another antibiotic, such as ciprofloxacin.[6] Other nomograms exist to optimize dose timing (DP Nicolau 1995 *Antimicrob Agents Chemother* **39** 650-5).

1 G Mawer 1974 *Br J Clin Pharm* 1 45 2 M Barza 1996 E-BM 1 144 & *Drug Ther Bul* 1997 35 36 3 R Hatala 1996 E-BM 1 145 4 PS Millard 1996 E-BM 1 144-5 5 RP Cooke 1996 BMJ ii 490

Drug therapeutic ranges

►Ranges should only be used as a guide to treatment.

A drug in an apparently too low concentration may still be clinically useful. Some patients require (and tolerate) levels in the 'toxic' range.

Amikacin Peak (½h post IV dose): 20–30mg/L. Trough: <10mg/L.

Carbamazepine Trough: 25–50µmol/L [6–12mg/L].

Clonazepam Trough: 0.08–0.24µmol/L [0.025–0.075mg/L].

Digoxin# (6–12h post dose) 1–2.6nmol/L [0.8–2µg/L]. <1.3nmol/L may be toxic if there is hypokalaemia. Signs of CVS toxicity: arrhythmias, heart block. CNS: confusion, insomnia, agitation, seeing too much yellow (xanthopsia), delirium. GI: nausea.

Ethosuximide Trough: 300–700µmol/L [40–100mg/L].

Gentamicin# Peak—½h post IV dose: 9–18µmol/L [5–10mg/L]. Trough (just before dose): ≤1.9µmol/L (<2mg/L). Toxic signs: tinnitus, deafness, nystagmus, vertigo, renal failure. See opposite.

Lithium# (12h post dose). Guidelines vary: 0.4–0.8mmol/L is reasonable. *Early* signs of toxicity (Li⁺ ~1.5mmol/L): tremor, agitation, twitching. *Intermediate:* lethargy. *Late:* (Li⁺ >2mmol/L) spasms, coma, fits, arrhythmias, renal failure (haemodialysis may be needed). See *OHCS* p354.

Netilmicin Peak—½h post IV dose: 7–12mg/L. Trough <2mg/L.

Phenobarbitone (and primidone) Trough: 45–130µmol/L [10–30mg/L].

Phenytoin# Trough: 40–80µmol/L [10–20mg/L]. Signs of toxicity: ataxia, nystagmus, sedation, dysarthria, diplopia.

Theophylline 10–20µg/mL (55–110µmol/L). (►see p777) Take sample 4–6h after starting an infusion (which should be stopped for ~15 mins just before the specimen is taken). Signs of toxicity: arrhythmias, anxiety, tremor, convulsions.

Tobramycin Peak (½h post IV dose): 11–21µmol/L [5–10mg/L]. Trough: ≤4.3µmol/L <2mg/L.

=Drugs for which *routine* monitoring is indicated.

*Trough levels should be taken just before the next dose.

The time since the last dose should be specified on the form.

Some important drug interactions

Note: '↑' means the effect of the drug in italics is increased (eg through inhibition of metabolism or renal clearance). '↓' means that its effect is decreased (eg through enzyme induction).

Adenosine ↓ by: Aminophylline. ↑ by dipyridamole.

Aminoglycosides ↑ by: Loop diuretics, cefalosporins.

Antidiabetic drugs (any) ↑ by: Alcohol, β-blockers, monoamine oxidase inhibitors, bezafibrate. ↓ by: Corticosteroids, diazoxide, diuretics, contraceptive steroids, (possibly also lithium).
  Sulfonylureas ↑ by: Azapropazone, chloramphenicol, clofibrate, co-trimoxazole, miconazole, sulfinpyrazone.
  Sulfonylureas ↓ by: Rifampicin, (nifedipine occasionally).
  Metformin ↑ by: Cimetidine. With alcohol: lactic acidosis risk.

Antiretroviral agents (HIV): See p218.

Angiotensin-converting enzyme (ACE) inhibitors ↓ by: NSAIDs.

Antihistamines (eg terfenadine) Avoid anything which ↑concentrations and risk of arrhythmias, eg erythromycin, other macrolides (eg azithromycin), antifungals, halofantrine, tricyclics, antipsychotics, SSRIs (p13), cisapride, protease inhibitors (p218), diuretics, β-blockers, antiarrhythmics.

Azathioprine ↑ by: Allopurinol.

β-blockers All ↑ by verapamil; ↓: NSAIDs. Lipophilic β-blockers (eg propranolol) are metabolized by the liver, and concentrations are ↑ by cimetidine. This does not happen with hydrophilic β-blockers (eg atenolol).

Carbamazepine ↑ by: Erythromycin, isoniazid, verapamil.

Cimetidine: Theophylline↑, warfarin↑, lignocaine (lidocaine)↑, amitriptyline↑, propranolol↑, pethidine↑, phenytoin↑, metronidazole↑, quinine↑.

Contraceptive steroids ↓ by: Antibiotics, barbiturates, carbamazepine, phenytoin, primidone, rifampicin.

Cyclosporin (=ciclosporin) ↑ by: Erythromycin. ↓ by: Phenytoin.

Digoxin ↑ by: Amiodarone, carbenoxolone and diuretics (as K⁺ levels lowered), quinine, verapamil.

Diuretics ↓ by: NSAIDs—particularly indomethacin (=indometacin).

Ergotamine ↑ by: Erythromycin (ergotism may occur).

Fluconazole: Avoid concurrent astemizole or terfenadine.

Lithium ↑ by: Thiazide diuretics.

Methotrexate ↑ by: Aspirin, NSAIDs.

Phenytoin ↑ by: Chloramphenicol, cimetidine, disulfiram, isoniazid, sulfonamides. ↓ by: carbamazepine.

Potassium-sparing diuretics with ACE inhibitors: (Hyperkalaemia).

Theophyllines ↑ by: Cimetidine, ciprofloxacin, erythromycin, contraceptive steroids, propranolol. ↓ by: barbiturates, carbamazepine, phenytoin, rifampicin. See p777.

Valproate ↓by: Carbamazepine, phenobarbitone, phenytoin, primidone.

Warfarin and *nicoumalone* (=acenocoumarol) ↑ by: Alcohol, allopurinol, amiodarone, aspirin, chloramphenicol, cimetidine, ciprofloxacin, co-trimoxazole, danazol, dextropropoxyphene, dipyridamole, disulfiram, erythromycin (and broad spectrum antibiotics), gemfibrozil, glucagon, ketoconazole, metronidazole, miconazole, nalidixic acid, neomycin, NSAIDs, phenytoin, quinidine, simvastatin (but not pravastatin), sulfinpyrazone, sulfonamides, tetracyclines, thyroxine (=levothyroxine).

Warfarin and *nicoumalone* (=acenocoumarol) ↓ by: Aminoglutethimide, barbiturates, carbamazepine, contraceptive steroids, dichloralphenazone, griseofulvin, rifampicin, phenytoin, vitamin K.

Zidovudine (AZT) ↑ by: Paracetamol (increased marrow toxicity).

IVI solutions to avoid *Dextrose:* Avoid frusemide (=furosemide), ampicillin, hydralazine, insulin, melphalan, quinine.

0.9% saline IVI: Avoid amphotericin, lignocaine (=lidocaine), nitroprusside.

Haematology—reference intervals

(For B$_{12}$, folate, Fe, and TIBC, see p754–5) **753**

Measurement	Reference interval	Your hospital
White cell count (WCC)	4.0–11.0 × 10^9/L	
Red cell count	♂ 4.5–6.5 × 10^{12}/L	
	♀ 3.9–5.6 × 10^{12}/L	
Haemoglobin	♂ 13.5–18.0g/dL	
	♀ 11.5–16.0g/dL	
Packed red cell volume (PCV)	♂ 0.4–0.54 L/L	
or haematocrit	♀ 0.37–0.47 L/L	
Mean cell volume (MCV)	76–96fL	
Mean cell haemoglobin (MCH)	27–32pg	
Mean cell haemoglobin concentration (MCHC)	30–36g/dL	
Neutrophils	2.0–7.5 × 10^9/L;	
	40–75% WCC	
Lymphocytes	1.3–3.5 × 10^9/L;	
	20–45% WCC	
Eosinophils	0.04–0.44 × 10^9/L;	
	1–6% WCC	
Basophils	0.0–0.10 × 10^9/L;	
	0–1% WCC	
Monocytes	0.2–0.8 × 10^9/L;	
	2–10% WCC	
Platelet count	150–400 × 10^9/L	
Reticulocyte count	0.8–2.0%* 25–100 × 10^9/L	
Erythrocyte sedimentation rate	depends on age (p618)	
Prothrombin time (factors I, II, VII, X)	10–14 seconds	
Activated partial thromboplastin time (VIII, IX, XI, XII)	35–45 seconds	

*Only use percentages as reference interval if red cell count is normal; otherwise use the absolute value. Express as a ratio versus control.

Proposed therapeutic ranges for prothrombin time See p596

Reference intervals—*biochemistry*

See p624 for the philosophy of the normal range; see OHCS p292 for children.
Drugs (and other substances) may interfere with any chemical method;
as these effects may be method-dependent, it is difficult for the clinician to be aware of all the possibilities. If in doubt, discuss with the lab.

Substance	Specimen	Reference interval	Your hospital
Adrenocorticotrophic hormone	P	<80ng/L	
Alanine aminotransferase (ALT)	P	5–35iu/L	
Albumin	P¶	35–50g/L	
Aldosterone	P✳	100–500pmol/L	
Alkaline phosphatase	P	30–300iu/L (adults)	
α-amylase	P	0–180 Somogyi u/dL	
α-fetoprotein	S	<10ku/L	
Angiotensin II	P✳	5–35pmol/L	
Antidiuretic hormone (ADH)	P	0.9–4.6pmol/L	
Aspartate transaminase	P	5–35iu/L	
Bicarbonate	P¶	24–30mmol/L	
Bilirubin	P	3–17μmol/L	
Calcitonin	P	<0.1μg/L	
Calcium (ionized)	P	1.0–1.25mmol/L	
Calcium (total)	P¶	2.12–2.65mmol/L	
Chloride	P	95–105mmol/L	
*Cholesterol (see p654)	P	3.9–7.8mmol/L	
VLDL (see p654)	P	0.128–0.645mmol/L	
LDL	P	1.55–4.4mmol/L	
HDL	P	0.9–1.93mmol/L	
Cortisol	P	a.m. 450–700nmol/L	
		midnight 80–280nmol/L	
Creatine kinase (CK)	P	♂ 25–195iu/L	
		♀ 25–170iu/L	
Creatinine (related to lean)	P¶	70–≤150μmol/L	
Ferritin	P	12–200μg/L	
Folate	S	2.1μg/L	
Follicle-stimulating hormone	P/S	2–8u/L(luteal) ↑ 18	
Gamma-glutamyl transpeptidase	P	♂ 11–51iu/L	
		♀ 7–33iu/L	
Glucose (fasting)	P	3.5–5.5mmol/L	
Glycated (glycosylated) Hb	B	2.3–6.5%	
Growth hormone	P	<20mu/L	
HbA1c (= glycosylated Hb)	B	2.3–6.5%	
Iron	S	♂ 14–31μmol/L	
		♀ 11–30μmol/L	
Lactate dehydrogenase (LDH)	P	70–250iu/L	
Lead	B	<1.8mmol/L	
Luteinizing hormone (LH) (pre-menopausal)	P	3–16u/L (luteal)	
Magnesium	P	0.75–1.05mmol/L	
Osmolality	P	278–305mosmol/kg	
Parathyroid hormone (PTH)	P	<0.8–8.5pmol/L	
Phosphate (inorganic)	P	0.8–1.45mmol/L	
Potassium	P	3.5–5.0mmol/L	

Prolactin	P	♂ <450u/L; ♀ <600u/L	
Prostate specific antigen	P	0–4 nanograms/mL, p653	**755**
Protein (total)	P	60–80 g/L	
Red cell folate	B	0.36–1.44 µmol/L (160–640 µg/L)	
Renin (erect/recumbent)	P✲	2.8–4.5/1.1–2.7 pmol/mL/h	
Sodium	P¶	135–145 mmol/L	
Thyroid-binding globulin (TBG)	P	7–17mg/L	
Thyroid-stimulating hormone (TSH) NR widens with age, p538	P	0.5–5.7mu/L	
Thyroxine (T4)	P	70–140nmol/L	
Thyroxine (free)	P	9–22pmol/L	
Total iron binding capacity	S	54–75µmol/L	
Triglyceride	P	0.55–1.90mmol/L	
Tri-iodothyroinine (T3)	P	1.2–3.0nmol/L	
Urate	P¶	♂ 210–480µmol/L ♀ 150–390µmol/L	
Urea	P¶	2.5–6.7mmol/L	
Vitamin B$_{12}$	S	0.13–0.68nmol/L (>150ng/L)	

ARTERIAL BLOOD GASES—*reference intervals*

pH:	7.35–7.45	P_aCO_2:	4.7–6.0 kPa
P_aO_2:	>10.6 kPa	Base excess:	± 2 mmol/L

Note: 7.6mmHg = 1kPa (atmospheric pressure ≈ 100kPa)

URINE reference intervals	Reference interval	Your hospital
Cortisol (free)	<280nmol/24h	
Hydroxy-indole acetic acid	16–73µmol/24h	
Hydroxymethylmandelic acid (HMMA, VMA)	16–48µmol/24h	
Metanephrines	0.03–0.69µmol/mmol creat- inine (or <5.5µmol/day)	
Osmolality	350–1000mosmol/kg	
17-Oxogenic steroids	♂ 28–30µmol/24h ♀ 21–66µmol/24h	
17-Oxosteroids (neutral)	♂ 17–76µmol/24h ♀ 14–59µmol/24h	
Phosphate (inorganic)	15–50 mmol/24h	
Potassium	14–120 mmol/24h	
Protein	<150mg/24h	
Sodium	100–250 mmol/24h	

---

* Desired upper limit of cholesterol would be ~6mmol/L.
✲ The sample requires special handling: contact the laboratory.
¶ See *OHCS* p81 for reference intervals in pregnancy
P=plasma (eg heparin bottle); S=serum (clotted; no anticoagulant); B=whole blood (edetic acid EDTA bottle)

Useful addresses (for those in the UK)

For *addresses of disease-specific organizations*, see the Health Information Line (below, or http://www.patient.org.uk/); for *poisons information services* see p792

British Diabetic Association 10 Queen Ann St, London w1m 0bd (0171 323 1531)

British Medical Association (BMA) BMA House, Tavistock Square, London wc1h 9jp (0171 387 4499)

Bureau of Hygiene and Tropical Medicine Keppel St, London wc1e 7ht (0171 636 8636)

Central Public Health Lab 61 Colindale Av, London nw9 5ht (0181 200 4400)

Committee on Safety of Medicines Freepost, London sw8 5br (0171 273 3000)

Communicable Disease Surveillance Centre (for up-to-date advice on travel health needs) 61 Colindale Avenue, London nw9 5ht (0181 200 6868)

Disabled Living Foundation (Advice on aids and equipment to help the disabled) 380–384 Harrow Rd, London w9 2hu (0171 289 6111)

Evidence-based medicine Cochrane Centre 01865 516300
NHS Centre for Reviews and Dissemination 01904 433707
Central Health Outcomes Unit DoH 0171 972 2000
Centre for Health Economics 01904 433645
King's Fund Centre 0171 267 6111
Centre for Evidence-based Medicine 01865 221321
Bandolier 01865 226863; *INTERNET:* www.jr2. ox.ac.uk/Bandolier
UK clearing house—Health Outcomes 0113 233 3940

General Medical Council 44 Hallam St, London w1n 6ae (0171 580 7642)

Health Information Line (for a wide range of information for doctors and patients, and addresses of disease specific organizations) 0800 665544

Liverpool School of Tropical Medicine Pembroke Place, Liverpool l3 5qa (0151 708 9393)

Malaria Reference Laboratory (for advice on malaria prophylaxis) 0171 636 8636 (for advice on treatment ring 0171 387 4411)

Medic-Alert Foundation 12 Bridge Wharf, 156 Caledonian Rd, London, n1 9ud (0171 833 3034)

Medical Defence Union (UK) 3 Devonshire Place, London w1n 2ea (0171 486 6181 and 0800 716376, fax 0161 491 1420)

Medical and Dental Defence Union 144 West George St, Glasgow (0141 332 6646)

Medical Foundation for the Care of Victims of Torture 96–98 Grafton Rd, Kentish Town, London nw5 3ej (0171 284 4321)

Medical Protection Society 50 Hallam St, London w1n 6de (0171 637 0541)

Multiple Sclerosis Society 25 Effie Road, London sw6 1ee (0171 736 6267)

Narcotics Abusers' Register Chief Medical Officer, Drugs Branch, Queen Anne's Gate, London sw1h 9yn (0171 273 2213)

National Counselling Centre for Sick Doctors 0171 935 5982

The Patients' Association (an advice service for patients) 18 Victoria Park Square, London e2 9pf (0181 981 5676)

Transplant service (UK) (Can these organs be used?) 0117 9507 777

Using the Internet for medicine

The Internet is a worldwide network of computer networks [see item number 1, on the table opposite]. Co-operation between networks allows the sharing of information resources and global communications for the cost of a local telephone call. *Access:* Most computers are connected to the Internet using an ordinary phone line, modem, and a commercial Internet access provider. Others connect via academic, hospital, or other networks. *E-mail:* Electronic mail involves 'posting' a text message (or computer file) to a unique e-mail address, which can be stored on the network until the recipient clears their 'mailbox'. *World-Wide Web:* www 'pages' may contain text, pictures, programs, other media, and links to further pages. To locate a page, simply type its Web address into your browser.

Education Consumer-oriented disease and self-help information is available online from academic [2], government [3], commercial [4], and non-profit [5] sources. Tutorials for undergraduates [6] and physicians [7] join multimedia case presentations [8], lectures [9], and information on postgraduate examinations [10].

Clinical care Current awareness is aided by digests of new medical research [11] and access to evidence-based reviews [12]. Information can be quickly gleaned from online versions of traditional journals [13], textbooks [14], practice guidelines [15], and databases [16]. Downloadable updates to electronic [17] and print publications [18] offer unrivalled currency. The Internet is being used experimentally for teleconsultation [19] and clinical information systems [20].

Research The Internet offers researchers MEDLINE [21], e-mail alerting services [22], the Cochrane Database [23], a place to present findings [24], details on grant availability [25], and even purchasing of equipment and supplies [26].

Communication Aside from the many advantages of e-mail, the Internet offers special-interest mailing lists [27], press releases [28], help finding employment [29], 'virtual' conferences [30], and information regarding local health-care services [31]. In the near future it is likely to expedite routine and alert-type medical communications; the UK government intends to link every GP surgery and hospital to NHSnet, permiting Internet access [32].

Caveats It can be difficult to filter information, but catalogues like OMNI [33] help. Other concerns are lack of agreed quality standards, often slow and unreliable connections, confidentiality of patient data, and the dangers of online advice. Some of these issues are being pursued by organizations such as the British Healthcare Internet Association [34].

If you have never had the experience of play on the internet leading to a mind-broadening event—perhaps inaccessible by any other route—you may shy away from the enormity of it all. This is a pity: so. . . *if in doubt, communicate* (a good rule-of-life for all of us, perhaps, except for spies and secret agents). For the internet is simply a collection of minds past and present: all the great thinkers are there, living on, forever, in their own words.

We thank Dr Bruce McKenzie for providing this page and choosing the addresses opposite.

Where to find information on the internet

1 BC McKenzie, Medicine and the Internet (2e). 1997; OUP: Oxford
2 Virtual Hospital: http://www.vh.org/
3 Health Education Board (Scotland): http://www.hebs.scot.nhs.uk/
4 PILS database of self-help groups: http://www.mentor-update.com/
5 CancerHelp UK: http://medweb.bham.ac.uk/cancerhelp/index.html
6 Online Course in Medical Bacteriology:
   http://www.qmw.ac.uk/~rhbm001/intro.html
7 Reuters clinical challenge: http://www.reutershealth.com/clinchal/
8 MedRounds:http://www.uchsc.edu/sm/pmb/medrounds/index.html
9 Radiation Therapy for Pediatric Brain Tumors:
   http://goldwein1.xrt.upenn.edu/ASTRO95/framed.htm
10 Royal College of General Practitioners: http://www.rcgp.org.uk/
11 Journal Watch: http://www.jwatch.org/
12 Bandolier: http://www.jr2.ox.ac.uk:80/Bandolier/index.html
13 http://www.bmj.com/ & http://www.thelancet.com/ & http://nejm.org/
14 Merck Manual: http://www.merck.com
15 CPG Infobase: http://www.cma.ca/cpgs/
16 Clinical Pharmacology Online: http://www.cponline.gsm.com/
17 *Oxford Clinical Mentor* online updates: http://www.mentor-update.com/
   (if access fails, try http://www.zyworld.com/ohcm/new.htm)
18 Online Updates: http://www.oup.co.uk/scimed/
19 All-in-one meta-analysis finder: http://www.gwent.nhs.gov.uk/trip/
20 Electronic Medical Record Systems Demonstration on the Web:
   http://www.cpmc.columbia.edu/edu/medinfoemrs.html
21 MEDLINE Resource Centre: http://omni.ac.uk/general-info/inter-
   net_medline.html; also http://www.nlm.nih.gov
22 UnCover Reveal: http://www.carl.org/reveal/
23 Cochrane Database of Systematic Reviews (CDSR) Online:
   http://www.hcn.net.au/cochrane/intro.htm
24 PosterNet: http://pharminfo.com/poster/pnet_hp.html
25 Medical Research Council: http://www.mrc.ac.uk/home.html
26 BioMedNet: http://BioMedNet.com/
27 GP-UK: http://www.mailbase.ac.uk/lists/gp-uk/
28 Department of Health Press Releases:
   http://www.coi.gov.uk/coi/depts/GDH/GDH.html
29 BMJ Classifieds: http://www.bmj.com/classified/index.html
30 MEDNET Conference: http://www.mednet.org.uk/mednet/vc.html
31 Buckinghamshire Health Authority: http://www.buckshealth.com/
32 'The new NHS' White Paper:
   http://www.open.gov.uk/doh/newnhs.htm
33 OMNI: http://omni.ac.uk/
34 British Healthcare Internet Association: http://www.bhia.org/

21. Emergencies†

Sources: Lancet; вмј; отм; D Sprigings et al 1995 Acute Medicine, Blackwell

Emergencies covered in other chapters See front end-papers.
In OHCS—Paediatrics: Life support and cardiac arrest (*OHCS* p310–11); is he seriously ill? (*OHCS* p175); epiglottitis (*OHCS* p276). *Adults:* Trauma (*OHCS* p678–738); drowning (*OHCS* p682); ectopic pregnancy (*OHCS* p24); eclampsia (*OHCS* p96); amniotic fluid embolus (*OHCS* p143); obstetric shock (*OHCS* p106); glaucoma (*OHCS* p494); pre-hospital care/first aid (*OHCS* p780–804).

†The word *emergency* has an illuminating history. It started out life being applied to the surfacing of submerged bodies. Next, astronomers took over the word, reserving it for those trying night watches when the heavenly body of interest was hidden behind the clouds, and etymologists assure us that we are to think of these ancient characters waiting in their night-time gardens for the hoped for emergency of the moon from behind clouds. (For analysis of other varieties of lunatic emergencies, see *the acutely psychotic* and *violent patient, OHCS* p354 and 360.) So now these ancient associations of bodies rising to the surface, and of dramatic events in the night, rise up like self-quickening ghosts*, to occupy the tiny spaces between those insistent bleeps forever summoning us to a new emergency ◆ ◆ ◆ ...

*S*uddenly I saw the cold and rook-delighting heaven
That seemed as though ice burned. . .
With the hot blood of youth, of love crossed
long ago . . .

When the ghost begins to quicken
Confusion of the death-bed over, is it sent
Out naked on the roads, as the books say, and stricken
By the injustice of the skies for punishement? (WB Yeats)

An approach to the very ill patient: how to buy time

►*Don't go so fast: we're in a hurry!* (Talleyrand to his coachman.)

What makes the topics listed opposite *emergencies* is that prompt action saves lives or prevents irreparable organ failure. Even within emergencies there are gradations, so that for most, there is time to assess your patient in some detail. But other emergencies demand the promptest action, such that when summoned from sleep, there is no time even to dress: for example, cardiac arrest, acute stridor, shock and tension pneumothorax. So when one is the doctor who is to be called first should such emergencies arise, not only have you to choose your night-wear carefully, but you need to know *by instinct* what to do when you arrive, bleary eyed, at the bedside. This means that no opportunity is to be lost in watching experts deal with emergencies. Our aim here is to allow the reader to prepare his mind so that he can make the most of such observations.

To the inexperienced, the following treatments may look easy; but this is rarely so as emergencies do not present themselves in the tidy compartments listed opposite. The problem is that a life is slipping through your fingers, and you must find out what the matter is to save the life—but the patient is too ill to survive a detailed history and examination. The trick is to buy time by supporting vital functions, as follows.

Preliminary assessment (primary survey):[1]

Airway   Protect cervical spine
Assessment: any signs of obstruction? Ascertain patency
Management: establish a patent airway

Breathing   Assessment: determine respiratory rate, check bilateral chest movement, percuss and auscultate
Management: if no respiratory effort, treat as arrest[2] (p770), intubate and ventilate. If breathing compromised, give high concentration O_2, manage according to findings, eg relieve tension pneumothorax

Circulation Assessment: check pulse and BP; is he peripherally shutdown?; look for evidence of haemorrhage
Management: –if no cardiac output, treat as arrest (p770)
–if shocked, treat as on p766–768

Disability   Assessment: determine level of consciousness using the AVPU score (p764); check pupils: size, equality and reaction

Exposure   Undress patient but cover to avoid hypothermia

Quick history from relatives may assist with diagnosis:
Events surrounding onset of illness, evidence of overdose/suicide attempt, any suggestion of trauma?
Past medical history especially diabetes, asthma/COPD, alcohol, opiate or street drug abuse, epilepsy or recent head injury; recent travel
Medication: current drugs. *Allergies*

Once ventilation and circulation are adequate, you may have bought enough time to carry out history, examination, investigations, and appropriate management in the usual way.

1 Advanced Trauma Life Support 1993 Am. Col. Surg. 2 CPR Guidelines 1997 Resus Council (UK)

⚕ Coma

Ask an experienced nurse to help. Place semi-prone, then: ●ABCs of life support ●Are pupils equal?* ●Stabilize cervical spine ●IV access ●Ward glucose test ●Do blood gases, FBC, U&E, LFT, ESR, ethanol, toxic screen (+urine, too), drug levels, blood cultures ●Have O₂, IV thiamine (p712), 50% glucose, and naloxone (p794) to hand (have a low threshold for giving these).

Quick history from family, ambulance staff, bystanders: Abrupt or gradual onset? How found—suicide note, seizure? If injured suspect cervical spinal injury and do not move spine (OHCS p726). Recent complaints—headache, fever, vertigo, depression? Recent medical history—sinusitis, otitis, neurosurgery, ENT procedure? Past medical history—diabetes, asthma, ↑BP, cancer, epilepsy, psychiatric illness? Drug or toxin exposure (especially alcohol or other recreational drugs)? Any travel?

Examination ●Vital signs are vital—obtain full set.
●Signs of trauma—haematoma, laceration, bruising, CSF/blood in nose or ears, fracture 'step' deformity of skull, subcutaneous emphysema.
●Stigmata of other illnesses: liver disease, alcoholism, diabetes, myxoedema.
●Skin for needle marks, cyanosis, pallor, rashes, poor turgor.
●Smell the breath (alcohol, hepatic fetor, ketosis, uraemia,) meningism (p420) ►but do not move neck unless cervical spine is cleared.
●Heart/lung exam for murmurs, rubs, wheeze, consolidation, collapse.
●Abdomen/rectal for organomegaly, ascites, bruising, peritonism, melaena.
●Are there any foci of infection (abscesses, bites, middle ear infection?)
●Note the absence of signs, eg no pin-point pupils in a known heroin addict, or a diabetic patient whose breath does not smell of acetone.

Taking stock The diagnosis may be clear, eg hyperglycaemia, alcohol excess, drug poisoning, uraemia, pneumonia, hypertensive or hepatic encephalopathy (p504). If there are localizing CNS signs and no history of trauma, and there is no fever, the diagnosis is only probably stroke. In all undiagnosed coma patients or in those with focal neurological signs, a CT scan is very helpful. A lumbar puncture may be needed for meningitis (p442) or subarachnoid haemorrhage (p438).

Causes of coma

Metabolic:	drugs, poisoning, eg carbon monoxide, alcohol	
	hypoglycaemia, hyperglycaemia (DKA, HONK)	
	hypoxia	
	CO₂ narcosis (COPD)	
	hypothermia	
	myxoedema, Addisonian crisis	
	hepatic/uraemic encephalopathy	
Neurological:	trauma	
	infection	meningitis (p442); encephalitis, eg Herpes simplex (give IV aciclovir if the slightest suspicion, p203) tropical: malaria (do thick films), typhoid, rabies, trypanosomiasis
	tumour	cerebral/meningeal tumour
	vascular	subdural/subarachnoid haemorrhage, stroke, hypertensive encephalopathy
	epilepsy	non-convulsive status or post-ictal state

---

*Check pupils every few minutes during the early stages, particularly if trauma is the likely cause. Doing so is the quickest way to find a localizing sign (so helpful in diagnosis, but remember that false localizing signs do occur)—and observing changes in pupil behaviour (eg becoming fixed and dilated) is the quickest way of finding out just how bad things are.

The neurological examination in coma

This is aimed at locating the pathology in one of two places. Altered level of consciousness implies either 1) a diffuse, bilateral, cortical dysfunction (usually producing loss of awareness with normal arousal) or 2) damage to the ascending reticular activating system (ARAS) located throughout the brainstem from the medulla to the thalami (usually producing loss of arousal with unassessable awareness). The brainstem can be affected directly (eg pontine haemorrhage) or indirectly (eg compression from trans-tentorial or cerebellar herniation secondary to a mass or oedema).

- Level of consciousness; describe using *objective* words (p764 as a guide).
- Respiratory pattern—Cheyne–Stokes (p40), hyperventilation (acidosis, hypoxia, or rarely, neurogenic), ataxic or apneustic (breath-holding) breathing (brainstem damage with grave prognosis).
- Eyes—almost all patients with ARAS pathology will have eye findings.

Visual fields—in light coma, test fields with visual threat. No blink in one field suggests hemianopsia and contralateral hemisphere lesion.

Pupils *Normal direct and consensual* = intact midbrain. *Midposition (3–5mm) non-reactive ± irregular* = midbrain lesion. *Unilateral dilated and unreactive ('fixed')* = third nerve compression. *Small, reactive* = pontine lesion ('pinpoint, pontine pupils') or drugs. *Horner's syndrome* (p700) = ipsilateral lateral medulla or hypothalamus lesion, may precede uncal herniation.

Extraocular movements (EOMs)—observe resting position and spontaneous movement then test the vestibulo-ocular reflex (VOR) with either the *Doll's-head manoeuvre* (normal if the eyes keep looking at the same point in space when the head is quickly moved laterally or vertically) or *ice water calorics* (normal if the eyes deviate towards the cold ear with nystagmus to the other side). If present, the VOR exonerates *most* of the brainstem from the VIIth nerve nucleus (medulla) to the IIIrd (midbrain). Do *not* move the head unless the C-spine is cleared.

Fundi—papilloedema, subhyaloid haemorrhage, hypertensive retinopathy, signs of other disease (eg diabetic retinopathy).
- Examine for CNS asymmetry (tone, spontaneous movements, reflexes).

The Glasgow coma scale (GCS)[1]

This gives a reliable, objective way of recording the conscious state of a person. It can be used by medical and nursing staff for initial and continuing assessment. It has value in predicting ultimate outcome. 3 types of response are assessed:

Best motor response This has 6 grades:

6 Carrying out request ('obeying command'): The patient does simple things you ask (beware of accepting a grasp reflex in this category).

5 Localizing response to pain: Put pressure on the patient's fingernail bed with a pencil then try supraorbital and sternal pressure: purposeful movements towards changing painful stimuli is a 'localizing' response.

4 Withdraws to pain: Pulls limb away from painful stimulus.

3 Flexor response to pain: Pressure on the nail bed causes abnormal flexion of limbs—decorticate posture.

2 Extensor posturing to pain: The stimulus causes limb extension (adduction, internal rotation of shoulder, pronation of forearm)—decerebrate posture.

1 No response to pain.

Note that it is the best response of any limb which should be recorded.

Best verbal response This has 5 grades:

5 Oriented: The patient knows who he is, where he is and why, the year, season, and month.

4 Confused conversation: The patient responds to questions in a conversational manner but there is some disorientation and confusion.

3 Inappropriate speech: Random or exclamatory articulated speech, but no conversational exchange.

2 Incomprehensible speech: Moaning but no words.

1 None.

Record level of best speech.

Eye opening This has 4 grades:
4 Spontaneous eye opening.

3 Eye opening in response to speech: Any speech, or shout, not necessarily request to open eyes.

2 Eye opening in response to pain: Pain to limbs as above.

1 No eye opening.

An overall score is made by summing the score in the 3 areas assessed. Eg: no response to pain+no verbalization+no eye opening=3. Severe injury, GCS ≤8; moderate injury, GCS 9–12; minor, injury GCS 13–15.

Note: an abbreviated coma scale, AVPU, is sometimes used in the initial assessment ('primary survey') of the critically ill:
●A = alert
●V = responds to vocal stimuli
●P = responds to pain
●U = unresponsive

Some centres score GCS out of 14, not 15, omitting 'withdrawal to pain'.

1 G Teasdale 1974 *Lancet* ii 81

►►Shock

Essence If the BP falls so that vital organs are not perfused adequately, the patient is shocked. Signs reflect peripheral or end-organ under-per-fusion (pallor, cold peripheries, faints, restlessness, capillary refill >2sec, oliguria). Also: pulse↑ (unless on β-blocker, or in spinal shock—*OHCS* p728) and hypotension (eg systolic BP <90mmHg). In the young and fit, the systolic BP may remain normal, although the *pulse pressure* will nar-row, with up to 30% blood volume depletion—making diagnosis difficult. The above end-organ signs are more reliable markers than BP and central venous pressure. Manage as follows. Get IV access and give oxygen.

Quickly examine BP; carotid pulse; pallor; cyanosis; jaundice; heart and chest (tension pneumothorax?). Aortic aneurysm? Melaena (do PR?). ►If BP fading, call the cardiac arrest team. Find the adrenaline (=epinephrine).

Causes *Anaphylaxis:* Type I IgE-mediated hypersensitivity eg to: penicillin, contrast media for radiology, latex, stings, eggs, fish, peanuts, semen. Release of histamine and other agents causes: capillary leak; wheeze; cyanosis; oedema (larynx, lids, lips); urticaria. ►►Secure the airway; remove the cause; give adrenaline (=epinephrine) 0.5–1mL of 1:1000 IM; repeat every 10min, until better. (If on β-blocker, consider salbutamol IV in place of adrenaline.) Also:
●Chlorpheniramine*10mg IV (may repeat)●Hydrocortisone 200mg IV
●O₂ ± IVI (0.9% saline eg 500mL over ¼ h) ●?IPPV + advanced life support
●If wheeze, treat for asthma, p776   ●Admit to ward. Monitor ECG
●Suggest a 'Medic-alert' bracelet naming the culprit allergen (p756).
● Teach about self-injected adrenaline (=epinephrine) to prevent fatal attack. Skin-prick tests showing specific IgE help identify which allergens to avoid.[1]

Septic shock: Gram –ve (or +ve) septicaemic shock from endotoxin-induced vasodilatation may be sudden and severe, with shock and coma but no signs of infection (fever, wcc↑). <u>Note warm peripheries</u>. *Specific rem-edy* (if no clue to source, p182): IV cefuroxime 1.5g/8h (after blood culture) or gentamicin (p750; do levels; reduce in renal failure) + antipseudomonal penicillin (eg ticarcillin 5g/8h IVI). Give <u>colloid, eg Haemaccel®</u>, by IVI. Refer to ITU if possible for intensive monitoring and <u>inotropes</u>. Consider dopamine in a 'renal' dose (2–5µg/kg/min IVI; but beware SEs, p110).

Hypovolaemic shock: Bleeding: Eg trauma, ruptured aortic aneurysm, ectopic pregnancy. Remedy: IVI until crossmatched blood arrives. Use group ORh –ve blood in severe bleeding (p102). Treat the underlying cause.
Fluid loss: Vomiting (eg GI obstruction), diarrhoea (eg cholera), burns, pools of sequestered (unavailable) fluids ('third spacing', eg in pancreati-tis). *Remedy:* IVI 0.9% saline until BP rises (p100). *Heat exposure (heat exhaustion)* may cause hypovolaemic shock (also hyperpyrexia, oliguria, rhabdomyolysis, consciousness↓, hyperventilation, hallucination, incon-tinence, collapse, coma, pinpoint pupils, LFTs↑, and DIC.) If this is present, do tepid sponging + fanning; avoid ice and immersion. Resuscitate with high-sodium IVI, such as 0.9% saline ± hydrocortisone 100mg IV. Dantrolene appears to be ineffective. Chlorpromazine 10–25mg IM may be used to stop shivering.[2] Stop cooling when core temperature <39°C.

Cardiogenic shock: p768. *Endocrine failure:* Addison's/hypothyroidism p786

Iatrogenic shock: Drugs, eg anaesthetics, antihypertensives.

Note Except for the first 3 causes given above, the immediate need is for fluid to be given IV quickly (see guidelines, p767).

1 P Ewan 1997 *Prescribers' J* 37(3) 125 2 E Lloyd 1994 *BMJ* ii 587 *New name: chlorphenamine

●Use the largest veins with which you are familiar, ie antecubital fossa—otherwise do a cut-down (p798) or central venous cannulation (p800). Rate of flow is inversely proportional to length of cannula, and CVP lines are long. Cut-downs are rarely used, but if you forget about them entirely, you stand to lose the occasional life.

●Use 2 large-bore cannulae (14G or 16G): it takes 20min to infuse 1 litre through a 18G cannula, but only 3min through one of 14G!*

●Raise the drip stand and squeeze the bag, or use an inflatable pressure device (like a sphygmomanometer cuff) to ↑infusion rate.

●Estimate and anticipate the blood loss from fractures:

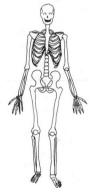

ribs   = 150 ml

pelvis = 2000 ml

femur = 1500 ml
(shaft)

tibia   = 650 ml

DOUBLE LOSSES IF COMPOUND FRACTURE

●Crystalloid (eg Hartmann's solution) has intravascular t½ of only 30–60 mins and must be given in 3 times the volume to that lost; colloid (eg Haemaccel®) lasts several hours and is replaced 1:1 with blood lost. Consider blood if haemorrhage and over 15% volume lost (adult blood volume = 70mL/kg; child = 80–90mL/kg)—crossmatched blood is ideal, but time-consuming; group compatible is a compromise, only takes 10mins to prepare and is preferable to ORh−ve.

●Give fluid *rapidly*; slow only when pulse falls, BP rises and urine flows (>30mL/h adult and >1mL/kg/h child). Catheterize the bladder. Consider CVP line to monitor progress. A satisfactory response might be a 2cm rise after IVI of 250mL colloid over 15mins.

●Don't forget to give O_2 (at 12L/min via tight-fitting face mask with reservoir in all trauma, unless strong contraindication); to ↓ peripheral blood loss by pressure and elevation; and to splint fractures (traction very important in reducing blood loss in fractured femur).

●Monitor pulse, BP, and ECG continuously. Remain at bedside.

►Ensure someone explains to the relatives that the illness is serious.

*The rate of flow (Q_1) of fluid along a tube of circular cross-section (of radius R), the fluid being under an axial pressure gradient P/L, obeys a fourth-power law: $Q_1 = \pi \, P/L \times R^4/8\mu$ where μ is the viscosity (G Hagen 1839 *Poggendorff's Ann d. Physik u. Chemie* XLVI, and verified by experiments by Poisseuille). This law is of interest to vascular surgeons: a small change in R has a dramatic effect, but if the cross-section becomes elliptical (with 2 axes of lengths 2a and 2b), the new flow (Q_2) only contains cubic, not 4th power terms: $Q_2 \approx \pi a^3 b^3/a^2 + b^2 \times P/4\mu L$ (Boussinesq 1868 & R Gibson, 1995[a]).

▶▶Cardiogenic shock

This has a 90% mortality. ▶Ask a senior physician's help both in formulating an *exact* diagnosis and in guiding treatment.

Cardiogenic shock is shock (p766) caused primarily by the failure of the heart to maintain the circulation. It may occur suddenly, or after progressively worsening heart failure.

Causes *Rapidly reversible:* Arrhythmias, cardiac tamponade, tension pneumothorax. *Others:* Myocardial infarction; myocarditis; myocardial depression (drugs, hypoxia, acidosis, sepsis); valve destruction (endocarditis), pulmonary embolus, aortic dissection.

Management Manage on Coronary Care Unit, if possible. Investigation and treatment may need to be done concurrently.
- Give O_2, with the patient placed in the most comfortable position.
- Give diamorphine 2.5–5mg IV for pain and anxiety.
- Monitor: ECG; urine output by catheter; blood gases (adjust O_2 accordingly); U&E; CVP. Do a 12-lead ECG every hour until the diagnosis is made.
- Consider monitoring: pulmonary wedge pressure (Swan–Ganz catheter); arterial pressure; cardiac output.
- Correct arrhythmias (p286–94), U&E imbalance, and acid–base balance.
- Give positively inotropic drugs: eg <u>dobutamine 2.5–10µg/kg/min</u> IVI, adjusted to keep systolic BP >80mmHg.
- ↑Renal perfusion with <u>low-dose dopamine: 2–5µg/kg/min</u> IVI (SE: p110).
- If pulmonary wedge pressure <15mmHg, give a plasma expander 100mL every 15mins IV. Aim at pressure 15–20mmHg.
- Look for and treat any reversible cause, eg myocardial infarction or pulmonary embolus. Consider thrombolysis (p282 and p774). Consider surgery for: acute VSD, mitral or aortic incompetence.
- Consider intra-aortic balloon pump if you expect the underlying condition to improve, or you need time awaiting surgery.

Cardiac tamponade *Essence:* Pericardial fluid collects → intrapericardial pressure rises → heart cannot fill → pumping stops. *Major causes:* Trauma, lung/breast <u>cancer</u>, <u>pericarditis, myocardial infarct</u>, <u>bacteria</u> eg TB. *Rare:* Urea↑, radiation, myxoedema, dissecting aorta, SLE, cardiomyopathy.

Signs: Falling BP, a rising JVP, and muffled heart sounds = Beck's triad; JVP↑ on inspiration (Kussmaul's sign); pulsus paradoxus (pulse fades on inspiration). Echocardiography may be diagnostic (is the echo separation >2cm?). CXR: globular heart; left heart border convex or straight; right cardiophrenic angle <90°. ECG: electrical alternans (p318).

Management: This can be very difficult. Everything is against you: time, physics, and your own confidence, as the patient may be too ill to give a history, and signs may be equivocal—but bitter experience has taught us not to equivocate for long. ▶▶Request the presence of your senior at the bedside (do not make do with telephone advice). With luck, prompt pericardiocentesis (opposite) brings swift relief. While awaiting this, give O_2, monitor ECG, and set up IVI. Take blood for group and save.

Emergency* needle pericardiocentesis

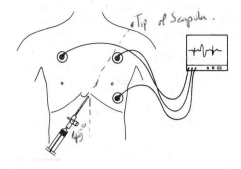

(*Procedures used by cardiologists for *elective* pericardiocentesis may differ, involving the use of guide-wires, screening, and catheters.)

- Get your senior's help (for whom this may serve as an *aide-mémoire*).
- Equipment: <u>20mL syringe, long 18G cannula, 3-way tap</u>, ECG monitor, skin cleanser.
- If time allows, use aseptic technique, and, if conscious, <u>local anaesthesia and sedation</u>, eg with midazolam: titrate up to 0.07mg/kg IV—start with 2mg over 30sec, max 1.5mg in elderly—antidote: flumazenil 0.2mg IV over 15sec, then 0.1mg every 60 seconds, up to 1mg in total.
- Ensure you have IV access and full resuscitation equipment to hand.
- Introduce needle at <u>45°</u> to skin just below and to <u>left of xiphisternum</u>, aiming for <u>tip of left scapula</u>. <u>Aspirate continuously</u> and watch ECG. Frequent <u>ventricular ectopics</u> or an injury pattern (<u>ST segment↓</u>) on ECG imply myocardium breached—<u>withdraw slightly</u>.
- Evacuate pericardial contents through the syringe and 3-way tap. Removal of only a small amount of fluid (eg 20mL) can produce marked clinical improvement. If you are not sure whether the fluid you are aspirating is pure blood (eg on entering a ventricle), <u>see if it clots (heavily bloodstained pericardial fluid does not clot)</u>, or measure its PCV.
- You can leave the cannula *in situ* temporarily, for repeated aspiration. If there is reaccumulation, <u>pericardiectomy</u> may be needed.
- <u>Send fluid for microscopy and culture, as needed, including tests for TB.</u>

Complications: laceration of ventricle or coronary artery (± subsequent haemopericardium); aspiration of ventricular blood; arrhythmias (ventricular fibrillation); pneumothorax; puncture of aorta, oesophagus (± mediastinitis) or peritoneum (± peritonitis).

▶▶Cardiorespiratory arrest

Causes MI; PE; trauma; electrocution; shock; hypoxia; <u>hypercapnia</u>; hypothermia; U&E imbalance; drugs, eg adrenaline (=epinephrine), digoxin.

Action Ensure safety of patient and yourself. Confirm diagnosis (unconscious, apnoeic, absent carotid pulse). Basic life support is as follows:

● **Shout for help.** Ask someone to call the arrest team and bring the defibrillator. <u>Note the time.</u>

● Give a praecordial thump if the arrest was witnessed. This may terminate ventricular arrhythmias. <u>Recheck</u> carotid pulse.

● Begin CPR (cardio-pulmonary resuscitation)
Airway: Extend the neck, lift the chin and clear the mouth. Ventilation: Use specialized bag and mask system (eg Ambu® system) with reservoir if available and two resuscitators present. Otherwise, use expired air ventilation with mask or direct mouth-to-mouth breathing. Give two rescue breaths. Each inflation should take about 2 seconds.

● Chest compressions should be centred over the <u>lower ⅓ of the sternum</u>. Use the heel of your hand and straight elbows. <u>Aim for 5cm</u> compression at 100/min. If alone, give 15 compressions to 2 breaths (15:2). In 2 person resuscitation, give 5 compressions to 1 breath (5:1). CPR should not be interrupted except to give shocks or to intubate.

Advanced life support Place defibrillator paddles on chest as soon as possible and set monitor to read through the paddles. Assess rhythm: is this VF/pulseless VT? In VF/VT, defibrillation must occur without delay. If the first 200J shock is unsuccessful, it should be repeated (200J), and if necessary, a third shock of 360J should be administered. <u>A pulse check is performed if an ECG rhythm compatible with a cardiac output is produced.</u>

Continue CPR for 1min while gaining IV access (peripheral or central). Consider intubation. Give adrenaline (epinephrine) 1mg IV followed by <u>20mL 0.9% saline flush.</u> Look for reversible causes of cardiac arrest: see box opposite. Treat accordingly.

Reassess ECG rhythm. Repeat defibrillation if still in VF/VT. All shocks 360J. Repeat cycles giving adrenaline every 3min. Consider antiarrhythmics.

If VF/VT is excluded, patient may be in asystole or electromechanical dissociation, rhythms with a poorer prognosis. These may, however, be due to remediable conditions (see box opposite), the treatment of which may be lifesaving. Continue CPR and give adrenaline. Search for a cause and treat accordingly. Consider atropine and antiarrhythmics.

Send someone to find the patient's notes and the patient's usual doctor. These may give clues as to the cause of the arrest.

If IV access fails, adrenaline (=epinephrine), atropine, and lignocaine (=lidocaine) may be given <u>down the tracheal tube</u> but absorption is unpredictable. Give 2–3 times the IV dose diluted in ≥10mL 0.9% saline followed by 5 ventilations to assist absorption. Intracardiac injection is not recomended.

When to stop resuscitation: There is no general rule as survival is influenced by the rhythm and the cause of the arrest. In patients without myocardial disease, do not stop until core temperature is >33°C and pH and potassium are normal. <u>Consider stopping resuscitation after 20 minutes if there is refractory asystole or electromechanical dissociation.</u>

After successful resuscitation: Do a 12–lead ECG; transfer to coronary care unit/ITU. Monitor vital signs; do CXR, U&E, glucose, blood gases, FBC, CK.

Whatever the outcome, explain to relatives what has happened.

Source: UK 1997 Guidelines, Resuscitation Council (UK) NB: adrenaline/epinephrine in large doses (eg 5mg, as above) has theoretical haemodynamic advantages, but studies have failed to show improved outcome (KA Ballew 1997 *BMJ* i 1462) P Baskett 1992 *Br J Anaesthesia* **69** 182

Cardiac arrest: *1997 adult advanced life-support algorithm*[1]

Each step assumes the previous one has been unsuccessful

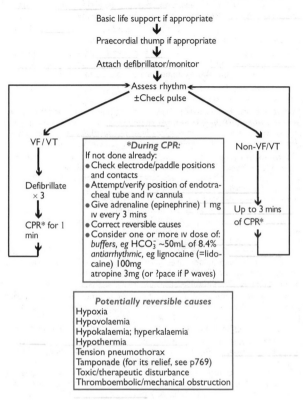

Basic life support if appropriate

↓

Praecordial thump if appropriate

↓

Attach defibrillator/monitor

↓

Assess rhythm
±Check pulse

VF / VT

↓

Defibrillate
× 3

↓

CPR* for 1
min

Non-VF/VT

↓

Up to 3 mins
of CPR*

*During CPR:
If not done already:
● Check electrode/paddle positions and contacts
● Attempt/verify position of endotracheal tube and IV cannula
● Give adrenaline (epinephrine) 1 mg IV every 3 mins
● Correct reversible causes
● Consider one or more IV dose of:
buffers, eg HCO_3^- ~50mL of 8.4% *antiarrhythmic, eg* lignocaine (=lidocaine) 100mg
atropine 3mg (or ?pace if P waves)

Potentially reversible causes
Hypoxia
Hypovolaemia
Hypokalaemia; hyperkalaemia
Hypothermia
Tension pneumothorax
Tamponade (for its relief, see p769)
Toxic/therapeutic disturbance
Thromboembolic/mechanical obstruction

Do not interrupt CPR for >10sec, except to defibrillate.

Resistant VF/VT: Consider: Lignocaine (=lidocaine) 100mg IV; can repeat once; then give 2–4mg/min IVI.
Different paddle position, eg antero–posterior Bretylium tosylate (tosilate) 5mg/kg IV; you must then continue CPR for 20 minutes.
Procainamide 100mg IV over 2min is an option.
Seek expert advice from a cardiologist.

Asystole with P waves: Start external pacing (percutaneous transthoracic pacing through special paddles). Use endocardial pacing if experienced pacer is available. If unavailable, use atropine 0.6mg/5min IV while awaiting further help.

Treat acidosis with good ventilation. Sodium bicarbonate may worsen intracellular acidosis and precipitate arrhythmias, so use it only in severe acidosis after prolonged resuscitation (eg 50mL of 8.4% solution by IVI).

1 Algorithm after the *UK Resuscitation Council Guidelines*, 1997

▶▶Severe pulmonary oedema

<u>Left ventricular failure</u> (post-MI, or ischaemic heart disease) is the usual cause. Other cardiac causes are <u>mitral stenosis</u>, <u>arrhythmias</u>, and <u>malignant hypertension</u>. Non-cardiac causes are given below.

Symptoms Dyspnoea, orthopnoea (eg paroxysmal), <u>pink frothy sputum</u>. Note: drugs; other illnesses (recent MI/COPD or pneumonia).

Signs Distressed, pale, sweaty, <u>pulse↑</u>, tachypnoea, pink frothy sputum, <u>pulsus alternans</u>, JVP↑, <u>fine lung crackles, triple/gallop rhythm</u>, <u>wheeze</u> (cardiac asthma). Quickly examine for possible causes (below).

Baseline tests and markers of progress: BP; heart rate; cyanosis; respiratory rate; JVP; peripheral oedema; enlarged liver.

Investigations CXR—cardiomegaly, signs of pulmonary oedema: look for shadowing (usually bilateral), <u>small effusions</u> at costophrenic angles, fluid in the lung fissures, and <u>Kerley B lines</u> (linear opacities, p718); ECG—signs of myocardial infarct; blood gases; U&E; 'cardiac' enzymes.

Management Begin treatment before investigations. Sit the patient up.
- Give O₂ by face mask: 100% if no pre-existing lung disease.
- Insert an IV cannula; monitor ECG (treat any arrhythmias, p286–294).
- Drugs: *Frusemide* (=furosemide) 40–80mg IV (more if renal failure) IV slowly. *Diamorphine* 2.5–5mg IV slowly, unless liver failure or COPD. Give *GTN* spray 2 puffs SL or 2 × 0.3mg tablets SL. If there is fast AF, give <u>digoxin 0.5mg PO</u> (or 0.5mg IV, slowly, if severely compromised).
- Complete investigations, examination, and history.
- Consider <u>isosorbide dinitrate (ISDN)</u> 2–7mg/h IVI if systolic BP >110mmHg or <u>dobutamine</u> 2.5–10μg/kg/min if BP <100mmHg. Inserting a Swan–Ganz catheter may help guide doses (aim for a pulmonary artery diastolic wedge pressure of 15–20mmHg with a systolic BP >100mmHg).[1]

Note: <u>if the BP is >180mmHg, treat for hypertensive LVF</u> (p302).

Continuing management: Frequent check of BP and pulse rate, heart sounds; restrict fluids; measure urine output; further IV frusemide (=furosemide) may be needed; U&E and ECG daily initially. *If improving:* Change to oral frusemide; sequential CXR; daily weight; BP and pulse/6h.

If the patient's worsening: <u>Consider venesecting 500mL blood ± ventilation (IPPV or CPAP, p354)</u> ± more ISDN, as above.* If shocked, call your senior and treat cardiogenic shock (p768). Adrenaline (=epinephrine) 0.5–1mg slowly IV may be advised, or dopamine IVI (start with 10μg/kg/min; ↑every ¼ h by 5μg/kg/min, until systolic BP >100mmHg; SE: p110).[1] Re-examine *often*; do serial ECGs. <u>Any new murmurs?</u> The infarction precipitating pulmonary oedema may also cause a VSD or mitral regurgitation.

Differential diagnosis Bronchospasm; pneumonia. It is often hard to make a definite diagnosis; all 3 conditions may co-exist, especially in the elderly. Do not hesitate to treat all 3 simultaneously (eg with salbutamol nebulizer, frusemide (furosemide) IV, diamorphine, amoxicillin—p176).

Non-cardiac causes of pulmonary oedema (rare):
- Allergic reactions, eg IV contrast agents (radiology, p726), venom, p795.
- Fluid overload, eg iatrogenic (too much IVI) or renal failure.
- <u>Smoke inhalation</u>: look for soot in the nostrils (OHCS p684)?
- ARDS (p350), look for predisposing factors eg trauma, post-op, sepsis.
- Infection: is there fever (eg malaria, Hanta virus, or trypanosomiasis)?
- Carbon monoxide poisoning (p794): coma, vomiting, and *no* cyanosis.
- Amniotic fluid embolus (OHCS p143): is she pregnant or post-partum?
- SLE (p672): is there a butterfly rash or proteinuria?
- *Is aspirin overdose or glue-sniffing/drug abuse likely?* Ask friends/relatives.

---

*Some say that IV nitrates should be used earlier (eg as a bolus), and are more helpful than diuretics (which stimulate renin, hence ↑ afterload), but large-scale trials are awaited. They certainly help those who don't respond to standard Rx: see G Cotter 1998 *Lancet* 351 389 1 D Sprigings 1995 *Acute Medicine*, Blackwell

►► Massive pulmonary embolism (PE)

► Always suspect pulmonary embolism (PE) in sudden collapse 1–2 weeks after surgery. Death rate in England and Wales: 30,000–40,000/year.[1]

Mechanism Venous thrombi, usually from DVT, pass into the pulmonary circulation and block blood flow to lungs. The source is often occult.

Prevention ●Mobilize early post-op. ●Anti-thrombo-embolic stockings. ●Heparin prophylaxis 5000u/8h sc. ●Avoid contraceptive pill if at risk, eg major or orthopaedic surgery. ●Recurrent PEs are prevented by anticoagulation or transjugular placing of a vena caval filter (non-ferromagnetic, to avoid MRI problems).[1]

The Patient Classically, PE presents 10 days post-op, with collapse and sudden breathlessness while straining at stool—but PE may occur after any period of immobility, or with no predisposing factors. Common presenting features: acute dyspnoea, pleuritic pain, hypotension, haemoptysis and syncope. Other signs: tachypnoea, cyanosis, gallop rhythm, JVP↑, pleural rub, right ventricular rub, loud P_2. Breathlessness may be the only sign. Multiple small emboli may present less dramatically with pleuritic pain, haemoptysis, and gradually increasing breathlessness.

Look for a source of emboli—especially DVT (is a leg swollen?)—but DVT signs may occur only *after* the embolism.

Tests ECG (commonly normal or sinus tachycardia); may be deep S-waves in I, Q-waves in III, inverted T-waves in III ('S$_I$ Q$_{III}$ T$_{III}$'), strain pattern V1–3 (p266), right axis deviation, RBBB, AF.
CXR—often normal; decreased vascular markings, small pleural effusion.
Blood gases (hyperventilation and impaired gas exchange, ie P_aO_2↓, P_aCO_2↓, pH often↑; see p328).
Lung ventilation–perfusion (V/Q) scan (p732). Look for ventilation–perfusion mismatch. If V/Q scan equivocal, pulmonary angiography may help.

Diagnosis Usually clinical. Most deaths from major PE occur within 1 hour, so angiography is rarely a practical option. Echocardiography may be useful if immediately available. If good story and signs, make the diagnosis. Start treatment (see below) prior to confirmatory radiology.

Management If critically ill consider immediate surgery. Otherwise:
●Give up to 100% O_2.
●Morphine 10mg IV if the patient is in pain or very distressed.
●Get IV access and start heparin 5000u IV bolus, then 1000–2000u/h IVI as guided by APTT (p596) or low molecular weight heparin eg tinzaparin 175u/kg/24h sc.[2]
●If you suspect acute major embolism, and systolic BP <90mmHg, start rapid colloid infusion. If BP still↓ after 500mL colloid, start dobutamine 5µg/kg/min (increase up to 20µg/kg/min as needed, until systolic BP >90mmHg). If BP still↓, consider noradrenaline (=norepinephrine).
●Consider thrombolysis if there is a clinically definite embolism, if the systolic BP <90mmHg after 30–60min standard treatment and there are no contraindications to thrombolysis (p283). A standard regimen is:
    Loading dose: streptokinase 600,000u IVI over 30min
    Maintenance dose: streptokinase 100,000u/h IVI for 24h
●Begin warfarin: eg 10mg/24h PO (p596). Continue for 3 months (longer if recurrent emboli).
●Try to prevent further thrombosis with compression stockings.
●Look for a cause of thrombosis. If no obvious risk factors, consider an underlying disease, eg thrombophilic tendency (p620), malignancy (especially prostate, breast, or pelvic cancer), SLE or polycythaemia.

(margin note: Get BP up)

1 DN Redhead 1994 *Journal of Surgery* 1994 **81** 1089 2 MD Simonneau 1997 *NEJM* **337** 663.

> *Differential diagnosis of dyspnoea with a normal CXR*
>
>   Shock (causing air hunger)
>   Pulmonary embolism
>   Acute asthma
>   Preradiological pneumonia (usually viral or PCP)
>   Metabolic acidosis
>   Sepsis
>   Hyperventilation
>   Foreign body in respiratory tract
>   Anaphylaxis

Heparin - effect on Antithrombin III (inhibits thrombin)
        Inactivates 9, 10, 11, 12 + Thrombin
    APPT = Partial thromboplastin time.   Intrinsic system
(KCCT)

Vit K: 2, 7, 9 and 10   INR (Extrinsic system)

Acute severe asthma[1]

▶The severity of an attack is easily underestimated.
▶An atmosphere of calm helps cure the patient.

Presentation Acute breathlessness and wheeze.

History Ask about usual and recent treatment; previous acute episodes and their severity. Have they been admitted to ITU?

Differential diagnosis Acute infective exacerbation of COPD, pulmonary oedema, upper respiratory tract obstruction, pulmonary embolus, anaphylaxis.

Tests Peak expiratory flow rate (PEFR)—but may be too ill; arterial blood gases; CXR (to exclude pneumothorax, infection); FBC; U&E.

Immediate management[1]
Assess severity of attack (see opposite). Warn ITU if attack severe.
Start treatment immediately (prior to investigations).

• Sit up and give oxygen in high-dose, eg 60%.
• Salbutamol 5mg or terbutaline 10mg nebulized in O_2.
• Hydrocortisone 200mg IV or prednisolone 30mg PO (or both if very ill).

▶▶If life-threatening features (see opposite) are present:
• Add ipratropium 0.5mg to the nebulized β-agonist.
• Give aminophylline IV 250mg (5mg/kg) over 20mins. Omit this bolus if patient is on oral theophyllines but urgently check level is therapeutic. Alternatively, give salbutamol or terbutaline 0.25mg IV over 10min.

Further management
If improving   • 40–60% O_2 + prednisolone 30–60mg/24h PO.
                • Nebulized salbutamol every 4h.
                • Monitor peak flow and oxygen saturations.

▶▶If patient not improving after 15–30 minutes
                • Continue 60% O_2 and steroids.
                • Nebulized salbutamol, max every 15–30min.
                • Ipratropium 0.5mg nebulized every 6h.

▶▶If patient still not improving:
                • Aminophylline infusion—small adult: 750mg/24h
                  —large adult 1500mg/24h.
                • Do levels if infusion lasts >24h.
                  Alternatively, give salbutamol infusion, eg 3–20µg/min.
                • If no improvement, or life-threatening features present, consider transfer to ITU. Patient must be accompanied by a doctor prepared to intubate.

Monitoring the effects of treatment
Repeat PEFR 15–30min after initiating treatment.
Pulse oximeter monitoring: maintain S_aO_2 >92%.
Check blood gases within 2h if   initial P_aCO_2 was normal/raised
                                  initial P_aO_2 <8kPa (60mmHg)
                                  patient deteriorating.
Record PEFR pre- and post-β-agonist in hospital at least four times.

Once patient improving
• Wean down and stop aminophylline over 12–24h.
• Reduce nebulized salbutamol and switch to inhaled β-agonist.
• Initiate inhaled steroids and stop oral steroids if possible.
• Continue to monitor PEFR. Look for deterioration on reduced treatment and beware early morning dips in PEFR.
• Look for the cause of the acute exacerbation and admission.

1 British Thoracic Society 1997 Guidelines *Thorax* **52** supplement, page s1–s21

Assessing the severity of an acute asthmatic attack

Severe attack:
- Unable to complete sentences
- Respiratory rate >25/min
- Pulse rate >110 beats/min
- Peak expiratory flow <50% of predicted or best

Life-threatening attack:
- Peak expiratory flow <33% of predicted or best
- Silent chest, cyanosis, feeble respiratory effort
- Bradycardia or hypotension
- Exhaustion, confusion, or coma
- Arterial blood gases: normal/high P_aCO_2 >5kPa (36mmHg)
  P_aO_2 <8kPa (60mmHg)
  low pH<7.35

On discharge, patients should have:

Been on discharge medication for 24h
Had inhaler technique checked
Peak flow rate >75% predicted or best with diurnal variability <25%
Steroid and bronchodilator therapy
Own PEF meter and management plan
GP appointment within 1 week
Respiratory clinic appointment within 4 weeks

Drugs used in acute asthma:

Aminophylline: The amount of IVI aminophylline may need altering according to the individual patient: always check the *BNF*.
Factors which may necessitate reduction of dose: Cardiac or liver failure, drugs which increase the half-life of aminophylline eg cimetidine, ciprofloxacin, erythromycin, propranolol, contraceptive steroids.
Factors which may require ↑dose: Smoking, drugs which shorten the half-life, eg phenytoin, carbamazepine, barbiturates, rifampicin.
►Aim for plasma concentration of 10–20μg/mL (55–110μmol/L). Serious toxicity (BP↓, arrhythmias, cardiac arrest) can occur at concentrations ≥25μg/mL. Measure plasma K+: theophyllines may cause K+↓.

Salbutamol side-effects: Tachycardia, arrhythmias, tremor, K+↓.

▶▶Head injury: emergency care

Do the ABCs of basic life support (p761), protecting the cervical spine. Retinal vein pulsation at fundoscopy helps exclude ICP↑. ▶If the pupils are unequal, diagnose rising intracranial pressure (ICP), eg from extradural haemorrhage and summon urgent neurosurgical help. Burr holes (on the side of the dilated pupil) may be needed. Other signs of ICP↑: deepening coma (or a lucid interval, then relapse), a rising BP and a slowing pulse (Cushing reflex), Cheyne–Stokes breathing (p40), apnoea, fixed dilated pupils (ipsilateral at first) and extensor posture. Try mannitol 20% 5mL/kg IV over 15min. Enlist an anaesthetist's help with transfer to a neurosurgical centre for urgent CT ± craniotomy. Aim to offer the neurosurgeon a well-oxygenated, well-perfused brain.

Initial management Write careful notes. Record times accurately.
- High-flow inspired O_2 (F_1O_2 >0.85+ tight fitting mask with reservoir).
- Stop blood loss. Take BP; treat shock with Haemaccel® (p766).
- History: When? Where? How? Had a fit? Lucid interval? Alcohol?
- Search for other injuries. Do blood alcohol, gases, U&E, glucose, FBC.
- Assess level of consciousness with the Glasgow Coma Scale (GCS).
- If alert, record the most difficult thing he can do.
- Assess anterograde amnesia (loss from time of injury) and retrograde amnesia—for pre-injury events (its extent correlates with the severity of the injury, and it never occurs without anterograde amnesia).
- Examine the CNS. Chart pulse, BP, T°, respirations + pupils every 15min.
- Evaluate lacerations of face or scalp. Palpate deep wounds with sterile glove to check for step deformity. Note obvious skull/facial fractures.
- Periorbital (raccoon sign), or postauricular (Battle sign) ecchymoses.
- Check for CSF leak, from nose (rhinorrhoea) or ear (any blood behind the drum). If any present, suspect basilar skull fracture and do CT. Give tetanus and antibiotic prophylaxis, and refer at once to neurosurgeons.
- Palpate the neck posteriorly for tenderness and deformity. If detected, or if the patient has obvious head injury, or injury above the clavicle with loss of consciousness, obtain cervical spine radiographs.
- On skull x-ray (posterior/anterior, Townes', and lateral views): look for sinus fractures and intracranial air. If the pineal gland is shifted (visible if calcified) or fractures cross blood vessels (eg middle meningeal artery—the vessel of extradural haemorrhage), do a CT scan.
- Nurse semi-prone if no spinal injury. Meticulous care to bladder + airway.
- If not severely injured: sit up when headache allows (if severe, suspect a complication). Treat pain with aspirin. *Criteria for admission:* Difficult to assess (child; post-ictal; alcohol intoxication; CNS signs; severe headache or vomiting; fracture. Loss of consciousness does **not** require admission if well, and a responsible adult is in attendance.
- Complications: *early* extradural/subdural haemorrhage; fits. *Later:* subdural haemorrhage, fits, diabetes insipidus, parkinsonism, dementia.

Drowsy trauma patients (GCS < 15 to >8) smelling of alcohol Do skull x-ray (+CT if fracture or focal signs). Alcohol is an unlikely cause of coma if plasma alcohol <44mmol/L. If test unavailable, estimate alcohol from the osmolar gap (p636). (If blood alcohol ≈ 40mmol/L, osmolar gap ≈ 40mmol/L.)

Improvement following impairment of brain function (concussion) Increasing pulse volume→ deeper respirations→ return of brainstem reflexes→ eyes open→ vomiting→ consciousness→ restlessness→ complaint of headache→ amnesia→ post-concussional syndrome (headache, dizziness, inability to concentrate, headaches, poor memory).

Indicators of a bad prognosis Increasing age, decerebrate rigidity, extensor spasms, prolonged coma, hypertension, P_aO_2↓ (on blood gases), T° >39°C. 60% of those with loss of consciousness of >1 month will survive 3–25yrs, but may need daily nursing care.

For *Spinal cord injury* and the *Persistent vegetative state*, see OHCS p726–32 & 733.

Getting help in severe neurotrauma

Work out the Glasgow coma score (p764) and get expert help whenever patients are comatose after neurotrauma; special measures may be needed, such as monitoring intracranial pressure (± ventriculostomy).

When to ventilate immediately:
Coma ≤8 on Glasgow Coma Scale (GCS)
P_aO_2 <9kPa in air (<13kPa in O_2)
P_aCO_2 >6kPa
Spontaneous hyperventilation (P_aCO_2 <3.5)
Respiratory arrhythmia, ie irregularity
Ventilate before neurosurgical transfer if:
Deteriorating level of consciousness
Bilateral fractured mandible
Bleeding into mouth, eg skull base fracture
Seizures

Inform neurosurgeon of:
Patient's age; past history
Time and mechanism of injury
Talked or not post-injury?
GCS on admission, and now
Pupil and limb responses
BP, pulse, P_aO_2, P_aCO_2
Respiratory rate & pattern
Skull fracture/other injury
Management so far; drugs

Risk of intracranial haematoma in adults

Fully conscious, no skull fracture = <1:1000
Confused, no skull fracture = 1:100
Fully conscious, skull fracture = 1:30
Confused, skull fracture = 1:4

▶▶Rising intracranial pressure (ICP↑)

Presentation Headache; drowsiness; vomiting; seizures. Trauma.

Signs Listlessness; irritability; drowsiness; falling pulse; rising BP; coma; irregular breathing; pupil changes (constriction at first, later dilatation—do not mask these signs by using agents such as tropicamide to dilate the pupil to aid fundoscopy). Papilloedema is an unreliable sign, but venous pulsation at the disc may be absent.

Causes Primary or metastatic tumours; head injury; haemorrhage (subdural, extradural, subarachnoid; intracerebral, intraventricular); brain abscess; meningoencephalitis; hydrocephalus; cerebral oedema. There are 3 types of cerebral oedema:
- Vasogenic: ↑ capillary permeability—tumour, trauma, ischaemia, infection.
- Cytotoxic—cell death, from hypoxia.
- Interstitial (eg obstructive hydrocephalus).

Because the cranium defines a fixed volume, brain swelling quickly results in ↑ICP which may produce a sudden clinical deterioration. The oedema from severe brain injury is probably both cytotoxic and vasogenic.

Herniation syndromes *Uncal herniation* is caused by a lateral supratentorial mass which pushes the ipsilateral inferomedial temporal lobe (uncus) through the temporal incisura and against the midbrain. The third nerve, travelling in this space, gets compressed causing a dilated ipsilateral pupil, then ophthalmoplegia (a fixed pupil localizes a lesion poorly but is 'ipsi-lateralizing'). This may be followed (quickly) by contralateral hemiparesis (pressure on the cerebral peduncle) and coma from pressure on the ascending reticular activating system (ARAS) in the midbrain.

Cerebellar tonsilar herniation is caused by ↑pressure in the posterior fossa forcing the cerebellar tonsils through the foramen magnum. Ataxia, VIth nerve palsies, and +ve Babinskis occur first, then loss of consciousness, irregular breathing and apnoea. This syndrome may proceed very rapidly given the small size of, and poor compliance in, the posterior fossa.

Subfalcian (cingulate) herniation is caused by a frontal mass. The cingulate gyrus (medial frontal lobe) is forced under the rigid falx cerebri. It may be silent unless the anterior cerebral artery is compressed and causes a stroke—eg contralateral leg weakness ± abulia (lack of decision-making).

Treatment: The goal is to ↓ICP and avert secondary injury. Urgent neurosurgery is required for the definitive treatment of ↑ICP from focal causes (eg haematomas). This is achieved via a craniotomy or burr hole. Also, an ICP monitor (or bolt) may be placed to monitor pressure. Surgery is generally *not* helpful following ischaemic or anoxic injury.

The following are **temporizing measures** which may help avoid herniation prior to definitive neurosurgical intervention:
- Elevate the head of the bed to 30–40°. Slightly extend head in midline.
- Hyperventilate the intubated patient to ↓P_aCO_2 (eg to 3.5kPa). This causes cerebral vasoconstriction and reduces ICP almost immediately.
- Osmotic agents (eg mannitol) can be useful in anticipation of definitive treatment but can lead to rebound ↑ICP after prolonged use (~12–24 hours). Give 20% solution 1–2g/kg IV over 10–20mins (eg 5mL/kg). Clinical effect is seen after ~20 minutes and lasts for 2–6 hours. Follow serum osmolality—aim for about 300mOsm but don't exceed 310.
- Corticosteroids are *not* effective in reducing ICP except for oedema surrounding tumours. If indicated, give dexamethasone 10mg IV and follow with 4mg/6h IV/PO. Give with H2 blocker.

Cerebral abscess

Suspect this in any patient with ICP↑, especially if there is fever or ↑WCC.

It may follow ear, sinus, dental, or periodontal infection; skull fracture; congenital heart disease; endocarditis; bronchiectasis.

Signs: Seizures, fever, localizing signs, or signs of ↑ICP. Coma. Signs of sepsis elsewhere (eg teeth, ears, lungs, endocarditis).

Tests: CT/MRI (eg 'ring-enhancing' lesion); ↑WBC, ↑ESR; biopsy.

Treatment: Urgent neurosurgical referral; prompt attention to rising intracranial pressure (opposite). If frontal sinuses or teeth are the source, the likely organism will be *Str milleri* (micro-aerophilic), followed by oropharyngeal anaerobes. In abscesses from the ear, *B fragilis* or other anaerobes are most common. Bacterial abscesses are often peripheral; toxoplasma lesions (p214) are deeper (eg basal ganglia).

▶▶Status epilepticus

This means <u>seizures lasting for >30min, or repeated seizures without intervening consciousness.</u> Mortality and risk of <u>permanent brain damage</u> increase with the length of attack. Aim to terminate seizures lasting more than a few minutes as soon as possible (certainly within 20mins).

Status usually occurs in known epileptics. If the patient presents for the first time with status epilepticus, the chance of a structural brain lesion is high (>50%). ▶Always ask yourself: <u>*Is the patient pregnant* (any pelvic mass)?</u> If so, eclampsia is the likely diagnosis: <u>call a senior obstetrician</u>—immediate delivery may be needed (*OHCS* p96). Alert theatre.

Diagnosis of tonic–clonic status is usually clear. Non-convulsive status (eg absence status or continuous partial seizures with preservation of consciousness) may be more difficult: look for subtle eye or lid movement. An EEG can be very helpful here.

Treatment <u>Remove false teeth. Insert Guedel</u> or nasopharyngeal (if trismus) <u>airway.</u> Ask an experieced nurse for laryngoscope, endotracheal tubes, <u>O₂,+ suction</u> (use as needed). Request her undivided attention.

- Diazepam (as Diazemuls®, less risk of thrombophlebitis) <u>10mg IV over 2min</u> (most of this can be given as a bolus; <u>beware respiratory depression during the last few mg</u>). <u>Wait 5mins.</u> Use this time to prepare other drugs. The <u>rectal route is an alternative if IV access is difficult.</u>*
- <u>50mL of 50% glucose (IV bolus)</u> unless certain that glucose is >5mmol/L. Glucose loads make matters worse if the patient is an alcoholic with <u>Wernicke's encephalopathy; thiamine 100mg IV prevents this.</u>
- <u>Dexamethasone 10mg IV if vasculitis/cerebral oedema (tumour) possible.</u>
- If seizures continue, set up a <u>0.9% saline IVI,</u> wherever you can; if possible, avoid veins crossing joints: splints are likely to fail. <u>Monitor ECG.</u>
- <u>Give diazepam IVI (5mg/min) until seizures stop or 20mg has been given</u>—or significant respiratory depression occurs.
- If seizures <u>persist,</u> start <u>phenytoin 15mg/kg IVI,</u> at a rate of up to 50mg/min. (<u>Do not put diazepam via the same line: they do not mix.</u>) Beware <u>BP↓</u> and <u>do not use if bradycardic or heart block.</u>
- If seizures continue (rare), get expert help. <u>Give more diazepam:100mg in 500mL of 5% dextrose; infuse at 40mL/h.</u> It is most unusual for seizures to remain unresponsive. If they do, allow the idea to pass through your mind that they could be pseudoseizures (p706), particularly if there are odd features, such as pelvic thrusts, or resisting attempts to open lids and do passive movements, arms and legs flailing around.
- If status continues for 1h after it began, arrange for an anaesthetist to paralyse and ventilate (anaesthesia). <u>Monitor EEG continuously.</u>

Chlormethiazole (=clormethiazole) is a reliable alternative to phenytoin for use when diazepam alone has failed. Give 5–15mL (max 40–100mL) of 0.8% chlormethiazole infusion over 5–10mins IV, and then by IVI according to response, eg 10 drops/min (0.5–1mL/min). A significant advantage is that the solution is ready prepared. It needs to be kept in a fridge (check its whereabouts *before* you start your period on call: planning *does* pay off). Take care with prolonged administration as the solution contains no electrolytes. Monitor vital signs, <u>pulse oximetry</u> (it is a major respiratory depressor), and <u>state of consciousness</u> continuously.

Tests Pulse oximetry, cardiac monitor, <u>glucose, blood gases, U&E,</u> Ca²⁺, FBC, platelets, ECG. Consider anticonvulsant levels, <u>toxicology screen, LP, culture blood and urine, EEG, CT,</u> carbon monoxide level.

As soon as seizures are controlled, start oral drugs (p450). Ask what the cause was (p448, eg hypoglycaemia, pregnancy, alcohol, drugs, CNS lesion or infection, hypertensive encephalopathy, inadequate anticonvulsant dose).

*<u>Diazepam Rectubes®</u>: give 0.5mg/kg stat dose–eg ~ <u>three 10mg tubes PR</u> (respiratory problems at this dose are *very* rare: all survived). If your back's still against the wall with no response after 10mins, try one last 10mg tube. <u>Halve dose if elderly.</u> *For children's Stesolid® regimen* (it's different), see *OHCS* p266.

►►Diabetic emergencies

Hyperglycaemic ketoacidotic coma Risk is <u>only with insulin-dependent diabetes</u>: it <u>may be the mode of presentation</u>, eg with a 2–3-day history of gradual decline into dehydration, acidosis, and coma pre-cipitated by infection, surgery, MI, or wrong insulin dose). Signs: <u>hyperventilation</u>; breath <u>smells ketotic</u>. Dehydration is more life-threatening than any hyperglycaemia—so its correction takes precedence.

Management of ketoacidotic coma: ●Set up a 0.9% saline IVI. Give <u>1 litre (L) stat</u>, then, typically, <u>1L over the next hour</u>, then <u>1L over 2h, then 1L over 4h, then 1L over 6h</u>. Those over 65yrs or with CCF need less saline.
●Glucose ward test: <u>usually >20mmol/L</u>, if so give 10u soluble insulin IV.
●Blood samples: lab glucose, U&E, HCO₃⁻, osmolality, <u>blood gases</u> (give O₂ if P₃O₂ <10.5kPa), FBC, blood culture. Urine tests: <u>ketones, MSU</u>.
●Pass an NGT—prevents gastric dilatation/aspiration. Take to ITU; <u>do CXR</u>.
●History (from relatives) and examination. *What precipitated the coma?*
●<u>Insulin sliding scale (opposite)</u>, initially with <u>hourly blood glucose tests</u>.
●Unless oliguric or initial K⁺ >6, <u>add 20mmol KCl to all but first litre</u>, adjusted via <u>hourly U&Es</u> (aim for K⁺ of 4–5mmol/L; K⁺ will fall fast, as glucose enters cells). <u>Use dextrose saline for IVI when blood glucose is <15mmol/L.</u>
●Give <u>heparin 5000u/8h SC</u> until mobile.
●Flow chart of vital signs, blood glucose, coma level (p764), urine output and ketones (hourly entries); insert catheter if no urine passed for >4h. Monitoring CVP may be helpful in guiding fluid replacement.
●Find and treat infection (lung, skin, perineum, urine after cultures), eg IV cefuroxime or amoxicillin IV + flucloxacillin IV ± metronidazole PR (p177–81).
●Be <u>alert to shock, cerebral oedema</u> (use mannitol), DVT, DIC (p598).
●<u>Change to SC insulin when ketones are ≤1+ and he can eat.</u> Experiment to <u>find the 24h dose needed by giving soluble insulin before each meal</u>, and <u>longer-acting isophane insulin at bedtime. Get onto a twice-daily dose by giving ⅔ of the 24h requirement before breakfast, and ⅓ before supper.</u> Check blood glucose frequently.
  ►Talk with the patient to ensure that there are no more comas.

Note: If <u>acidosis is severe (pH <7)</u>, <u>some physicians give IV bicarbonate</u> (eg 1mL/kg of 8.4% over 1h, and recheck arterial pH); others never give it because of its effect on the oxyhaemoglobin dissociation curve.

Hyperglycaemic hyperosmolar non-ketotic coma Only those with <u>non-insulin dependent</u> diabetes are at risk of this. The <u>history is longer (eg 1 week)</u>, with <u>marked dehydration</u> and <u>glucose >35mmol/L</u>. <u>Acidosis is absent</u> as there has been no switch to ketone metabolism—the patient is <u>often old</u>, and presenting for the first time. The osmolality is <u>>340mmol/kg</u>. <u>Focal CNS signs</u> may occur. The <u>risk of DVT is high</u>, so give *full* heparin anticoagulation (p596).
  <u>Rehydrate over 48h with 0.9% saline IVI</u> eg at half the rate used in ketoacidosis. (0.45% saline can be dangerous as it is hypotonic). <u>Wait an hour before giving any insulin</u> (it may not be needed, and you want to avoid rapid changes). If it is needed, 1u/h might be a typical initial dose.

Hyperlactataemia is a rare but serious complication of DM (eg after septicaemia or biguanide use). Blood lactate: >5mmol/L. Seek expert help. <u>Give O₂</u>. Treat any sepsis vigorously.

Hypoglycaemia Presentation: <u>odd behaviour (eg aggression), sweating, pulse↑, seizures,</u> and coma of *rapid* onset. See p762. <u>Give 50–100mL 50% dextrose IV fast.</u> This harms veins, so follow by 0.9% saline flush. Expect prompt recovery. If not, give dexamethasone 4mg/4h IV to combat cerebral oedema after prolonged hypoglycaemia. Dextrose IVI may be needed for severe hypoglycaemia. <u>If IV access fails try glucagon (1–2mg IM).</u> <u>Once conscious, give sugary drinks.</u>

Sliding scale of insulin via IVI pump in diabetic ketoacidosis

Hourly glucose result	Soluble insulin	If infection/insulin resistance (p529)
0–3.9	0.5u/h	1u/h
4–7.9	1	2
8–11.9	2	4
12–16	3	6
>16mmol/L	4	8

If there is no pump, load with 10u IM, then give 4–6u/h IM while glucose is >14mmol/L

Pitfalls in diabetic ketoacidosis

1 **A high WCC** may be seen in the absence of infection.

2 **Infection:** often there is no fever. Do MSU, blood cultures and CXR. Start broad spectrum antibiotics early if infection is suspected.

3 **Creatinine:** some assays for creatinine cross-react with ketone bodies, so plasma creatinine may not reflect true renal function.

4 **Hyponatraemia** may occur due to the osmotic effect of glucose. If < 120mmol search for other causes, eg hypertriglyceridaemia.

5 **Ketonuria** does not equate with ketoacidosis. Normal individuals may have up to ++ketonuria after an overnight fast. Not all ketones are due to diabetes—consider alcohol if glucose normal. +++Ketonuria means diabetes mellitus. Test plasma with Ketostix® or Acetest® to demonstrate ketonaemia.

6 **Recurrent ketoacidosis:** blood glucose may return to normal long before ketones are removed from the blood, and a rapid reduction in the amount of insulin administered may lead to lack of clearance and return to DKA. This may be avoided by maintaining a constant rate of insulin eg 4–5u/h IVI, and co-infusing dextrose 10–20% to keep plasma glucose at 6–10mmol/L—the *extended insulin regimen.*[1]

6 **Acidosis** but without gross elevation of glucose may occur, but consider overdose (eg aspirin) and lactic acidosis (in elderly diabetics).

7 **Serum amylase** is often raised (up to × 10) and nonspecific abdominal pain is common even in the absence of pancreatitis.

To estimate plasma osmolarity: 2[Na+] + [urea] + [glucose] mmol/L. **1** *Lancet* 1997 **350** 787

Thyroid emergencies

Myxoedema coma

The Patient—on examination: Looks hypothyroid; >65 years old; hypothermia; hyporeflexia; glucose↓; bradycardia; coma; seizures.

History: Prior surgery or radioiodine for hyperthyroidism.

Precipitants: Infection; myocardial infarct; stroke; trauma.

Examination: Goitre; cyanosis; heart failure; precipitants.

Treatment: Preferably in intensive care.
- Take venous blood for: T3, T4, TSH, FBC, U&E, cultures.
- Take arterial blood for P_aO_2.
- Give high-flow O_2 if cyanosed. Correct any hypoglycaemia.
- Give T3 (triiodothyronine) 5–20µg 12h/iv slowly. Be cautious: this may precipitate undiagnosed angina.
- Give hydrocortisone 100mg/8h iv, especially important if pituitary hypothyroidism is suspected (ie no goitre, or previous radioiodine, or thyroid surgery).
- IVI 0.9% saline. Be sure to avoid precipitating LVF.
- If infection suspected give antibiotic, eg cefuroxime 1.5g/8h IVI.
- Treat *heart failure* as appropriate (p298).
- Treat *hypothermia* with warm blankets in warm room. Beware complications (hypoglycaemia, pancreatitis, arrhythmias). See p70.

Continuing therapy:
- T3 5–20µg/4–12h iv until sustained improvement (eg ~2–3 days) then thyroxine (=levothyroxine) 50µg/24h po. Continue hydrocortisone.
- iv fluids as appropriate (hyponatraemia is dilutional).

Hyperthyroid crisis (thyrotoxic storm)

The Patient: Severe hyperthyroidism: fever, agitation, confusion, coma, tachycardia, AF, D&V, goitre, thyroid bruit, 'acute abdomen' picture.

Precipitants: Recent thyroid surgery or radioiodine; infection; MI; trauma.

Diagnosis: Confirm with technetium uptake if possible, but do not wait for this if urgent treatment is needed.

Treatment: Enlist expert help.
- IVI 0.9% saline, 500mL/4h. NG tube if vomiting.
- Take blood for: T3, T4, cultures (if infection suspected).
- Sedate if necessary (chlorpromazine 50–100mg PO/IM).
- If no contraindication, give propranolol 40mg/8h po (maximum iv dose: 1mg over 1min, repeated up to ten times at ≥2min intervals).
- High-dose digoxin may be needed to slow the heart, eg 0.5mg iv over 30min, then 0.25mg iv over 30min every 2h, up to a max of ~1mg.
- Anti-thyroid drugs: carbimazole 15–25mg/6h po (or via NGT, if needed). After 4h give Lugol's solution 0.5mL/8h po for 1 week to block thyroid.
- Dexamethasone 4mg/6h po.
- Treat suspected infection with eg cefuroxime 1.5g/8h IVI.
- Adjust iv fluids as necessary. Cool with tepid sponging ± paracetamol.

Seek advice from an endocrinologist.

Continuing treatment: After 5 days reduce carbimazole to 15mg/8h po. After 10 days stop propranolol and iodine. Adjust carbimazole (p542).

►►Addisonian crisis ⓟ

The Patient may present in shock (tachycardia; peripheral vasoconstriction; postural hypotension; oliguria; weak; confused; comatose)—typically (but not always!) in a patient with known Addison's disease, or someone on long-term steroids who has forgotten to take their tablets.

An alternative presentation is with hypoglycaemia.

Precipitating factors: Infection, trauma, surgery.

Management: If suspected, treat before biochemical results.
- Take blood for cortisol (10mL heparin or clotted) and ACTH if possible (10mL heparin, to go straight to laboratory).
- Hydrocortisone sodium succinate 100mg IV stat.
- IVI: use a plasma expander first, for resuscitation, then 0.9% saline in 5% dextrose.
- Monitor blood glucose: the danger is hypoglycaemia.
- Blood, urine, sputum for culture.
- Give antibiotic (eg cefuroxime 1.5g/8h IVI).

Continuing treatment ●Glucose IV may be needed if hypoglycaemic.
- Continue IV fluids, more slowly. Be guided by clinical state.
- Continue hydrocortisone sodium succinate 100mg IM every 6h.
- Change to oral steroids after 72h if patient's condition good. The tetracosactrin (=tetracosactide) test is impossible while on hydrocortisone.
- Fludrocortisone is needed only if hydrocortisone dose <50mg per day and the condition is due to adrenal disease.
- Search for the cause, once the crisis is over.

Hypopituitary coma

Usually develops gradually in a person with known hypopituitarism. Rarely, the onset is rapid due to infarction of a pituitary tumour (pituitary apoplexy)—as symptoms include headache and meningism, subarachnoid haemorrhage is often misdiagnosed.

Presentation: Headache; ophthalmoplegia; consciousness↓; hypotension; hypothermia; hypoglycaemia; signs of hypopituitarism (p558).

Tests: T4; cortisol; TSH; ACTH; glucose. Pituitary fossa x-ray; CT.

Treatment:
- Hydrocortisone sodium succinate 100mg IV/6h.
- Only after hydrocortisone begun: T3 10µg/12h PO.
- Prompt surgery is needed if the cause is pituitary apoplexy.

►►Phaeochromocytoma emergencies

Stress, abdominal palpation, parturition, general anaesthetic, or contrast media used in radiography may produce dangerous *hypertensive crises* (pallor, pulsating headache, hypertension, feels 'about to die').

Treatment ●Phentolamine 2–5mg IV. Repeat to maintain safe BP.
●Labetolol is an alternative agent (p302). ●When BP controlled, give phenoxybenzamine 10mg/24h PO (increase by 10mg/day as needed, up to 0.5–1mg/kg/12h PO); SE: postural hypotension; dizziness; tachycardia; nasal congestion; miosis; idiosyncratic marked BP drop soon after exposure.

Propranolol (eg 20mg/8h PO) is also given at this stage. Prepare for surgery.

Acute poisoning—general measures

Emergency care Clear airway. Consider ventilation (if the respiratory rate is <8/min, or P_aO_2 <8kPa, when breathing 60% O_2, or the airway is at risk, see p354). Treat shock (p766). If unconscious, nurse semi-prone.

Assess the patient Diagnosis is mainly from history. The patient may not tell the truth about what has been taken. Use *MIMS Colour Index* or *BNF* description (or the computerized system 'TICTAC'—ask pharmacy) to identify tablets and plan specific treatment. Doing T°PR and BP can give valuable information. A *fast or irregular pulse* suggests salbutamol, antimuscarinics, tricyclic, quinine or phenothiazine poisoning. *Slow respirations* may indicate opiate toxicity. *Hypothermia* may be from phenothiazines, barbiturates, or tricyclics, while *hyperthermia* suggests amphetamines, MAOIs, cocaine, or antimuscarinics (p452). Next assess level of consciousness (p764) and CNS. *Coma* suggests benzodiazepines, alcohol, opiates, tricyclics, or barbiturates. *Seizures* suggest recreational drugs, hypoglycaemic agents, tricyclics, phenothiazines, or theophyllines. *Constricted pupils* suggest opiates or insecticides (organophosphates, p795); if *dilated*, suspect amphetamines, cocaine, quinine, or sympathomimetics. Check for papilloedema; recent head injury; signs of injury. Estimate blood glucose: *hyperglycaemia* suggests organophosphates, theophyllines, or MAOIs; *hypoglycaemia* suggests insulin, oral hypoglycaemics, alcohol, or salicylate. Do U&E (*renal failure* may be due to salicylate, paracetamol, or ethylene glycol; *metabolic acidosis* may be due to alcohol, ethylene glycol, methanol, paracetamol, or carbon monoxide poisoning—p794). ↑*Osmolality* causes: alcohols (ethyl or methyl); ethylene glycol. Do urine and plasma drug screen.

If you are not familiar with the poison Get more information. The *Data Sheet Compendium* is useful. If in doubt how to act, phone Poisons Information Service (p792). *Take blood* as appropriate (p792). Always check paracetamol and salicylate levels. *Empty stomach* if appropriate (p792). Freeze 20mL of aspirate, urine and blood if crime suspected.

Consider antidote (p794) or oral activated charcoal (p796).

Continuing care Measure temperature, pulse, BP, and blood glucose regularly. Use a continuous ECG monitor. If unconscious nurse semi-prone, turn regularly, keep eyelids closed. A urinary catheter will be needed if the bladder is distended, or renal failure is suspected, or forced diuresis undertaken. Take to ITU, eg if respirations↓. Do blood gases+U&E.

Psychiatric assessment Be sympathetic despite the hour! Interview relatives and friends if possible. Aim to establish:
●*Intentions at time:* Was the act planned? What precautions against being found? Did the patient seek help afterwards? Does the patient think the method was dangerous? Was there a final act (eg suicide note)? ●*Present intentions.* ●*What problems* led to the act: do they still exist? ●*Was the act* aimed at someone? ●Is there a *psychiatric disorder* (depression, alcoholism, personality disorder, schizophrenia, dementia)? ●What are his *resources* (friends, family, work, personality)?

The assessment of suicide risk: The following increase the chance of future suicide: original intention was to die; present intention is to die; presence of psychiatric disorder; poor resources; previous suicide attempts; socially isolated; unemployed; male; >50yrs old. See *OHCS* p338 & p339.

Referral to psychiatrist: This depends partly on local resources. Ask advice if presence of psychiatric disorder or high suicide risk.

Common law or the Mental Health Act: (in England and Wales) may provide for the detention of the patient against his or her will: see *OHCS* p398.

Acute poisoning—specific points

Poisons information services in the UK Belfast: 01232 240503; Cardiff: 01222 709901; Edinburgh: 0131 536 2300; Leeds: 0113 243 0715; London: 0171 635 9191; Newcastle 0191 232 5131.

Emergency blood drug level (in lithium-heparin tube) for all unconscious patients eg for paracetamol/aspirin (see later); digoxin (>4ng/mL, or >5mmol/L?); methanol (>500mg/L?); lithium (in plain tube, >5mmol/L?); iron (>3.5mg/L?); theophylline (>50mg/L?). Haemoperfusion, haemodialysis may be needed if level > that in brackets. (Digibind & digoxin, see p794).

When to empty a stomach If within 2–4h of poisoning unless only small dose of a 'safe' drug (eg benzodiazepine) is involved. It is worth doing up to 6h after ingestion of *opiates* and *anticholinergics,* up to 8h after tricyclics or long-acting theophyllines, and up to 12h after *salicylates.*

▶Do not empty stomach if petroleum products or corrosives such as acids, alkalis, bleach, descalers have been ingested (*exception:* paraquat) or if the patient is unconscious (unless you protect the airway).

Methods available for emptying stomachs
1 *Gastric emptying and lavage:* If unconscious, or no gag reflex, protect airway with cuffed endotracheal tube. If conscious, get verbal consent.
  • It may be wise to monitor O_2 by pulse oximetry. See p658.
  • Have suction apparatus to hand and working.
  • Position the patient in left lateral position.
  • Raise the foot of the bed by 20cm.
  • Pass a lubricated tube (14mm external diameter) via the mouth, asking the patient to swallow.
  • Confirm position in stomach—blow air down, and auscultate over the stomach.
  • Siphon the gastric contents. Check pH with litmus paper.
  • Perform gastric lavage using 300–600mL tepid water at a time. Massage the left hypochondrium.
  • Repeat until no tablets in siphoned fluid.
  • Leave activated charcoal (50g in 200mL water) in the stomach unless alcohol, iron, Li^+, or ethylene glycol ingested.
  • When pulling out tube, occlude its end (prevents aspiration of fluid remaining in the tube).

2 *Induce vomiting:* This is now no longer generally recommended in adults, and perhaps only has a rôle in children caught in the act of consuming tablets, who reach hospital very rapidly. Do not do if patient likely soon to lose consciousness. Dose example: 15–30mL syrup of ipecacuanha followed by 200mL water. Repeat after 20mins if there has not been any vomiting. (**Note:** this is not a very efficient way of reducing the absorption of poisons, and the use of *activated charcoal,* p796, is to be preferred.)

Note: if the patient is known to be unconscious because of alcohol intoxication and the use of only a small number of benzodiazepine tablets (the commonest agents), it is probably wisest to avoid gastric lavage, with its attendant risks of aspiration, and to allow the patient to sleep off the effects of the poison.

Some specific poisons and their antidotes

Benzodiazepines Flumazenil (for respiratory arrest) 200µg over 15sec; then 100µg at 60sec intervals if needed. Usual dose range: 300–600µg IV over 3–6mins (up to 1mg; 2mg if on ITU).

β-blockers Severe bradycardia or hypotension. Try atropine 0.3mg IV. Give glucagon 5–10mg IV bolus if atropine fails.

Botulinum toxin (eg from tinned foods *via Clostridia*), causing diplopia, blurred vision, photophobia, ataxia, pseudobulbar palsy, and sudden cardiorespiratory failure—eg with *no* GI signs. Nurse on ITU. Intubate early. Seek expert help. Give botulinum antitoxin IM (20mL diluted to 100mL with 0.9% saline IVI ± 10mL 3h later and then at 12–24h). *Treat as early as possible.* Also give 20mL IM to those who have ingested toxin but who are asymptomatic. In UK, phone 0171 2015371 if unable to get antitoxin.

Co-proxamol Dextropropoxyphene (opiate) and paracetamol (p796).

Cyanide is one of the fastest-killing poisons; it has affinity for Fe^{3+}, inhibits the cytochrome system, and stops aerobic respiration. *The 3 phases:* ●Anxiety ± confusion ●Pulse↑or↓, BP↓ ●Fits ± coma ± shock. *Treatment:* ►►100% O_2, GI decontamination; dicobalt edetate 300mg IV over 1–5min, then 50mL 50% dextrose IV. Repeat up to twice. *Get expert help.* See p805.

Carbon monoxide In spite of hypoxaemia the skin is pink (or pale), not cyanosed as carboxyhaemoglobin (COHb) displaces O_2 from Hb binding sites. Symptoms: headache, vomiting, tachycardia, tachypnoea, and, if COHb >50%, seizures, coma, and cardiac arrest. ►►Remove the source. Give 100% O_2 (± IPPV). Metabolic acidosis (do blood gases) usually responds to correction of hypoxia. If severe, anticipate cerebral oedema. Give mannitol IVI (p780). Confirm diagnosis with a heparinized blood sample (COHb >10%) quickly as levels may soon return to normal. Monitor ECG. *Hyperbaric O_2 may help, even many hours' post-exposure.●* Consider this if there is a history of coma, neuropsychiatric symptoms, CVS complications, pregnancy or COHb is >40%. In the UK, ring the Royal Navy to find a nearby compression chamber (01705 822351).

Digoxin (Cognition↓, yellow-green visual halos, arrhythmias, nausea.) If serious arrhythmias are present, inactivate with digoxin-specific antibody fragments. Give 60 × total digoxin load (antibody fragments are 60 × heavier than digoxin molecules). The load (mg) is plasma digoxin concentration (ng/mL) × body weight (kg) × 0.0056. If load or level is unknown, give 20 vials (800mg)—adult or child >20kg. Consult *Data Sheet*. Dilute in water for injections (4mL/40mg vial) and 0.9% saline (to make a convenient volume); give IV over ½h (bolus if desperate), *via* a 0.22µm-pore filter.

Heavy metals Dimercaprol eg 2.5–3mg/kg IM up to 6 doses/24h for 48h—then twice daily for 10 days. Enlist expert help.

Iron Desferrioxamine (=deferoxamine) 15mg/kg/h IVI; max 80mg/kg/day.

Oral anticoagulants If not normally on anticoagulants and not bleeding, give phytomenadione (vitamin K) 10mg/24h PO. If bleeding, give fresh frozen plasma (FFP) IV. If normally on warfarin and bleeding, give vitamin K, 5–10mg IV. But if it is vital that he remains anticoagulated, use FFP, and enlist expert help. Warfarin can normally be restarted within 2–3 days. Major bleeding should be treated with vitamin K ~10mg IV *slowly*; life-threatening bleeding with vitamin K ≤50mg IV, *slowly*; then infuse vitamin-K-dependent clotting factors. Cholestyramine 4g/6h PO aids elimination.

Opiates (Many analgesics contain opiates.) Give naloxone 0.4–1.2mg IV; repeat every 2min until breathing adequate (it has a short $t_{1/2}$, so it may need to be given often; max 10mg). Naloxone may precipitate features of opiate withdrawal—diarrhoea and cramps will normally respond to diphenoxylate and atropine (Lomotil®—eg 2 tablets/6h PO). Sedate with thioridazine 25–50mg PO as needed. High-dose opiate misusers may need methadone (eg 10–30mg/12h PO) to combat withdrawal. Register opiate addiction (OHCS p362), and refer for help.

795

Phenothiazine poisoning (eg chlorpromazine). There are no specific antidotes. Severe dystonia (torticollis, retrocollis, glossopharyngeal dystonia, opisthotonus) responds to procyclidine 5–10mg IM/IV or orphenadrine 20–40mg IM/IV (adults). Treat shock by raising the legs (± plasma expander IVI, or dopamine IVI if desperate). Restore body temperature. Monitor ECG. Avoid lignocaine (=lidocaine) in arrhythmias. Use diazepam IV for prolonged fits in the usual way (p782). Neuroleptic malignant syndrome consists of: hyperthermia, rigidity, extrapyramidal signs, autonomic dysfunction, mutism, confusion, coma, WCC↑, CPK↑; it may be treated with cooling. Dantrolene has been tried (p86).

Carbon tetrachloride poisoning This solvent, used in many industrial processes, causes vomiting, abdominal pain, diarrhoea, seizures, coma, renal failure, and tender hepatomegaly with jaundice and liver failure. IV acetylcysteine may improve prognosis. Seek expert help.

Organophosphate insecticides inactivate cholinesterase—the resulting increase in acetylcholine causes the SLUD response: salivation, lacrimation, urination, and diarrhoea. Also look for sweating, small pupils, muscle fasciculations, coma, and respiratory distress. *Treatment:* Wear gloves; remove soiled clothes. Wash skin. Take blood for RBC and serum cholinesterase activity. Give atropine IV 2mg every 30min until full atropinization (dry mouth, pulse >70). Up to 3 days' treatment may be needed. Also give pralidoxime 30mg/kg slowly IV (dilute with ≥10mL Water for Injections). Repeat as needed every 30min; max 12g in 24h. Even if fits are not occurring, diazepam 5–10mg IV seems to help.

Ecstasy poisoning Ecstasy is a semi-synthetic, hallucinogenic substance (MDMA, 3,4-methylenedioxymethamphetamine). Its effects range from nausea, muscle pain, blurred vision, confusion and ataxia to tachyarrhythmias, hyperthermia, hyper/hypotension, water intoxication, DIC, K⁺↑, acute renal failure, hepatocellular and muscle necrosis, cardiovascular collapse and ARDS. There is no antidote and treatment is supportive. Management depends on clinical and lab findings, but may include:

- Administration of activated charcoal and monitoring of BP, ECG and temperature for at least 12h (rapid cooling may be needed).
- Monitor urine output and U&E (renal failure p386), LFT, creatinine kinase, platelets and coagulation (DIC p598). Metabolic acidosis may benefit from treatment with sodium bicarbonate.
- Anxiety: diazepam 0.1–0.3mg/kg PO or IV can be used.
- Narrow complex tachycardias in adults: consider metoprolol 5–10mg IV.
- Hypertension can be treated with nifedipine 5–10mg PO or phentolamine 2–5mg IV. Treat hypotension conventionally.
- Hyperthermia: attempt to cool, if rectal T° >39°C consider dantrolene 1mg/kg IV (may need repeating: discuss with your senior and a poisons unit, p792). Hyperthermia with ecstasy is akin to serotonin syndrome, and propranolol, muscle relaxation and ventilation may be needed.[1]

Snake-bite *Signs of systemic envenoming:* BP↓ (vasodilatation, viper cardiotoxicity); D&V; swelling spreading proximally within 4h of bite; bleeding gums/venepuncture sites; anaphylaxis; ptosis (neurotoxicity); trismus; rhabdomyolysis; pulmonary oedema. *Tests:* WCC↑; clotting↓; platelets↓; urine RBC↑; CK↑; P_aO_2↓. *Management:* Avoid active movement of affected limb (∴ use splints/slings). *Avoid incisions and tourniquets.* ▶Get help.[3] Is antivenom indicated (IgG from venom-immunized sheep)?—eg 10mL IV over 15min (adults **and** children) of *Zagreb antivenom* for adder bites; have epinephrine to hand.

1 H Sternbach 1991 *Am J Psy* 148 705 2 D Warrell 1998 *Prescrib J* 38 10 3 UK tel: 01865 221332/220968/220279

Salicylate poisoning

Aspirin is a weak acid with poor water solubility. It is present in many over-the-counter preparations. Acute ingestion of 150–300mg/kg may lead to mild toxicity; 300–500mg/kg moderate toxicity; >500mg/kg severe toxicity. Anaerobic metabolism and the production of lactate and heat are stimulated by the uncoupling of oxidative phosphorylation.

Signs and symptoms: Patients present initially with respiratory alkalosis due to central hyperventilation, then develop a metabolic acidosis (anion gap↑). Also tinnitus, lethargy or coma, seizures, vomiting, ↓BP and heart block, pulmonary oedema, hyperthermia. *Treatment:* Do not expect the acute ingestion of 150mg/kg to produce significant toxicity other than GI irritation. Obtain quantitative level at 6h post ingestion. Empty the stomach (p792) if >15 tablets (=4.5g) have been taken within 12h. Beware hypoglycaemia. Do repeated plasma glucose. Also do INR (may be prolonged, and vitamin K may be needed).

If the level is <4.3mmol/L (600mg/L) simply increase oral fluids and measure urine output. If ≥4.3mmol/L, use alkaline diuresis (under expert guidance in ITU, as there is significant morbidity) and activated charcoal (the latter is a much safer means of enhancing the elimination of salicylates). However, charcoal is unpalatable—and patients may be vomiting after salicylate poisoning, so give it by NGT. A suitable regimen is 50g activated charcoal/4h, until recovery or until plasma drug levels are safe.

An alternative is urinary alkalinization (in ITU, eg with boluses of 50–100mL sodium bicarbonate 1.2% IV; do catheter urine pH every 15mins—aim for ~8). Monitor CVP and arterial pH. Seek expert help.

If these measures are impracticable, refer for haemodialysis or charcoal haemoperfusion, particularly if salicylate is >7.2mmol/L (1000mg/L).

Paracetamol poisoning

There may be vomiting ± RUQ pain. Later there is jaundice and encephalopathy from liver damage (the main danger) ± renal failure.
- Do an emergency blood level when 4h have elapsed since ingestion.
- Empty the stomach if >7.5g has been taken. If plasma paracetamol is above the line on the graph opposite, or if presentation is 8–15h after ingestion of 7.5g paracetamol, act to prevent liver damage, as follows:
- Give N-acetylcysteine by IVI, 150mg/kg in 200mL of 5% dextrose over 15mins. Then 50mg/kg in 500mL of 5% dextrose over 4h. Then 100mg per kg/16h in 1L of 5% dextrose. SE: shock, vomiting, wheeze (in ≤10%).
- An alternative is methionine 2.5g/4h PO for 16h (total: 10g), but absorption is unreliable if there is vomiting. Benefit is lessened by concurrent charcoal[1] (which may be beneficial within 8h of ingestion).
- Benefit of gastric lavage is unclear.[2] Do not wait for the 4h blood level before treatment if you know a large amount has been ingested.
- If ingestion time is unknown, or it is staggered, or presentation is >15h from ingestion treatment *may* help. ► Get advice. The graph may mislead if HIV+ve (hepatic glutathione↓), or if long-acting paracetamol has been taken, or if pre-existing liver disease or induction of liver enzymes has occurred.[3] ► Beware glucose↓; ward-test hourly; INR/12h.

Do not hesitate to get expert advice. *Criteria for transfer to a specialist unit:*
- *Encephalopathy* or *ICP↑*. Signs of CNS oedema: BP >160/90 (sustained) or brief rises (systolic >200mmHg), bradycardia, decerebrate posture, extensor spasms, poor pupil responses. ICP monitoring can help, p780.
- *INR* >2.0 at <48h—or >3.5 at <72h (so measure INR every 12h). Peak elevation: 72–96h. LFTs are *not* good markers of hepatocyte death. If INR is *normal* at 48h, the patient may go home.
- *Renal impairment* (creatinine >200μmol/L). Monitor urine flow. Daily U&E and serum creatinine (use haemodialysis if >400μmol/L).
- *Blood pH* <7.3 (lactic acidosis → tissue hypoxia). • *Systolic BP* <80mmHg.

Graph for deciding who should have *N*-acetylcysteine

▶One tablet of paracetamol=500mg

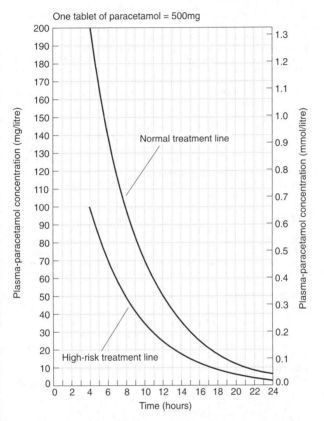

One tablet of paracetamol = 500mg

Patients whose plasma-paracetamol concentrations are above the **normal treatment line** should be treated with acetylcysteine by intravenous infusion (or, provided the overdose has been taken **within 10–12 hours**, with methionine by mouth). Patients on enyzme-including drugs (e.g. carbamazepine, phenobarbitone, phenytoin, rifampicin, and alcohol) or who are malnourished (e.g. in anorexia, in alcoholism, or those who are HIV-positive) should be treated if their plasma-paracetamol concentrations are above the **high-risk treatment line**. We thank Dr Alun Hutchings for permission to reproduce this graph.

NB: if paracetamol ingestion has been staggered (over some hours) serum levels may mislead: treat regardless, if significant amounts have been taken.
1 J Vale 1995 *Lancet* **346** 547 2 P Connor 1995 *Lancet* **346** 1236 3 SJ Ward 1995 *Lancet* **346** 1236

►►Emergency procedures: 1

There is no substitute for learning by experience. Often it is wiser to wait for someone to come and carry out an urgent procedure than to try for the first time by oneself—but some procedures must occasionally be performed at once. They are:

Cut-down onto a vein ●Indication: shock, eg exsanguination, when veins are collapsed, and IV access fails.

●Aim: to expose a vein and cannulate it under direct vision.

●Equipment: scalpel, artery forceps, cannula, dressing pack.

●Procedure: use the long saphenous vein as it courses anterior to the medial malleolus. Make a 3cm transverse skin incision. Free the vein using fine artery forceps. Insert and secure the cannula. It does not matter if you cannot use stitches: haemostasis can be achieved by pressure and elevation of the leg.

Note: experts may choose a CVP line rather than do a 'cut-down'. However, the insertion of CVP lines is hazardous, and should not be attempted without prior supervision. But a 'cut-down' should certainly be attempted if expert help is not immediately available and there is exsanguination. In these circumstances, they have saved many lives.

Relieving a tension pneumothorax

●Aim: to release air from the pleural space. (In a tension pneumothorax air is drawn in, intrapleurally, with each breath, but cannot escape due to a valve-like effect of the tiny flap in the parietal pleura. The increasing pressure progressively embarrasses the heart and the other lung.)

●Equipment: IV cannula (eg Venflon®), three-way tap, syringe.

●Insert the cannula through an intercostal space anywhere on the affected side. The three-way tap is connected between the syringe and the cannula. By aspirating on the syringe and expelling the intrapleural air through the three-way tap, the tension is relieved, and the lung is able to re-expand.

●Proceed to formal chest drainage (p800).

Note that if a 3-way tap is not immediately to hand, simply insert the cannula, and allow the air to escape, and then place a chest drain.

Cardioversion/defibrillation ●Indications: ventricular fibrillation or tachycardia, fast AF, supraventricular tachycardias if other treatments (p290–p294) have failed.

●Aim: to completely depolarize the heart using a direct current.

●Procedure: do not wait for a crisis before familiarizing yourself with the defibrillator.

  – Set the energy level (eg 200 joules for ventricular fibrillation or ventricular tachycardia; 100J for atrial fibrillation; 50J for atrial flutter).

  – Place conduction pads (eg Littmann™ Defib Pads) on chest, one over-apex (p40) and one below right clavicle (less chance of skin arc than jelly).

  – Make sure no one else is touching the patient or the bed.

  – Press the button(s) on the electrode to give the shock.

  – Watch ECG. Repeat the shock at a higher energy if necessary.

●Note: for AF and SVT it is necessary to synchronize the shock on the R wave of the ECG (by pressing the 'SYNC' button on the machine). This ensures that the shock does not initiate a ventricular arrhythmia. *If the SYNC mode is engaged in VF the defibrillator will not discharge!*

●It is only necessary to anaesthetize the patient if conscious.

●After giving the shock, monitor ECG rhythm. Consider anticoagulation, as the risk of emboli is increased. Get an up-to-date 12-lead ECG.

►In children use 2J/kg in VF/VT; if >10kg use *adult* paddles; *OHCS* p310–11.

Cricothyroidotomy

Essence An emergency procedure to <u>overcome upper airway</u> <u>obstruction above the level of the larynx.</u>

Indications Upper airway obstruction when endotracheal intubation not possible, eg <u>irretrievable foreign body</u>; facial oedema (burns, angio-oedema); <u>maxillofacial trauma</u>; <u>infection</u> (epiglotittis).

Procedure Lie the patient supine with neck extended (eg pillow under shoulders). Run your index finger down the neck anteriorly in the midline to find the <u>notch in the upper border of the thyroid cartilage</u>: just below this, between the thyroid and cricoid cartilages, is a <u>depression</u>—the <u>cricothyroid membrane.</u>

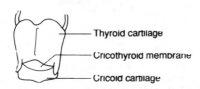

— Thyroid cartilage

— Cricothyroid membrane

— Cricoid cartilage

a. *Needle cricothyroidotomy:* <u>Pierce the membrane with large-bore cannula (14G)</u> attached to syringe: <u>withdrawal of air confirms position.</u> Slide cannula over needle at 45° to skin in sagittal plane. Use a Y-connector or improvise <u>connection to O$_2$ supply</u> and give 15L/min: use thumb on Y-connector to allow O$_2$ in over 1sec and CO$_2$ out over 4sec ('transtracheal jet insufflation'). Preferred method in children <12yrs. Will only sustain life for 30–45 mins before CO$_2$ builds up.

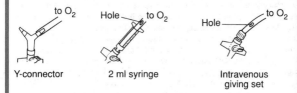

to O$_2$

Y-connector

Hole ——   to O$_2$

2 ml syringe

Hole ——   to O$_2$

Intravenous giving set

b. *Mini-Trach II®:* This contains a guarded blade, introducer, 4mm uncuffed tube (slide over introducer) with ISO connection and binding tape. Patient can breathe spontaneously or be ventilated via bag (high resistance). Will sustain for 30–45mins.

c. *Surgical cricothyrotomy:* Smallest tube for prolonged ventilation is 6mm. Introduce high volume low pressure cuff tracheostomy tube through horizontal incision in membrane.

Complications <u>Local haemorrhage</u>; posterior perforation of trachea ± <u>oesophagus</u>; laryngeal stenosis if membrane over-incised in childhood; tube blockage; subcutaneous tunnelling.

►Note: needle and Mini-Trach® are temporary measures pending formal tracheostomy.

▶▶Emergency procedures: 2

Inserting a chest drain (Also see p356 and p358.)

- Preparation: trolley with dressing pack, iodine, needles, 10mL syringe, 20mL 1% lignocaine (=lidocaine), scalpel (N°15), suture, chest drain (eg 28F, smaller ones block or kink), drainage bottle, connection tubes, sterile H_2O, tape). Incontinence pad under patient. Swab extensively.
- Choose insertion site:[1] <u>4th–6th intercostal space, mid-axillary line</u>; if you <u>need to drain fluid also, use the 7th space posteriorly</u>.
- Infiltrate down to pleura with 10–20mL of 1% lignocaine. Wait 3mins.
- Make <u>2cm incision above 6th rib</u>, to avoid neurovascular bundle under 5th rib. <u>Bluntly dissect with forceps down to pleura. Puncture pleura with scissor/forceps</u> then <u>sweep a finger inside chest to clear adherent lung</u> and exclude (eg in blunt abdominal trauma) stomach in the chest!
- Before inserting the drain <u>withdraw metal trochar 2cm</u>; <u>introduce the drain *atraumatically*. There is often no need for a trochar at all.</u>
- <u>Advance the tip upwards to the apex. Stop when you meet resistance.</u> Then withdraw the introducer completely and <u>attach the drain</u> via the tubing to the bottle. Ensure the longer tube within the bottle is under-water and bubbling with respiration. If patient is to be moved to another hospital substitute Heimlich flutter valve or drainage bag with flap valve for underwater drain. You should <u>never clamp chest drains</u>.[2]
- Fix the drain with a second suture tied around the tube like a 'Roman gaiter'. Bandage the drain to prevent it slipping.
- Request CXR to check the position of the drain. Give analgesia (PO/IM).

Note that before puncturing the pleura, some operators insert 2 horizontal sutures over the hole, or a purse-string suture, leaving the ends free to make a seal once the drain is finally removed.

Inserting a subclavian venous cannula Set a trolley (dressing pack, iodine, needles, scalpel (N°15), CVP pack, suture, Opsite® dressing); put incontinence pad under patient who should be lying flat. <u>Tilt bed 10° head down</u>. Swab chest and neck and surround area with green towels.

- Choose your insertion point: <u>1cm below the right clavicle, 2/3 of the way along its length from the sternoclavicular joint</u>. If available, ultra-sound can help find the insertion point and reduces complication rates (it allows visualization of the vein, and its position relative to the artery, and demonstrates how anatomy changes with posture).▶[3]
- Infiltrate with lignocaine. Wait 3 min. <u>Puncture skin with scalpel</u>.
- Insert the CVP pack's large needle into the hole. <u>Advance in the direction of the suprasternal notch</u>, under the clavicle, <u>exerting mild continuous suction on the syringe. Keep the needle parallel with the floor to minimize the risk of pneumothorax</u>.
- You may require several passes at slightly different angles to enter the vein. Stop when you can easily aspirate blood.
- What to do now depends on the type of CVP pack. <u>If there is a sheath over the large needle, advance it</u>, remove the needle and secure the sheath. If not, keep the needle very still and remove syringe. There will be a trickle back of blood. <u>Insert the guide wire</u> (soft end first) into the needle. It should advance easily. Remove the needle. There will be a sheath which comes mounted on a tapering dilator. Advance this over the wire into the vein. Holding the sheath, remove wire and dilator. Secure the sheath. ▶<u>During insertion, *never* completely let go of</u> the wire. It can travel fully into the vein and to the heart and require urgent surgical or transvenous removal.
- CXR: check end of the line is in the SVC; exclude pneumothorax.

1 Br Thoracic Soc. 1993 BMJ ii 114 2 PS Wong 1993 BMJ ii 443 ▶3 E Gualtieri 1995 *Crit Car Med* 23 692 (With inexperienced operators the success rate was 92% *vs* 44% if ultrasound was not used; N=52; randomized.)

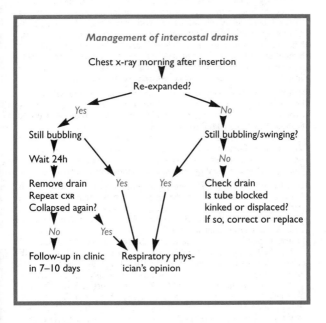

Management of intercostal drains

Chest x-ray morning after insertion

Re-expanded?

Yes — No

Still bubbling

Wait 24h

Remove drain
Repeat CXR
Collapsed again?

No — Yes

Follow-up in clinic
in 7–10 days

Yes

Yes

Still bubbling/swinging?

No

Check drain
Is tube blocked
kinked or displaced?
If so, correct or replace

Respiratory phys-
ician's opinion

Inserting a temporary cardiac pacemaker

Indications in the acute phase of myocardial infarction
- Complete AV block: −with inferior MI (right coronary artery occlusion) pacing may only be needed if symptomatic; *spontaneous recovery may occur.* −with anterior MI (representing massive septal infarction).
- Second degree block: −Wenckebach (p287) implies decremental AV node conduction; may respond to atropine in inferior MI; pace if anterior MI. −Type 2 block is usually associated with distal fascicular disease and carries high risk of complete heart block, so pace in both types of MI.
- First degree block: observe carefully: 40% develop higher degrees of block.
- Bundle branch block: pace prophylactically if evidence of trifascicular disease (p266) or non-adjacent bifascicular disease.
- Sino-atrial disease + serious symptoms: pace unless responds to atropine.

Other indications where temporary pacing may be needed
- Pre-op: if surgery is required in patients in any of the categories above (whether or not MI has occurred), do 24h ECG; liaise with the anaesthetist.
- Drug poisoning, eg with β-blockers, digoxin, or verapamil.
- Symptomatic bradycardia, uncontrolled by atropine or isoprenaline.
- Suppression of drug-resistant VT and SVT (overdrive pacing; do on ITU).
- Asystolic cardiac arrest with P-wave activity (ventricular standstill).
- During or after cardiac surgery—eg around the AV node or bundle of His.

Method and technique for temporary pacing Learn from an expert.
- Preparation: check that a defibrillator is at hand, that the patient is connected to an ECG monitor, and that a radiographer with screening equipment is present. Create a sterile field and ensure that the pacing wire fits down the cannula easily.
- Insertion: place the cannula into the subclavian or internal jugular vein as on p800. If this proves difficult, access to the right atrium can be achieved via the femoral vein. Pass the pacing wire through the cannula into the right atrium. It will either pass easily through the tricuspid valve or loop within the atrium. If the latter occurs, it is usually possible to flip the wire across the valve with a combined twisting and withdrawing movement. Advance the wire slightly. At this stage the wire may try to exit the ventricle through the pulmonary outflow tract. A further withdrawing and rotation of the wire will aim the tip towards the apex of the right ventricle. Advance slightly again to place the wire in contact with the endocardium. Remove any slack to decrease the risk of subsequent displacement.
- Checking the threshold: connect the wire to the pacing box and set the 'demand' rate slightly higher than the patient's own heart rate and the output to 3 volts. A paced rhythm should be seen. Find the pacing threshold by slowly reducing the voltage until the pacemaker fails to stimulate the heart (pacing spikes are no longer followed by paced beats). The threshold should be less than one volt, but a slightly higher value may be acceptable if it is stable—eg after a large infarction.
- Setting the pacemaker: set the output to 3 volts or over 3 times the threshold value (whichever is higher) in 'demand' mode. Set the rate as required. Suture the wire to the skin, and fix with a sterile dressing.
- Check the position of the wire (and exclude pneumothorax) with a CXR.
- Recurrent checks of the pacing threshold are required over the next few days. The formation of endocardial oedema can be expected to raise the threshold by a factor of two to three.

►Burns

Most hospitals do not have their own burns unit. Resuscitate and organize expeditious transfer for all major burns. Always assess site, size, and depth of the burn; small burns in the young, the old, or at specific sites may still require specialist help.

Assessment The size of the burn must be estimated to calculate fluid requirements. Ignore erythema. <u>Consider transfer to a burns unit if >10% burn in children or elderly, or >20% in others</u>. Use a Lund and Browder chart or the <u>'rule of nines'</u>:

Arm (all over) 9%	Front 18%	Head (all over) 9%	Palm 1%
Leg (all over) 18%	Back 18%	Genitals 1%	

(In children, head = 14%; leg = 14%)

Estimating burn thickness: **Partial thickness is** <u>painful, red, and blistered;</u> <u>full thickness is painless and white/grey.</u>

Refer <u>full thickness burns >5% of body area or full/partial thickness burns involving face, hands, eyes, genitalia to a burns unit.</u>

Resuscitation ●*Airway:* **Beware of upper airway obstruction developing if inhaled hot gases** (<u>only superheated steam will cause thermal damage distal to trachea</u>)—**suspect if** <u>singed nasal hairs or hoarse voice.</u> <u>Consider early intubation or surgical airway (p799).</u>

●*Breathing:* Give 100% O_2 if you suspect <u>carbon monoxide poisoning</u> (may have cherry-red skin, but often not) as t½ carboxyhaemoglobin (COHb) falls from 250min to 40min (consider <u>hyperbaric oxygen if pregnant</u>; CNS signs; >20% COHb). SpO_2 measured by pulse oximeter is unreliable (falls eg 3% with up to 40% COHb). Do <u>escharotomy bilaterally</u> in anterior axillary line if <u>thoracic burns impair chest excursion</u> (*OHCS* p689).

●*Circulation:* >10% burns in a child and >15% burns in adults require <u>IV fluids.</u> <u>Put up 2 large-bore (14G or 16G) IV lines.</u> Do not worry if you have to put these through burned skin. Secure them well: they are literally lifelines. It does not matter whether you give <u>crystalloid or colloid;</u> the volume is what is important. Use a 'Burns Calculator' flow chart[1] or a formula, eg:

Muir and Barclay formula (popular in UK):
<u>[weight (kg) × %burn] /2 =mL colloid</u> (eg Haemaccel®) per unit time. <u>Time periods are 4h, 4h, 4h, 6h, 6h, 12h.</u>

●*Parkland formula* (popular in USA):
4 × weight (kg) × %burn=mL Hartmann's solution in 24h, half given in first 8h (unsatisfactory in children, so use a 'Burns Calculator').

►You must replace fluid from the time of burn, not from the time first seen in hospital. You must also give 1.5–2.0mL/kg/h <u>5% dextrose</u> if Muir and Barclay formula is used. Formulae are only guides: adjust IVI rate according to clinical response and <u>urine output</u> (aim for >30mL/h in adults; >1mL/kg/h in children). <u>Catheterize</u> the bladder.

Treatment ►Do *not* apply cold water to extensive burns: this may intensify shock. Do not burst blisters. <u>Covering extensive partial thickness burns with sterile linen prior to transfer to a burns unit will deflect air currents and relieve pain.</u> Use <u>morphine</u> in 1–2mg aliquots IV. Suitable dressings include <u>Vaseline® gauze</u>, or <u>silver sulfadiazine</u> under absorbent gauze; change every 1–2 days. <u>Hands</u> may be covered in silver sulfadiazine inside a <u>plastic bag.</u> Ensure <u>tetanus immunity.</u> <u>Give 50mL whole blood for every 1% of full-thickness burn, half in the second 4h of IV therapy, and half after 24h.</u>

1 SM Milner 1993 *Lancet* 342 1089

Lund & Browder charts

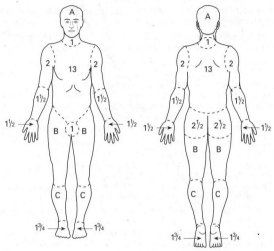

Relative percentage of body surface area affected by growth

Area	Age 0	1	5	10	15	Adult
A: half of head	9½	8½	6½	5½	4½	3½
B: half of thigh	2¾	3¼	4	4¼	4½	4¾
C: half of leg	2½	2½	2¾	3	3¼	3½

Smoke inhalation

In addition to thermal injury, the problems are carbon monoxide poisoning (p794) and *cyanide poisoning*—common from smouldering plastics. Cyanide binds reversibly with ferric ions in enzymes, so stopping oxidative phosphorylation, causing dizziness, headaches, and seizures. Tachycardia and dyspnoea soon give way to bradycardia and apnoea. The aim is to detach cyanide from cytochrome oxidase by making attractive ferric opportunities by producing methaemoglobin (each molecule has 3 ferric haem groups) from Hb—using amyl nitrate 0.2–0.4mL via an Ambu bag. Less safe alternatives are sodium nitrite solution (10mL of 3% IV over 3min; dimethylaminophenol (5mL of 5% IV over 1min). Also give sodium thiosulfate (25mL of 50% IV over 10min) to provide an extra source of sulfur to augment cyanide conversion to non-toxic thiocyanate. Alternatively, chelate cyanide with dicobalt edetate (20mL of 1.5% IV over 1min), followed by 50mL of glucose IV infusion 50%. (These are adult doses.)

The major disaster

Planning All hospitals have a detailed *Major Accident Plan*, but additionally the tasks of key personnel can be distributed on individual *Action Cards*.

At the scene Call the police; tell them to take command.

Safety: Is paramount—your own and others. Be visible (luminous monogrammed jacket) and wear protective clothing where appropriate (safety helmet; waterproofs; boots; respirator in chemical environment).

Triage: See *OHCS* p786. Label RED if will die in a few mins if no treatment. YELLOW = will die in ~2h if no treatment; GREEN = can wait. (BLUE = dead).

Communications: Are essential. Each emergency service will dispatch a control vehicle and will have a designated incident officer for liaison. Support medical staff from hospital report to the medical incident officer—he is usually the first doctor on the scene: his job is to assess then communicate to the receiving hospital the number and severity of casualties, to organize resupply of equipment and to replace fatigued staff. He must resist temptation to treat casualties as this compromises his rôle.

Equipment: Must be portable and include: intubation and cricothyrotomy set; intravenous fluids (colloid); bandages and dressings; chest drain (+flutter valve); amputation kit (when used ideally 2 doctors should concur); drugs—*analgesic:* morphine; *anaesthetic:* ketamine 2mg/kg IV over >60sec (0.5mg/kg is a powerful analgesic without respiratory depression); limb splints (may be inflatable); defibrillator/monitor; ± pulse oximeter.

Evacuation: Remember: with immediate treatment on scene, the priority for evacuation may be reduced (eg a tension pneumothorax—RED—relieved can wait for evacuation—becomes YELLOW), but those who may suffer by delay at the scene must go first. Send any severed limbs to the same hospital as the patient, ideally chilled—but not frozen.

At the hospital a 'major incident' is declared. The *first receiving* hospital will take most of the casualties; the *support* hospital(s) will cope with overflow and may provide mobile teams so that staff are not depleted from the first hospital. A control room is established and the medical coordinator ensures staff have been summoned, nominates a triage officer and supervises the best use of in-patient beds and ITU/theatre resources.

Blast injury may be caused by domestic (eg gas explosion) or industrial (eg mining) accidents or by terrorist bombs. Death may occur without any obvious external injury (air emboli). Injury occurs in six ways:

1 **Blast wave** A transient (milliseconds) wave of overpressure expands rapidly producing cellular disruption, shearing forces along tissue planes (submucosal/subserosal haemorrhage) and re-expansion of compressed trapped gas—bowel perforation, fatal air embolism.

2 **Blast wind** This can totally disrupt a body or cause avulsive amputations. Bodies can be thrown and sustain injuries on landing.

3 **Missiles** Penetration or laceration from missiles are by far the commonest injuries. Missiles arise from the bomb or are secondary, eg glass.

4 **Flash burns** These are usually superficial and occur on exposed skin.

5 **Crush** Injuries: beware sudden death or renal failure after release.

6 **Psychological** injury eg post-traumatic stress disorder (*OHCS* p347).

Treatment Approach the same as any major trauma (p761). Rest and observe any suspected of exposure to significant blast but without other injury. Gun-shot injury: see *OHCS* p679.

Principal source: SG Mellor Blast injury. In: I Taylor, CD Johnson (eds) *Recent Advances in Surgery 14*, Churchill Livingstone, London 1991 53–68; S Miles 1990 Major accidents BMJ **301** 923

Index

Manual indexes have limitations: use our *'intelligent' electronic index* (p17) for exploring and explaining *combinations* of signs, symptoms, and test results.
(For drugs, consult the disease you want to treat rather than the drug name.)

1997 UK adult basic life-support algorithm[1]

This algorithm assumes that only one rescuer is present, with no equipment. (If a defibrillator is to hand, get a rhythm readout, and defibrillate, as opposite, as soon as possible.)

Remove yourself and the casualty
from obvious dangers

⬇

Check responsiveness *(shake & shout)*

⬇

Open the airway *(head tilt/chin lift)*

⬇

Check breathing *(look, listen, feel; if breathing, place in recovery position)*

⬇

Give 2 breaths *(have up to 5 goes at giving 2 rescue breaths sufficient to raise the chest)*

⬇

Assess for signs of life for 10sec only *(look for signs of circulation; now phone for help at once)*

↙   ↘

Circulation present: No circulation: *(100 compressions/min at*
Continue rescue breathing   Compress chest *ratio of 15:2 with ventilat-*
                            & give breaths *ions if single rescuer; 1:5*
                                            if two. Spend <10sec to
                                            check circulation, eg car-
                                            otid pulse, every minute)

Managing the airway
- You open the airway by tilting the head and lifting the chin—but only do this if there is no question of spinal trauma.
- Use a close-fitting mask if available, held in place by thumbs pressing downwards either side of the mouthpiece; palms against cheeks.

Chest compressions
- Cardiopulmonary resuscitation (CPR) involves compressive force over the lower sternum with the heel of the hands placed one on top of the other, directing the weight of your body through your vertical, straight, arms.
- Depth of compression: ~4cm.
- Rate of compressions: 100/min.

Remember that these are guidelines only, and that the exact circumstances of the cardiorespiratory arrest will partly determine best practice. The guidelines are also more consensus-based than evidence based (p742), and are likely to be adapted from time to time, for example, as consensus develops about the best recovery position—eg semi-lateral position, with under-most arm either straight at the side, in dorsal position, or in the ventral position cradling the head with the upper-most arm crossing it (more stable, but possible risk to arm blood flow).[2]

1 A Handley 1997 *British Journal of Anaesthesia* **79** 151 2 A Handley 1993 *Resuscitation* **26** 93–95